P9-DIF-967

Medical Emergencies in

DENTISTRY

DATE DUE

R C
86.7
.B464
2002

Medical Emergencies in
DENTISTRY

JEFFREY D. BENNETT, DMD

Associate Professor, Department of Oral and Maxillofacial Surgery
School of Dental Medicine
University of Connecticut
Farmington, Connecticut

MORTON B. ROSENBERG, DMD

Professor, Department of Oral and Maxillofacial Surgery;
Head, Division of Anesthesia and Pain Control
Tufts University School of Dental Medicine
Boston, Massachusetts

WB SAUNDERS COMPANY

A Harcourt Health Sciences Company
Philadelphia   London   Montreal   Sydney   Tokyo   Toronto

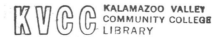
KVCC KALAMAZOO VALLEY
COMMUNITY COLLEGE
LIBRARY

APR 1 8 2002

W.B. SAUNDERS COMPANY
A Harcourt Health Sciences Company

The Curtis Center
Independence Square West
Philadelphia, Pennsylvania 19106

Senior Publishing Director: John Schrefer
Acquisitions Editor: Penny Rudolph
Developmental Editor: Jaime Pendill
Project Manager: Linda McKinley
Production Editor: Rich Barber
Designer: Julia Ramirez

NOTICE

Pharmacology is an ever-changing field. Standard safety precautions must be followed, but as new research and clinical experience broaden our knowledge, changes in treatment and drug therapy may become necessary or appropriate. Readers are advised to check the most current product information provided by the manufacturer of each drug to be administered to verify the recommended dose, the method and duration of administration, and contraindications. It is the responsibility of the treating physician, relying on experience and knowledge of the patient, to determine dosages and the best treatment for each individual patient. Neither the publisher nor the editor assumes any liability for any injury and/or damage to persons or property arising from this publication.

Library of Congress Cataloging in Publication Data

Bennett, Jeffrey, DMD.
Medical emergencies in dentistry/Jeffrey Bennett, Morton Rosenberg.

p.   cm.

Includes bibliographical references and index.

ISBN 0–7216–8481–5

1. Medical emergencies. 2. Dental emergencies.   I. Rosenberg, Morton (Morton B.)   II. Title.
  [DNLM: 1. Emergencies. 2. Dentistry. WU 105 B471m 2002]

RC86.7.B464 2002   616.02'5'0246176—dc21   2001044680

MEDICAL EMERGENCIES IN DENTISTRY

ISBN: 0-7216-8481-5

Copyright © 2002 by W.B. Saunders Company

All rights reserved. No part of this publication may be reproduced or transmitted in any form or by any means, electronic or mechanical, including photocopy, recording, or any information storage and retrieval system, without permission in writing from the publisher.

Printed in the United States of America

Last digit is the print number: 9   8   7   6   5   4   3   2   1

Contributors

A. Omar Abubaker, DMD, PhD
Associate Professor, Department of Oral and
    Maxillofacial Surgery
School of Dentistry, Division of Oral and
    Maxillofacial Surgery, Department of Surgery
School of Medicine
Virginia Commonwealth University
Richmond, Virginia

Eric M. Alltucker, DDS, MD
Private Practice
San Luis Obispo, California

Leon A. Assael, DMD
Professor and Dean, Department of Oral Health
    Science
University of Kentucky College of Dentistry
Lexington, Kentucky

Roger S. Badwal, DMD, MD
Assistant Clinical Professor, Department of Oral
    and Maxillofacial Surgery
University of Connecticut Health Center
John Dempsey Hospital
Farmington, Connecticut;
Attending Physician, Department of Surgery
Division of Oral and Maxillofacial Surgery
Danbury Hospital
Danbury, Connecticut

O. Ross Beirne, DMD, PhD
Professor, Chair, and Director of Residency
    Training, Department of Oral and
    Maxillofacial Surgery
University of Washington School of Dentistry
Seattle, Washington

George Blakey III, DDS
Assistant Clinical Professor, Department of Oral
    and Maxillofacial Surgery
University of North Carolina School of Dentistry
Chapel Hill, North Carolina

Remy H. Blanchaert, Jr., MD, DDS
Assistant Professor, Department of Oral and
    Maxillofacial Surgery;
Director, Postgraduate Residency Program
Baltimore College of Dental Surgery
University of Maryland Dental School;
Baltimore, Maryland

Robert Bona, MD
Professor of Clinical Medicine and Director,
    Hemophilia and Thrombosis Treatment
    Center, Department of Medicine
Division of Hematology-Oncology
University of Connecticut Health Center
Farmington, Connecticut

Martin R. Boorin, DMD
Assistant Professor, Department of Dental
    Medicine
Stony Brook School of Dental Medicine
Stony Brook, New York;
Attending Anesthesiologist, Departments of
    Dental Medicine and Anesthesiology
Long Island Jewish Medical Center
New Hyde Park, New York

Michael J. Buckley, DMD, MS, MBA
Associate Professor and Director of Research,
    Department of Oral and Maxillofacial
    Surgery;
Associate Dean for Clinical Affairs;
Chief, Division of Surgical Dental Science;
Director, Department of Dental Medicine
University of Pittsburgh Medical Center
Pittsburgh, Pennsylvania

Kevin J. Butterfield, DDS, MD
Resident, Department of Oral and Maxillofacial
    Surgery
University of Connecticut Health Center
Farmington, Connecticut

Albert E. Carlotti, Jr., DDS
Associate Clinical Professor, Department of
    Surgery (Oral and Maxillofacial)
Brown University School of Medicine
Providence, Rhode Island;
Private Practice
Warwick, Rhode Island

Thomas B. Dodson, DMD, MPH
Associate Professor, Department of Oral and
    Maxillofacial Surgery
Harvard School of Dental Medicine
Boston, Massachusetts;
Director of Resident Training, Department of
    Oral and Maxillofacial Surgery
Massachusetts General Hospital
Boston, Massachusetts

**James R. Hupp, DMD, MD, JD,
    MBA, FACS**
Professor and Chair, Department of Oral and
    Maxillofacial Surgery
Baltimore College of Dental Surgery
University of Maryland Dental School;
Chair, Department of Dental and Maxillofacial
    Surgery
University of Maryland Medical Center
Baltimore, Maryland

Roger L. Eldridge, DDS, JD
Associate Professor and Director, Special
    Patient Program/Oral Health Care Delivery
Baltimore College of Dental Surgery
University of Maryland Dental School
Baltimore, Maryland

Alan L. Felsenfeld, DDS
Adjunct Professor and Director of Clinical
    Affairs, Department of Oral and Maxillofacial
    Surgery
University of California–Los Angeles School of
    Dentistry
Los Angeles, California

Stephen E. Feinberg, DDS, MS, PhD
Professor, Department of Oral and Maxillofacial
    Surgery
University of Michigan School of Dentistry
Ann Arbor, Michigan

Earl G. Freymiller, DDS, MD
Associate Clinical Professor and Chair,
    Department of Oral and Maxillofacial Surgery
University of California–Los Angeles School of
    Dentistry;
Chief of the Dental Service
University of California–Los Angeles Medical
    Center
Los Angeles, California

Steven Ganzberg, DMD, MS
Associate Professor, Department of
    Anesthesiology
The Ohio State University College of Dentistry
    and College of Medicine and Public Health
Columbus, Ohio

Michael T. Goupil, DDS, MEd, MBA
Assistant Dean of Dental Student Affairs;
Assistant Professor, Department of Oral and
    Maxillofacial Surgery
University of Connecticut School of Dental
    Medicine
Farmington, Connecticut

James E. Kennedy, DDS, MS
Dean Emeritus and Professor, Department of
    Periodontology
University of Connecticut School of Dental
    Medicine
Farmington, Connecticut

Robert J. Lesny, DDS
Private Practice
Burlington, Vermont

Stuart E. Lieblich, DMD
Associate Clinical Professor, Department of
    Oral and Maxillofacial Surgery
University of Connecticut School of Dental
    Medicine
Farmington, Connecticut;
Senior Attending and Director of Ambulatory
    Anesthesia, Department of Oral and
    Maxillofacial Surgery
Hartford Hospital
Hartford, Connecticut

Mark D. Litt, PhD
Professor, Department of Behavioral Sciences
    and Community Health
University of Connecticut School of Dental
    Medicine
Farmington, Connecticut

Howard I. Mark, DMD, FACD
Clinical Professor, Department of Oral and
    Maxillofacial Surgery
University of Connecticut School of Dental
    Medicine
Farmington, Connecticut

Samuel J. McKenna, DDS, MD
Associate Professor, Department of Oral and
    Maxillofacial Surgery
Vanderbilt University School of Medicine
Nashville, Tennessee

Daniel McNally, MD
Division Chief, Pulmonary Division, Depart-
    ment of Medicine
University of Connecticut School of Dental
    Medicine
Farmington, Connecticut

Paul A. Moore, DMD, PhD, MPH
Professor, Department of Dental Public Health
University of Pittsburgh School of Dental
    Medicine;
Adjunct Professor, Department of
    Pharmacology
University of Pittsburgh School of Pharmacy;
Adjunct Professor, Department of
    Epidemiology
University of Pittsburgh Graduate School of
    Public Health
Pittsburgh, Pennsylvania

Anthony R. Petito, DDS, MD
Clinical Instructor, Department of Surgery (Oral
    and Maxillofacial)
Brown University School of Medicine
Providence, Rhode Island;
Private Practice
Warwick, Rhode Island

James C. Phero, DMD
Professor, Departments of Anesthesia,
    Pediatrics, and Surgery
University of Cincinnati College of Medicine
Cincinnati, Ohio

Joseph F. Piecuch, DMD, MD
Clinical Professor, Department of Oral and
    Maxillofacial Surgery
University of Connecticut School of Dental
    Medicine
Farmington, Connecticut;
Director, Department of Oral and Maxillofacial
    Surgery Service

Hartford Hospital
Hartford, Connecticut

Lorraine A. Rosenthal, RN, BSN
Department of Critical Care Nursing
University of Pittsburgh Medical Center
Pittsburgh, Pennsylvania

Marc S. Rosenthal, DMD, MD
Private Practice
Providence, Rhode Island

Steven M. Roser, DMD, MD, FACS
Georg Guttman Professor of Clinical
    Craniofacial Surgery, Division of Oral
    and Maxillofacial Surgery
Columbia University School of Dental and Oral
    Surgery;
Director, Graduate Medical Education
New York Presbyterian Hospital
New York, New York

Steven N. Saef, MD, FACEP
Assistant Professor, Division of Emergency
    Medicine, Department of Anesthesia and
    Peri-Operative Medicine
Medical University of South Carolina;
Emergency Physician, Department of
    Emergency Medicine
Medical University Hospital and Charleston
    Memorial Hospital
Charleston, South Carolina

Noah A. Sandler, DMD, MD
Assistant Professor, Department of Oral and
    Maxillofacial Surgery
University of Minnesota School of Dentistry
Minneapolis, Minnesota

Daniel S. Sarasin, DDS
Adjunct Assistant Professor, Department of
    Oral Pathology, Radiology, and Medicine
University of Iowa College of Dentistry
Iowa City, Iowa;
Private Practice
Cedar Rapids, Iowa

Steven J. Scrivani, DDS, MD, DSc
Edward Zegarelli Assistant Professor,
    Department of Oral and Maxillofacial Surgery
The Center for Oral, Facial and Head Pain
New York Presbyterian Hospital
Columbia University
Columbia-Presbyterian Medical Center
New York, New York

David M. Shafer, DMD
Associate Professor, Department Head, and
  Residency Program Director,
Department of Oral and Maxillofacial Surgery
University of Connecticut School of Dental
  Medicine;
Assistant Professor, Department of Surgery
University of Connecticut School of Medicine
Farmington, Connecticut;
Clinical Chief and Associate Chief of Staff, Department of Dentistry
John Dempsey Hospital
Farmington, Connecticut;
Division Chief, Oral and Maxillofacial Surgery,
  Department of Dentistry
Connecticut Children's Medical Center;
Attending Staff, Department of Dentistry
Hartford Hospital
Hartford, Connecticut

Bertrand Sorel, DMD, MD
Private Practice
West Palm Beach, Florida

James Q. Swift, DDS
Associate Professor and Director, Division of
  Oral and Maxillofacial Surgery
University of Minnesota School of Dentistry
Minneapolis, Minnesota

Reuben N. Turner, DDS
Private Practice
Provo, Utah

Patrick J. Vezeau, DDS, MS
Adjunct Associate Professor, Department of
  Oral and Maxillofacial Surgery
Southern Illinois University School of Dentistry
Alton, Illinois;
Adjunct Assistant Professor, Department of
  Oral and Maxillofacial Surgery
University of Iowa College of Dentistry
Iowa City, Iowa;
Private Practice
Davenport, Iowa

Brent B. Ward, DDS, MD
Adjunct Lecturer, Department of Surgery,
  Section of Oral and Maxillofacial Surgery
University of Michigan School of Dentistry
Ann Arbor, Michigan

K. Jeff Westlund, DDS, MS
Adjunct Associate Professor, Department of
  Oral and Maxillofacial Surgery
University of Iowa College of Dentistry
Iowa City, Iowa;
Private Practice
Cedar Rapids, Iowa

William H. Wood, DDS
Associate Professor and Director of Undergraduate Education of Oral and Maxillofacial
  Surgery
Louisiana State University School of Dentistry
New Orleans, Louisiana

John A. Yagiela, DDS, PhD
Professor and Chair, Division of Diagnostic and
  Surgical Sciences
University of California-Los Angeles School of
  Dentistry;
Professor, Department of Anesthesiology
University of California–Los Angeles School of
  Medicine
Los Angeles, California

Vincent B. Ziccardi, DDS, MD
Assistant Professor and Residency Program
  Director, Department of Oral and
  Maxillofacial Surgery
University of Medicine and Dentistry of New
  Jersey
Newark, New Jersey

This book is dedicated to our teachers, students, and patients who have taught us more than we can ever teach them.

Foreword

Modern health care has dramatically increased life expectancy of patients in the United States and other industrialized nations through enhanced understanding of the etiology and pathogenesis of disease, improved diagnostic capability, advanced surgical procedures, and new pharmacologic agents. Today's dental patient, both young and old, often presents with a complex medical history that includes several medications. The dentist's challenge is not the development of a dental treatment plan but a plan for the patient's medical management, including the anticipation of potential medical emergencies and the appropriate treatment.

The effective management of a medical emergency requires integration of knowledge from a variety of disciplines, including human physiology and pathophysiology, internal medicine and pharmacology. Drs. Bennett and Rosenberg and their co-authors have recognized this complexity, as well as the need to present medical emergency management in a way that is equally appropriate for the dental student as for the experienced practitioner concerned with the training of office staff or defining the supportive role of the dentist in the management of a systemic disease.

Unfortunately, patients do not always follow classic patterns, and the practitioner must avoid the trap of assuming that just because the patient has a specific disease, the present difficulty must be associated with that disease. By emphasizing a problem-based approach to the management of medical emergencies, a conceptual framework is provided that facilitates understanding, early recognition, and prompt response.

This book on medical emergencies is a valuable addition to the dentist's library. Most importantly, it can serve as the basis for the development and execution of formal ongoing training directed at enhancing the office staff's awareness of the presentation of emergencies and of each person's role in emergency management.

James E. Kennedy, DDS, MS
Dean Emeritus
University of Connecticut
School of Dental Medicine
Farmington, Connecticut

Preface

The concept of this book has evolved over many years from the experience of teaching the management of medical emergencies to both undergraduate dental students and practicing general dentists and specialists. Fundamental concepts began to emerge, and these provide the framework of this text.

Part I provides the reader with the foundation for the management of medical emergencies. These chapters discuss basic emergency drug therapy and review the use of emergency equipment as well as the specific skills required to treat different types of patients in the dental environment from pediatric to elderly populations. The second and third parts of the text address the diagnosis and management of medical emergencies by concentrating on early recognition of signs and symptoms and the implications of preexisting medical conditions. Part II discusses the significance of these signs and symptoms and the protocols that the dental team should follow in emergency management, from assessment and initial intervention to definitive diagnosis and more directed treatment.

Many patients have significant medical diseases that can impact dental treatment and cause or complicate medical emergency treatment. Part III discusses the onset of the medical emergency for patients who have preexisting medical conditions. Many medical emergencies are not easily diagnosed in these patients. For example, a simple syncopal episode in a healthy patient initiated by fear and apprehension may actually be a life-threatening event in a diabetic patient if caused by hypoglycemia.

Part IV discusses special patient populations and issues. Topics of interest include the management of the pregnant patient, herbal medications and their potential systemic effects and dental treatment implications, recognition of child and elder abuse, and medicolegal considerations.

With the comprehensive framework used to present this material, our goal is to allow the dentist and the dental team to recognize the subtle changes of an evolving medical emergency and to determine an appropriate level of intervention. To become a knowledgeable health care professional, it is also necessary to understand what considerations and treatments may be instituted after transfer to a medical facility. Preparation and treatment of a medical emergency in the dental office cannot be relegated to the dentist alone. The successful management of a medical emergency depends on a well-trained, collaborative dental team.

Our guiding principle has been the safety and well-being of the patients entrusted to our care. Medical training does not cease at the end of dental school. We are all lifelong learners. Only through constant review and study can we attain the proficiency necessary to diagnose and treat medical emergencies, understand the impact of underlying disease, and provide the safe environment our patients deserve.

Jeffrey D. Bennett
Morton B. Rosenberg

Acknowledgments

We wish to acknowledge the overwhelming commitment for this project from its inception to completion from WB Saunders, especially Jaime Pendill, Penny Rudolph, and Rich Barber; Carol Weis at Top Graphics; our colleagues who contributed their time, patience, and expertise; and our families for their continued support, forbearance, and love.

Many thanks for the individuals who have been there for me: JHB, SJB, LMR, LAA, JBD, DMS, MTG, RGT, CB, SAA, DPL, and MS.

JDB

I continue to stand on the shoulders of giants: Ken Stern, Lonnie Norris, Heinrich Wurm, Maria Papageorge, and Thomas Quinn.

MBR

Contents

Medical Emergencies in
DENTISTRY

Patient Assessment

I

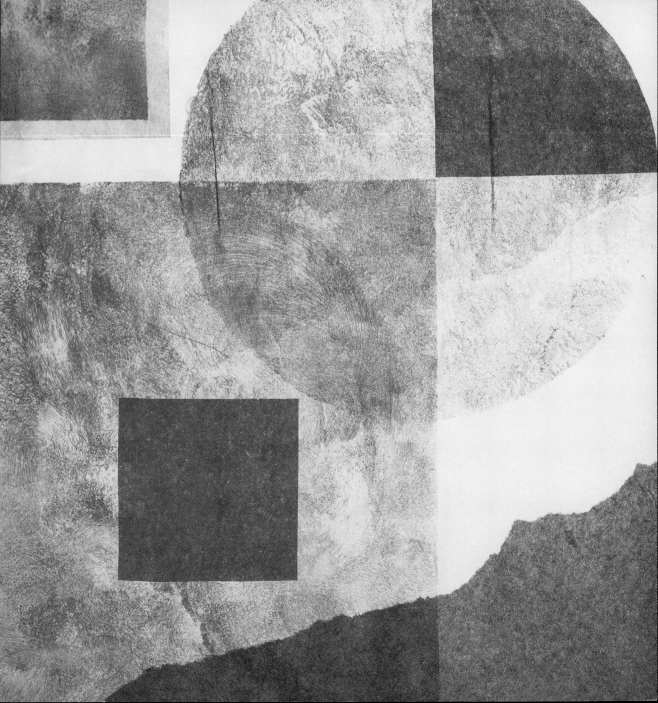

Basic Principles and Resuscitation

Steven N. Saef

Jeffrey D. Bennett

When a medical emergency occurs in the dental office, the dentist and staff must be organized and proficient in providing appropriate care to the patient. In making a diagnosis, clinicians can use a problem-oriented approach or a system-oriented approach.

The *problem-based approach* provides the dentist and staff with the methodology of proceeding from signs and symptoms to diagnosis and management of a disease. This approach to managing an emergency event in the dental office is "hands on" and concise. It emphasizes the necessity (1) to recognize and identify the significant features, (2) to define the problem and develop a likely diagnosis, and (3) to intervene imminently and stabilize the immediate event.

The *system-based approach* is a more traditional methodology for patient assessment and management. The practitioner is aware of the patient's medical history and, when encountering an adverse event, addresses the most likely etiology—the patient's known medical disorder. Understanding the medical disorders encountered in the dental office allows the practitioner to modify dental treatment, prevent medical emergencies, and recognize abnormal changes that warrant further assessment and possible intervention.

This chapter reviews the basic philosophy on how to approach a patient who develops a medical emergency while in the dentist's office. A standardized approach to emergency situations involves ascertaining the magnitude of illness, the appropriate treatments that can be provided in the office, and the need to transfer a patient to a hospital emergency department (ED).

The dentist and staff must adopt a particular way of thinking in emergency situations to obtain the best outcomes. They must be psychologically prepared to slip into "emergency mode." When suspected, problems must be presumed present and treatment instituted. An axiom of emergency situations is widely acknowledged: "More patients will do well when you act than when you don't act." This in turn leads to the maxims "err on the side of aggression" and "when in doubt, do." Clinicians must know their limitations, however, and only intervene to the limits of their competence. The appropriate principle here is the first rule of medicine: "First, do no harm."

PREPARATION
Office Planning

Techniques can be applied in office emergencies to save lives and moderate disease. Health care providers have the responsibility to become knowledgeable about such techniques and provide them to their patients as effectively as possible when needed.

To be prepared, a dentist must be familiar with both abnormal signs and symptoms suggestive of medical emergencies and medical illnesses likely to occur in the office setting and must know their "antidotes." Such manifestations of disease are predictable based on previous experience and the incidence of medical illness in dental patients. The dentist should become familiar with common clinical features and medical illnesses (Boxes 1-1 and 1-2).[1-3] The practicing dentist should have a working knowledge of these disorders and how they can cause a patient to become acutely ill in the office. The response to acute illness in the dental patient should include (1) anticipation of its presence based on the patient's medical history and the clinical situation, (2) a search for illness or injury likely to be present, and (3) readiness to provide appropriate treatment. Preparation for a cardiac arrest requires a course in *basic life support* (BLS) that meets the standards of the American Heart

3

Box 1-1	Classification of Common Medical Disorders Seen in Dental Emergencies

CATEGORY	DISORDERS
Cardiac	Angina, myocardial infarction, dysrhythmias, cardiac arrest
Vascular	Hypertension, hypotension, hemorrhage
Pulmonary	Obstructed airway, asthma, chronic obstructive pulmonary disease
Metabolic	Hypoglycemia, adrenal insufficiency, hyperthyroidism
Neurologic/central nervous system	Seizure, cerebrovascular accident (stroke)/transient ischemic attack, vasodepressor syncope, hyperventilation
Poisoning/toxicity	Reactions to local anesthetics, drug interactions, acetaminophen/aspirin side effects, alcohol intoxication
Allergy	Anaphylaxis, urticaria, airway edema, bronchospasm

Box 1-2	Common Clinical Features of Dental Emergencies and Differential Diagnosis

CLINICAL FEATURE	DISORDERS
Unconsciousness	Vasodepressor syncope, myocardial infarction (MI), cardiac arrest, cerebrovascular accident (stroke)/transient ischemic attack (CVA/TIA), hypoglycemia, adrenal insufficiency, drug overdose
Altered mental status	Hypoxia, CVA/TIA, seizure, hypoglycemia, drug overdose
Hyperventilation	Anxiety (hyperventilation syndrome), asthma (bronchospasm), allergic reaction, MI, congestive heart failure (CHF), hyperglycemia, hyperthyroidism
Hypoventilation/apnea	Adverse drug reaction/overdose, airway obstruction, bronchospasm
Wheezing	Asthma, aspiration, foreign body obstruction, allergic reaction/anaphylaxis
Dyspnea	CHF, anxiety, asthma, aspiration, foreign body obstruction
Hypertension	Anxiety, adverse drug effect/interaction
Hypotension	Adverse drug effect, vasodepressor syncope, myocardial decompensation (MI, CHF), adrenal insufficiency, hypothyroidism
Tachycardia	Adverse drug effect/interaction, illicit drugs, congenital abnormalities, hyperthyroidism, hyperglycemia
Bradycardia	Vasovagal/vasodepressor syncope, cardiac decompensation (e.g., sick sinus syndrome), adverse drug effect/interaction
Chest pain	Angina, MI, mitral valve prolapse, anxiety, musculoskeletal disease, gastroesophageal reflux disease, pulmonary pleuritis

Association (AHA). Additional classes in *advanced cardiac life support* (ACLS) can also be sought. Such courses are available throughout the United States and internationally. Psychologically, the dentist should be as ready to provide glucose to the diabetic patient with a low blood sugar level or sublingual nitroglycerin to the patient with angina as to apply BLS techniques to the patient in cardiac arrest. Some basic treatment measures can prove invaluable to patients in office medical emergencies (Box 1-3).

Finally, the dentist must identify when problems cannot be managed in the office and when 911 must be called, activating the *emergency medical services* (EMS) system. Effective preparation for office emergencies includes attention to each of the categories discussed next.[4]

History

Every patient should have a medical history obtained as part of the preliminary process to dental care. The history should specifically screen for underlying illness that could dictate modification in the delivery of care. An appropriate medical assessment will identify disorders that can result in an office emergency.

The history can be obtained in part through the use of forms distributed to the patient before the office visit. A patient interview then establishes personal contact and rapport as well as providing more salient information about the likelihood of disease than reviewing a form. Taking a relevant history also serves to keep important features of the history clearly in mind. Patients may forget important information while

---

> **Box 1-3   Basic Treatment Measures in Dental Emergencies**
>
> I. Airway management
>   A. Perform maneuvers to open airway.
>   B. Assess ventilatory effort.
>   1. If ventilation is spontaneous and unobstructed, proceed to C.
>   2. If ventilation is obstructed:
>   a. Consider inserting oral or nasal airway.
>   b. If necessary, apply maneuvers for foreign body obstruction (Heimlich maneuver).
>   3. If no spontaneous ventilations:
>   a. Provide rescue breathing with bag-valve-mask device or pocket mask with protective filter and oxygen inlet.
>   b. Consider inserting esophageo-tracheal tube (Combitube) or endotracheal tube.
>   C. Provide supplemental oxygen.
> II. Cardiovascular management
>   A. Palpate carotid, femoral, and radial pulses; if pulseless, initiate chest compressions.
>   B. Obtain blood pressure measurement.
> III. General management
>   A. Position patient.
>   B. Measure finger-stick blood glucose level.
>   C. Administer medications (oral, sublingual, inhalational, intramuscular).
>   D. If skilled, establish intravenous access and administer fluids and drugs as appropriate.

> **Box 1-4   Reasons for Medical Consultation in Dental Practice**
>
> 1. Clarify information pertaining to patient's medical history.
> 2. Request further information pertaining to patient's medical condition (e.g., echocardiogram, stress test, or cardiac catheterization report for patient with atherosclerotic heart disease before proceeding with treatment).
> 3. Determine if patient is in optimal condition for treatment.
> 4. Request that patient's condition be optimized before treatment (e.g., dentist may note repeated hypertension and inform treating physician of continued abnormality).
> 5. Arrange assistance in management of patient during perioperative period as necessary (e.g., insulin regimen for diabetic patient).

completing a form and may not consider important facts unless asked specifically about them.

Depending on the patient's response to the medical history, the practitioner may seek further information from the patient's physician or a hospital discharge summary. Although the dentist should not hesitate to contact the patient's physician, there should be a specific purpose for requesting medical consultation (Box 1-4). Consultation with a physician is insignificant if it seeks only patient clearance for treatment. Also, the dentist who does not request the appropriate information probably will not receive the desired information.

The more complex the patient's medical history, the more medications the patient usually takes. A patient may be unable to provide a complete list of medications and dosages during the medical history appointment. If a medical colleague is treating the patient, the patient's medication list may be obtained from this office. However, patients are often under the care of several physicians, who may be prescribing medications for a specific condition, unaware of their colleagues' prescriptions. Since patients frequently acquire all their medications from one pharmacy despite having prescriptions from several physicians, clarification of the patient's medications may be obtained by calling the pharmacy. The dentist must then associate each medication with a component of the patient's medical history. Understanding the patient's medications frequently provides further insight into the patient's medical disorder (Box 1-5).

The history obtained during the initial consultation precedes dental care, with opportunity to obtain more comprehensive information. The history taken at the time of an office emergency is by necessity more brief and directed.

Physical Examination

A physical examination appropriate to the screening assessment should check for signs of important underlying illness. The first component is the patient's general appearance; patients can appear well or unwell, acutely ill or chronically ill. The examiner then documents the patient's vital signs, including heart rate, respiratory rate, blood pressure, and temperature.

Box 1-5	Primary Medications for Common Systemic Diseases

DISEASE	MEDICATIONS
Arrhythmia/palpitation	Amiodarone, digoxin, procainamide, quinidine, β-blockers, anticoagulants
Asthma	β-Agonists (e.g., albuterol), inhaled steroids (e.g., fluticasone), leukotriene inhibitors (e.g., montelukast), theophylline
Atherosclerotic heart disease	Nitrates (e.g., isosorbide), antiplatelets (e.g., aspirin, ticlopidine)
Congestive heart failure	Digoxin, ACE inhibitors, furosemide
Diabetes	Sulfonylureas (e.g., glipizide, glyburide), thiazolidinediones (e.g., pioglitazone, rosiglitazone), metformin, acarbose
GERD	Omeprazole, lansoprazole, H2 antagonists (e.g., cimetidine), pantoprazole, rabeprazole
Hypertension	Angiotensin II antagonists (e.g., irbesartan), ACE inhibitors (e.g., enalapril/enalaprilat), calcium channel blockers (e.g., amiodipine), adrenergic agonists/antagonists (e.g., clonidine), β-blockers (e.g., metoprolol), diuretics (e.g., hydrochlorothiazide)
Seizure disorder	Phenytoin, carbamazepine, valproic acid, primidone, phenobarbital, clonazepam

GERD, Gastroesophageal reflux disease; *ACE,* angiotensin-converting enzyme.

Box 1-6	Clinical Observations of Potential Systemic Disease

CLINICAL OBSERVATION	DISEASE PROCESS
Slow gait	Impaired cardiovascular or pulmonary reserve, musculoskeletal disease
Orthopnea	CHF, atherosclerotic heart disease
Barrel chest	Chronic obstructive pulmonary disease
Jugular venous distinction	CHF
Peripheral edema	CHF
Petechiae/ecchymoses	Hepatic disease, coagulation abnormality, anticoagulant therapy

CHF, Congestive heart failure.

Office staff should know how to take, record, and interpret vital signs. Vital signs should be recorded for every patient, and the dentist should be alerted to abnormal readings. Indirect indicators of medical instability (e.g., clamminess, confusion) should be reported as well. The dentist should also note any other important findings (Box 1-6).

Dental Care Plan

Once an appropriate medical history and examination are complete, the dentist must determine an appropriate manner in which to deliver dental treatment. Most patients require no modification; they will present on the day of dental care exactly as they would on any other day. They will take all doses of normal medications as planned.

Select groups of patients, however, require modification in their routine schedule and med- ication consumption or in delivery of dental care (Box 1-7). If required, many patients are sufficiently familiar with their medical regimens to make dose adjustments. If not, or if any doubt exists about how to proceed with scheduled doses of medication, a call to the patient's general practitioner is warranted to receive recommendations about altering the doses. Such recommendations are routine for most medical internists, who regularly provide consultation on patients scheduled for inpatient surgery. Patients who depend on prescribed "as-needed" (prn) medications (e.g., nitroglycerin for angina, albuterol for asthma) should bring the medicines with them and should be encouraged to use them when perceived necessary, as they would at any other time.

The physical and mental stress associated with dental treatment may cause hemodynamic changes and contribute to the development of many potential emergency situations. Modifying

Box 1-7	Treatment Modifications for Common Conditions and Interventions

CONDITION/INTERVENTION	MODIFICATION
Asthma	Depending on severity of disease, be aware of possible sensitivity to the antioxidant contained in local anesthetics with a sympatho-mimetic agent.
Cardiovascular disease	Consider supplemental oxygen, continuous monitoring, and short appointments (e.g., patient may not tolerate supine positioning). Ensure that patient has taken prescribed medications; be cognizant of interaction of epinephrine with medications. Consider sedation.
Corticosteroid regimen	Consider increasing steroids that depend on adrenal suppression; however, stress associated with most dental procedures does not mandate altering corticosteroid dose.
Dental anxiety,* dental phobia	Consider use of sedative technique (e.g., nitrous oxide, oral anxiolytic, parenteral sedation).
Diabetes mellitus	Alter medications based on the patient's dietary restriction before treatment and ability to eat after treatment. Ensure that patient has eaten, and consider obtaining a blood glucose reading (depending on planned treatment and severity of disease).
SBE	Prescribe antibiotic prophylaxis. Rick factors can include cardiac valve disease and connective tissue disorders.
Spina bifida	Individuals who have had frequent exposure to latex products are at risk for developing a latex allergy. Many products used in the dental office contain latex, including vials of local anesthetics and many emergency drugs.
Sedation, anesthesia	Ensure patient receives nothing by mouth (NPO) for up to 8 hours before treatment.
Substance abuse	These patients may be prescribed a long-acting opioid antagonist (e.g., naltrexone). If indicated, manage pain with a nonopioid agent.

SBE, Subacute bacterial endocarditis.
*Mental stress and anxiety can contribute to the development of an emergency.

the patient's stress with behavioral or pharmacologic methods may decrease the incidence of medical emergencies.

Occasionally the screening history and physical examination will lead the dentist to arrange for a dental procedure in a hospital, which may mean referring the patient to a colleague who practices in this setting. Even if the dentist is not providing the actual care, referral to a hospital-based provider is a valuable service to the patient.

Finally, if medical illness seems sufficiently unstable to prohibit safe dental care, the procedure may need to be postponed pending further medical stabilization. Routine referral practices with the patient's regular physician usually provide eventual clearance, with instructions on safely managing the patient.

Staff Training

All staff should be trained and current in basic cardiopulmonary resuscitation (CPR) and first-aid procedures. The AHA courses in BLS can provide all staff members with adequate instruction on the recognition of emergencies and initiation of lifesaving measures while awaiting EMS arrival. Courses should be offered to the entire office staff on an annual or semiannual basis. Training the staff as a group can foster a more effective team response than separate outside courses and can identify those members who are more likely to respond automatically and those who might need guidance.

Basic first-aid measures, such as controlling bleeding with direct pressure, elevating the head of a patient who is having respiratory difficulty, and positioning a lightheaded patient supine, are detailed at first-responder classes, many of which include BLS training. Many skills needed to provide first aid to a patient in the office are similar to those needed in the home; therefore a staff member with good common sense can become a valuable emergency provider if encouraged and trained.

If pediatric patients are regularly seen in the practice, pediatric resuscitation skills should also be addressed. Airway assessment and CPR for infants and children are covered in BLS courses. Advanced skills are taught in pediatric advanced life support courses.

Practice drills should be scheduled regularly. As with a fire drill, simulated emergencies may be arranged periodically (e.g., heart attack, allergic reaction, or seizure). Regular practice helps ensure a state of readiness, and the staff will be less stressed when responding to a real emergency.

Emergency Kit

Two principles to use when creating an emergency kit are (1) ensure familiarity with the kit's contents and organization and (2) keep it simple. A kit should be stocked and ready with the necessary medications and equipment to respond to an emergency. The purpose of the emergency kit is to sustain life (BLS armamentarium) and to stabilize and prevent medical *urgencies* from becoming medical *emergencies*. The kit should contain equipment and medications that the dental team is fully trained and competent in using (Box 1-8). The level of sophistication of the emergency kit will reflect the EMS system and the availability of and distance to more advanced medical care (Figure 1-1). Maintenance of such a kit requires the scheduled replacement of drugs or devices with expiration dates and the assignment of this responsibility to office personnel (see discussion below).

Written Emergency Plan

A written description of the procedures to follow in an office emergency should be prepared in advance. Role designations for the staff should be clearly described. Individuals should be familiar with different roles and their respective responsibilities depending on who is present in the office (Box 1-9). No individual should be excluded. Medical emergencies do not occur as expected. For example, the first person in the office to encounter the patient having an allergic reaction to their prophylactic antibiotics could be the receptionist. This individual should be able to recognize that a problem exists and report it directly to the dentist or activate the emergency protocol.

Phone numbers and local resources should be clearly described. If an internist and oral surgeon have practices nearby, their numbers should be on file, and staff should know when

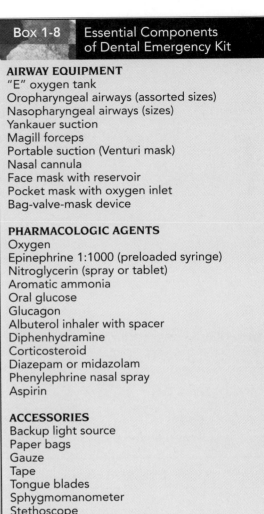

Box 1-8 Essential Components of Dental Emergency Kit

AIRWAY EQUIPMENT
"E" oxygen tank
Oropharyngeal airways (assorted sizes)
Nasopharyngeal airways (sizes)
Yankauer suction
Magill forceps
Portable suction (Venturi mask)
Nasal cannula
Face mask with reservoir
Pocket mask with oxygen inlet
Bag-valve-mask device

PHARMACOLOGIC AGENTS
Oxygen
Epinephrine 1:1000 (preloaded syringe)
Nitroglycerin (spray or tablet)
Aromatic ammonia
Oral glucose
Glucagon
Albuterol inhaler with spacer
Diphenhydramine
Corticosteroid
Diazepam or midazolam
Phenylephrine nasal spray
Aspirin

ACCESSORIES
Backup light source
Paper bags
Gauze
Tape
Tongue blades
Sphygmomanometer
Stethoscope
Syringes (tuberculin, 3 ml)
Needles (25 and 20 gauge)
Alcohol wipes
Pillow
Blanket
Surgilube
Glucometer

and how to contact them. The numbers for the local EDs should be available so that the dentist can notify the ED physician that a patient is en route. It is helpful for the dentist to have established a relationship with the medical director of the local EMS system (usually a physician associated with a local ED). This is a contact that can also familiarize the dentist with colleagues in the local ED, a relationship that could prove invaluable if a difficult situation arises.

A code word is helpful for initiating an emergency response. A "code blue" or a "911" in a par-

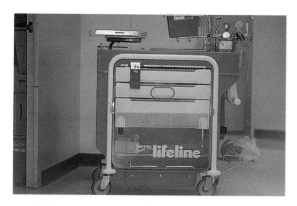

Figure 1-1. Full crash cart for advanced cardiac life support. A similar cart may be used for a dental office. Each drawer can be appropriately labeled to identify its contents. Alternatively, an emergency cart can be assembled and contained in a smaller, more portable container.

Box 1-9	Designated Roles in Office Emergency Management

1. Recognize a problem and activate the office emergency system.
2. Obtain the emergency kit (medications and equipment).
3. Record vital signs (blood pressure, pulse, respiratory rate) and provide continuous monitoring.
4. Open airway, administer supplemental oxygen, and perform rescue breathing as necessary.
5. Perform chest compressions.
6. Prepare and administer medications.
7. Document the event.
8. Request outside assistance.*
9. Clear the immediate area of other patients.
10. Inform family and obtain information relevant to current situation.

*Person requesting outside assistance should stay on the phone until emergency personnel have all the necessary information. Person should inform the dentist that emergency personnel are en route to the office.

ticular treatment room can assist in coordinating the response and delivering efficient care. Staff should not hesitate to contact the dentist at any time if they believe a problem exists. New staff should receive written material about the emergency plan, should be shown the location of all equipment, and should have their role in an emergency assigned and explained.

RECOGNITION AND ASSESSMENT

The capacity to respond to an emergency requires recognition of a problem. Occasionally an emergency situation is obvious; frequently it is not. Surprisingly, patients who are in cardiopulmonary arrest, despite being more seriously ill, can be easier to identify and manage than patients with more subtle signs, such as anxiety, confusion, or pallor. The trigger that leads to "emergency mode" may be a patient complaint or a change in patient condition. Patients who require resuscitation must be differentiated from those with less serious medical problems who require specific therapy. Clinicians must be able to gauge levels of illness and make specific diagnoses.

Levels of Illness

To determine the level of illness, a physician must be able to interpret the signs and symptoms that indicate life is in danger. The earliest signs of serious illness arise from the central nervous system (CNS). Anxiety, fear, and even slight nausea (difficult to discriminate in the dentist's chair) can be the brain's first response to the lack of an adequate blood supply or of a vital nutrient such as oxygen or glucose. If the process inducing the deficiency progresses, the patient will become openly anxious, sure that "something is wrong." This will progress to confused, agitated, and even violent behavior; the patient may not allow anyone to help and may require restraint. Lethargy eventually develops, followed by coma.

The next most visible measures of serious illness are skin changes. The skin possesses a rich blood supply and many accessory structures that can yield signs of acute internal derangements. The most prominent sign is *diaphoresis*, or sweating, particularly of the brow. In an emergency setting, when sweat repeatedly accumulates on the brow despite frequent wiping, serious metabolic failure is proceeding. *Pallor* and even grayness of the face and limbs are signs of extreme sympathetic nervous system activation in an attempt to preserve core (heart and brain) circulation. *Capillary refill*, the time required for pink color to return after pushing against the palm of the hand, becomes prolonged as peripheral circulation is sacrificed. Normally, color should return in the time one can say, "capillary refill."

Vital signs are checked next in determining the level of illness. Ranges can be used to judge the seriousness of the patient's condition (Table 1-1). Vital signs must always be interpreted in

Table 1-1	Ranges of Normal, Borderline, and Abnormal Vital Signs		
Vital Sign	Normal	Borderline	Abnormal
Heart rate (beats per minute)	60-100	50-60 100-120	<50 >120
Systolic blood pressure (mm Hg)	90-140	80-90 140-190	>200 <60
Diastolic blood pressure (mm Hg)	60-90	50-60 90-110	<50 >120
Respiratory rate (breaths per minute)	12-20	10-12 24-36	<10 >36
Capillary refill (seconds)	<2	2	>2

Box 1-10 Symptoms and Signs of Potentially Serious Illness

SYMPTOMS
Chest pain
Shortness of breath
Restlessness
Apprehension
Nausea and vomiting
Thirst
Weakness
Feeling of impending doom

SIGNS
Skin cool and pale
Diaphoresis
Pupils dilated
Lips blue
Pulse rapid and weak
Breathing rapid and shallow
Worsening mental status:
Confusion →
combativeness → lethargy

the context of the clinical situation. Many healthy young women have blood pressure (BP, in millimeters of mercury, or mm Hg) in the range of 80 systolic and 60 diastolic. Athletes can have a heart rate (HR, in beats per minute, or beats/min) in the low 50s, which even dips into the 40s and high 30s during sleep. On the other hand, if a 55-year-old man is complaining of chest pain and is diaphoretic, nauseous, and pale with a BP of 90/60 and an HR of 120, he is critically ill.

Symptoms that represent early signs of an emergency include chest pain or pressure, shortness of breath, dizziness, headache, and abdominal pain. These symptoms should be given particular attention when they are associated with CNS or skin changes or abnormal vital signs (Box 1-10). If any of these findings is present

when assessing a patient with an emergency, immediate transfer to an ED should be considered.

RESUSCITATION PLAN

Emergency assessment and management strategies known as the primary and secondary surveys can be used to resuscitate any acutely ill or injured person. These surveys originated in 1966 with the National Highway Safety Act, which authorized the Department of Transportation to fund ambulances, communications, and training programs for prehospital medical services. The National Highway Traffic Safety Administration (NHTSA) was created and charged with the development of a curriculum that would teach how to assess and manage acutely ill and injured people in our increasingly industrial and technical society. Physicians with resuscitation experience in the military and at academic medical centers met at consensus conferences and laid the foundation for the highly evolved surveys currently used. Their efforts have resulted in such familiar phrases as 911, CPR, and the ABCs. Through trial and error, innovation, and basic scientific study, the present techniques of the primary and secondary surveys have become widely accepted and applied.

The Primary and Secondary Surveys provide a framework for organizing a purposeful resuscitation. Fast, intuitive, and dynamic, they detect and treat problems that compromise the fundamental needs of life (oxygenation and circulation). Operating principles serve as ground rules to the surveys and guide the clinician in interpreting historical and physical findings during the initial assessment and management. Since the surveys are organized according to the basic requirements of life, clinicians should adhere to their sequences to properly address immediately and potentially life-threatening problems in the order of their importance.

When doubt exists about whether to treat, generally the clinician should err on the side of action rather than inaction. Seriously ill patients are more likely to do poorly if nothing is done than if something is done. The risk of a complication is grossly outweighed by the risk of disease progression.

The dentist must know what to look for, how to find it, and how to treat it once found. This aspect of the survey takes the most time to develop. Each clinician has a different level of experience and knowledge; ability to recognize and treat depends on prior education, training, and involvement with resuscitations. Nevertheless, specific illnesses can be predicted in certain clinical settings. If a disease is not treatable, there is no point in spending valuable time looking for it. Finally, the clinician must know the specific "antidote" for each illness sought.

The four parts to the overall resuscitation plan are the primary survey, resuscitation, secondary survey, and definitive care[5] (Box 1-11). The *primary survey* and *resuscitation* are by nature simultaneous. The primary survey is geared toward *immediately* life-threatening injuries (i.e., will kill within seconds to minutes), whereas the secondary survey seeks *potentially* life-threatening injuries (i.e., will kill within hours to days). When found, an immediately life-threatening injury must be treated, according to the rules of the primary survey, before proceeding with the sequence of resuscitation. If the primary survey is completed and the patient remains unstable, the clinician must repeat the survey, again looking for immediately life-threatening injuries that can be treated.

When the primary survey is successfully completed, with appropriate intervention by the clinician and positive response from the patient, the patient's life is no longer in danger. This allows a thorough *secondary survey*, which includes a more extensive history and physical examination as well as diagnostic testing and treatment. The *definitive care* phase of the resuscitation plan refers to focused interventions designed to return the patients to their previous condition before injury or illness. This can extend up to and include rehabilitation. Although it may not be possible to restore the patient to his or her previous level of health, this should always remain the goal.

Box 1-11 Emergency Management and Resuscitation Plan

PRIMARY SURVEY
1. ABCDE: airway, breathing, circulation, disability, expose
2. Purpose: identification and treatment of *immediately* life-threatening problems
3. History: "AMPLE" (see Box 1-8)
4. Resuscitation: measures are instituted during primary survey to treat problems as they are found

SECONDARY SURVEY
1. Head to toe by region: head, neck, chest, abdomen, skeletal, neurologic
2. Purpose: identification and treatment of *potentially* life-threatening problems
3. History: data gathering
   a. Find quick sources of information.
   b. Interview the patient.
   c. Interview the family and bystanders.
   d. Look over the scene.
   e. Check for medical identification bracelet.
   f. Call the patient's physician.
4. System-specific tests and therapy
5. Reevaluation: repeat primary and secondary surveys until help arrives.
6. Definitive care: additional care needed to restore patient to preinjury or preillness condition

---

Primary Survey

The primary survey is a fast, choreographed procedure that draws on rote memory, intuition, and clinical judgment. The dentist must make quick, definitive decisions based on the circumstances surrounding the illness or injury, the resources available to treat the problems at hand, and personal capabilities. If the dentist decides, "This problem is here," action is taken. If the dentist says, "This problem is not here," the survey continues. For example, when assessing an airway in a victim of a potential heart attack, the dentist might ask the patient, "How are you? Can you speak?" The patient might say, "I feel bad. I have chest pain." The patient also might appear ill: cold, clammy, and diaphoretic. The dentist would determine, "This patient can speak. He has an unobstructed, functional larynx and trachea. I don't need to intervene and provide ventilatory support." On the other hand, if the patient does not answer, the dentist would need to presume an airway problem and apply maneuvers to establish an airway (e.g., head tilt, chin lift, jaw thrust). If in doubt about the airway, the dentist should err on the side of instituting airway techniques.

The primary survey has eight tenets (Box 1-12), as follows:

1. *Proceed rapidly.* The survey is fast; the rate of change in an emergency is high and does not permit extensive consideration. Lengthy deliberation about the "right" action is impossible. If you *do* know what to do, *do it.* If you do *not* know what to do and a patient is in trouble, do not think. *Call for help.*

2. *Err on the side of aggression.* Generally, there is a deliberative process regarding the risks and benefits of any medical intervention. When illness or injury is acute or severe, however, the pace of the process requires a decision.

3. *When in doubt, do.* Widely supported by the experience of caring for emergency patients is the concept that more patients will do well when you act than if you do not act. All physicians are concerned about possibly doing more harm than good when initiating treatment. This leads to questions about whether to intervene, and often the questions remain when the time arrives to implement treatment. If you are uncertain, for instance, about whether a patient is having an allergic reaction, you will do more harm by *not* treating it than by treating it. If a "heart attack" is in question, you will be of more help to the patient by activating the EMS system and calling 911 than by worrying about overreacting.

4. *Stay in sequence.* The dentist should adhere to the order of the "ABCs." *Airway* comes first because without a patent tube connecting the oropharynx to the lungs, oxygen delivery is impossible. *Breathing* comes second because without a functioning bellows, oxygen cannot be supplied to hemoglobin. *Circulation* comes third because without it, vital organs cannot be perfused. The dentist should not work on the lungs unless oxygen (or room air) can reach them or on the circulation unless hemoglobin can be saturated with oxygen. These intuitive priorities seem obvious, but even the obvious can become blurred when a patient is dying in the chair.

5. *Know what to look for, how to recognize it, and how to treat it when present.* Each of the steps in the surveys can reveal findings that represent disease. You are unlikely to recognize a finding, however, unless you are familiar with it.

> ### Box 1-12 Tenets of Primary Survey
>
> 1. Proceed rapidly.
> 2. Err on the side of aggression.
> 3. When in doubt, "do."
> 4. Stay in sequence.
> 5. Know what to look for, how to recognize it, and how to treat it when present.
> 6. Look only for likely, treatable problems.
> 7. Use only eyes, ears, and stethoscope.
> 8. Initiate only simple tests or treatments.

---

6. *Look only for treatable problems.* These problems can be tagged to each step of the primary survey. A discrete list of illnesses and injuries can be identified as likely to occur in the population seeking dental care (see Table 1-1).

7. *Use only eyes, ears, and stethoscope.* The primary survey is a "seat of your pants" survey involving the history and physical examination, both of which must be very brief and focused. All decisions being made are based on direct examination of the patient for signs of compromised vital functions.

8. *Initiate only simple tests or treatments.* Simple tests include finger-stick glucose check and pulse oximeter reading, if available. Basic treatments include oxygen, an albuterol inhaler, glucose-containing solutions, and sublingual nitroglycerine.

Airway

The airway refers to the pathway from the atmosphere to the lungs and comprises the mouth, pharynx, larynx, and trachea. Obstruction at any of these points can compromise airway patency. The airway assessment involves determining if obstruction is present. The most basic method of airway assessment is to ask the patient a simple question (e.g., "Are you okay?"). An appropriate answer demonstrates an intact functional airway, with normal pharyngeal and laryngeal muscle function. The clinician also can judge airway patency by looking at the patient. If the victim of illness or injury is sitting in a relaxed state, appears to be thinking clearly, and has warm and well-perfused skin, the airway is probably intact.

On the other hand, if the patient appears in an abnormal posture and does not respond to a question or shake, further assessment is indicated. First, lie the victim down on the floor or set the dental chair to its most posterior position. Next, place one hand on the patient's forehead and apply gentle backward pressure while simultaneously lifting the chin upward with your other hand placed under the anterior mandible (Figure 1-2). Look, listen, and feel for the movement of air at the mouth and nose. Turn your head sideways and look down the patient's torso to check for chest wall movement as you listen and feel with your ear over the patient's face. If air movement is not detected, presume that your positioning is off and reposition the head and neck. Repeat your head-tilt, chin-lift maneuver. Try grabbing the lower incisors and pulling the jaw forward (Figure 1-3). Move behind the patient and apply a jaw thrust (Figure 1-4). Tools to assist at this point include a nasopharyngeal airway and an oropharyngeal airway. Many likely, treatable causes exist for a nonpatent airway (see Box 1-1).

If the airway cannot be established, assume that it is obstructed by a foreign body. Attempt the Heimlich maneuver, as recommended by the AHA. Consider a dislodged tooth, an instrument, or a piece of aspirated surgical material. Remember, if you think it is possible, err on the side of aggression and attempt to treat it.

If a foreign body appears unlikely, continue to work on airway positioning. Consider an inflammatory disorder of the airway, such as allergic edema, maxillofacial space infection, epiglottitis, or croup. These may be treated with mist, oxygen, epinephrine, or steroids and require patient transport to a hospital ED for continued treatment. Attempt to ventilate with a bag-valve-mask device, insert a Combitube, or perform endotracheal intubation if you are capable and have the necessary equipment. Activate the EMS system to ensure help is on the way.

Before moving on from the airway step of the primary survey, you should be confident that a patent tube from the atmosphere to the patient's lungs is established.

Breathing

Breathing refers to the ability of the lungs to inhale and exhale. This is a function distinct from having a patent airway. Observe and communicate with the patient. In the unconscious victim, look, listen, and feel to assess breathing during the primary survey. *Look* for the chest to rise symmetrically, *listen* for inspiration, and *feel* for the exhaled breath of air. Next, assess the work of breathing: respiratory depth, rate, and effort. Inspect the chest wall for retractions of the intercostal muscles. Ordinarily the movement of these muscles should not be apparent

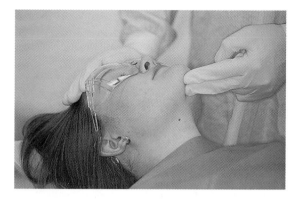

Figure 1-2. Jaw-forehead lift. Note that the hand on the chin should be on the inferior border of the mandible and should not displace the soft tissue of the submental or submandibular region posteriorly, which could contribute to upper airway obstruction.

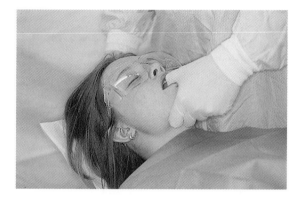

Figure 1-3. Tongue-jaw lift.

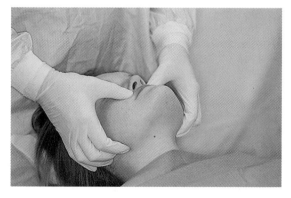

Figure 1-4. Jaw thrust. Anterior displacement of the jaw is an effective maneuver to open the airway. The maneuver is uncomfortable for the conscious patient.

as they move with the ribs while the thoracic cage expands and contracts. In the patient with respiratory distress the action of these muscles becomes noticeable because they sink into the intercostal spaces as the thorax expands and they billow as the thorax contracts to induce exhalation. The action of the sternocleidomastoid muscles also becomes much more apparent when respirations become labored, standing out as muscular bands connecting the mastoid process behind the ear to the medial clavicle.

Using a stethoscope, auscultate the chest listening for air movement. A clean blowing sound is usually heard as the lung alveoli fill with air, termed *vesicular* breath sounds. When fluid accumulates in the tiny alveoli, they pop open as the surface tension of the fluid holding them shut is overcome, producing a crackling sound referred to as *rales*. If the patient has spasm or swelling of the bronchi, as occurs with asthma and sometimes heart failure, *wheezing* occurs.

Indirect but very effective indicators of respiratory insufficiency are changes in the patient's mental status and skin. The patient who cannot breathe often becomes anxious. If this progresses to true hypoxia, confusion and agitation will develop as the brain loses its reasoning capacity. This is followed by an increasing lethargy, which progresses to stupor and then coma. Use the patient's level of consciousness (LOC) as a means of assessing effective respiration. The skin will also change with worsening hypoxia, progressing through alterations in color, temperature, and texture. Healthy skin is warm and dry. Vital organ dysfunction results in diaphoresis, with pallor caused by vasoconstriction. Ultimately, cold clammy skin is produced, which suggests metabolic stress.

The causes of respiratory insufficiency or distress are protean, but for the purposes of the primary survey, you should search for, know how to identify, and know how to treat a discrete number of illnesses or injuries (see Box 1-1). Consider the clinical setting. In a patient who has just received a medication and complains of shortness of breath, for example, think of an allergic reaction or asthma attack resulting in bronchospasm. In a middle-aged or elderly patient complaining of chest pain and shortness of breath, consider congestive heart failure.

Circulation

The circulatory assessment focuses on the differential diagnosis of shock. *Shock* refers to a final common pathway of vital organ failure resulting from inadequate delivery of essential nutrients, most frequently oxygen and glucose. The circulatory system delivers these nutrients to the tissues and therefore is usually the source of the cause when delivery is inadequate to meet demands. Shock can have cardiovascular, hemorrhagic, neurologic, and septic causes. The most likely precipitants in an office setting are cardiogenic, caused by pump failure; allergic, caused by profound dilation of the vascular tree in response to chemical mediators released by mast cells and basophils; or hypovolemic, caused by bleeding or volume depletion.

Cardiogenic shock would typically occur in a patient at risk for cardiac disease. Fortunately, such patients are usually known in advance. They have either a history of heart disease or risk factors (hypertension, diabetes, high cholesterol, tobacco use, family history.) If such a patient has a sudden episode of deterioration, assume it is of cardiac etiology.

Allergic shock also presents in a clinical context, which can facilitate diagnosis. If the patient is a previously healthy younger person who deteriorates after administration of a medication, presume allergic reaction to the medication. If the symptoms of malaise and signs of deterioration are accompanied by a rash (usually urticarial, characterized by wheals) and itching, err on the side of treating an allergic reaction (see Chapter 11).

Hypovolemic shock results from bleeding, which may be associated with a variety of procedures, including odontectomy or periodontal flaps and grafts. GI bleeding can occur in a patient with a history of peptic ulcer disease and presents with signs of circulatory insufficiency accompanied by black or bloody stools.

Circulatory failure is assessed by looking for both indirect and direct signs of inadequate circulation. Indirect signs are seen in the CNS and the skin. As the brain receives less and less of its oxygen and nutrient requirements, it responds with changes in behavior and LOC. Apprehension develops; the patient may feel frightened for no reason. Next, LOC starts to deteriorate, resulting in agitation and resistance. This progresses to lethargy, followed by complete unresponsiveness or coma.

If the patient is conscious, even if you do not feel a pulse, chest compressions are not necessary. Position the patient supine with the head slightly elevated. When a conscious patient appears to be in shock, assume that, despite the difficult circumstances, a basic minimal flow to the brain is taking place. Any level of circulation that produces consciousness is better than the level that can be achieved with the best CPR. If the patient is not in respiratory distress, the legs can be elevated to help move fluid back toward the heart. A warm blanket may help the patient conserve energy and feel better.

In performing the direct circulatory assessment, begin by checking for a central pulse. If pulses are not felt and the patient is unresponsive, the patient is in cardiac arrest. The most frequent rhythm in the adult with cardiac arrest is *ventricular tachycardia* or *ventricular fibrillation*. The most effective intervention for ventricular fibrillation/ventricular tachycardia is early defibrillation. Within minutes the heart converts to asystole, and survival is poor. Survivability depends on early defibrillation, with a 10% decline in survival rate for each minute that passes before defibrillation. This explains the immediate call for "help" (activation of EMS system) as taught in BLS. Chest compressions combined with ventilations should be initiated until defibrillation capabilities are available. Properly performed CPR temporarily provides oxygen to the cells and appears to prolong ventricular fibrillation. This is a temporary measure until the patient can be defibrillated.

The use of an *automatic external defibrillator* (AED) allows early defibrillation and thus is incorporated into BLS courses. If a dental facility is equipped with an AED, the device should be immediately applied and a shock delivered before implementation of chest compressions. The significance of early defibrillation is best exemplified by the instructions for the sole health care rescuer to administer three defibrillations before activating the EMS system when a defibrillator is available. If a defibrillator is not available and *the patient is an adult*, one does not even begin CPR unless the EMS has been activated to be sure a defibrillator is on the way.

In children, respiratory illness is the most likely cause of a cardiac arrest. The likelihood of resuscitating a child depends more on the rate of recovery of a patent airway and respirations than on defibrillation. The young heart is relatively immune to acute ischemia and malignant arrhythmia. For this reason, airway maneuvers and CPR are recommended for 1 minute by the sole rescuer before activating the EMS system. Activation should not be delayed in a multistaffed dental facility.

If a pulse is present, assess for rate, rhythm, and quality. An alteration in the pulse may be attributed to impaired cardiac output or a dysrhythmia. *Dysrhythmias* may occur in a variety of dental patients and have both cardiac and noncardiac causes, including anxiety, iatrogenic administration of epinephrine in the local anesthetic agent, illicit drugs, congenital abnormalities (e.g., paroxysmal supraventricular tachycardia), and myocardial disease states. Assess the effect of the dysrhythmia. Measure the BP to assess the full impact that the impaired cardiac output or dysrhythmia is producing on circulatory function. Palpation of the pulse provides an indication of the systolic pressure. In general a systolic BP of 80 mm Hg or higher is necessary to produce a radial pulse. Femoral pulses require 70 mm Hg, and for carotid pulses to be palpable, 60 mm Hg must be present. Simultaneously note the temperature and texture of the patient's skin. The skin shows a gradually progressive spectrum of change suggestive of inadequate cardiac output. This manifests as diaphoresis, which usually begins on the brow and becomes more diffuse with increased severity of circulatory impairment. Capillary refill takes longer than 1 or 2 seconds, and pallor of the extremities increases as perfusion is lost.

Disability

Disability refers to the neurologic assessment for immediately life-threatening disease. The clinician is looking at only two easily measurable parameters of the neurologic function: LOC and pupils. *Level of consciousness* is assessed using the "AVPU" method. The patient either is alert or responds to voice or to pain, or the patient is labeled unresponsive. After the AVPU score is assigned, the *pupils* are classified as equal or unequal, reactive or unreactive. Any decreased LOC not explainable by the ordinary use of anesthesia is abnormal and could be caused by neurologic injury. Conditions in earlier parts of the survey, including respiratory failure or circulatory failure, can also cause decreased LOC. Pupillary asymmetry is a definite indicator of focal neurologic injury and mandates further evaluation in a hospital ED unless it is previously documented.

Usually, in the patient with a neurologic event, the dentist can only make the diagnosis. If the neurologic examination is abnormal, the patient must go to the ED. Proper treatment entails supporting the ABCs and activating the EMS system.

Expose

Expose means to disrobe the patient as necessary to ensure an adequate assessment, not missing or misdiagnosing any injury or illness. The patient does not need to be entirely undressed, but the clinician should be able to evaluate the heart, lungs, or extremities as needed to perform the ABCD assessment.

History

History taking during the primary survey is scant. Frequently the patient is unable to give a history at the time of the emergency, and the current circumstances constitute the largest portion of the history. The clinician obtains only the "AMPLE" history,[6] a simple checklist to acquire relevant data (Box 1-13). A more detailed history will be obtained during the secondary survey as part of the data-gathering process.

Summary

The primary survey is suited to seriously ill patients. Any patient who can pass a primary survey without requiring treatment, by definition, does not have an immediate threat to life. If such a threat has been identified, treatment has been initiated. The primary survey does *not* need to be completed before calling for help. One of the most powerful tools to treat illness identified during the primary survey is to call 911.

Secondary Survey

By definition, the secondary survey is not initiated unless the primary survey has been completed, treating immediately life-threatening illness or injury. Compared with the primary survey, the secondary survey is (1) a more methodical assessment, which usually is more time consuming and focuses on potentially life-threatening injuries; (2) a systematic evaluation moving from head to toe; and (3) a more careful physical examination and more thorough history. The situation remains critical, however, and most information must be solicited from available sources. The sources include (1) talking to the patient if possible, (2) interviewing family members or individuals who may have accompanied the patient, (3) interviewing witnesses of the event, (4) reviewing the patient's chart, (5) contacting the patient's physician, and (6) noting the circumstances of the event.

The secondary survey is a compartmentalized history and physical examination. The six compartments are head, neck, chest, abdomen, skeletal, and neurologic (Box 1-14). As in the primary survey, each compartment has its repertoire of likely, detectable, and treatable illnesses (see Box 1-1). Some conditions are also found in the primary survey but present in a less severe or not imminently life-threatening form. A fine line exists between the primary and secondary surveys, and the distinction may not be clear. For example, a patient with an asthmatic attack might pass the primary survey without any intervention; however, on secondary survey, careful inspection might identify an abnormality and indicate the need for intervention. Clinically, this patient would be having a bronchospastic attack, which would be typical for the patient and not life threatening.

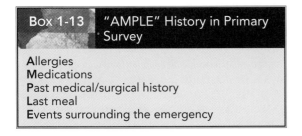

Box 1-13	"AMPLE" History in Primary Survey

Allergies
Medications
Past medical/surgical history
Last meal
Events surrounding the emergency

Box 1-14	Compartments of Secondary Survey

REGION	COMMON ILLNESSES
Head	Sinusitis, pharyngitis, odontogenic infection, avulsed tooth, facial bone fracture
Neck	Stridor, space infection, hemorrhage with hematoma, neoplasm with airway compromise, cervical injury
Chest	Angina, myocardial infarction, palpitations, asthma, emphysema, chronic bronchitis, congestive heart failure, hyperventilation, pneumonia
Abdomen	"Acute abdomen"
Skeletal	Fracture (fractured hip can result in significant blood loss), dislocation
Neurologic	Stroke, seizure, mental status changes secondary to metabolic or circulatory derangements

Head

Palpate the head carefully, looking for abnormalities. These abnormalities may have either contributed to or resulted from the initial emergency. Maxillofacial space infections can compromise the upper airway. Infections involving regions associated with the muscles of mastication result in trismus. Assess the patient's speech. Inquire about a change in voice quality, and listen for a "raspy" voice, which may indicate extension of the infection toward the larynx. Assess for contusions, lacerations, and bleeding from the ears, nose, mouth or throat, as well as for alveolar fractures, subluxed and avulsed teeth, and facial fractures. A dentist must account for avulsed teeth, displaced restorations, and dental instruments. If all objects cannot be found, chest and abdominal radiographs are indicated. If at risk for injury, the eyes should be examined. If primary intracranial disease is suspected, or if the patient sustained a significant fall or impact to the head, a computed tomography (CT) scan may be indicated. Radiography requires patient transfer to a hospital ED.

Injuries to the facial region are common in the abused patient. Any of the previous injuries, including lacerations, contusions, periorbital ecchymoses, areas of avulsed hair, fractures, and facial pain, are characteristic of abuse and warrant further investigation.

Neck

Examine the neck systematically using inspection, palpation, and auscultation. Inspect the external contours for symmetry, swelling, and erythema. Palpate for any tenderness, crepitus, or irregularities. Examine the external jugular veins for distention. Distended veins require further investigation into illnesses causing increased right ventricular pressures. If heart disease is suspected, venous distention can support a diagnosis of heart failure. Auscultate the neck for *stridor*, a high-pitched inspiratory sound. Look for retractions of the sternal notch or of the sternocleidomastoid muscles, which are recruited to assist when additional force is necessary to expand the thorax for inspiration or expiration.

Chest

Examination of the chest assesses both pulmonary function and cardiac function and is subjective as well as objective. Inquire about chest pain, palpitations, and shortness of breath. A complaint of chest pain or shortness of breath may be of cardiac or pulmonary etiology. Assessment of cardiac function is a continuous process from the primary survey. Palpate the rate, rhythm, and quality of a peripheral pulse. Record the BP. Observe respiratory rate, depth, and work of breathing. Assess the movement of the chest and abdomen; a disjointed movement between the thoracic and abdominal movements is consistent with respiratory distress. Evaluate the work of breathing by noting if the intercostal muscles retract, descending into the spaces between the ribs with inspiration. Normally, minimal to no visible movement of these muscles should occur.

Auscultate for wheezes, rales, rhonchi, and diminished breath sounds, seeking the specific diagnoses of asthma, congestive heart failure, or aspirated foreign body. Inspect the thoracic cavity for symmetry and size; a barrel-shaped chest suggests chronic obstructive pulmonary disease. If the patient is unconscious and further inspection is warranted, note any surgical scars and their significance. A midsternal scar suggests a coronary artery bypass graft. A scar in the upper chest suggests a pacemaker or an automatic implantable defibrillator. Palpate the region for these objects.

Although rare, nontraumatic pneumothorax may be related to aspects of dental treatment (e.g., irritation of pharynx causing patient to cough, rupture of bullae secondary to nitrous oxide). Hyperinflation resulting from a pneumothorax can make one hemithorax appear slightly larger.

Abdomen

The various causes of abdominal distress may have gastrointestinal pathology or may be a symptom of cardiovascular, pulmonary, genitourinary, or gynecologic pathology. The abdominal pain may be a direct consequence of dental treatment (e.g., gastric irritation associated with prescribed NSAIDs), may be an indirect consequence of dental treatment (e.g., gastroesophageal reflux from supine positioning), or may have no association with dental treatment (e.g., ruptured aortic aneurysm). Initial assessment seeks to find a basis for the complaint. This initial approach is based on the patient's history. For example, in the patient with a history of gastroesophageal reflux disease the situation may have been avoided by taking precautions with the patient's initial positioning. With the complaint of abdominal pain, however, positioning the patient upright may be of benefit. If the symptoms cannot be attributed and explained by the patient's medical history, further examination is required.

Inspect the skin for external signs of injury, such as bruising or swelling. Notice the contour of the abdomen and whether it appears distended or flat. Palpate gently and systematically, gradually covering the entire anterior abdominal wall, seeking tenderness and masses. In particular, look for a pulsatile mass in an elderly patient who clinically appears in shock and is complaining of abdominal pain. This could represent an abdominal aortic aneurysm and is a surgical emergency.

When symptoms and signs of abdominal illness are present in association with a general deterioration in the patient's condition, the dental treatment should be interrupted and the patient referred for further evaluation of the abdominal situation. Making a definitive diagnosis often presents a difficult challenge to the ED physician. Dentists are not required to make a definitive diagnosis but should know when immediate medical referral is indicated.

Skeletal

Skeletal assessment is directed at the spine and the large bones, which can be associated with bleeding or neurologic injury. In the ED the patient presenting with a facial fracture will be questioned and examined, possibly with radiographs to assess for a cervical spine injury. The injured patient, especially with a dental injury (e.g., alveolar fracture, avulsed tooth), may believe the injury is more appropriate for the dentist to treat and present to the dental office. The treating physician must always be suspicious of associated injuries in the trauma patient. The more likely scenario in the dental office is for the patient to fall secondary to a multitude of problems (e.g., vasodepressor syncope, orthostatic hypotension). The dentist needs to have a basic knowledge of cervical spine assessment to make an educated decision when the situation is not obvious (Box 1-15). If spinal injury is suspected, the most appropriate action is to call EMS. Placing a patient in full spinal immobilization is beyond the capability of most dental offices.

When the dentist becomes suspicious of a *cervical injury*, the patient should be appropriately positioned. When presenting with an associated traumatic event, the patient may be asked to lie supine in the dental chair or on the floor. If the incident occurred within the office and the patient has fallen to the floor, intervention depends on whether the patient is conscious or uncon-

---

Box 1-15   Cervical Spine Assessment

1. Palpate the neck.
   a. Areas of tenderness
   b. Irregularities
   c. Crepitus
2. Assess for subcutaneous emphysema.
3. Assess for peripheral paresthesias.
   a. Assess for sensation and response to painful stimuli.
   b. Note lack of sensation and response.
4. Assess for paresis.
5. Assess tracheal deviation.
6. Assess respiratory pattern.

---

scious. If the patient is unconscious, the dental team should adhere to the basic ABCDEs. Often, patients "slump" to the floor without risk of cervical injury. If the incident was witnessed, cervical spine precautions may not be necessary. If cervical spine injury is suspected, however, appropriate precautions must be taken when assessing the airway. If the airway is patent and the patient is breathing, the patient should be left in the position until the arrival of EMS personnel, who are familiar with managing cervical trauma. If the airway is obstructed, any maneuver to open the airway must minimize movement of the neck.

The dental team may not be able to immobilize the cervical spine, but they should employ techniques to minimize neck mobility and achieve airway patency. A mandibular jaw thrust minimizes neck movement. If the patient is completely obtunded, an oropharyngeal airway may also be beneficial. However, insertion of an adjunct airway (nasopharyngeal, oropharyngeal) in the partially obtunded individual may result in coughing and vomiting, which may have adverse effects on cervical stability. If an airway cannot be established or positive-pressure ventilation is required, the patient must be positioned supine. The recommended technique involves in-line stabilization of the head, cervical spine, and thoracic spine.

If conscious and able to cooperate, allow the patient to assume a position of comfort. With suspected cervical injury, however, high movement should be minimal. For example, the patient resting against a wall should remain in that position until a preliminary examination is done. If suspicion remains high after an initial examination, the patient should remain in this position until emergency personnel arrive. The dentist should err on seeking emergency assistance if there is any question regarding the extent of injury, since the consequences of not detecting an injury are significant.

The other component of the skeletal examination pertains to inspection of the *long bones*. Injuries to the wrist and upper extremity may result from attempts to brace and protect oneself. Geriatric patients may be more susceptible to a hip fracture. If associated with a fracture, these injuries may bleed heavily. Palpate the bones for irregularities, tenderness, mobility, crepitance, or hematoma formation. Examine the pelvis by applying a compressive force, either by squeezing the pelvis from the sides or by pressing both sides of the pelvis against the underlying surface. Rotate the patient's hips internally and externally to assess for pain or limitation of movement, which could indicate a fracture in the elderly patient. A classic hip fracture produces external rotation and shortening of the leg at the hip joint.

Neurologic

The neurologic portion of the secondary survey is designed to look for evidence of CNS injury beyond that which causes decreased LOC or unequal pupils. Inspect the face for symmetry. Ask the patient to repeat a simple phrase. Ask the patient to smile, and note if both sides of the mouth lift. Ask the patient to close the eyes and wrinkle the forehead. Check extraocular mobility by asking the patient to look up and down and then side to side; the eyes should move equally. Check if the tongue protrudes symmetrically and if the soft palate elevates symmetrically, indicating an intact gag reflex. Lightly touch each extremity to check for sensory deficits, then assess motor strength in the arms and legs. Any asymmetry or positive finding on neurologic assessment is abnormal and indicates a need for medical evaluation, probably in the ED.

Continuing Care and Reassessment

Repeat the surveys until the emergency resolves or EMS arrives. To determine how the patient is responding to treatments, examine the same features of the clinical picture used to gauge the level of illness. Try to ascertain if the patient is doing one of three things: getting better, getting worse, or staying the same. If the situation is not improving or remains unchanged, further emergency care is required. Provide continued assessment and intervention until EMS personnel arrive to assume care and transport the patient to the hospital.

Definitive Care

The goal of intervention is to reverse the emergency completely and restore the patient to a preinjury or a preillness condition. If the condition remains critical without evidence of improvement, further care is required and the patient should be transported to the hospital ED. If the patient's condition improves but does not return to a normal physiologic state, further care also is required. The management decision may not be as clear in these patients, but using common sense may be sufficient.

The dentist should consult with the patient and family regarding definitive care. The situation may not always warrant that the patient be transported to an ED. Patients may seek further care from their regular physician to optimize their medical condition. The dentist may need to discuss the situation with the patient's physician and direct the patient to the physician's office for further assessment. This may be an acceptable alternative in the patient with chronic obstructive pulmonary disease who has increased bronchospasm associated with a respiratory infection. Alternatively, if the patient has improved and is in satisfactory condition, a direct referral may not be required. The patient may still require medical examination and optimization of the medical condition before further dental treatment. An anxious patient who had a vasodepressor episode and loss of consciousness may not require further medical assessment but will require assisted transportation home. These are *recommendations* only, and the actual decision must be made based on the clinician's best judgment and discussion with the patient.

A difficult situation develops when the dentist determines that the patient requires transportation to the ED and the patient refuses to be transported. The dentist should activate the EMS system and request emergency personnel to the office. It would best serve the patient if the dental team had the assistance of the emergency personnel. The emergency personnel will help to determine the patient's capability to refuse further medical intervention and transportation to the ED. The EMS team also may alter the patient's perspective on the situation and subsequently convince the patient to allow transport with subsequent medical transportation to the ED. If the patient ultimately is not transported to the ED, definitive care should be arranged with the family and physician. Also, it should be documented that emergency assistance was offered and declined by the patient.

NEED TO TRANSFER

All cases require a decision about the patient's transfer to the local hospital's ED. Often this decision is straightforward. When uncertain, the dentist should fall back to the tenet of emergency medicine that states, "When in doubt, do," and arrange transfer. If a patient must be transferred, this determination should be made as soon as possible. A decision *not* to transfer should be made only when the vital signs are normal and the patient has no signs or symptoms of serious disease.

The transfer decision is based on "hard" findings and general impressions. Hard findings are signs encountered in the primary and secondary surveys that indicate major organ dysfunction, including abnormal vital signs, altered mental status, diaphoresis, changes in pulse (absent, irregular, rapid, or weak), cyanosis, and pallor. The hard category also includes symptoms such as chest pain, shortness of breath, and the patient's feeling of "impending doom." General impressions of serious illness are intuitive; the dentist may not "like the way this one looks" and may want to act aggressively.

The question of transfer may be a common-sense decision and the plan with which the dentist and patient feel most comfortable. The clinician may say, "I'm familiar with this constellation of signs and symptoms. They add up to a pattern that I recognize, which is not serious and is within my ability to treat." These patients can be treated in the office, and the dental care can be resumed. At other times the dentist concludes, "I am concerned that this patient has an illness I am unable to confidently diagnose," or, "Although I am able to make the diagnosis, it is beyond my ability to treat." In these situations the patient must be transferred to an ED, even if this means activating the EMS system (calling 911). Many lives have been saved because a clinician used common sense or acted on intuition.

Presenting the Case

When paramedics arrive, or when an ED physician calls to hear what happened, the dentist should be prepared to present the case in an organized way. Recounting the findings and treatments as they occurred during the primary and secondary surveys serves as a guide to an accurate description of the office emergency. This is an excellent way of organizing thoughts and not forgetting important information.

Box 1-16   Documentation in Dental Emergency Management

1. Brief history of event
2. Positive findings on primary survey
3. Positive findings on secondary survey
4. Treatments provided and responses to treatment
5. Time of important events
6. Disposition

Emergency Department Management

The ED of a modern hospital is a receiving center for all patients who need emergency assistance. It can be used for *any* emergency, no matter how minor. In the ED the process initiated in the dental office can be continued, with invasive diagnostic and therapeutic procedures, advanced medical and surgical therapy, and intensive care.

Procedures that seem major in an office setting are routine in the ED. A seizure that does not stop in the office may be controlled with general anesthesia in the ED. A stroke (cerebrovascular accident) can be confirmed by CT scan and consideration given to anticoagulation. A myocardial infarction can be treated with thrombolytic drugs and cardiac catheterization. An airway can be controlled surgically by cricothyroidotomy if necessary.

Documentation

Documentation of the events during an office emergency is important for the patient's health because it affects future care. Documentation is instrumental in properly informing other health care providers about the circumstances of the emergency. Finally, it is a key part of the medical record, which may be necessary to explain the dentist's actions. Important information should be recorded in a description of the emergency (Box 1-16). Forms should be available to record office emergencies (Figure 1-5).

BASIC AIRWAY MANAGEMENT
Anatomy and Physiology

The respiratory system consists of a passageway from outside the body to the alveoli within the lungs. It is divided into an upper and a lower airway. The *upper airway* is composed of the mouth and nose, the pharynx, and the larynx. Patency

Name		Age	Weight	Height
Medications		Allergies		
Past medical health		History of event		

Time	BP	HR	RR	Findings/interventions (e.g., medications)

Figure 1-5. Form for documenting an emergency.

of the upper airway depends on maintaining muscle tone of the tongue, soft palate, and pharynx. The nose, mouth, and pharynx of the upper airway are shared with the upper component of the gastrointestinal (GI) tract.

The *lower airway* is separated from the GI tract by the epiglottis. However, the contiguous structure of the lower airway with the GI tract puts the patient at risk for contamination of the lower airway. In the healthy dental patient, intact muscle tone and reflexes maintain patency of the upper airway and protect the lower airway from GI contamination and aspiration of foreign debris. In the obtunded or unconscious patient, loss of muscle tone and protective reflexes compromises airway patency and increases the risk of aspiration. The lower airway is composed of the trachea, bronchi, bronchioles, and alveoli. These structures do not deform and become obstructed as do structures in the upper airway. However, mucous secretions and smooth muscle spasm of the bronchi decrease the size of the airway conduit and can compromise airflow through the respiratory tract.

The function of the respiratory system is to bring oxygen from the atmosphere into the alveoli, where it can diffuse into the blood and be distributed to the cells of the body. Simultaneously the blood carries carbon dioxide, the byproduct of metabolism, from the cells to the lung, where CO_2 diffuses into the alveoli and is exhaled through the airway into the atmosphere. The stimulus to breathe is controlled by the respiratory center and depends on both hypoxemia and CO_2 levels. In the patient without pulmonary disease the primary stimulus is increasing levels of CO_2. Chronic pulmonary and cardiovascular diseases may impair gaseous exchange at the level of the alveoli; these patients have a hypoxic respiratory drive.

Airway Assessment

Airway assessment is performed in a systematic manner to ensure that critical components are not overlooked. Airway management protocol entails an assessment of airway patency, breathing (ventilatory effort), and oxygenation. If the airway is not patent, the patient cannot exchange gas. If the patient is not breathing, oxygenation is not occurring. First, assess LOC. An obstructed airway causes hypoxia, which causes anxiety and agitation. A conscious patient who is relaxed and comfortable is unlikely to have an obstructed airway. The corollary is that agitation is an airway problem until ruled out.

Obstruction of the upper airway in the conscious dental patient may have resulted from an

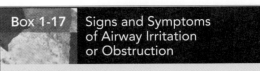

| Box 1-17 | Signs and Symptoms of Airway Irritation or Obstruction |

1. Agitation
2. Universal distress signal
3. Coughing
4. Crowing (partial obstruction)
5. Silence (complete obstruction)
6. Wheezing
7. Cyanosis
8. Oxygen desaturation (if pulse oximeter available)

aspirated dental instrument, dental appliance, crown, or tooth. Aspiration may occur in the conscious patient when an object slips from the dentist's hand or passes behind a pharyngeal barrier (e.g., rubber dam). In this situation the loss and displacement of the object is the primary event contributing to the medical emergency. Aspiration of an object usually results in airway irritability, frequently manifested as coughing (Box 1-17); this may be transient. An aspirated object that becomes lodged within the upper airway causes either poor air exchange or complete airway obstruction. The Heimlich maneuver is recommended for relieving a foreign body obstruction (see later discussion).

Alternatively, the object may pass through the trachea and into the right or left bronchus. This may or may not result in bronchospasm; after the initial event the patient may not have signs or symptoms of aspiration. Suspicion of an aspirated object requires further evaluation. Even if an object was swallowed and has passed into the stomach, further medical evaluation may be indicated (see Chapter 18).

In the obtunded or unconscious patient, airway obstruction is most frequently associated with loss of muscle tone. Airway maneuvers are designed to compensate for this lost muscle tone (Figures 1-6 and 1-7; see also Figures 1-2 to 1-4). If a patent airway cannot be achieved, foreign body obstruction must be considered. Aspiration of a foreign body may have gone unnoticed and may be the etiology of the emergency. Alternatively, displacement of an object, aspiration, and airway obstruction may have resulted from the medical emergency, such as loss of a dental instrument when a patient had a seizure. The obtunded or unconscious patient also has impaired pharyngeal and laryngeal reflexes and is at risk for aspiration of gastric contents. Although most medical emergencies are not associated with active regurgitation, airway man-

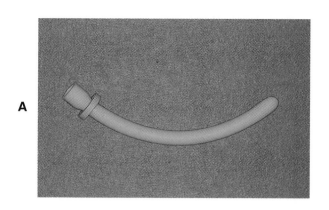

A

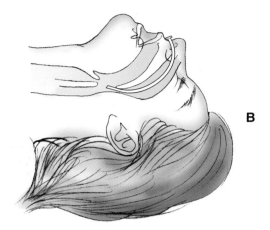

B

Figure 1-6. **A,** Nasopharyngeal airway. This soft, pliable, hollow rubber tube passes through the nasal chamber into the pharynx between the tongue and the posterior pharyngeal wall. The hollow passage serves as a conduit for ventilation. **B,** Nasopharyngeal airway in place.

Technique for Insertion of Nasopharyngeal Airway

1. Administer nasal spray (e.g., phenylephrine, 0.25% or 0.5%).
2. Identify appropriate-size airway, approximately the length from tip of the nose to meatus of the ear.
3. Lubricate airway.
4. Insert airway along floor of the nose with a gentle motion.
5. Slight rotation of airway may facilitate its passage when resistance is encountered.

---

agement may result in gastric distention and increase the incidence of vomiting.

Oxygenation

Once a patent airway has been established, the next step in airway management is to assess whether the patient is breathing. If the patient is breathing, whether conscious or unconscious, assessment is directed toward determining the adequacy of oxygenation. Impaired oxygenation may be secondary to inadequate ventilation (respiratory rate and depth) or inadequate gas exchange, which in turn may be caused by many acute and chronic conditions, such as asthma, myocardial infarction (MI), and congestive heart failure (CHF). Intuitively, administration of supplemental oxygen is beneficial. The only situation in which oxygen is not indicated is for management of hyperventilation syndrome. Otherwise, oxygen should never be withheld. If there is concern that the administration of supplemental oxygen will impair the hypoxic respiratory drive in a patient with chronic obstructive pulmonary disease (COPD), the rescuer should be prepared to provide assisted ventilation.

Administration of oxygen requires a portable O_2 source. Often emergencies occur in practice settings that do not have access to wall-mounted oxygen sources. An "E" tank measures 29½ inches high and 4½ inches wide and weighs about 25 pounds (Figure 1-8). When full, this tank contains 2000 pounds per square inch (psi). The psi should be checked and recorded daily. Because oxygen is stored as a compressed gas, the amount of gas remaining in the cylinder is easily calculated. The following formula provides a general guide when determining how long a supply of oxygen will last during an emergency:

Duration of administration = (Pounds per square inch × 0.28)/Liters per minute

A full E tank that has a flow rate of 10 liters per minute (L/min) will last approximately 60 minutes.

Oxygenation can be administered with a nasal cannula, face mask, or face mask with reservoir. The selection of an appropriate device depends on the patient's oxygenation problem or respiratory distress, as well as the underlying medical condition. A *nasal cannula* delivers a low oxygen flow of 2 to 6 L/min. It is designed for individuals with minimal or no oxygenation problem and is

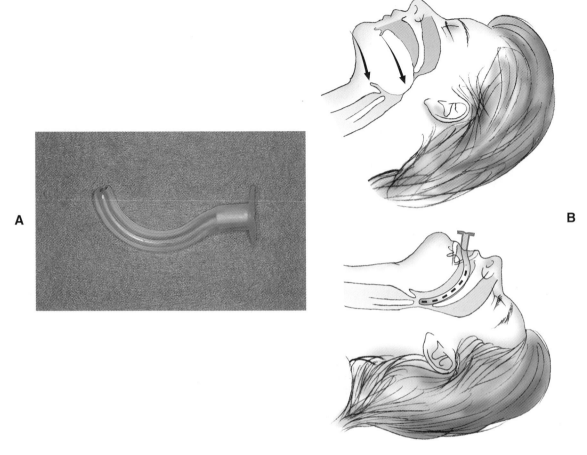

A

B

Figure 1-7. **A,** Oropharyngeal airway. This semicircular device has a hollow center channel or two side channels. The airway holds the tongue anterior to the posterior pharyngeal wall. **B,** Oropharyngeal airway in place.

Techniques for Placement of Oropharyngeal Airway

FIRST TECHNIQUE
1. Select the appropriate-size airway, approximately the length from commissure of the mouth to tragus of the ear.
2. Place a tongue blade distal to the circumvallate papillae.
3. Displace the tongue anteriorly and toward floor of the mouth.
4. Insert airway with the concave side toward the tongue.
5. Position airway posterior to the tongue, displacing the tongue away from the posterior pharyngeal wall.

SECOND TECHNIQUE
1. Insert airway with the concave side toward roof of the mouth.
2. Rotate airway into correct position when the tip is in proximity of the posterior pharyngeal wall.
3. Position airway posterior to the tongue, displacing the tongue away from the posterior pharyngeal wall.
4. Tip of the tongue may be pulled anteriorly to confirm correct placement of airway.

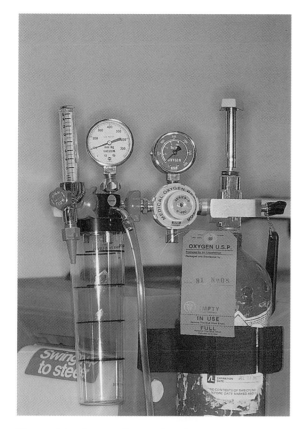

Figure 1-8. Oxygen "E" tank with Venturi suction. An office should be equipped with a portable oxygen tank. The availability of suction is essential whenever managing a patient with a compromised airway. The suction device attached to the oxygen tank provides portable suction that is always accessible when the tank is in use. The suction is created by flow of oxygen; thus it works in the event of an electrical failure. However, its use can rapidly deplete the oxygen reserve from the tank, and it should be used only when typical suction devices are not available. The wrench on the top should be secured to the oxygen tank so that it is always available when the tank is required. Without the wrench the tank cannot be opened, and no oxygen can be administered.

not intended to provide a high inspired oxygen content. The nasal cannula consists of narrow-gauge, pliable tubing with short pliable prongs that minimally extend into the nasal passages (Figure 1-9). It is nonconfining and may be more readily accepted by a patient who feels constricted by a face mask. Dry gaseous flow from the nasal cannula can be irritating to the nasal mucosa. At the upper flow rate, patients may find the stream of oxygen uncomfortable; it is more comfortable if the nasal cannula is positioned and secured before initiating oxygen flow.

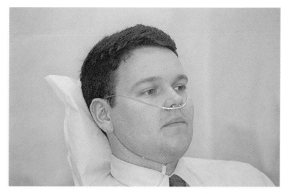

Figure 1-9. Nasal cannula.

Oxygen supplementation from a nasal cannula does not depend on whether the patient is breathing through the mouth or nose. The nasopharynx becomes a reservoir of oxygen-supplemented gas. Each inspiration mixes with this reservoir of oxygen, providing a tidal volume with an increased oxygen concentration. The percent of oxygen supplementation depends on the liter-per-minute flow of oxygen and the patient's tidal volume. The percentage of oxygen delivered by a nasal cannula can easily be approximated. For each L/min of oxygen flow increase, an additional 4% of oxygen is administered, as follows:

Percent oxygen administered = Room air (20.96%) + [4% × Oxygen flow (L/min)]

The maximum oxygen concentration supplied by a nasal cannula approximates 44%.

Oxygen administration in the COPD patient carries the risk of eliminating the hypoxic respiratory drive. A *Venturi mask* allows the oxygen concentration to be adjusted to 24%, 28%, 35%, and 40%. Oxygen delivery is initiated at 24% and titrated upward as required, observing the patient for respiratory depression. The ability to provide appropriate intervention for hypoxia is crucial, although the dental office will not have unlimited equipment. The nasal cannula can be used in a manner comparable to a Venturi mask to provide increasing concentrations of oxygen delivery.

A *face mask* is a transparent triangular mask that covers both the nose and the mouth. It is designed with and without an oxygen reservoir. The face mask without an oxygen reservoir provides an oxygen content of 40% to 60% at the recommended flow of 8 to 10 L/min. As with the nasal cannula, the face mask is not designed to provide

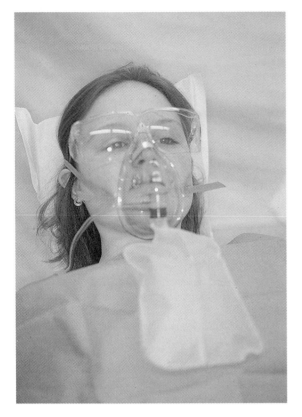

Figure 1-10. Face mask with reservoir.

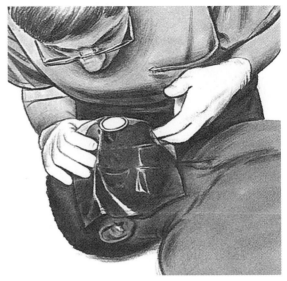

Figure 1-11. Mouth-to-mouth ventilation with barrier technique. *From American Heart Association:* Guidelines 2000 for CPR and ECC, *Dallas, 2000, The Association.*

sufficient oxygen for an entire inspired tidal volume, and the inspired oxygen is diluted with room air. A lesser oxygen flow will result in both delivery of lower oxygen content and rebreathing of exhaled air. The face mask thus provides minimal, if any, advantages over the nasal cannula.

A *face mask with reservoir* provides a significant advantage over the nasal cannula (Figure 1-10). At an oxygen flow of 10 L/min, the device delivers approximately 100% oxygen. To minimize rebreathing and to optimize oxygenation, the flow rate should be set such that the reservoir bag remains inflated. The face mask should be moderately tight fitting.

Face masks are transparent to allow visualization and monitoring of secretions and possible gastric regurgitation. The high oxygen content is appropriate for the patient who is experiencing moderate to severe oxygen desaturation or respiratory distress.

Ventilation

If the patient is not breathing after the establishment of airway patency, efforts are directed toward providing positive-pressure ventilation.

Mouth-to-mouth ventilation is the simplest technique of ventilating a patient. Since it is taught in most BLS courses, office personnel will probably be familiar with this technique. To maintain appropriate infection control, emergency kits should contain barrier devices for mouth-to-mouth resuscitation (Figure 1-11). The technique is limited in both its esthetic appeal and its ability to provide high inspired oxygen concentrations. Room air contains approximately 21% oxygen. The oxygen content of a rescue breath is 5% less than that of the rescuer's inspiration. Placing a nasal cannula with a flow of 6 L/min on the rescuer may increase the amount of oxygen delivered to the victim.

The *pocket mask* with a one-way valve and an oxygen inlet has several advantages over mouth-to-mouth ventilation (Figure 1-12). The mask provides a more effective barrier between the victim and the rescuer because of its microfilter and the diversion of the victim's exhalations away from the rescuer. The oxygen inlet allows the administration of higher oxygen concentrations. A flow of 10 L/min provides oxygen content of approximately 50%. The pocket mask may be more effective than the bag-valve-mask (BVM) device in providing positive-pressure ventilation. Familiarity with performing positive-pressure ventilation using a pocket mask can be incorporated into BLS instruction.

A *bag-valve-mask* device with oxygen inlet is the recommended equipment to provide positive-pressure ventilation. The BVM is available in adult

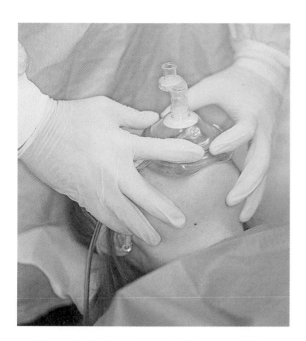

Figure 1-12. Pocket mask with oxygen inlet.

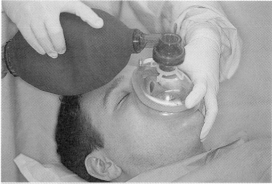

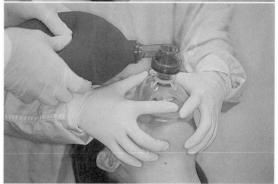

Figure 1-13. **A,** Bag-valve-mask device. **B,** Achieving a satisfactory seal may be difficult in select individuals. Allowing one rescuer to secure the mask to the patient's face with both hands may minimize an air leak and optimize ventilation. Second rescuer is required to squeeze the reservoir bag and provide positive-pressure ventilation. Slow, gentle ventilations and continuous observation to ensure chest movement minimizes the risk of gastric insufflation and resultant regurgitation.

and pediatric sizes, and an office should have one of each, with an appropriate selection of masks. The mask should be transparent and capable of making a tight seal against the face. However, many rescuers will have difficulty achieving a tight seal. The bag should thus be self-inflating, avoiding the need to have a tight seal between the mask and face. It should have an adjustable pop-off valve and a nonrebreathing valve to improve the rescuer's ability to provide positive-pressure ventilation with high oxygen content. A flow of 15 L/min is suggested to ensure adequate tidal volume and oxygen delivery (Figure 1-13).

Complications of positive-pressure ventilation include insufficient tidal volume and gastric distention. The insertion of an oropharyngeal airway may increase the ease and quality of ventilation and may minimize the incidence of gastric distention. Gastric distention promotes gastric regurgitation, which increases the risk of aspiration. Gastric distention also displaces the diaphragm superiorly, compromising ventilatory effort.

Emergency personnel often insert an *endotracheal* (ET) *tube* shortly after initiating resuscitation efforts. The insertion of an ET tube establishes a direct and patent conduit into the lower airway, which isolates the lower airway from the GI tract. The ET tube (1) facilitates ventilations with a

high inspired oxygen concentration, (2) allows suctioning of the lower airway, (3) protects against aspiration, and (4) provides a route for drug delivery. Most important, the ET tube maintains a patent protected airway and delivers a high inspired oxygen content. With the tube in place, the patient can be more aggressively hyperventilated with less concern about a synchronous rhythm of cardiac compression to ventilation. However, ET intubation requires advanced training. Complications occur even in experienced hands. Airway manipulation in the semiconscious patient can aggravate the gag reflex and promote vomiting and aspiration of gastric contents. Unrecognized intubation of the esophagus can obstruct ventilation and oxygenation. Trauma to the airway is also a risk. The inclusion of a laryngoscope and ET tubes in most prepackaged medical emergency kits for dentists is unrealistic.

The *esophageotracheal tube* (Combitube) is an alternative to the ET tube that is acceptable for the dental facility. In this double-lumen tube, one lumen is open at both ends. The other lumen is closed at the tip and is perforated along its lower half. The Combitube has two inflatable cuffs: a smaller cuff at the distal end of the tube and a much larger cuff approximately one third of the way from the distal end. The perforated area of the tube is between the small and large cuffs (Figure 1-14).

The Combitube is blindly inserted with the head in a neutral position. In more than 95% of cases the tube is inserted into the esophagus. The small cuff and then the large cuff are inflated. After insertion and inflation of both cuffs, positive-pressure ventilation is attempted. If the device is placed within the esophagus, ventilation is accomplished through the lumen with the closed tip. The small cuff inflated within the esophagus seals the stomach, preventing gastric distention and gastric regurgitation resulting in aspiration. The large cuff inflated in the pharynx acts as an obturator; oxygen is directed from the lateral perforations toward the trachea. Auscultation of breath sounds over the lung fields or absence of epigastric sounds confirms esophageal placement and indicates acceptable ventilation.

After confirmation of effective ventilation, the stomach can be decompressed by passing a nasogastric tube through the open lumen into the stomach. If no breath sounds are auscultated over the lung fields, ventilation is attempted through the other lumen. Successful ventilations indicate that the tube has been inserted into the trachea and is thus equivalent to ET intubation. If adequate ventilation is not achieved through either lumen, the Combitube must be removed. Management of the airway is reassessed. The BVM may be used, the Combitube reinserted, or an alternative technique attempted.

The primary principle of management of the patient in respiratory distress is *ventilatory support with supplemental oxygen*. Unlike an ET tube, the Combitube does not require advanced training. Compared with a face mask the Combitube has a better seal, with improved ventilation, and the ability to isolate the lower airway from the GI tract. The Combitube is contraindicated in pediatric patients (generally less than 10 years of age) because it is too large and in patients with pharyngeal or esophageal pathology.

When the patient is unable to be ventilated with any of the previous devices, *transtracheal ventilation* can provide an alternative means of airway management. The goal is to oxygenate and possibly ventilate the patient. The transtracheal

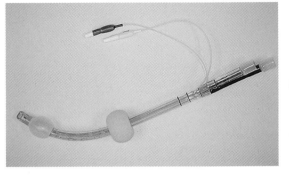

A

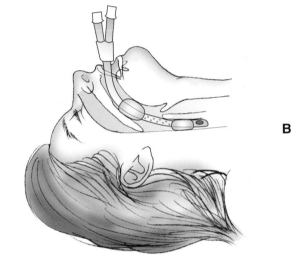

B

Figure 1-14. **A,** Esophageotracheal tube (Combitube). **B,** Combitube in place.

technique entails the placement of a catheter through the cricothyroid membrane of the larynx. First the cricoid cartilage is palpated; it is easily palpable and a reliable landmark. A catheter attached to an empty syringe is inserted in the midline just above the cricoid cartilage through the cricothyroid membrane into the trachea. Continuous negative pressure is applied with the syringe during percutaneous insertion of the catheter. Aspiration of air confirms placement within the trachea. The trocar is removed from the catheter. An oxygen source is attached to the adapter, and the patient is subsequently oxygenated. Depending on the catheter's size, ventilation may be possible (Figure 1-15).

Heimlich Maneuver
Obstruction and Aspiration

Airway obstruction is most often associated with relaxation of the upper airway musculature and can usually be corrected by applying airway

A

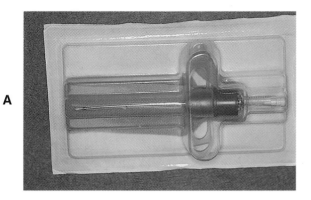

B

Cricothyroid membrane

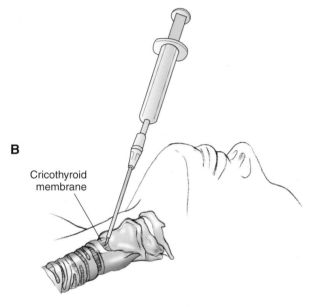

Figure 1-15. **A,** Transtracheal ventilation set. **B,** Insertion of catheter into trachea.

A

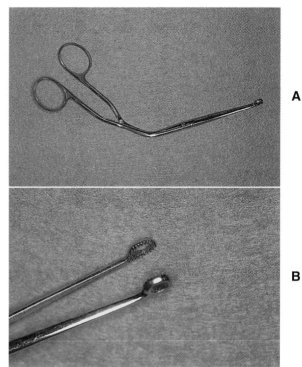

B

Figure 1-16. McGill forceps. **A,** The angulation and blunt tip are designed to facilitate directing an endotracheal tube through the glottis. However, the design provides the dentist with an instrument that can be used to retrieve a foreign object in the pharynx. **B,** The blunt tip minimizes iatrogenic injury to the mucosal tissue.

maneuvers such as the chin-forehead lift or mandibular jaw thrust. If these are ineffective, adjunctive devices such as an oral or a nasopharyngeal airway may provide relief of the obstruction (Figures 1-16 to 1-20).

If airway obstruction persists, the dentist must consider potential factors that could cause the obstruction. Airway obstruction may be secondary to an oral and maxillofacial infection, postsurgical bleeding into the soft tissues, or an allergic reaction. These conditions may cause narrowing of the airway secondary to pharyngeal swelling and lingual displacement. Foreign body aspiration can also cause airway obstruction. Patients with select neurologic disorders or elderly patients with dysphagia may be at increased risk of aspiration from either a

foreign object or gastric regurgitation from pharyngeal stimulation. Alternatively, a fixed prosthesis may become dislodged secondary to a seizure and aspirated because of diminished laryngeal reflexes. When the patient develops an acute respiratory problem, the dentist looks for the obvious etiology. Loss of an object or the potential for regurgitation (of solid material) and subsequent aspiration with the onset of inadequate air exchange suggests a foreign body obstruction.

Much dental treatment is now performed with the patient in the supine position. However, patients in respiratory distress usually feel more comfortable in and reposition themselves into a more upright position. The repositioning to the more erect position may be unfavorable gravitationally by promoting further apical passage of the object. However, the most important aspect is to allow patients to position themselves so that they can produce a forceful and effective cough.

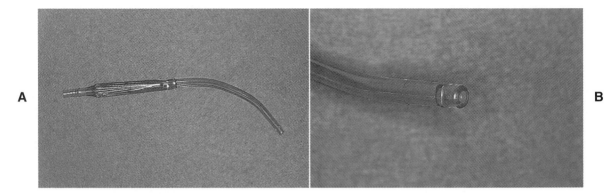

Figure 1-17. Yankauer suction device. **A,** Tonsillar suction tube is attached to a high-speed evacuator. **B,** Blunt tip allows the instrument to pass blindly into the pharynx, minimizing the risk of iatrogenic perforation. The large channels allow the suction to evacuate globular material that may have been regurgitated or displaced into the pharynx.

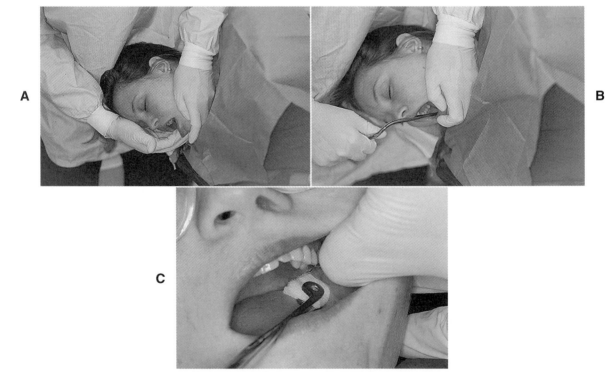

Figure 1-18. Despite the potential for numerous objects to be displaced into the airway, foreign body obstruction or aspiration is an uncommon occurrence in the dental office. When an object is displaced, however, quick action may prevent a potential problem. **A,** The patient is repositioned to the side facing the dentist in a slight Trendelenburg position. **B** and **C,** If visualized, the object may be retrieved using a McGill forceps or Yankauer suction device. Immediate availability of these instruments will optimize the chances for a successful intervention.

A

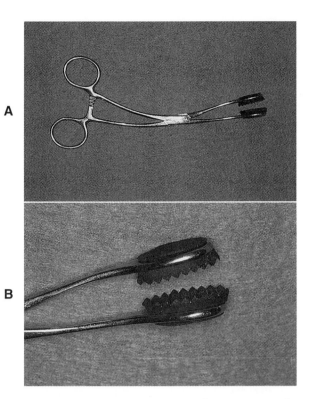

B

Figure 1-19. **A,** Tongue-grasping forceps. **B,** Appliance has serrations that allow the tongue to be held firmly without causing iatrogenic injury and to be pulled forward.

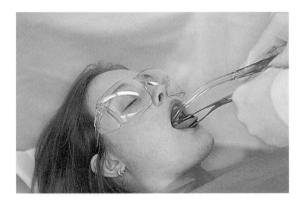

Figure 1-20. If an object is displaced from the mouth into the pharynx, or if the patient has excessive secretions or fluid in the back of the throat, the tongue may be gently pulled forward and a tonsillar (Yankauer) suction device gently inserted to evacuate the debris.

Aspiration of a foreign body may cause partial or complete airway obstruction. The dentist must differentiate between good and inadequate air exchange. Signs of inadequate air exchange include agitation, retraction at the sternal notch,

flaring of the nares, paradoxical movement of the thoracic and abdominal walls, high-pitched noise while inhaling (stridor), and ineffective cough. The patient with poor air exchange from partial or complete obstruction will become hypoxic, and if untreated, brain damage may occur within 4 to 6 minutes.

Technique

The Heimlich maneuver is the recommended method to alleviate a foreign body obstruction of the airway in persons over 1 year of age. The Heimlich *abdominal thrust* elevates the diaphragm, increasing tracheobronchial airway pressure, which forces air from the lungs to expel the obstructive object.[7] The dental patient who is semi-supine or sitting upright should be turned slightly to the side away from the dentist. As the dentist wraps the arms around the victim's waist, the iliac crest is identified bilaterally. The umbilicus is midline at the level of the height of the iliac crest. A thumb from one hand is placed in the umbilicus. The thumb side of the fist of the other hand is placed firmly against the midline of the abdomen just cephalad to the thumb identifying the umbilicus so that a closed fist with the folded thumb is against the abdomen in the epigastric area. The fist is now grasped with the other hand. Up to five upward and inward thrusts are performed, after which the patient is reassessed.

If the patient remains supine in the chair, the dentist should straddle the patient's thighs. The dentist identifies the umbilicus and positions the palmar surface of one hand just cephalad to the umbilicus in the epigastric area. The other hand is then placed on top of the initial hand, and the fingers are interlocked. Up to five abdominal thrusts are similarly performed, after which the patient is reassessed.

The process continues until the patient becomes unconscious or the object is expelled. If emergency medical assistance was not requested earlier, it should be requested once the obstruction persists despite initial intervention. If the patient becomes unconscious, a tongue-jaw lift with blind finger sweep is performed in the adult patient. In the pediatric patient, however, the tongue-jaw lift is performed and the object removed only if seen. The pediatric airway differs anatomically from the adult airway. The narrowest part of the adult airway is the glottis. Apical displacement of an object will relieve the obstruction, and survival depends on ventilation of at least one lung. Subsequent bronchoscopy may be required to remove the object. In the pediatric patient the airway is conical with the narrowest part at the level of the cricoid cartilage. Apical displacement of an object will result in further impaction of the object within the narrowest part of the airway, resulting in an inability to alleviate the obstruction (Figure 1-21).

Sellick Maneuver

The Sellick maneuver (*cricoid pressure*) consists of backward pressure of the cricoid cartilage causing temporary esophageal occlusion between the cartilage and the cervical vertebrae. The maneuver is effective in preventing both gastric regurgitation and gastric insufflation during positive-pressure ventilation. Efficacy depends on adequate pressure applied to the cricoid cartilage. A Combitube cannot be inserted when cricoid pressure is being applied. Although the Sellick maneuver is effective against passive regurgitation, its application should cease during active vomiting, when application of cricoid pressure can result in esophageal rupture.

Management of Regurgitation

Gastric distention and subsequent regurgitation is a known risk associated with positive-pressure

ventilation in the unprotected airway. The patient who vomits should be placed into a Trendelenburg position (see later discussion), which gravitationally protects against aspiration. This provides an interval during which the upper airway may be suctioned. Patients may also be turned into the left lateral decubitus position. This positioning takes advantage of the upward angulation of the left bronchi, which minimizes the risk of aspirate passing into the left lung. The right bronchi forms less of an acute angle from the trachea but is equally susceptible to aspiration regardless of the patient's lateral positioning. Therefore the patient in the left lateral decubitus position may have less risk of the aspirate contaminating both lung fields. Regardless of positioning, if the upper airway is not adequately suctioned before a ventilatory effort in the obtunded patient or before implementation of positive-pressure ventilation, the vomitus may pass or may be pushed into the tracheobronchial tree despite the Tredelendburg position.

Simultaneous with positioning the patient, the pharynx needs to be suctioned. Although the need for rapid and thorough suctioning is intuitive, iatrogenic injury must be avoided. Perforation of the pharyngeal mucosa has both immediate and delayed consequences. Acute com-

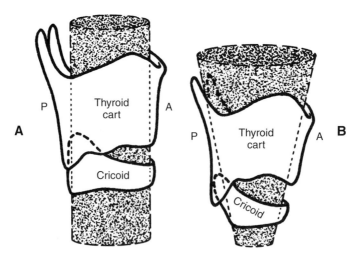

Figure 1-21. **A,** Adult airway (larnyx). The narrowest component is at the level of the glottis. Apical displacement of a foreign object will result in the object passing into one of the bronchi. Although the object will need to be retrieved, the patient will be able to be ventilated despite the potential for obstruction of one lung. **B,** Pediatric (infant) airway. The narrowest component is at the level of the cricoid cartilage. Apical displacement will lodge the foreign object into the airway, worsening the obstruction and making it more difficult to retrieve the object. *From Coté CJ, Todres ID: The pediatric airway. In Cote CJ, Ryan JF, Todres ID, et al, editors:* A practice of anesthesia for infants and children, *ed 2, Philadelphia, 1992, WB Saunders.*

plications associated with pharyngeal perforation include hemorrhage complicating airway management and emphysema of the cervical tissue planes potentially extending into the mediastinum secondary to positive-pressure ventilation. Perforation of the carotid arteries or branches of the carotid arteries, which are located behind the posterior pharyngeal wall, can result in life-threatening hemorrhage. Effective suctioning thus requires a blunt-tipped device with large openings. The blunt tip allows placement of the device into the pharynx with minimal risk of iatrogenic injury. The large openings facilitate suctioning of particulate material.

The suction should be able to be connected to the high-speed evacuation system located in each dental operatory. A backup device should be available because the device may be needed in another area or an electrical failure may occur. Auxiliary suction devices are battery powered, manually operated, or gas driven.

Cervical Spine Injury

Hospital dentists and oral/maxillofacial surgeons are usually confronted with the possibility of a cervical spine injury when they are asked to consult on a trauma patient who has sustained a facial fracture. The incidence of a cervical injury in the presence of a facial fracture varies from approximately 1% to 6%. The highest incidence of cervical injuries in the facial trauma patient is associated with the forces in vehicular accidents. However, cervical injuries in facial trauma patients have also resulted from a fall when the individuals lost their balance and were unable to appropriately protect themselves. Therefore the dentist must always be attentive and suspicious, although the likelihood of a patient sustaining a cervical injury associated with a fall in the dental office is low.

The dentist should have a low threshold for consideration of a cervical injury in the patient who (1) sustained a facial fracture (including an alveolar fracture) at the time of the fall, (2) remains obtunded, (3) complains of neck pain or tenderness, (4) complains of paresthesia below the neck, (5) demonstrates altered motor function below the neck, or (6) has a gross anatomic deformity. The child or the mentally impaired patient presents a special situation in that the person may be unable to vocalize the complaint.[8,9]

Patients suspected of cervical injury are routinely immobilized. This is usually accomplished using a combination of a rigid cervical collar, sandbags, and spine board. It cannot be expected

that the dentist will have this equipment or level of expertise. Therefore, if such an injury is suspected, it is prudent to activate the EMS system. If breathing, the patient should be maintained in the same position until emergency personnel arrive. A face mask may be held close to the patient's mouth and nose to administer supplemental oxygen. It would also be advantageous to have tonsillar suction available in both the awake and the obtunded patient. The awake patient, who will inevitably be quite anxious, may have difficulty swallowing and will appreciate the assistance of the suction in clearing the oral cavity of secretions. If the patient is obstructed, the airway must be repositioned to overcome the obstruction, with the least amount of movement. If the patient is supine, the airway may be opened using the mandibular jaw thrust. If ineffective, the dentist may consider inserting a nasopharyngeal or an oropharyngeal airway. Care must be taken so that insertion of the device does not stimulate the patient's airway, which may result in violent coughing and significant patient movement.

Establishing a patent airway in the patient who is awkwardly positioned secondary to a fall presents a significant challenge to the dental team. First an attempt should be made at opening the airway as previously discussed. If this is unsuccessful, survival may depend on ventilation and oxygenation. The head, neck, and upper body must be aligned and stabilized. The inclusion of a soft cervical collar in the emergency cart provides minimal benefit in the management of this injury because it permits approximately 75% of neck movement.[10] If the head and neck are twisted, they should be gently aligned as the patient is moved. Once the patient is repositioned, attention should be directed to using airway maneuvers to establish a patent, nonobstructed airway.

A Combitube may be inserted with the patient in any position. It may be the considered first-line intervention for establishing a patent airway in the completely obtunded patient who is awkwardly positioned.

Airway Monitoring and Pulse Oximetry

Pulse oximetry is the standard of care in monitoring the sedated patient. Although oximetry is readily available in offices where sedation is provided, it may not be available in the typical dental facility. Because many offices are acquiring automated monitoring equipment, however, specifically for pulse and BP, pulse oximetry is a component or an option of the equipment

(Figure 1-22). The pulse oximeter is a noninvasive device that provides rapid measurements of pulse rate and oxygen saturation. Monitoring the patient's *oxygen saturation* is an effective tool in assessing the need for and efficacy of respiratory intervention and support.

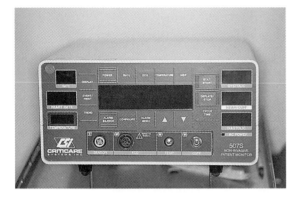

Figure 1-22. Automated monitoring units with pulse oximeter can record blood pressure, oxygen saturation, and pulse rate.

The pulse oximeter is limited in that it monitors oxygen saturation. Adequacy of or need for respiratory intervention is best ascertained by knowing the *partial pressure of oxygen in arterial blood* (PaO_2). PaO_2 can be assessed directly, but this requires arterial cannulation and laboratory equipment. Therefore, adequacy of PaO_2 is inferred from the oxygen saturation measurements. The relationship between PaO_2 and arterial hemoglobin oxygen saturation is nonlinear. When the PaO_2 is greater than 100 mm Hg, changes in PaO_2 will not be detected by oxygen saturation. Also, as the oxygen saturation approaches 85% to 90%, small changes in PaO_2 are associated with significant decreases in oxygen saturation.

The practitioner should never depend solely on the pulse oximeter for assessing and detecting changes in the patient's respiratory status without directly observing the patient. For example, a patient receiving supplemental oxygen may have a PaO_2 well above 100 mm Hg. If the patient develops respiratory distress, the PaO_2 will initially and ominously decline without any initial change in the oxygen saturation. There is a very narrow window of acceptable oxygen sat-

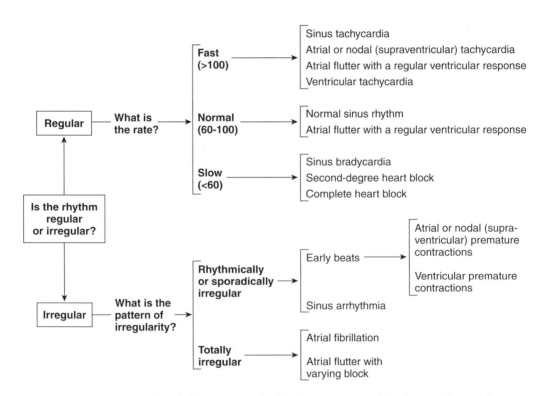

Figure 1-23. Approach to differentiation of select heart rates and rhythms. *Adapted from Bickley LS, Hoekelman RA: Bates' guide to physical examination and history taking, ed 7, Philadelphia, 1998, Lippincott.*

uration. For the patient receiving supplemental oxygen, the oxygen saturation alarm should be set at 94%. If the patient cannot maintain an oxygen saturation of 94% or higher, consideration should be given to increasing the percent of oxygen delivered. The decrease in oxygen saturation may also indicate a ventilatory problem. Oxygen saturation is only one measurement, to be used with other indicators to determine the need for assisted ventilation.

The data from all monitors must be carefully interpreted. False-negative results can occur. Excessive patient movement, cold extremities, and ambient light adversely affect the instrument performance and contribute to errors with pulse oximetry.

Basic Cardiac Maneuvers
Palpation of Pulse

The arterial pulse is palpated to determine rate, rhythm, and quality. The pulse may be fast or slow, regular or irregular, bounding or weak (Figure 1-23 and Box 1-18). The pulse is most often palpated in one of three locations: carotid, femoral, or radial. In most situations the practitioner will palpate the radial pulse. All office staff should be familiar with assessing a radial pulse. This can be easily accomplished by incorporating it into the regular office routine. Once the patient is seated, a staff member records vital signs (BP and pulse). The dentist can then repeat these measurements as indicated (Figures 1-24 to 1-26).

Blood Pressure

BP should be a routine measurement obtained from all patients at the initial consultation. If BP is not recorded at each subsequent appointment, it should be at least monitored when a

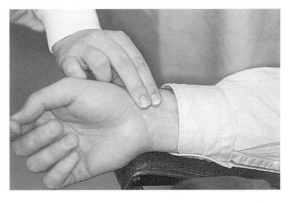

Figure 1-24. Radial pulse. The radial artery can be palpated just proximal to the wrist. Pressure is applied over the radial artery with the pads of the index and middle fingers.

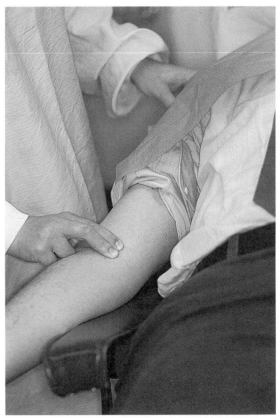

Figure 1-25. Brachial pulse. With the palms up and the elbow slightly extended, the brachial artery can be palpated in the antecubital fossa just medial to the biceps tendon. Familiarity with brachial artery palpation should be acquired with routine blood pressure monitoring. The artery is usually palpated and the stethoscope placed over it.

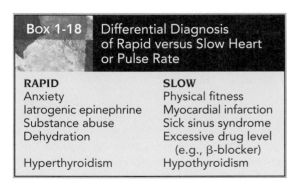

Box 1-18	Differential Diagnosis of Rapid versus Slow Heart or Pulse Rate
RAPID	**SLOW**
Anxiety	Physical fitness
Iatrogenic epinephrine	Myocardial infarction
Substance abuse	Sick sinus syndrome
Dehydration	Excessive drug level (e.g., β-blocker)
Hyperthyroidism	Hypothyroidism

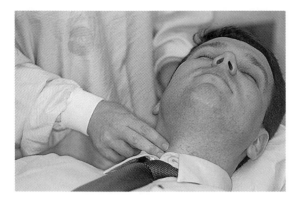

Figure 1-26. Carotid pulse. The ipsilateral carotid pulse is assessed by moving the hand from the midline laterally. The carotid pulse is palpated just inside the medial border of the sternocleido-mastoid muscle. Palpation of the artery should be just below the level of the thyroid cartilage that corresponds to the carotid sinus.

procedure is performed. Standard instrumentation includes a sphygmomanometer and a stethoscope. Automatic units are becoming more common. At times, however, such as in an emergency, the automatic BP machine may not function. The dentist and staff should know how to take a BP reading using a sphygmomanometer and stethoscope. If the office adheres to a policy of obtaining baseline vital signs at each appointment, the staff should be familiar with and have acquired the skill to take BP measurements.

For BP readings the patient should ideally have been seated for about 5 minutes. The patient's arm should be free of restrictive clothing. The examiner should palpate the brachial artery, which is just medial to the biceps tendon. The BP cuff can then be placed around the arm, with the inflatable bladder centered over the brachial artery. Cuffs of automatic machines generally indicate the part of the cuff that should be placed over the brachial artery. The cuff should fit firmly, and the examiner should be able to insert one or two fingers between the cuff and the patient's arm. The cuff is placed approximately 2 to 3 cm (1 inch) above the antecubital fossa, and then the patient's arm should be stabilized at heart level. This is most easily accomplished by having the patient rest the arm on a table or an arm board attached to the chair. When performing the skill manually, the examiner now identifies the radial artery. The BP cuff is inflated until the pulsatile flow through the radial artery is no longer palpable. The cuff is inflated to a pressure approximately 30 mm Hg greater than that noted

when the radial pulse disappeared. The examiner now firmly places and holds the diaphragm of the stethoscope over the brachial artery. The pressure in the cuff is then deflated at a rate of 2 to 3 mm Hg per second. The systolic pressure is the BP when the sounds appear. The sound will change in character as the pressure in the cuff is deflated. It eventually becomes muffled and then ceases. The examiner should allow the cuff to deflate an additional 10 to 20 mm Hg while continuing to listen before allowing the cuff to deflate rapidly. The diastolic pressure is the BP when the sound ceases completely. The sound may persist despite being muffled for several mm Hg after its initial change in character, or it may never cease. If the sound persists, the diastolic measurement is the BP when the sound changed significantly in character and became muffled.

When measuring BP with an automatic unit, the examiner usually needs to ensure only that the appropriate cuff is selected and that it is appropriately attached to the patient. At times, especially when obtaining a measurement is urgent, the unit cannot obtain a reading. Several units present the mm Hg as the unit is cycling. The examiner can obtain an estimate of palpable systolic pressure by palpating the radial artery as the unit is either deflating or inflating. The palpable systolic pressure is the measurement when the radial pulse first appears as the cuff is deflating.

Common to both the sphygmomanometer and the automatic units is the basic principle pertaining to cuff size and placement and arm position. A small cuff or an excessively loose cuff will result in artificial elevation of BP. An excessively tight cuff will also result in falsely elevated BP (diastolic rather than systolic). A large cuff will result in an artificial decrease in pressure. The office should have at least three different sizes of cuff (pediatric, adult, large adult) to avoid this problem. Artificially high BP readings will also occur if the arm is below the level of the heart or if the patient is forced to assist in stabilizing the arm at a specific height. Artificially low BP measurements will result if the arm is held above the level of the heart.

Precordial Thump

The precordial thump is a forceful blow applied to the midsternal region that may convert a patient out of ventricular fibrillation or ventricular tachycardia into a life-sustaining rhythm. Controversy surrounds its efficacy, and some have stated that it has detrimental effects. Therefore

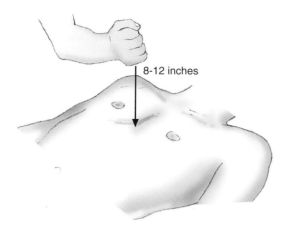

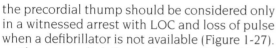

Figure 1-27. Precordial thump.

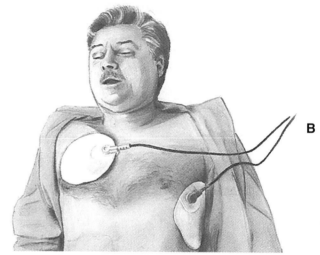

Figure 1-28. **A,** Automatic external defibrillator (AED). **B,** Placement of AED electrode pads. *From American Heart Association:* Guidelines 2000 for CPR and ECC, *Dallas, 2000, The Association.*

the precordial thump should be considered only in a witnessed arrest with LOC and loss of pulse when a defibrillator is not available (Figure 1-27).

The precordial thump begins about 20 cm (8 inches) above the chest. Many practitioners have difficulty in determining the exact height and force to employ. The practitioner may consider placing the fist firmly on the midsternal region and allowing the forearm to lay across the chest until the elbow comes in contact with the abdomen. With the elbow placed passively on the abdomen, the practitioner can fully elevate the forearm, then provide a forceful thump.

If the thump is unsuccessful, cardiac compressions should begin immediately after reassessment of the patient.[11-13]

Automatic External Defibrillator

An AED should be available and should be used by the first responder to an adult cardiac arrest. The AED is important because the most likely, treatable cause of sudden unresponsiveness with cardiac etiology in the adult patient is ventricular fibrillation. The most successful treatment for ventricular fibrillation in the adult patient is early defibrillation. Without early intervention, neurologic compromise occurs in as quickly as 10 minutes. The goal is survival without neurologic deficit. Survivability with early CPR (within 2 minutes) and early defibrillation (within 6 to 7 minutes) is reported to approach 20%. If defibrillation is administered within 4 minutes and ACLS within 8 minutes, the survival rate approaches 30%. However, delayed defibrillation (beyond 10 minutes) has a dismal 2% to 8% survival rate.[14,15]

An AED is designed for the adult patient (Figure 1-28). The device consists of the actual defibrillator and a set of two adhesive pads that attach to the patient. These pads read and analyze the cardiac rhythm as well as deliver the electrical shock. A diagram on each pad identifies where it should be placed. One pad is placed along the upper right sternal border; the other pad is placed along the lower left ribs over the apex of the heart, which facilitates lead II monitoring. The pads should be directly adherent to the skin. The patient may need to be shaved if direct contact cannot be made and maintained with the skin. Any transdermal delivery devices or medications should be removed or wiped clear of the area where the pad will be placed. The pads should not be placed directly over an implantable device, such as a pacemaker.

There are two types of AEDs: a fully automatic unit and a semiautomatic unit. For the *fully automatic unit* the pads are attached and the device turned on. If the patient has a rhythm amenable to defibrillation, the unit delivers an electrical charge. The unit will reassess the rhythm and repeat the defibrillation up to three times. The primary benefit of the *semiautomatic unit* is that the operator must press a button, once so advised, to deliver the electrical charge. This is an additional safety factor; before delivering the electrical charge, the operator must ensure that all individuals are clear of the patient. The standard phrase ingrained in ACLS is, "I'm clear, you're clear, everybody clear." After the shock is delivered, the unit will either automatically reanalyze the rhythm or prompt the operator to press an analyze button. The need to press a button to analyze the rhythm is a further safety feature because the unit will not charge until the rhythm is analyzed.

In addition to the automatic and semiautomatic features, the units are available in either monophasic or biphasic waveforms. The biphasic waveform represents newer technology. Both units are designed to give energy levels consistent with ACLS protocol: 200, 300, and 360 joules, then 360 joules thereafter. Some units allow the operator to set the energy level.

Once either unit is made operational, CPR and all physical contact with the patient must be discontinued while the AED analyzes the rhythm and delivers the shock. It takes up to 15 seconds for the device to analyze the rhythm. Conventional defibrillators require the operator to interpret the rhythm. The AED eliminates the need for training in rhythm recognition. Health care providers can be trained in the use of AEDs by participating in the AHA's Healthcare Provider course. The newer units are becoming more sophisticated and, once turned on, will prompt the operator as to appropriate action. This entails (1) ensuring that the defibrillator cables are plugged in, (2) making sure the defibrillator pads are properly placed, and (3) alerting the operator to avoid physical contact with the patient so that the unit can analyze the rhythm. AEDs also indicate when the operator should check for pulses, when CPR should begin, and when repeat rhythm assessment and defibrillation should be initiated.

Both failure to shock and inappropriate shocks have been reported with the AEDs. The primary errors have been those of omission, in which the unit failed to recognize a rhythm that was amenable to defibrillation. The incidence of inappropriate shocks is less than 0.1%. The potential for inappropriate shocks may be reduced by not activating the analysis mode until cardiac arrest has been confirmed.

It cannot be expected that each dental facility will have personnel who are competent in ACLS. However, the accessibility to AEDs within public areas eliminates a major deterrent to successful resuscitative efforts. The availability of AEDs in private offices is controversial. Equipping each office may be unreasonable, but it may be reasonable to equip an office building or medical facility of a specified size with a centrally located AED. It would be the responsibility of dental office personnel to know the unit's location and operation.

Chest Compressions

The purpose of chest compressions is to increase intrathoracic pressure and compress the heart so that circulation to the vital organs is restored. Properly performed compressions achieve a cardiac output 25% to 33% of the normal value, with the efficacy decreasing over time. Therefore it is critical to be able to defibrillate early. This readdresses the issue of whether a dental office should have access to an AED.

Another area of controversy is the reluctance of individuals to administer mouth-to-mouth ventilation. This conflict developed secondary to concerns about acquiring an infectious disease. Literature on this controversy suggests that chest compressions without ventilations are efficacious for the first several minutes.[16,17] However, all dental offices should be equipped to administer positive-pressure ventilation.

Patient Positioning
Trendelenburg Position

The patient is supine in the dental chair in an inclined position, with the head placed below and the feet elevated slightly above the level of the heart (Figure 1-29). The Tredelenburg position promotes the return of blood in the lower extremities to the core circulation. This is of benefit in managing the hypotensive patient. The Trendelenburg position also places the pharynx below the trachea. If an object has been displaced into the pharynx, or if the unconscious patient has regurgitated, the trachea and lower airway are now in a more gravitationally favorable position to minimize the risk of aspiration.

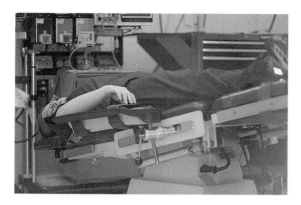

Figure 1-29. Trendelenburg position.

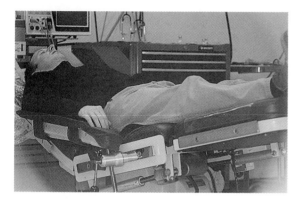

Figure 1-30. Syncopal position.

Syncopal Position

In the conscious patient the downward position of the head can be uncomfortable. In the syncopal position, placing the patient with the head and heart at the same level and the feet elevated approximately 20 degrees can minimize pooling of blood in the periphery and improve circulation to the brain. The dental chair should be positioned so that the head and heart are at the same level. A pillow can be placed under the feet to achieve appropriate elevation of the lower extremities (Figure 1-30).

CINCINNATI STROKE SCALE

The Cincinnati stroke scale is a modification of the 15-item National Institutes of Health stroke scale. The scale was developed to provide an easy, reliable, and reproducible method of diagnosing a stroke (cerebrovascular accident) out of hospital to expedite optimal care within the limited time to administer thrombolytic medications. The scale evaluates for facial palsy, arm

Box 1-19	Cincinnati Stroke Scale

FACIAL DROOP
Patient shows teeth or smiles.
Normal: Both sides of face move equally.
Abnormal: One side of face does not move as well as other side.

ARM DRIFT
Patient closes eyes and extends both arms straight out for 10 seconds.
Normal: Both arms move the same, or both arms do not move at all.
Abnormal: One arm does not move, or one arm drifts downward.

SPEECH
Patient repeats, "The sky is blue in Cincinnati."
Normal: Patient says the correct words with no slurring of speech.
Abnormal: Patient slurs words, says the wrong words, or is unable to speak.

From Kothari RU, Pancioli A, Liu T, et al: *Ann Emerg Med* 33:373-378, 1999.

weakness, and speech abnormalities[18,19] (Box 1-19). A positive finding for any of the tests suggests that the patient has sustained a stroke and that the EMS system should be activated.

VASCULAR ACCESS AND ROUTES OF DRUG ADMINISTRATION

Several factors must be considered when choosing the route of drug delivery, including (1) the patient's LOC, (2) the drug's ability to be absorbed, (3) the rapidity of onset required, (4) the risk/benefit ratio of administration via a specific route, and (5) the clinician's technical skill. Each of these considerations depends partly on the others.

Intravenous Route

Intravenous (IV) cannulation provides direct access into the venous circulation. The advantages include the ability to administer both IV fluids and drugs. The IV route circumvents the potential limitations of absorption that may be associated with other routes of administration. Direct access into the bloodstream provides almost immediate drug delivery to the specific end-organ sites. The most rapid onset and peak effect are accomplished with IV administration. However, the severity of the side effects may be most extreme when the drug is administered intravenously.

Cannulation of the venous circulation may be accomplished peripherally or centrally. Proficiency in *peripheral venous cannulation* is well within the realm of the dentist. IV access, however, should not be used during an emergency if the dentist is not proficient with this technique. During an emergency, peripheral IV access should be established in the upper extremity. The most accessible anatomic sites include the dorsum of the hand (Figure 1-31), forearm, and antecubital fossa (Figure 1-32). There is anatomic variation within the antecubital fossa, where the median cephalic, median basilic, or median cubital vein should be accessible.

Cannulation of a peripheral vein should be accomplished with an indwelling plastic catheter inserted over a hollow needle. After the plastic catheter is inserted and the needle withdrawn, the upper extremity can be moved without jeopardizing the vessel's integrity. Fluid resuscitation depends on the gauge and length of the needle. The larger the gauge and shorter the length of catheter, the more rapidly fluid can be adminis-

tered. The larger the gauge of catheter, the greater the likelihood the vessel may be traumatized, resulting in a failed cannulation. Availability of 20-gauge and 18-gauge catheters 5 cm (2 inches) in length is appropriate for an emergency kit. The 5-cm 20-gauge and 18-gauge catheters will allow a fluid infusion of approximately 40 and 80 milliliters per minute (ml/min), respectively (Boxes 1-20 and 1-21; Figures 1-33 and 1-34).

Potential complications include hematoma (most common), intraarterial injection, nerve injury, embolism, and phlebitis. If a *hematoma* develops during catheter insertion, remove the catheter unit and apply pressure to the site. Withdrawing the catheter from the vessel but not totally removing it from the arm prevents bleeding from the puncture site. While the catheter is allowed to remain partially within the patient, the needle is completely removed. Pressure applied to the site may be required to prevent hematoma formation. Select an alternative site for cannulation that is not immediately distal to the site of failed cannulation.

Because the veins, especially those within the antecubital fossa, are close to the arteries, care should be taken to avoid the intraarterial cannulation. Pressures in an artery are usually higher than in a vein, which results in a pulsatile backflow from the catheter into the IV tubing. If this occurs, withdraw the catheter and apply pressure. If the tourniquet was not removed after the catheter was successfully inserted, it may also result in a significant backflow of blood into the

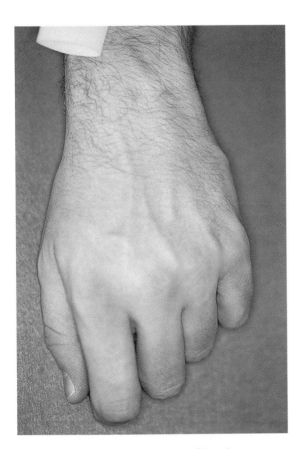

Figure 1-31. Dorsum of hand.

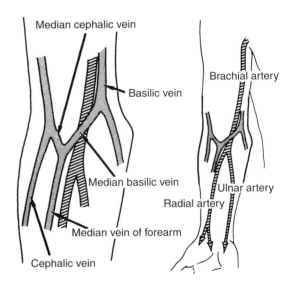

Figure 1-32. Antecubital fossa. *From Topazian RG: J Am Dent Assoc 81:409-412, 1970.*

Box 1-20   Steps in Intravenous (IV) Infusion Setup

1. Adhere to sterile technique. Although speed is essential, sterility can be maintained without compromising speed.
2. Obtain a bag of fluid and remove from external packaging. Hang it on an IV pole or similar device at an approximate height of 5 or 6 feet. The IV bag has an adapter that will accept the drip chamber component of the infusion set. A removable cap maintains sterility of this adapter.
3. Open the infusion set. The infusion set at one end has a drip chamber. The drip chamber has a sharp, rigid, hollow adapter (spike) that is capable of engaging the bag of IV fluid. The other end has a standard adapter that attaches to the indwelling catheter. The adapters have removable caps that maintain their sterility. The infusion set also has at least one drug administration port and a flow regulator. Close the flow regulator.
4. Remove the caps from the IV bag adapter and infusion set spike, maintaining their sterility. Insert the spike from the infusion set into the IV bag.
5. Gently squeeze and release the drip chamber. This will allow fluid from the IV bag to flow into the drip chamber. Repeat this until the drip chamber is half full.
6. Open the fluid regulator and allow the fluid to infuse completely through the IV line. Ensure that there is no air in the IV line. Frequently the line may be flushed without removing the sterile cap on the distal adapter. If the adapter must be removed to flush the line with IV fluid, maintain sterility of the tip.

Box 1-21   Steps in Peripheral Cannulation Technique

1. Apply a tourniquet proximal to the site of cannulation.
2. Examine the intended site, locating a satisfactory vein for cannulation. A good site to insert a catheter is where two feeding veins form a "Y." Allowing the arm to hang below the level of the heart facilitates this. Slightly tapping the intended site of cannulation may also assist in venodilation of the vein.
3. Cleanse the site with alcohol.
4. Stabilize the vein by pulling the skin distal to the penetration site taut.
5. Penetrate the skin either distal or lateral to the intended site of venous puncture. With the needle bevel side up, the catheter is initially inserted through the skin. The angle of insertion should vary between 15 and 30 degrees, depending on whether the vein is superficial or deep. Penetration of tougher skin is facilitated by a more acute angle.
6. Penetrate the vein with the needle, which results in a flow of blood into the indwelling catheter "flash" chamber. The needle is longer than the catheter. This is not an indication that the catheter has entered the vein. The needle must be advanced to allow the catheter to enter the vessel. Although there is some variability, the catheter unit should be almost flush with the skin as it is advanced into the vessel. Once the catheter unit has been inserted to a depth in which it is felt that the catheter has entered the vein, the catheter may be advanced.
7. Advance the catheter using one of two techniques:
   a. Stabilize the flash chamber, and advance the catheter into the vein without risk of perforating the vessel.
   b. Stabilize the catheter, and withdraw the needle/flash chamber approximately one-third to one-half its distance. The catheter now extends beyond the needle tip, preventing the needle from penetrating the vessel, but the needle still provides some rigidity to the catheter. The catheter unit is advanced until the catheter is fully inserted.
8. Remove the tourniquet.
9. Palpate the catheter tip and place a finger just beyond it. This will prevent blood from escaping from the catheter when the infusion set is connected to the catheter.
10. Completely remove the flash chamber with needle. Attach the infusion tubing. Ensure that the intravenous tubing has been infused with fluid. Open the flow regulator to observe for flow of fluid. This will ensure that the catheter is appropriately placed. Inadequate flow may indicate that the catheter is lodged against a valve or is not within the vein. If fluid is infusing, check to ensure that there is no evidence of infiltration into adjacent tissue.
11. Secure the catheter to the patient using one of numerous ways. A carefully placed but poorly secured catheter can become dislodged at the most inappropriate time.

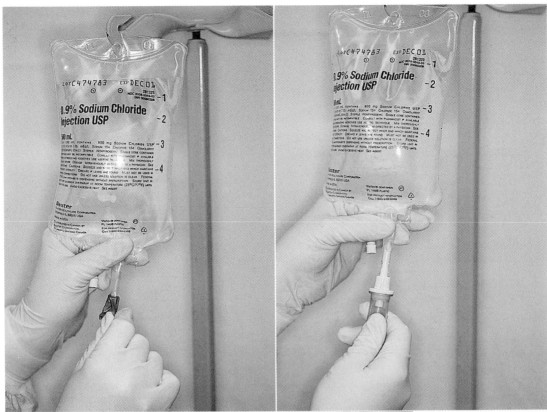

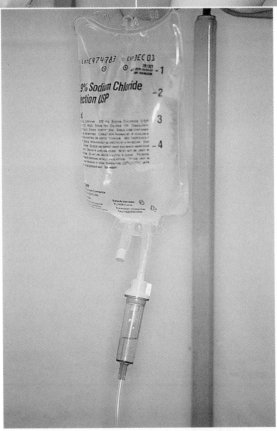

Figure 1-33. Intravenous (IV) infusion setup.

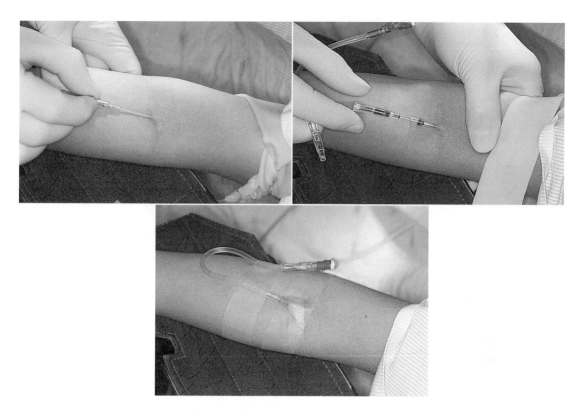

Figure 1-34. Peripheral cannulation.

infusion tubing. Be sure to check that the tourniquet has been removed before rapidly removing the catheter. Complications associated with intraarterial injections can be avoided by attaching an IV infusion line to the catheter rather than injecting directly into the catheter.

Nerve injury is rare with IV cannulation. However, the superficial radial vein and the median cubital and median basilic veins are in proximity to the radial nerve and median nerve, respectively. The incidence of *embolism* is low with the catheter-over-the-needle technique. Once the catheter has been advanced, however, it should never be withdrawn back over the needle.

Intraosseous Route

Intraosseous (IO) puncture is an alternative technique to IV cannulation. It is most frequently employed in the pediatric patient. The IO technique should be considered when peripheral cannulation has failed or is deemed difficult. It is an effective manner for administering drugs and initiating IV therapy until tertiary personnel can establish an alternative venous access site. All resuscitative medications may be delivered via the IO route.

The two most common sites used for IO cannulation are in the tibia. The proximal tibia is used in children less than 6 years of age. The distal tibia may be used in the pediatric as well as the adult patient. IO infusion has been used for resuscitation of the adult patient in cardiac arrest[20] (Box 1-22 and Figure 1-35).

Complications associated with IO puncture include subcutanoeus or subperiosteal infiltration of fluid, physeal plate injury or tibial fracture, hematoma, local abscess, osteomyelitis, and sepsis.

Intramuscular Route

Intramuscular (IM) injection produces a predictable and relatively fast drug level when the ability to establish IV access is not an option. Four anatomic regions are typically used for the IM administration of drugs: (1) deltoid area (shoulder), (2) vastus lateralis region (anterolateral thigh), (3) ventrogluteal area (lateral hip), and (4) dorsogluteal area (upper outer quadrant of buttock). These sites have minimal numbers of nerves and large blood vessels, as well as adequate bulk to accommodate the injectate.

Box 1-22   Steps in Intraosseous Puncture

1. Ensure that patient is in the supine position.
2. Place a pad under the knee to create a bend of about 30 degrees.
3. Locate the puncture site, which is the antero-medial surface 1 to 3 cm distal to the tibial tuberosity.
4. Use sterile technique. Wear sterile gloves and cleanse the skin with alcohol or povidone-iodine (Betadine).
5. Introduce the needle into the bone using a rotary motion. A large-caliber bone marrow aspiration needle (with stylet) should be used. The angle of insertion should be 60 to 90 degrees away from the epiphyseal plate. Penetration through the cortex should result in decreased resistance.
6. Remove the stylet, and attach a 12-ml syringe containing saline to the needle. The use of

the stylet will minimize the risk of a core of bone occluding the needle. Positive aspiration of bone marrow confirms intraosseous placement of the needle. Despite being in the intraosseous cavity, there may not be a positive aspirate.

7. If the needle is felt to have penetrated the cortex and to be within the intraosseous cavity, inject approximately 5 ml of saline to flush the needle. If the saline flushes easily without any evidence of infiltration, the needle is most likely in the correct location.
8. Attach the infusion set to the needle. Gently insert the needle until the hub is in contact with the skin and is secure.

Muscle selection depends on several factors. Of the various sites, the *dorsogluteal* muscle is the least accessible in an acute emergency. The *vastus lateralis* and *ventrogluteal* muscles are well developed in children and recommended for pediatric IM injections. The vastus lateralis muscle should be used in children less than 1 year of age. The volume of injectate for a child under age 2 years should not exceed 2 ml into the vastus lateralis.

The *deltoid* area has a few advantages. The rapidity of onset of a drug is affected by the ionization of the drug and the vehicle in which it is dissolved, as well as being dependent on the perfusion of the muscle. The highest perfusion rate of the administration sites is seen in the deltoid muscle. Absorption and onset may occur as rapidly as 4 to 5 minutes. The rate of absorption is approximately 30% more rapid in the deltoid muscle compared to the vastus lateralis muscle. The deltoid site is also easily accessible in the upper third of the upper arm and does not require disrobing. The superior aspect is delineated by the lower edge of the acromion process. The inferior boundary is a line with the axillae. The deltoid area is acceptable for both the child and the adult. The volume of injectate in the deltoid muscle should not exceed 4 ml in the adult patient. However, a dose of 1 ml is recommended as the safest volume.

Potential complications of IM injection include nerve injury, sterile abscess, infection, hematoma, and inadvertent intravascular injection. The potential of experiencing a *nerve injury* associated with a correctly administered IM in-

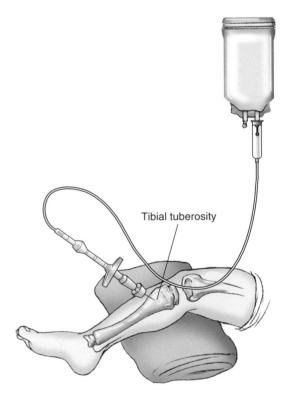

Figure 1-35. Intraosseous cannulation in proximal tibia.

Tibial tuberosity

jection in the deltoid region is low. Inappropriate injection into the middle third of the upper arm may risk injury of the radial nerve. Inadvertent *intravascular administration* of an intended IM agent may result in adverse side effects. Different concentrations of drugs are frequently used for different routes of administration; the quantity of injectate is decreased for an IM injection. An inadvertent intravascular injection can be avoided by aspirating before injecting the drug.

The dentist must be comfortable and confident with IM injection techniques (Boxes 1-23 and 1-24; Figures 1-36 and 1-37).

Intralingual Route

An alternative to IM injection is intralingual injection of a drug. Absorption and distribution of a drug depend on the blood flow through the injection site. The tongue provides a highly vascular bed, which facilitates rapid absorption and distribution of the drug. Absorption has been shown to be greater than 30% more rapid than a comparable injection into the deltoid muscle.[21] The peak effect of sympathomimetic drugs administered via an intralingual injection occurs as rapidly as 30 seconds after administration. However, some variability in onset is associated with both intralingual and IM injections but not with IV administration.

An intralingual injection can be accomplished intraorally with direct access into the lateral or ventral surface of the tongue. Alternatively, in an emergency when this may not be practical, intralingual administration can be established through the submental triangle. *Submental injection* involves a few basic principles (Figure 1-38). The needle penetration should be in the midline; this applies to intralingual administration as well. The primary benefit of the midline position is that it avoids vessels. Nerves and salivary glands are also avoided because they are located laterally. The submental technique is similar to an IM injection. The skin is prepared with alcohol and pulled taut. The needle is inserted 90 degrees to the skin and passed to the selected depth. Aspiration of blood indicates that the needle is within a vessel. Aspiration of air suggests entry into the mouth.

The submental approach has several advantages compared with the intra-oral-lingual approach. Unless unconscious, the patient is unlikely to open and keep the mouth open voluntarily, allowing the injection. The tongue is vascular, and any trauma during administration may result in intraoral hemorrhage, which could precipitate laryngospasm. Hemorrhage may also result in a hematoma that could increase in size and compromise the airway; this may occur from either the intraoral or the submental approach. An additional benefit to the submental approach is that

---

Box 1-23 Equipment for Intramuscular (IM) Injections

NEEDLE
Adult patient: 3.5-4 cm (1½ inch), 21-23 gauge
Pediatric patient: 2.5 cm (1 inch), 21-23 gauge

SYRINGE
Size should correspond to amount administered.
Consider using a tuberculin syringe for a dose less than 1 ml.

Box 1-24 Steps for Intramuscular (IM) Injections into Deltoid Muscle

1. Cleanse the site with alcohol.
2. Grasp deltoid muscle with the nondominant hand.
3. Gently squeeze the muscle, making it bulge; this may cause mild discomfort.
4. Introduce the needle at a 90-degree angle to the skin using the dominant hand. The insertion should be a quick, directed motion to the desired depth. The appropriate length of insertion depends on the patient's size. Never insert the needle to its hub.
5. Aspirate to ensure that the needle is not within a vessel.
6. Inject the drug into the muscle, and quickly withdraw the needle.

---

the face mask does not have to be removed and thus interrupt oxygenation and ventilation.

In a medical emergency associated with potential circulatory compromise, the intralingual administration provides an excellent alternative to IV administration when the intravenous route is not available. Intralingual injection is considered one of the easiest, least risky, and fastest nonintravenous methods of drug administration.

Subcutaneous Route

For subcutaneous (SC) injection a 25-gauge needle is used to deposit the pharmacologic agent just beneath the skin into the subcutaneous tissue. The needle is inserted at a 45-degree angle to the skin. SC administration provides slow, sustained release of an agent. Controlled delayed absorption of the agent retards onset while providing a prolonged therapeutic effect. The peak

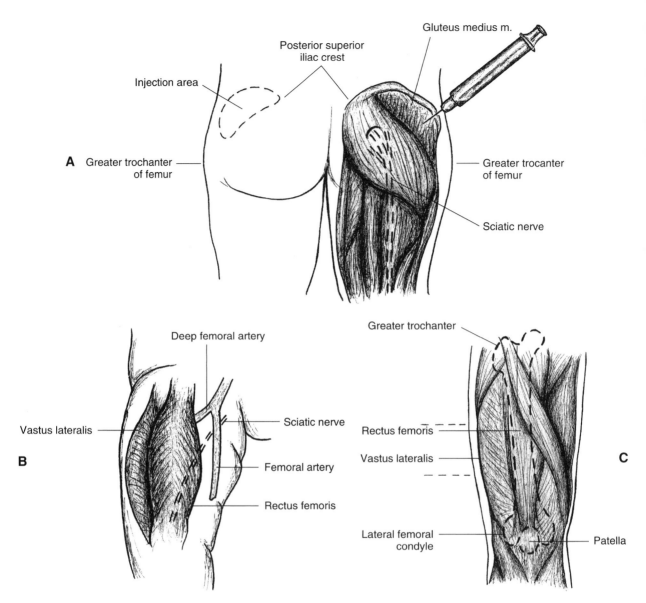

Figure 1-36. Sites of intramuscular (IM) injection. **A,** Dorsogluteal area. **B,** Vastus lateralis muscle of upper thigh, for children. **C,** Vastus lateralis muscle, for adults.

Continued

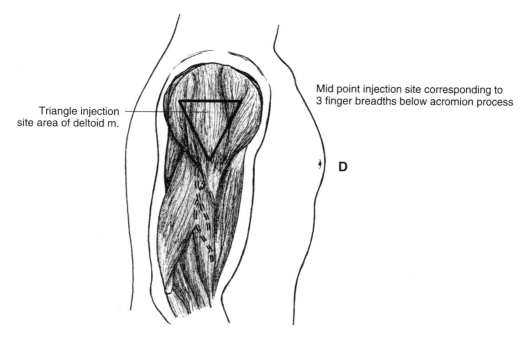

Triangle injection site area of deltoid m.

Mid point injection site corresponding to 3 finger breadths below acromion process

D

Figure 1-36, cont'd. D, Deltoid muscle. *From Dym H, Ogle OE:* Atlas of minor oral surgery, *Philadelphia, 2000, WB Saunders.*

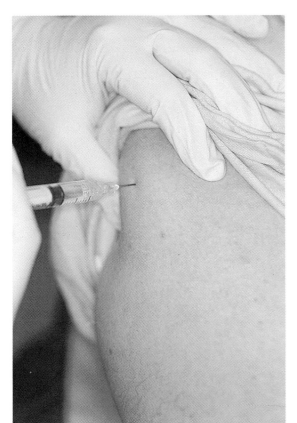

Figure 1-37. Intramuscular injection into deltoid muscle.

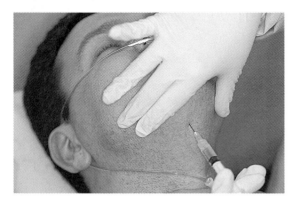

Figure 1-38. Submental injection.

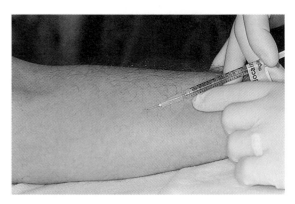

Figure 1-39. Site of subcutaneous injection.

drug level is less than that achieved with IV or IM administration. Therefore the SC route may avoid the adverse effects seen with more rapid and higher drug levels. The drug's absorption in SC administration is affected by tissue perfusion. Decreased cardiac output (e.g., hypotension) or a cool extremity decreases the rapidity of absorption. The SC route is contraindicated in states of circulatory compromise (Figure 1-39).

Inhalational and Endotracheal Routes

The inhalational route of administration provides rapid absorption because of the large surface area of respiratory mucosa and the high blood flow. In the nonintubated patient, dispersement of an aerosol allows direct delivery of an agent to the terminal branches of the respiratory tree. However, the efficacy of the medication depends on the aerosol reaching the terminal site. Placing the inhaler into the mouth and closing the lips around the tip result in a significant percentage of the aerosol coating the oral mucosa and upper airway, not reaching the lower airway. Devices called *spacers* prevent the medication from coating the upper airway and optimize the delivery of the inhalant to the lower airway.

Modifications of spacer devices should allow medications to be administered to the conscious or unconscious patient and the spontaneously breathing or respiratory compromised patient. For the spontaneously breathing patient, the devices have a mouthpiece similar to a traditional inhaler or a face mask. The aerosol dispenser is attached to the spacer (Figure 1-40). The patient is instructed to take a breath and ex-

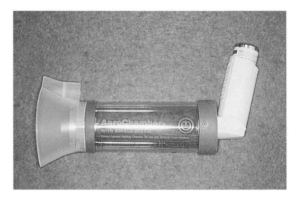

Figure 1-40. Inhaler inserted into spacer, which will fit securely over a patient's nose and mouth.

hale fully. The device is then placed firmly over the patient's mouth and nose. The inhaled medication is dispersed into the spacer, from which the patient now takes a deep breath, holds it for a few seconds, and exhales. The patient then takes a second maximal inspiration, holds, and exhales. For the impaired patient the medication should be administered through the circuit used in ventilating the patient.

In the intubated patient, three drugs are traditionally administered through an endotracheal (ET) tube: atropine, epinephrine, and lidocaine. The medication dosage is approximately 2 to 2½ times that of an IV dose. The drug should be diluted with saline to a volume of 10 ml. Medications administered by ET tube have a rate of onset comparable to IV administration. During ACLS the ET tube provides the second route of administration if IV access has not yet been established.

Table 1-2	Hypoglycemic Agents		
Agent	**Dose**	**Route**	**Onset**
Oral glucose source	15-gram glucose load (simple carbohydrate)	Oral	15-20 minutes
Glucagon	Adult: 1 mg Pediatric: 0.5 mg (0.025-0.1 mg, not to exceed 1 mg)	IM	10-20 minutes
Dextrose 50% in water (D50W)	Adult: 25 grams (1 ampule) Pediatric: 0.5-1 g/kg of diluted solution (D25W)	IV	5-10 minutes

Sublingual Route

The permeability of the sublingual mucosa allows rapid absorption, and the vascularity of the tissue provides for a rapid onset of drug effect. The buccal mucosa provides an alternative route of administration. The buccal mucosa, however, is not as permeable as the sublingual tissue. The drug absorbed sublingually or buccally avoids GI degradation and first-pass metabolism by the liver.

For the agent to be effective, the patient must be able to maintain the drug sublingually, allowing its complete dissolution and absorption. Xerostomia (dryness of mouth) may prolong dissolution of a tablet. Adding a few drops of water may facilitate dissolution of the tablet. The patient must be informed to avoid swallowing. Any quantity of a drug swallowed is absorbed through the GI route and is subject to GI degradation.

Oral Route

In the nonemergency situation, oral (PO) administration of a drug is the most common route to achieve therapeutic action. The absorption and bioavailability of a drug may be variable, incomplete, and affected by multiple factors, including gastric pH, gastric emptying time, presence of food in the stomach, and inactivation by the GI system through destruction by enzymes or metabolism within the hepatic portal circulation. Absorption also depends on perfusion of the GI system, which may be compromised during a medical emergency. Administration of an elixir or suspension achieves a more rapid onset than tablet form.

Oral administration requires a conscious patient with intact reflexes to avoid the risk of aspiration. Nausea and vomiting interfere with the ability to take a drug orally. Patients with medical urgencies (e.g., delayed allergic reaction, conscious patient with hypoglycemia) may respond to oral agents.

EMERGENCY DRUG AND FLUID THERAPY
Hypoglycemic Agents

The purpose of oral hypoglycemic agents is to increase the blood glucose level in the hypoglycemic patient (Table 1-2). In the patient who is conscious and able to swallow, an oral glucose-containing agent usually reverses the progression of the symptoms. It is important to have a palatable agent that will not induce the sensation of nausea or vomiting. The minimal glucose load should be no less than 10 grams (g), but 15 g is recommended. An increase in plasma glucose level and clinical relief will occur within 15 to 20 minutes.[22]

Many diabetic patients can assess when they are becoming hypoglycemic. They also will be able to assess the clinical relief associated with the administration of an oral carbohydrate. A degree of patience is required. Repeating the administration of the oral carbohydrate more frequently than every 15 minutes will likely result in hyperglycemia. Oral solutions are absorbed more rapidly than solids. The sugar source should be a *simple carbohydrate* that is supplied for the management of hypoglycemia and that accurately reflects the grams of carbohydrate. Many offices have refrigerated juices as their sugar source. Unfortunately, the sugar content of fruit juices varies, so the amount of carbohydrate administered will not be known. In one investigation an orange juice labeled with 15 g of carbohydrate actually contained an average of 11.5 g.[22] This was reflected in the delayed recovery when compared to both glucose and sucrose solution and tablets. The sugar source should *not* be a complex carbohydrate. Patients who are taking acarbose

(Precose) for their diabetes are unable to absorb complex carbohydrates.

Dextrose

If decreased LOC has impaired the patient's ability to swallow, an alternative route to PO administration must be used. If IV access can be established, the recommended treatment for hypoglycemia is the administration of *dextrose 50% in water* (D50W). Emergency personnel consider this the standard of care. The adult patient should receive 1 or 2 ampules of D50W (25 to 50 g of dextrose), which should restore the circulating glucose levels to a satisfactory therapeutic range; the increase in blood glucose may approach 75 milligrams per deciliter (mg/dl). The onset of effect should be within 5 to 10 minutes; however, complete neurologic recovery may lag 30 minutes behind the increase in blood glucose. The solution should be diluted 1:1 with sterile water to make a 25% solution (D25W) before administering the dextrose solution to the pediatric patient. The suggested initial dose is 0.5 to 1 milligram per kilogram of body weight (mg/kg).

Few risks are associated with administration of D50W. Extravasation of the D50W into the skin adjacent to the IV catheter can cause necrosis. Slow administration is advised to avoid this complication. There is also concern about administering dextrose to an alcohol-dependent patient. A thiamine deficiency in these patients can cause Wernicke's encephalopathy; 100 mg of IV thiamine should be administered before dextrose. Since hyperglycemia can compound neurologic injury, D50W should not be administered to the patient with a suspected neurologic injury.

Glucagon

The ability to establish IV access is not considered a standard of care within a dental facility. This necessitates an alternative route of administration. *Glucagon* is a pancreatic hormone that stimulates hepatic glycogenolysis and hepatic gluconeogenesis. It is available as a lyophilized powder (1 mg), which is mixed with 1 ml of normal saline for injection. The agent can be administered via the SC, IM, or intralingual route. In the dental office the route of administration will be IM. The dose for the adult is 1 mg; the child receives 0.5 mg. The dose can be repeated in 20 minutes. Onset of action of IM glucagon occurs in 10 to 20 minutes in 98% of patients.[23]

The efficacy of glucagon depends on hepatic glycogen stores; states of nutritional deprivation decrease its effectiveness. An oral glucose source should be administered once consciousness returns.

The primary adverse effect associated with the administration of glucagon is nausea with vomiting. Although manageable, nausea interferes with resumption of oral intake. In the type II diabetic patient the administration of glucagon may initially exacerbate the hypoglycemia.[24] Glucagon stimulates the release of insulin, which may be available in the type II diabetic patient.

Regardless of the agent administered, a fingerstick glucose test should be performed before or after administration to confirm the diagnosis.

For patients taking beta-adrenergic blocking agents (β-blockers), epinephrine therapy may be relatively ineffective in the management of an allergic or anaphylactic reaction. Glucagon has sympathomimetic activity and may be effective in these patients at a dose of 1 mg intralingually (preferably intravenously), which can be repeated in 5 minutes if necessary (Box 1-25).[25]

Antihistamines

Various signs and symptoms of allergic reactions are initiated and maintained as a result of the release of histamine. The emergency kit should contain an H_1-receptor antagonist (e.g., diphenhydramine), which blocks the receptor's response to histamine, with both oral and parenteral forms available (Box 1-26). An H_2-receptor antagonist

Box 1-25	Management of Anaphylaxis in Patient Taking a ß-Blocker	
AGENT	**DOSE**	**ROUTE**
Glucagon	1 mg	IV, IM

Box 1-26	Antihistamines	
CONDITION	**AGENT/DOSE**	**ROUTE**
Allergic reaction	Diphenhydramine (Benadryl)	
	25 mg tablets	PO
	50 mg/ml	IM
	(25-50 mg)	

(e.g., cimetidine) may also be administered, although it is of less importance and often is not included in an emergency kit.

Mild allergic reactions consisting of pruritus, erythema, and urticaria can be managed with an oral antihistamine, which can be administered in the office with a prescription provided to the patient. For a mild allergic reaction the patient should be instructed to take the medication for the first 24 hours and then as necessary to relieve the symptoms. Moderate, non-life-threatening conditions can be treated with a parenteral antihistamine. The IV route is preferred because of the rapid onset of action, although IM administration is a viable option. If the dentist wants the patient's physician to participate in the management of the allergic reaction, the dentist should directly consult with the physician before the patient leaves the office. Follow-up care and examination by the physician can be determined during this phone consultation. Antihistamines are not indicated and should not be administered in the management of an acute asthmatic attack because they thicken the bronchial secretions.

Diphenhydramine (Benadryl) may produce sedation, impairing the patient's ability to perform various tasks; the patient's transportation home must be considered. *Chlorpheniramine* (Chlor-Trimeton), *cetirizine* (Zyrtec), and *loratadine* (Claritin) are alternative antihistamines that have less CNS effect, resulting in less sedation. When a fast onset of the H_1-blocking action is required, however, diphenhydramine remains the recommended treatment.[26,27]

Aromatic Ammonia

The primary inclusion of aromatic ammonia in the emergency kit is for the treatment of vasodepressor syncope (Box 1-27). The agent is available as a *vaporole*. When the vaporole is cracked or crushed, a noxious odor is released that stimulates the respiratory and vasomotor centers of the medulla. In the patient with syncope the

cracked vaporole is placed under the nose (Figure 1-41). In conjunction with placing the patient into a syncopal position and providing supplemental oxygen, aromatic ammonia should result in a return of consciousness and an increase in both heart rate and blood pressure. A failure to respond may be suggestive of a cardiovascular, neurologic, or metabolic cause for the syncopal episode.

Since vasodepressor syncope is the most common medical urgency in the dental office, it has been widely suggested that it may be beneficial to secure the vaporole to the dental chair. However, the vaporoles should be contained within the emergency kit. First, it is a basic principle to maintain all emergency drugs and armamentarium in one location. Second, when attached to the dental chair, the vaporole becomes a fomite. It is continuously contaminated by daily dental procedures and cannot be disinfected.

Aspirin

The American College of Cardiology (ACC) and the AHA recommend that patients presenting with an acute myocardial infarction (MI) chew an aspirin (Box 1-28).[28] This recommendation is based on the data from the second International

Box 1-28	Aspirin
CONDITION	**DOSE/ROUTE**
Acute myocardial infarction	Chew and swallow 160-325 mg tablet

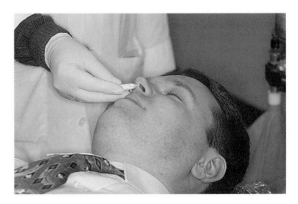
Figure 1-41. Administration of aromatic ammonia vaporole.

Box 1-27	Aromatic Ammonia
CONDITION	**ROUTE**
Vasopressor syncope	Crack or crush and hold under patient's nose

Study of Infarct Survival, which demonstrated a 23% reduction in mortality when aspirin was administered to a patient with an acute MI.[29] The reduced mortality from acute MI is associated with aspirin's antithrombotic effect. Aspirin irreversibly inhibits the synthesis of thromboxane A_2, which is responsible for platelet aggregation and vasoconstriction.[30] A single 100-mg dose of aspirin is effective in inhibiting the production of thromboxane A_2 and achieving this antiplatelet effect.[31] The cumulative effect of repeated daily doses allows the administration of a lower daily dose of aspirin to obtain maximal antithrombotic benefit while minimizing the adverse effects.

In the patient with an acute MI the objective is to achieve a rapid effective plasma level. Doses of 160 to 325 mg have been recommended. The ACC/AHA recommend chewing the aspirin rather than swallowing a whole aspirin or taking a solution (e.g., Alka-Seltzer). One study showed that chewing buffered aspirin (325 mg) for 30 seconds and then swallowing with water provided the most rapid and sustained effect.[32] Significant platelet inhibition occurred within 5 minutes, with maximal antithrombotic effect in 13 to 14 minutes (range, 7 to 28 minutes). These values represent the absorption in a fasted patient; slower absorption and onset may result from factors such as food in the GI tract.

No increase in major complications has been associated with the administration of an aspirin to the patient having an acute MI.[33]

Benzodiazepines

Most seizures are spontaneous and unpredictable. Although they are usually self-limiting, episodes of prolonged seizures and status epilepticus may develop. The risk of morbidity and mortality associated with status epilepticus escalates as the duration of the seizure increases. The ability to intervene if necessary is essential (Table 1-3). The first-line drug in the management of active seizures is an IV benzodiazepine. IV access can be difficult to establish in the patient with a seizure, however, and is not available in most dental facilities. An alternate route of administration must be selected.

The IV benzodiazepine usually administered is *diazepam* (Valium). Diazepam is available for parenteral administration in a propylene glycol solvent because it is poorly water soluble. This results in erratic absorption and delayed onset of activity when the drug is administered intramuscularly. Onset of action may be faster with oral administration, which is not a viable alternative during an active seizure. Rectal administration of diazepam is an acceptable alternative route for the treatment of seizures. The rectal gel facilitates administration; high lipid solubility results in rapid absorption. Peak drug level occurs in 3 to 30 minutes, with bioavailability of 80% to 100%.[34] Cessation of fast activity on the electroencephalogram (EEG) with rectal administration is comparable to that associated with IV diazepam.[35] Recent studies report no cases of serious respiratory depression and suggest that caregivers can administer the treatment in a nonmedical setting.[34]

Midazolam (Versed) is a water-soluble, highly lipophilic benzodiazepine that is rapidly and almost completely absorbed after IM administration. IM midazolam has been shown to be as efficacious in abolishing seizure activity as IV diazepam.[36,37] The recommended IM dose is 0.2 to 0.3 mg/kg. Onset of action usually occurs in 10 minutes. The intranasal route may be considered as an alternative to IV administration. The

Table 1-3	Benzodiazepines		
Agent	**Availability**	**Route**	**Dose**
Diazepam gel (Diastat, Athena Neurosciences, San Francisco)	5 mg/ml (preloaded syringes in 5, 10, 15, and 20 mg)	Rectal	Child (2-6 years): 0.5 mg/kg Child (6-12 years): 0.3 mg/kg Adult (12 years and older): 0.2 mg/kg Maximum: 20 mg
Midazolam	5 mg/ml (parenteral preparation)	IM	0.2 mg/kg Maximum: 10 mg

suggested dose for intranasal midazolam is also 0.2 mg/kg.[38]

Respiratory depression is a potential risk after the administration of diazepam or midazolam. Some have questioned the potential for respiratory depression with these medications at the recommended doses. The dentist must be equipped to administer positive-pressure ventilation.

Corticosteroids

Corticosteroids are used as replacement therapy in patients with insufficient hormone production (e.g., Addison's disease) and as antiinflammatory agents for acute and chronic conditions (Table 1-4). Patients taking corticosteroids for inflammatory conditions in the previous 2 years may also have adrenal insufficiency, which may be exacerbated under certain conditions. The inclusion of corticosteroids in the emergency kit is for the management of acute adrenal insufficiency, asthma, allergy, and anaphylaxis.

Corticosteroids suppress acute inflammation. In the patient with an acute asthmatic or anaphylactic reaction, these agents are beneficial in suppressing airway edema and bronchospasm. Corticosteroids have a delayed onset (longer than 1 hour) and are not the primary drug class used to manage the emergency. However, corticosteroids are beneficial in providing long-term stabilization once the emergency has resolved. Administering the agent in the office initiates the interval before onset of action and benefit of agent seen.

Corticosteroids also potentiate the cardiovascular (e.g., vasoconstriction, inotropy/chronotropy) and pulmonary (e.g., bronchodilation) effects of catecholamines. This is beneficial in the management of asthma and anaphylaxis, but it is critical in managing acute adrenal insufficiency. Recognizing the problem, making the correct diagnosis of adrenal insufficiency, and rapidly administering corticosteroids constitute lifesaving therapy.

Epinephrine

Epinephrine is included in the emergency kit for the treatment of both severe bronchospasm refractory to β_2-agonist inhaler therapy and severe allergic or anaphylactic reaction with pulmonary and cardiovascular compromise (Table 1-5). For the treatment of anaphylaxis or laryngeal edema, epinephrine is the agent of choice. Epinephrine is also indicated for the management of ventricular fibrillation. Of the various drugs employed in ACLS, epinephrine has the greatest effect on increasing the heart's susceptibility to converting to a normal sinus rhythm from ventricular fibrillation after defibrillation. Administration of epinephrine during cardiac arrest is by the IV route or ET tube. Neither technique is a standard skill mastered or required of dental personnel.

Table 1-4	Corticosteroids	
Condition	Dexamethasone (Decadron, 4 mg/ml)	Methylprednisolone (Solu-Medrol, 125 mg/2 ml)
Laryngeal edema, bronchospasm	8 mg IM	125 mg IV/IM
Anaphylaxis	8 mg IM	125 mg/ml
Adrenal insufficiency	8 mg IM	125 mg/ml

Table 1-5	Epinephrine	
Diagnosis	Dose	Frequency*
Bronchospasm	Adult: 0.1-0.5 mg SC/IM (1:1000)	Every ½ hour
	Pediatric: 0.01 mg/kg SC (1:1000)	Every ½ hour
Anaphylaxis	Adult: 0.1-0.25 mg IV (1:10,000) *or*	Every 5-15 minutes
	0.3-0.5 mg IM (1:1000)	
	Pediatric: 0.01 mg/kg IM (not to	Every 10-15 minutes
	exceed 0.5 mg in a single dose)	Every 15 minutes

*As necessary (prn).

Epinephrine is a sympathomimetic agent that stimulates both α_1-adrenergic and β_1-/β_2-adrenergic receptors. The primary beneficial effects are bronchodilation, vasoconstriction, and increased rate and force of cardiac contraction. In addition, epinephrine reduces the release of histamine and other mediators from mast cells and basophils.

Epinephrine also has significant cardiovascular and CNS effects, including an increased myocardial dysrhythmogenic potential, tachycardia, hypertension, increased myocardial oxygen demand precipitating angina, nervousness, and restlessness. Drug interactions may occur with nonselective β-blockers, α-blocking agents, and tricyclic antidepressants. Patients with a history of cardiovascular disease (e.g., hypertension, arrhythmias, angina, MI), cerebral arteriosclerosis, or hyperthyroidism are more susceptible to the adverse effects of epinephrine. Caution must be exercised with the administration of epinephrine in the gravid female. Sympathomimetic agents such as epinephrine and phenylephrine (Neo-Synephrine) can decrease placental blood flow, resulting in adverse fetal consequences. Epinephrine also increases the blood glucose level; the diabetic patient may require monitoring and secondary management by emergency personnel. Because of the potential for severe adverse effects, epinephrine should not be considered the first-line agent for the management of hypoglycemia.

Anaphylaxis or laryngeal edema may develop rapidly, which necessitates the immediate availability of the drug. An epinephrine 1:1000 solution in a preloaded syringe (Figure 1-42) and several ampules should be a component of the emergency kit. The 1:1000 concentration contains 1 mg of epinephrine in 1 ml of solution; this concentration is contraindicated for intravascular administration. The SC or IM/intralingual route is used, depending on the peripheral perfusion. When the patient has adequate peripheral perfusion, the SC route should be used. Epinephrine is absorbed more slowly after SC injection. Onset of action occurs within a few minutes, with less potential for significant adverse cardiovascular effects. The dose amount will depend on the severity of the emergency and the patient's medical history. Vital signs should be continuously assessed, and if available, monitors should be attached to the patient. The dentist should anticipate the need to administer more than one dose.

An EpiPen autoinjector (Center Laboratories, Port Washington, NY) is a disposable prefilled automatic injection device designed to deliver a single dose of epinephrine. The EpiPen is avail-

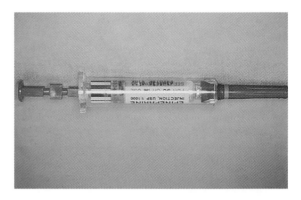

Figure 1-42. Preloaded epinephrine syringe (1 cc = 1:1000). Rectangular shape of the plunger limits the dose of epinephrine unless the plunger is rotated.

able in both an adult (0.3 ml of a 1:1000 epinephrine solution) and a pediatric (EpiPen Jr., 0.3 ml of a 1:2000 epinephrine solution) dosage. The EpiPen is generally prescribed to an allergic individual who may need to self-administer the epinephrine during an emergency. The autoinjector is not a good alternative for the emergency cart to replace the preloaded 1-ml epinephrine 1:1000 syringe. The IM injector delivers the medication into the thigh. The injector eliminates control over dose amount and injection site.

Inhaled β_2-Agonists

Bronchodilators are the mainstay of treatment for wheezing. Several medications are available. The primary agents are the β-adrenergic agonists (Table 1-6). These agents relax the smooth muscles of the bronchial tree. Both selective and nonselective agents are available; a selective agent is preferable. The use of a selective β_2-agonist minimizes the adverse effects, including tachycardia, arrhythmia, hypertension, angina, restlessness, flushing, and tremor. The β_2-agonists should be administered as an aerosol. This route of delivery allows the agent to be delivered directly to the effector site, achieving rapid onset, good effects, and minimal dose delivered to other organs, which reduces the adverse effects associated with adrenergic stimulation.

Bronchodilator therapy can be given using either a *metered-dose inhaler* (MDI) or a nebulizer. An MDI is appropriate for the dental office. Administering the medication using a spacer optimizes the delivery of the aerosol to the bronchial tree. In an emergency the patient should take one puff

Table 1-6	Management of β_2-Agonists	
Agent (Trade Name)	**Onset**	**Mechanism of Action**
Albuterol (Proventil, Ventolin)	5-15 minutes	β_2- agonist (most selective); preferred agent
Metaproterenol (Alupent, Metaprel)	5-15 minutes	β_2-agonist
Terbutaline (Brethaire, Brethine)	5-30 minutes	β_2-agonist
Ipratropium* (Atrovent)	5-15 minutes	Anticholinergic agonist

*Consider after β_2-agonist and before SC epinephrine. Role in acute setting is not clear.

each minute up to a total of four puffs. In the patient who is refractory to treatment, the dosing may need to be repeated several times. The risk associated with multiple administrations is excessive adrenergic stimulation. However, the lack of a response may result from the lack of medication reaching the effector site during the initial puffs. Separation of the inhalations by a few minutes may allow initial improvement, maximizing the effect of the subsequent doses. The alternative to repeating the bronchodilator therapy is the administration of SC epinephrine. Dependent on the severity of the situation, the dentist will have to consider the risks, benefits, and necessity to proceed to this step.

Albuterol, epinephrine, metaproterenol, isoproterenol, and terbutaline are inhaled bronchodilators. *Albuterol* is the preferred choice because it is the most selective of the β_2-agonists. It provides rapid onset within 5 to 15 minutes and has a duration of 4 to 6 hours. The asthmatic patient who carries an inhalant should place the MDI in an accessible area. *Metaproterenol* and *terbutaline* are less selective but are acceptable alternatives to manage bronchospasm in the office. Over-the-counter medications such as Primatene Mist (epinephrine), which are nonselective, are associated with increased side effects. The self-administering patient may be lacking medical supervision; the practitioner must assess each situation. Consideration should be given to administering the selective β_2-agonist in the emergency kit. Patients may also be taking long-acting β-agonists, such as salmeterol (Serevent). Salmeterol has a slow onset and is not appropriate for the treatment of an acute bronchospasm.

Bronchial smooth muscle has parasympathetic innervation in addition to the sympathetic innervation. The parasympathetic innervation causes bronchoconstriction. Patients may be prescribed and using an anticholinergic bronchodilator such as *ipratropium* or a combination of albuterol and ipratropium (Combivent). These drugs block the action of acetylcholine at the parasympathetic sites in bronchial smooth muscle, causing bronchodilation. Onset of action occurs in 5 to 15 minutes. The role of anticholinergic bronchodilators in the acute emergency is not clearly delineated, but they have minimal side effects. The dentist should consider administering an anticholinergic agent after the β-agonist.

The administration of inhaled steroids is not a primary treatment for an acute event because of their slow onset of action over hours.

Intravenous Fluids

The establishment of IV cannulation provides the ability to administer both fluids and drugs. Fluid administration provides the ability to (1) correct a preexisting deficit, (2) replace ongoing fluid losses, and (3) expand the intravascular compartment of the extracellular space. In dental offices where sedation is routine, common crystalloid solutions include dextrose 5% in water (D5W), D5/0.45% normal saline (NS), D5/0.9% NS, 0.45% NS, and 0.9% NS. The dentist must understand the concept of fluid compartmentalization so that the solution most appropriate for infusion can be selected.

Total body water exists in two major compartments, intracellular and extracellular. The *intracellular* compartment represents about two thirds of the total body water and the *extracellular* compartment about one third. The extracellular compartment is further subdivided into *intravascular* (one fourth) and *extravascular* (three fourths) compartments. Free water is constantly redistributed among these compartments, as dictated by ionic, osmotic, and hydrostatic pressure. The primary extracellular electrolytes are sodium and chloride. These electrolytes are not freely diffusible between compartments. Any alteration in the concentration of these electrolytes in a specific compartment will result in a compensatory shift of free water.

A physiologic choice for the replacement of a fluid deficit is 0.45% NS solution. Infused over 24 hours, this would provide the daily sodium requirement (1 to 2 mEq/kg). The advantage of an isotonic solution (e.g., 0.9% NaCl) in an emergency is the preferential distribution of the fluid within the extracellular space. This fluid will remain within the intravascular space for the first 15 to 30 minutes before equilibration within the extracellular compartment. This provides the advantage of countering the vasodilation and subsequent hypotension that may occur as a primary effect of a medical emergency or secondary to the administration of medicines (e.g., nitroglycerin).

D5W, a hypotonic solution, is rapidly redistributed and leaves the intravascular space; it thus does not provide a physiologic benefit comparable to that of the saline solutions. In addition, the normal hormonal response to stress produces an increase in blood glucose. Furthermore, the infusion of a dextrose solution may intensify this hyperglycemia, which may worsen the neurologic injury in the patient with hypoxemia.[39,40] Although this problem is unlikely during a dental sedative procedure, the administration of a dextrose solution is contraindicated for the management of medical emergencies, except hypoglycemia, for which a high concentration of dextrose is administered.

Nitroglycerin

The administration of nitroglycerin results in a peripheral venous and arterial vasodilation, with the venous effect predominating (Table 1-7). The beneficial effects include a reduced preload, decreased myocardial oxygen demand, and improved perfusion to the ischemic myocardium. Nitroglycerin is used to treat angina and perioperative hypertension.

Nitroglycerin is available as a 0.4-mg sublingual tablet and as a 0.4-mg metered lingual aerosol. Comparative evaluation between the spray and the tablet has been equivocal. Some studies, however, have demonstrated a more rapid effect from the spray.[41] The decreased initial efficacy of the tablet may be associated with its need to dissociate in the mouth before absorption. Although dissociation and absorption occur simultaneously, at times the tablet may not dissociate in the patient's mouth; this is usually discovered during administration of a second tablet. Moistening the patient's mouth will minimize this problem. Nitroglycerin spray eliminates this problem and has improved stability (Figure 1-43). The spray does not require special storage and has a shelf life of 3 years. Nitroglycerin tablets require storage in a light-resistant container and lose their potency within 12 weeks once opened.

Many patients with a history of angina are taking a form of nitroglycerin. The administration of sublingual nitroglycerin or lingual aerosol is relatively safe. Side effects include headaches, flushing, dizziness, and postural hypotension. In one study the average drop in systolic blood pressure after the first 0.4-mg sublingual nitroglycerin tablet was 8.8% (14 mm Hg; range, 11 to 16 mm Hg), with an additional 7% decrease after the second tablet.[42] Therefore the patient should rest in a sitting or supine position during administration. The change in heart rate is variable, although minimal. Potential bradycardia with hypotension has been reported, but the mechanism is not understood. The incidence of bradycardia is unknown.

Nitroglycerin is recommended for relief of angina in patients with prescribed formulations as well as those with new-onset angina and suspected MI. Doses of a sublingual tablet or lingual aerosol can be repeated every 5 minutes. Blood pressure should be taken after each dose; an additional dose should not be administered if the systolic pressure is less than 90 mm Hg.

Hypotension is managed by placing the patient supine with the heart and brain at the same level and the feet elevated approximately 15 degrees. If the office is equipped and staffed to es-

Table 1-7	Nitroglycerin		
Condition	**Dose**		**Comments**
Angina	One tablet or spray every 5 minutes until symptoms resolve or patient becomes hypotensive		If symptoms persist after three tablets, consider emergency to be myocardial infarction and call 911.
Myocardial infarction	One tablet or spray every 5 minutes until symptoms resolve or patient becomes hypotensive		Call 911.

tablish IV access, the hypotension can be managed by infusing a balanced salt solution.

Nitrous Oxide

Nitrous oxide was first used as an anesthetic in medicine and dentistry in 1844. It provides anxiolysis, sedation, and analgesia. The practitioner should be aware that many adverse events are aggravated by mental stress and anxiety. Incorporating a sedative technique into a dental practice may be beneficial in select situations.

Nitrous oxide may also provide some benefit in an emergency. Administration of nitrous oxide requires simultaneous delivery of at least 30% oxygen. More frequently the concentration of nitrous oxide is 20% to 50% when used in emergency care, with 50% to 80% oxygen administered through the nasal hood. The analgesic potency of 20% nitrous oxide has been equated to 15 mg of morphine.[43] Nonanesthetic administration of nitrous oxide significantly decreases ischemic pain of myocardial origin.[44,45]

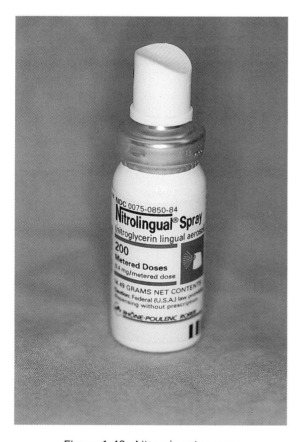

Figure 1-43. Nitroglycerin spray.

Oxygen

An imbalance of oxygen supply and demand can have catastrophic neurologic and cardiovascular effects. Most dental emergencies involve impaired oxygen supply or demand. The level of impairment is directly related to the adverse event. The etiology may be primarily *respiratory*, as in bronchospasm, resulting in diminished oxygen delivery within the lungs; *cardiovascular*, as in angina, resulting in diminished oxygen delivery to the myocardium; *neurologic*, as in a seizure, potentially resulting in a central apnea or an impaired ability to maintain an open airway; or *iatrogenic*, such as an adverse drug effect to the epinephrine in the local anesthetic causing tachycardia, resulting in both increased demand and decreased supply of oxygen.

Oxygen therapy is beneficial for essentially all medical emergencies. The concern of oxygen toxicity does not become evident until after 3 to 5 days of ventilatory support with inspired concentrations of oxygen. Oxygen therapy is even indicated for the patient with COPD, whose correction of hypoxemia may reduce the respiratory drive necessitating assisted ventilation. Oxygen therapy is contraindicated in one dental office emergency, *hyperventilation syndrome*; the delivery of the oxygen flushes away the carbon dioxide and counters the desired treatment of increasing the CO_2 level.

SUMMARY

In an office emergency the dentist must be able to slip into "emergency mode" and act aggressively when necessary. Preparations include learning and practicing the standard resuscitation plan, including the primary and secondary surveys. The physician must be familiar with likely, treatable medical problems, must know how to recognize them, and must be able to provide treatment. A course in basic life support is requisite. A decision must be made for every patient about activating the EMS system and whether the patient should be transferred to the ED. The dentist must be able to present the patient's case to other health care providers and properly document the office emergency.

The dental office staff can handle the management of an unanticipated medical event. Treatment requires a dentist and dental staff who are familiar with the pharmacologic agents and the emergency equipment necessary to intervene in such a situation. A lack of familiarity will result in the unanticipated medical episode progressing into a medical emergency.

REFERENCES

1. Stewart CM, Lado E: Preparation of office emergencies: equipment, skills, and attitudes of general dentists and specialists, *Gen Dent* 36:211-214, 1988.

2. Moore PA: Review of medical emergencies in dentistry. Part 1. Staff training and prevention, *Gen Dent* 36:14-17, 1988.

3. Fast TB, Martin MD, Ellis TM: Emergency preparedness: a survey of dental practitioners, *J Am Dent Assoc* 112:499-501, 1986.

4. Protzman S, Clark J: The dental assistant's management of medical emergencies, *Dental Assistant*, May/June 1996, p 7.

5. American College of Surgeons Committee on Trauma: *Advanced trauma life support manual*, Chicago, 1993, American College of Surgeons.

6. Sanders MJ: *Mosby's paramedic textbook*, St Louis, 1994, Mosby.

7. Heimlich HJ: A life-saving maneuver to prevent food choking, *JAMA* 234:398-401, 1975.

8. Bayless P, Ray VG: Incidence of cervical spine injuries in association with blunt head trauma, *Am J Emerg Med* 7:139-142, 1989.

9. Beirne JC, Butler PE, Brady FA: Cervical spine injuries in patients with facial fractures: a 1 year prospective study, *Int J Oral Maxillofac Surg* 24:26-29, 1995.

10. Gisbert V, Hollerman J, Ney A, et al: Incidence and diagnosis of C7-T1 fractures and subluxations in multiple trauma patients: evaluation of advanced life support guidelines, *Surgery* 106:702-708, 1989.

11. Robertson C: The precordial thump and cough techniques in advanced life support: a statement for the Advanced Life Support Working Party of the European Resuscitation Council, *Resuscitation* 24:133-135, 1992.

12. Caldwell G, Millar G, Quinn E, et al: Simple mechanical methods for cardioversion: defence of the precordial thump and cough version, *Br Med J* 291:627-630, 1985.

13. Miller J, Trasch D, Horwitz L, et al: The precordial thump, *Ann Emerg Med* 13:791-794, 1984.

14. Cummins RO, Ornato JP, Thies WH, et al: Improving survival from cardiac arrest: the "chain of survival" concept—a statement for health care professionals from the Advanced Cardiac Care Life Support Subcommittee and the Emergency Cardiac Care Committee, American Heart Association, *Circulation* 83:1832-1847, 1990.

15. Eisenberg MS, Cummins RO, Damon S, et al: Survival rates from out of hospital cardiac arrest: recommendations for uniform definitions and data to report, *Ann Emerg Med* 19:1249-1253, 1990.

16. American Heart Association: Guidelines 2000 for cardiopulmonary resuscitation and emergency cardiovascular care, *Circulation* 102(8):I22-59, 2000.

17. Noc M, Weil MH, Sun SJ, et al: Mechanical ventilation may not be essential for initial cardiopulmonary resuscitation, *Chest* 108:821-827, 1995.

18. Kothari RU, Hall K, Brott T, et al: Early stroke recognition: developing an out-of-hospital NIH stroke scale, *Acad Emerg Med* 4:986-990, 1997.

19. Kothari RU, Pancioli A, Liu T, et al: Cincinnati prehosptial stroke scale: reproducibility and validity, *Ann Emerg Med* 33:373-378, 1999.

20. Iserson KV: Intraosseous infusions in adults, *J Emerg Med* 7:587-591, 1989.

21. Sullivan KJ, Berman LS, Koska J, et al: Intramuscular atropine sulfate in children: comparison of injection sites, *Anesth Analg* 84:54-58, 1997.

22. Slama G, Traynard P-Y, Desplanque N, et al: The search for an optimized treatment of hypoglycemia: carbohydrates in tablets, solution, or gel for the correction of insulin reactions, *Arch Intern Med* 150:589-593, 1990.

23. Vukmir RD et al: Glucagon: prehospital therapy of hypoglycemia, *Ann Emerg Med* 20:375-381, 1991.

24. Marri G et al: Glucagon in sulfonylurea hypoglycemia? *Lancet* 1:303-304, 1968.

25. Perkin RM et al: Mechanisms and management of anaphylactic shock not responding to traditional therapy, *Ann Allergy* 54:202-203, 1985.

26. Ballmer-Weber BK, Gex-Collet C, Wuthrich B: Inhibition of histamine or allergen-induced wheals by a single dose of acrivastine, fexofenadine, or cetirizine, *J Investig Allergol Clin Immunol* 9:351-355, 1999.

27. Grant JA, Danielson L, Rihoux JP, et al: A double-blind, single-dose, crossover comparison of cetirizine, ebastine, epinastine, fexofenadine, terfenadine, and loratadine versus placebo: suppression of histamine-induced wheal and flare response for 24 h in healthy male subjects, *Allergy* 54:700-707, 1999.

28. Ryan TJ, Anderson JL, Antman EM, et al: ACC/AHA guidelines for the management of patients with acute myocardial infarction: a report of the American College of Cardiology/American Heart Association Task Force on Practice Guidelines (Committee on Management of Acute Myocardial Infarction), *J Am Coll Cardiol* 28:1328-1419, 1996.

29. Second International Study of Infarct Survival Collaborative Group: Randomised trial of intravenous streptokinase, oral aspirin, both, or neither among 17,187 cases of suspected acute myocardial infarction: ISIS-2, *Lancet* 2:349-360, 1988.

30. Fitzgerald GA: Mechanisms of platelet activation: thromboxane A_2 as an amplifying signal for other agonists, *Am J Cardiol* 68:11B-15B, 1991.

31. Patrono C, Ciabattoni G, Patrignani P, et al: Clinical pharmacology of platelet cyclooxygenase inhibition, *Circulation* 72:177-184, 1985.

32. Feldman M, Cryer B: Aspirin absorption rates and platelet inhibition times with 325-mg buffered aspirin tablets (chewed or swallowed intact) and with buffered aspirin solution, *Am J Cardiol* 84:404-409, 1999.

33. Baigent C, Collins R, Appleby P, et al: ISIS-2: 10 year survival among patients with suspected acute myocardial infarction in randomized comparison of intravenous streptokinase, oral aspirin, both, or neither, *Br Med J* 316:1337-1343, 1998.

34. Kriel RL, Cloyd JC, Pellock JM, et al: Rectal diazepam gel for treatment of acute repetitive seizures, *Pediatr Neurol* 20:282-288, 1999.

35. Franzoni E et al: Rectal diazepam: a clinical and EEG study after a single dose in children, *Epilepsia* 24:35-41, 1983.

36. Chamberlain JM, Altieri MA, Futterman C, et al: A prospective, randomized study comparing intramuscular midazolam with intravenous diazepam for the treatment of seizures in children, *Pediatr Emerg Care* 13:92-94, 1997.

37. Yakinci C, Mungen B, Sahin S, et al: Midazolam in treatment of various types of seizures in children, *Brain Dev* 19:571-572, 1997.

38. O'Regan ME, Brown JR, Clark M: Nasal rather than rectal benzodiazepines in the management of acute childhood seizures, *Dev Med Child Neurol* 38:1037-1045, 1996.

39. Bush GH, Steward DJ: Can persistent cerebral damage be caused by hyperglycemia? *Pediatr Anaesth* 5:385-387, 1995.

40. Nicolson SC: Glucose: enough versus too much, *J Cardiothorac Vasc Anesth* 11:409-410, 1997.
41. Laslett LJ et al: Sublingual nitroglycerin administered by spray versus tablet: comparative timing of hemodynamic effects, *Cardiology* 77:303-310, 1990.
42. Brandes W et al: Nitroglycerin-induced hypotension, bradycardia, and asystole: report of a case and review of the literature, *Clin Cardiol* 13:741-744, 1990.
43. Chapman WP, Arrowood JG, Beecher HK: The analgesic effects of low concentrations of nitrous oxide compared in man with morphine sulfate, *J Clin Invest* 22:871-875, 1943.
44. Stewart RD, Paris PM, Stoy WA, et al: Patient controlled inhalational analgesia in prehospital care: a study of side effects and feasibility, *Crit Care Med* 11:851-855, 1983.
45. Thompson PL, Lown B: Nitrous oxide as an analgesic in acute myocardial infarction, *JAMA* 235:924-927, 1976.

Pediatric Considerations

Morton B. Rosenberg
James C. Phero

The treatment of the pediatric patient with an acute emergency has only recently been recognized as distinct from that of the adult patient. Pediatric health care is not merely the application of adult medical principles to smaller patients.[1] Pediatric emergency care requires an understanding of how pediatric anatomy and physiology influence a child's response to the acute manifestations of pediatric pathophysiology. The pediatric patient requires a totally different approach, ranging from choice of drugs to resuscitative techniques and equipment.

DEVELOPMENTAL CONSIDERATIONS

A child's development includes the *newborn stage* (first 30 days of life), *infant stage* (first year of life), and *pediatric stage* (first 12 years of life). Each stage has its own unique subset of anatomic and physiologic considerations. This chapter focuses on the pediatric stage and reviews the effects of pediatric growth and development on physiologic, anatomic, and pharmacologic responses to acute medical emergencies.

Understanding the importance of physiologic and anatomic differences between adults and children begins with the realization that although differences in size are readily apparent, differences in body proportions are not as obvious but are just as significant. The child's greater body surface areas translates into greater heat loss, resulting in hypothermia, and increased fluid requirements, which can easily lead to relative or absolute hypovolemia during medical emergencies. Most importantly, because of the child's higher metabolic rate and oxygen consumption, any emergency that interferes with oxygen delivery (e.g., soft tissue airway obstruction, upper airway edema, foreign body in airway, bronchospasm) quickly becomes life threatening. Because children are so susceptible to hypoxia, immediate evaluation and management of the pediatric airway represent the priority in every pediatric medical emergency.

AIRWAY MANAGEMENT

The numerous anatomic differences between the adult and pediatric airway have a dramatic impact on emergency care.

Primary Survey

In any medical emergency the first step is determining that the *airway* (A) is open, followed by evaluation of *breathing* (B) and *circulation* (C), the "ABCs" of cardiopulmonary resuscitation (CPR). Clinically, this evaluation includes (1) assessing the work of breathing, (2) monitoring respiratory rate, (3) observing mucous membrane color, and (4) establishing the patient's level of consciousness (LOC). Airway management can be as simple as observation or as complex and invasive as endotracheal intubation or cricothyrotomy.

After an initial determination of rate and depth of respiration, pediatric airway evaluation focuses on the overall *work of breathing*. Nasal flaring, manifested as widening of the nostrils on inspiration, is an early sign of increased work. Retractions of the accessory muscles of respiration (suprasternal, infraclavicular, subdiaphragmatic, intercostal) are more serious signs. Auscultation of the chest in the pediatric patient should always be attempted but can be misleading because the child's chest wall transmits sounds so easily that interpretation is often difficult. Wheezing is an important finding, however, especially in children with a history of bronchospastic disease or past respiratory response to a known allergen. Signs of impending respiratory failure include decreased breath sounds, listlessness, altered LOC, diminished

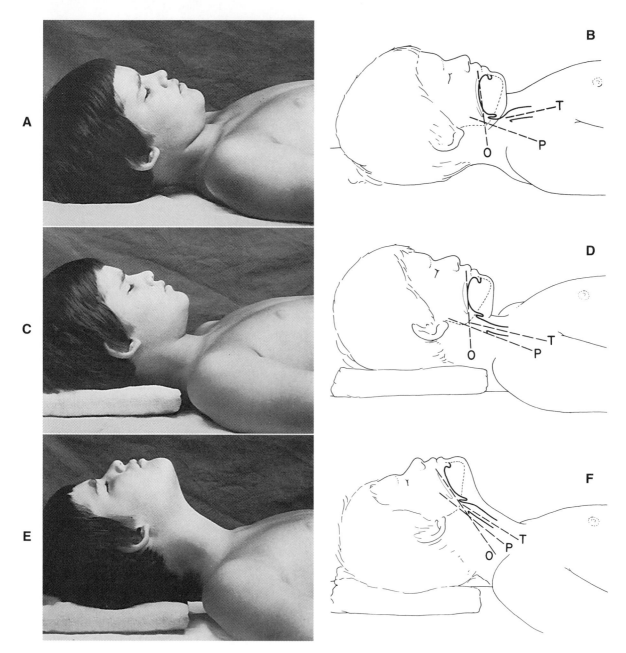

Figure 2-1. Positioning for ventilation and tracheal intubation. With patient supine **(A)** the oral *(O)*, pharyngeal *(P)*, and tracheal *(T)* axes pass through three divergent planes **(B)**. Folded sheet or towel under occiput of the head **(C)** aligns the pharyngeal *(P)* and tracheal *(T)* axes **(D)**. Folded towel under the occiput plus extension of the atlanto-occipital joint **(E)** results in alignment of the oral *(O)*, pharyngeal *(P)*, and tracheal *(T)* axes **(F)**. *From Coté CJ, Ryan JF, Todres ID, et al, editors: A practice of anesthesia for infants and children, Philadelphia, 1993, WB Saunders.*

responses to pain, decreased muscle tone and cyanosis.[2]

Head Position

Proper positioning of the pediatric airway to ensure an open airway differs from adult positioning because children have larger heads. The child's head occupies a larger total body surface area, and the occiput is more prominent. One of the most common problems in pediatric airway management is the failure to position the child's head properly to allow for adequate ventilation. The child should be first placed in the *sniffing position*, which consists of flexion of the neck on the long axis of the body and slight extension of the head (Figure 2-1). This can be achieved by placing a towel or a hand under the child's occiput. This maneuver accompanied by a jaw thrust can often open the obstructed airway and also aids in visualization of the vocal cords if laryngoscopy and endotracheal intubation become necessary.

Anatomy and Airway Obstruction

Airway obstruction may occur during any pediatric medical emergency when LOC is altered or totally obtunded. Obstruction may be caused by relatively large *tonsils* and *adenoids*, which reach their greatest size from ages 4 to 10 years. The enlarged tonsils and adenoids may be associated with a positive history of obstructive sleep apnea or snoring elicited from the child's parents. These lymphoid tissues often cause airway obstruction during deep sedation or general anesthesia and may play a role in other situations that result in unconsciousness and the inability to maintain an open airway. Large tonsils and adenoids along with a relatively large *tongue*, as is often seen in infants and young children, can create total soft tissue airway obstruction that may be deadly if not rapidly diagnosed and treated.

Another important factor creating difficulties for the pediatric patient in overcoming soft tissue airway obstruction is the *respiratory muscles* themselves. The chest wall and diaphragm are much more compliant in children than adults. In a young child the ribs are more horizontal and are oriented at right angles to the vertebrae, compared to the more caudal direction of adult ribs. Coupled with underdeveloped intercostal muscles that cannot elevate these horizontal ribs efficiently, children tend to use abdominal and diaphragmatic breathing. Therefore they have difficulty overcoming airway obstruction and are more effected by gastric distention and abdominal splinting than adults.[3]

The upper and lower portions of a child's airway are significantly smaller than those in an adult, resulting in increased airway resistance. The child's airway is easily obstructed by debris, blood, pus, edema, or even active smooth muscle constriction. The *larynx* is higher in the neck of a child than in an adult, extending from the second to the fourth cervical vertebrae and positioned more anteriorly. The epiglottis is more spoon shaped and cartilaginous and sits at a 45-degree angle. These anatomic features contribute to making laryngoscopy, visualization of the vocal cords, and intubation more difficult unless special considerations are observed.

Correct choice of endotracheal (ET) tube must be based on the diameter of the child's *cricoid ring*, the narrowest portion in the pediatric upper airway, rather than the glottic opening, the narrowest portion in the adult upper airway (Table 2-1). An ET tube passes easily through the vocal cords of a child but may fit too tight in the subglottic region. For this reason, uncuffed tubes are generally used in pediatric patients until ages 8 to 10. The loose, areolar, columnar epithelium of the pediatric upper airway is not only highly reactive, but also quite sensitive to both traumatic injury and infection, especially in the area of the cricoid cartilage. This explains why upper respiratory tract infections, such as croup and epiglottitis, can be life threatening. The angulation of pediatric right mainstem bronchus can often lead to inadvertent right endobronchial intubation when an ET tube is placed during resuscitation.

Aspiration of Foreign Bodies

Foreign body aspiration is a major cause of acute airway obstruction in infants and children. Many foreign objects will lodge at the cricoid ring. Infants under 1 year of age should be turned upside down and four sharp back blows delivered to dislodge the object. If this maneuver fails, the child should be turned prone and four chest thrusts performed. In older children the optimal method for relief of complete airway obstruction due to a foreign body remains controversial. At this time, the Heimlich maneuver, a series of subdiaphragmatic abdominal thrusts designed to increase intrathoracic pressure and dislodge the foreign body, is recommended (Figure 2-2).[4]

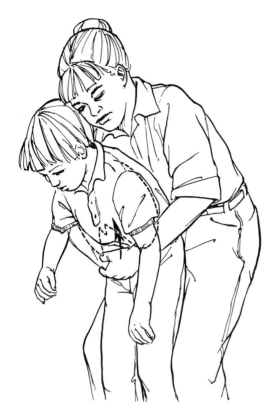

Figure 2-2. Abdominal thrusts with victim standing or sitting (conscious). *From American Heart Association:* BLS for healthcare providers, *Dallas, 1997-1999, The Association.*

Table 2-1	Anatomic Differences Between Adult and Pediatric Airways	
	Pediatric	**Adult**
Position of larynx	C2-C4	C4-C6
Narrowest portion of airway	Cricoid cartilage	Glottis
Shape of epiglottis	Ω (Omega)	V
Angulation of right mainstem bronchus	Less vertical	More vertical

Positive-Pressure Ventilation and Advanced Techniques

Every dental office should have the ability to administer oxygen to a spontaneously breathing patient and should have the equipment and staff training to deliver positive-pressure ventilation.

Because of inadequate oxygen reserves due to anatomic and physiologic factors, oxygen should be considered for all pediatric emergencies. Oxygen has few if any side effects in pediatric patients. It may be delivered to the spontaneously breathing patient via a nasal cannula, nasal hood, or face mask.

The easiest form of assisted ventilation in a child is *bag-valve-mask ventilation*. Proper airway seal and sufficient pressures to generate adequate tidal volumes are easily accomplished if the correct-size equipment is available. A proper mask fit provides a tight seal on the face and will extend from the bridge of the nose to the midpoint of the symphysis of the mandible, avoiding compression of the eyes. Rescue breaths should be delivered slowly over 1 to 1.5 seconds. Attention should be directed in ensuring adequate ventilation, as evidenced by bilateral symmetric chest rise with each breath, while avoiding excessive inspiratory pressure, which can result in gastric distention. Besides increasing the risk of aspiration and regurgitation of gastric contents, gastric distention often prevents adequate ventilation in the pediatric patient. During assisted or controlled ventilation, gastric distention can be reduced by the application of cricoid pressure (*Sellick maneuver*), which occludes the proximal esophagus.[5]

The practitioner should be aware of the volume a child requires for adequate ventilation and the appropriate pressure required to ventilate the patient (Table 2-2). Resuscitation bags come in pediatric and adult sizes to assist the practitioner with delivering the appropriate volume with each squeeze.

Endotracheal intubation is an advanced technique that requires training and practice. Practitioners who use this approach to airway management during resuscitative maneuvers must be aware of appropriate sizes of ET tubes for the pediatric patient. Again, uncuffed tubes are generally used because the tube may be too tight in the subglottic region, with the potential for inflammation and swelling of the subglottic region on extubation. Tonsils and adenoids should always be suspected if airway obstruction develops in the unconscious child. Also, these lymphoid tissues can be sheared off or traumatized during endotracheal intubation. Uncontrolled bleeding may result in decreased visualization during laryngoscopy or obstruction of the ET tube lumen by lymphoid tissue.

Table 2-2	Respiratory Differences between Pediatric and Adult Patients			
	3 Years	5 Years	12 Years	Adult
Tidal volume (ml, cc)	112	270	480	575
Minute ventilation (liters per minute)	2.46	5.5	6.2	6.4
Vital capacity (ml, cc)	870	1160	3100	4000
Functional residual capacity (ml, cc)	490	680	1970	3000

Table 2-3	Reference Values for Cardiovascular Measurements in Pediatric Patients		
Age	Heart Rate (beats/min)	Systolic Blood Pressure (mm Hg)	Diastolic Blood Pressure (mm Hg)
Neonate	140	65	40
1 year	120	95	64
3 years	100	100	70
12 years	80	110	60

CARDIOVASCULAR MANAGEMENT

By the end of the postnatal period, most major developmental changes in the cardiovascular system have occurred. The pediatric cardiovascular system is more fragile than the adult's, as evidenced by less muscle mass and less contractility. However, the pediatric system has a compensatory mechanism to increase cardiac output through increasing the heart rate (Table 2-3). The response of a normal pediatric heart to any condition or medical emergency that increases metabolic rate and oxygen consumption (e.g., fever, stress, anxiety, hypoxia, hypovolemia, hypercarbia) is tachycardia. Blood pressure is also highly rate dependent, and bradycardia will result in hypotension and later cardiac arrest. Progressive bradycardia during a medical emergency is an ominous sign that usually indicates a hypoxic state and impending arrest.

Cardiopulmonary Arrest

Cardiopulmonary arrest in the pediatric patient is rarely of sudden onset. In the adult population, cardiopulmonary arrest predominantly results from a primary cardiac event, precipitated by the presence of coronary artery disease. Adults often have primary cardiac arrest secondary to myocardial infarction, whereas children have primary cardiac arrest secondary to a prolonged period of respiratory compromise. The adage that "adults drop dead but children *droop* dead" reflects the fact that respiratory failure resulting in hypoxia, hypercarbia, and acidosis is the primary initiator of the progressive nature of cardiopulmonary arrest in children. Thus, by the time cardiac arrest occurs, multiple vital organs have undergone serious, often irreversible injury. Outcomes for children worsen significantly once cardiac arrest occurs during any medical emergency. Many investigators have confirmed that survival rates after respiratory arrest alone, whether in or outside the hospital, are significantly higher than after cardiac arrest.[6,7]

Early recognition and prompt, aggressive intervention of respiratory failure to prevent further hypoxemia and respiratory acidosis may be the most important factors in averting cardiac arrest and improving survival for the pediatric patient. Causes of respiratory deterioration in children can include allergic reactions, hypoglycemia, congenital heart disease, infection, poisoning, drowning, airway obstruction from foreign bodies or soft tissue, and drug overdose (Box 2-1). As respiratory failure worsens, a progressive bradycardia may ensue that if left untreated, ultimately results in *asystole*, the most common presenting rhythm for pediatric cardiopulmonary arrest. Resuscitation at this point usually fails.[8]

Box 2-1	Common Causes of Pediatric Cardiopulmonary Arrest

Airway mismanagement
Anesthetic/sedative overdose
Drug induced (e.g., succinylcholine-induced hyperkalemia)
Embolism
Hypovolemia
Metabolic disturbances (e.g., diabetic ketoacidosis)
Respiratory infections
Sepsis
Airway obstruction (e.g., foreign body aspiration)

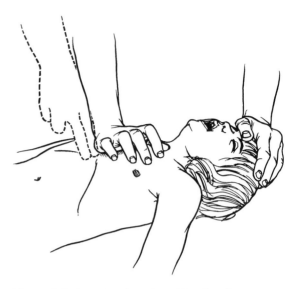

Figure 2-3. Locating hand position for chest compression in child. Rescuer's other hand is used to maintain head position to facilitate ventilation. *From American Heart Association:* BLS for healthcare providers, *Dallas, 1997-1999, The Association.*

Circulatory Compromise

Circulatory compromise in the pediatric patient can be difficult to assess because children have substantial compensatory mechanisms. In the infant and young child the pulse is most easily palpated in the brachial or femoral artery. In older children and adults the carotid artery provides the best pulse in evaluating the adequacy of circulation. External chest compression should be initiated with artificial ventilation when the heart rate is less than 80 beats per minute in the infant or less than 60 in the child or when palpable peripheral pulses are absent. Chest compression ratios have been simplified for infants and children. A compression rate of 100 per minute is recommended for the child. The ratio of compressions to ventilation is 5:1. The infant's chest should be compressed with two or three fingers, just below the intermammary line where it intersects the sternum, to a depth of 1.25 to 2.5 cm (½ to 1 inch) and at a rate of 100 times per minute. The chest of a child older than 1 year is compressed with the "heel" of the hand, two fingerbreadths above the intersection of the ribs' costal margins with the sternum, to a depth of 2.5 to 3.75 cm (1 to ½ inches) and at a rate of 80 to 100 times per minute (Figure 2-3). Adult CPR procedures should be used in children over 8 years old.[9]

Intravascular Volume and Fluid Administration

Children have a greater percentage of body water than an adult has and a smaller circulating blood volume (Box 2-2). Even small amounts of fluid loss can compromise the pediatric circula-

Box 2-2	Reference Values for Pediatric Blood Volumes

GROUP	BLOOD VOLUME (mg/kg)
Neonates (<1 month)	90
Infants (<2 years)	80
Children (prepubescent, <12 years)	75

tion, quickly leading to hypovolemic shock, tissue hypoxia, and if left untreated, cardiac arrest. Hypotension in children is a late clinical manifestation of shock, and blood pressure should not be the sole determinant of perfusion. Even with a loss of 20% of blood volume, blood pressure in the pediatric patient may remain unchanged. It is important to check for other signs in order to detect hypovolemic shock such as cool clammy extremities, peripheral capillary refill time longer than 2 seconds, rapid respirations, mottled skin, weak or absent peripheral pulses, listlessness, and decreased LOC. On detection of hypotension, aggressive and early fluid resuscitation and expansion of the circulating blood volume are important to avert progressive shock and subsequent cardiac arrest.

Vascular Access

As in adult resuscitation, establishment of vascular access is imperative in order to infuse medications and fluids for circulatory support. Routine intravenous (IV) techniques are the routes of choice but can often be technically difficult and time consuming during pediatric resuscitation. The insertion of an IV cannula is a basic skill for the treatment of many pediatric medical emergencies. If inserted during emergency treatment, an ET tube may also serve as an alternate route for the administration of nonlipid drugs into the central circulation if IV access is unobtainable or delayed. Epinephrine, atropine, lidocaine, and naloxone may be safely administered through the ET tube after being diluted in 1 to 2 ml of normal saline.

Intraosseous techniques have also been advocated as a means of providing immediate vascular access to pediatric patients less than 6 years of age within the first 5 minutes of an emergency. Injections into the bone marrow are absorbed almost immediately into the circulation. Pediatric specialists should consider training in this advanced, lifesaving technique.[10] A spinal needle with stylet or a bone marrow needle is inserted into the anterior surface of the tibia 1 to 3 cm (about ½ to 1 inch) below the tibial tuberosity and directed slightly inferiorly to avoid the epiphyseal plate. Proper placement is confirmed by lack of resistance after passage through the cortex of the tibia. The needle stands erect in the tibia without support, blood or bone marrow freely aspirates from the needle, and the IV infusion flows freely without subcutaneous infiltration.

Box 2-3	Drugs Used in Pediatric Advanced Life Support
DRUG	**DOSE**
Adenosine	0.1-0.2 mg/kg (maximum: 12 mg)
Atropine	0.02 mg/kg per dose Minimum dose: 0.1 mg Maximum single dose: 0.5 mg (child), 1.0 mg (adolescent)
Bretylium	5 mg/kg; may be increased to 10 mg/kg
Calcium chloride	20 mg/kg per dose
Dopamine	2-20 µg/kg/min
Dobutamine	2-20 µg/kg/min
Epinephrine (bradycardia)	IV/IO, 0.01 mg/kg (1:10,000)
Epinephrine (asystole or pulseless arrest)	First dose: IV/IO, 0.01 mg/kg (1:10,000); doses as high as 0.2 mg/kg may be effective Subsequent doses: IV/IO, 0.1 mg/kg (1:1000); doses as high as 0.2 mg/kg may be effective
Epinephrine infusion	Initial: 0.1 µg/kg/min
Lidocaine	1 mg/kg per dose
Lidocaine infusion	20-50 µg/kg/min
Sodium bicarbonate	1 mEq/kg per dose, or 0.3 × kg × base deficit

Modified from American Heart Association: *JAMA* 268: 2251-2275, 1992.
IV, Intravenous; *IO,* intraosseous.

Resuscitation Measures

Recent changes in pharmacologic therapeutic recommendations during CPR based on new experimental data in pediatric resuscitation are important additions to the treatment of cardiac arrest and supraventricular tachycardia (Box 2-3).[11]

Epinephrine

The efficacy of epinephrine, a potent α- and β-adrenergic receptor agonist, has been well established in helping to restore spontaneous circulation after cardiac arrest.[1] Epinephrine is the first-line therapy for asystole. After ventilation has been established in these patients, as well as in those with bradycardia associated with severe cardiac compromise, epinephrine should be administered before atropine. Finally, as a continuous infusion, epinephrine may be preferable to dopamine in the treatment of shock that is unresponsive to fluid resuscitation.

Since 1980 the recommended dose of epinephrine for asystolic arrest in children has been 0.01 mg/kg of a 1:10,000 solution, intravenously or by the intraosseous route. High doses of epinephrine may be beneficial in children with cardiac arrest.[13] Current American Heart Association (AHA) guidelines are to increase the second and subsequent doses for unresponsive asystolic and pulseless arrest 10 times the initial dosage, or 0.1 mg/kg of a 1:1000 solution, intravenously. The higher dose of epinephrine should be administered within 3 to 5 minutes of the initial standard dose and may be repeated every 3 to 5 minutes. Doses as high as 0.2 mg/kg may be effective.

Supraventricular Tachycardia

Supraventricular tachycardia (SVT) is the most common symptom-producing tachydysrhythmia in children. The mechanism of action of most cases of SVT is the development of a reentrant circuit that self-perpetuates the arrhythmia. Whenever a child's heart rate exceeds 200 beats per minute, diastole shortens, decreasing the ventricular filling time, which leads to a fall in stroke volume and cardiac output. Synchronized *cardioversion* is still considered the treatment of choice for hemodynamically unstable SVT. The recommended strength of the initial shock for cardioversion is 0.5 joules (J)/kg. In the stable child with SVT the administration of IV *adenosine* (0.1 mg/kg) is the treatment of choice.[14] Verapamil was previously recommended, but it caused cardiovascular collapse in several cases and is no longer listed for the pediatric patient.[15]

ALLERGIC REACTIONS

Immediate allergic reactions are attributed to release of several mediators from mast cells and basophils through immunoglobulin E (IgE). These regulators and other autacoids can also be synthesized and released by non-IgE-mediated mechanisms and can produce a similar clinical syndrome. Because an IgE mechanism cannot always be confirmed, the terms *pseudoallergic* and *anaphylactoid* are often used when describing these reactions.

Minor allergic or pseudoallergic reactions involve only the skin, presenting as pruritus, maculopapular rash, and urticaria. Cutaneous reactions are mediated primarily by histamine and can be counteracted by antihistamines such as diphenhydramine.

Anaphylactoid reactions may also present with cutaneous signs but are distinguished by a syndrome of systemic complications, including acute bronchospasm, laryngeal edema, and hypotension. In addition to histamine, other autacoids contribute to the pathogenesis of anaphylactoid reactions. These include prostaglandins, leukotrienes, and a variety of proteases for which no specific antagonists exist. Glucocorticoids produce a more generalized inhibitory effect on inflammatory autacoids, but this influence is not seen for several hours after administration and limits their value for managing the acute event. Any child who experiences an anaphylactoid event will require emergency medical services (EMS) transport to an emergency department. Steroid administration may be held until that time, or at least until the acute syndrome is stabilized.

Management of an acute anaphylactoid event requires oxygen supplementation and administration of epinephrine. Both the α- and β-receptor stimulation of epinephrine are required to reverse the anaphylactoid syndrome. The α-receptor-induced vasoconstriction reduces laryngeal edema and increases blood pressure. Stimulating the β-receptors relieves bronchospasm and improves cardiac output.

Many doses and routes for administration have been suggested, but an initial subcutaneous (SC) or IV dose of 0.01 mg/kg is recommended most consistently. A 1:1000 concentration is preferred for SC and a 1:10,000 concentration IV administration. The duration of epinephrine's effect may be as brief as 5 to 10 minutes. Additional doses may be required before EMS arrival at the office. If IV access is available, hypotension may be managed with fluid challenge, which should correct the hypovolemia that accompanies increased permeability of the vascular bed.[16]

COMPLICATIONS OF DIABETES

Diabetes mellitus is a disorder of carbohydrate metabolism that results from defects in insulin secretion, insulin action, or both.[17] *Type* 1 (or I) diabetic patients have an absolute insulin deficiency, whereas *type* 2 (or II) diabetics produce inadequate amounts of insulin and exhibit tissue resistance. Type 2 diabetic patients are generally managed with diet or oral hypoglycemic agents, but some may require insulin replacement. Only type 1 diabetics experience acute diabetic coma, which manifests not only as hyperglycemia with subsequent hyperosmolar coma, but also as ketoacidosis from lack of insulin's inhibitory influence on lipolysis. This complication is highly unlikely and usually occurs in the undiagnosed patient.

Regardless of classification, *hypoglycemia* is the most common acute event in diabetic patients and can be attributed to excessive medication and inadequate carbohydrate intake. As serum glucose dips below 60 mg/dl, compensatory hormones are released, including epinephrine, which accounts for the early warnings of tachycardia, shakiness, and diaphoresis. As the concentration drops further, generally to less than 50 mg/dl, cognitive and additional central nervous system (CNS) functions become impaired. Hypoglycemic reactions must be taken seriously because brain tissue relies on glucose exclusively as an energy substrate. In addition to the standard "syncope protocol," the child must be given concentrated glucose. If they remain conscious, patients can be permitted to drink a sweetened beverage, but a viscous glucose concentrate should be available for more severe episodes. The concentrate should be placed in the buccal mucosa and permitted to dissolve and seep down the esophagus and into the stomach. Research has shown that glucose cannot diffuse through oral mucosa.[18]

If an IV line is in place, a 50% dextrose solution can be infused slowly, keeping in mind that its osmolarity leads to venous irritation. The IV route is mandated in the unconscious patient. Glucagon is a less desirable alternative. After intramuscular administration, glucagon elevates blood glucose by stimulating glycogenolysis. This action requires 10 to 20 minutes and may be ineffective in children with limited stores of glycogen, such as from poor nutrition or dieting.

CONVULSIVE SEIZURES

Convulsive seizures are attributed to excessive synchronous discharge of large numbers of cortical neurons and may be caused by drug toxicity or a variety of injuries and diseases. Events are designated as *epileptic seizures* only if they have a chronic pattern of recurrence. Typical *grand mal seizures* last a minute or less and require only protecting the child from physical harm. After a seizure, patients are tired and require the supportive measures included in a standard syncope protocol. The patient's physician should be notified of the event and will generally want to obtain a serum level of the child's anticonvulsant medication.

Status seizures continue unabated for 20 to 30 minutes or repeat without full recovery. This definition is based on the time required until injury to CNS neurons and is impractical for clinical practice. A more operational definition is a seizure that continues for 5 minutes unabated or repeats without complete recovery.[19] Despite brief periods of apnea and cyanosis, most children breathe adequately, provided their airway is maintained.

Benzodiazepines are the preferred agents for terminating seizure activity. If IV access is available, diazepam or lorazepam are the conventional choices. Alternatively, midazolam (0.2 to 0.3 mg/kg) can be administered intramuscularly and generally takes effect in 10 minutes.

DRUG OVERDOSE AND INTERACTIONS

Two common elements appear to be the principal contributing factors in serious drug reactions among children: high drug dosage and drug interactions. In many case reports describing pediatric dental mortality and morbidity involving sedation, general anesthesia, and local anesthesia, the dosage of one drug or multiple agents exceeded the recommended maximum level.[20] The dentist must be aware of the maximum recommended doses of all drugs administered to children and must realize that a reduction in these recommendations is warranted to avoid the toxic effects of additive drug combinations. Drug dosages must also be based on the patient's general health. Fixed doses of drugs based on age are not as accurate as *dosages* based on weight or body surface area. Since local anesthesia is often used alone and in combination with other CNS depressants, the dentist must be familiar with the specific local anesthetic used and dosage recommendations based on body weight.

MONITORING

Constant vigilance and observation are mandatory during dental procedures in pediatric patients. This approach may be as routine as assessment of the efficacy of local anesthesia and verbal assessment of the patient's well-being. It also may be as sophisticated as use of electronic monitors to determine cardiovascular and respiratory parameters during treatment utilizing sedative techniques and during the care of severely compromised patients. The introduction of *pulse oximetry* into clinical practice has resulted in the ability to obtain real-time data, simply and noninvasively, regarding hemoglobin saturation. Pulse oximetry should be used routinely as a primary monitoring device whenever possible during sedation and is an extremely important adjunct in the emergency management of children with respiratory compromise.[2]

EMERGENCY PREPAREDNESS

The goal must be to institute simple resuscitative measures before full cardiopulmonary arrest develops. Regardless of the medical emergency, caring for a child under these circumstances is challenging and terrifying. Those specializing in the treatment of infants and children should consider *pediatric advanced life support* (PALS) and continual review of the AHA guidelines. This training will bolster confidence and enable the practitioner to respond effectively to any pediatric emergency.

Dental office preparedness must be tailored according to the *type of patient* (e.g., young healthy patients in an orthodontic practice versus medically compromised children in a special needs clinic), *practice location* (an urban setting where emergency help is nearby versus a rural location where there may be a significant delay until help arrives), *training* (whether the dentist and staff are capable of performing advanced emergency procedures and protocols), and whether *sedation/anesthesia* is utilized. At a minimum, all pediatric offices should be equipped with oxygen and equipment specific for the patient population of the office and have the capacity to deliver oxygen under positive pressure. Pediatric-size monitoring equipment, IV catheters, and airway adjutants are also necessary. Pediatric drug dosages should be readily assessed and administered as appropriate (Box 2-4).

Box 2-4	Emergency Preparedness Checklist

All staff members have specific assigned duties.

Contingency plans have been made in case of a missing staff member.

All staff members have appropriate training in the management of medical emergencies.

The dental office is equipped with emergency equipment and supplies appropriate for that practice.

Periodic, unannounced emergency drills are conducted at least quarterly.

Appropriate emergency phone numbers are placed prominently by each phone.

Oxygen tanks and oxygen delivery systems are checked regularly. Other emergency respiratory support equipment is present, in good working order, and located according to the emergency plan.

All emergency medications are checked monthly to ensure that expired drugs are replaced.

All emergency supplies are restocked immediately after use.

A specific individual has been assigned to ensure that the above measures have been completed and to document this checklist review.

Modified from Fast TB, Martin MD, Ellis TM: Emergency preparedness: a survey of dental practitioners, *J Am Dent Assoc* 112:449-501, 1986.

SUMMARY

Fortunately, the incidence of cardiopulmonary arrest and major medical emergencies is extremely low during pediatric dental treatment. Because most cardiopulmonary arrests in children result from a progressive deterioration in respiratory function, outcome is critically dependent on rapid diagnosis and evaluation of the adequacy of ventilation and the pediatric airway. Medically compromised children are best treated in facilities equipped for their care and staffed by personnel trained in emergency treatment. Iatrogenic complications can be reduced by strict adherence to recommended pediatric drug and local anesthesia dosages, with a critical eye regarding drug interactions and the additive effects of CNS depressants.

REFERENCES

1. Seidel JS: Emergency medical services and the pediatric patient: are the needs being met? II. Training and equipping emergency medical services providers for pediatric emergencies, *Pediatrics* 78:808-812, 1986.
2. Mayer T: Initial evaluation and management of the injured child. In Mayer T, editor: *Emergency management of pediatric trauma*, Philadelphia, 1985, WB Saunders.
3. American Heart Association: Pediatric airway management. In *Textbook of pediatric life support*, Dallas, 1990, The Association.
4. Heimlich HJ: A life-saving maneuver to prevent food choking, *JAMA* 234:415-417, 1975.
5. Salem MR, Wong AY, Mani M, Sellick BA: Efficacy of cricoid pressure in preventing gastric inflation during bag-mask ventilation in paediatric patients, *Anesthesiology* 40:96-99, 1974.
6. Thompson JE, Bonner B, Lower GM: Pediatric cardiopulmonary arrests in rural populations, *Pediatrics* 86:302-306, 1990.
7. Schoenfeld PS, Baker MD: Management of cardiopulmonary and trauma resuscitation in the pediatric emergency department, *Pediatrics* 91:726-729, 1993.
8. Torphy DE, Minter MG, Thompson BM: Cardiorespiratory arrest and resuscitation of children, *Am J Dis Child* 138:1099-1102, 1984.
9. American Heart Association: Basic life support. In *Textbook of pediatric life support*, Dallas, 1990, The Association.
10. Rossetti VA, Thompson BM, Miller J: Intraosseous infusions: an alternative route of pediatric intravascular access, *Ann Emerg Med* 14:885-887, 1985.
11. American Heart Association: Standards for cardiopulmonary resuscitation and emergency cardiac care, *JAMA* 268:2251-2275, 1992.
12. Zaritsky A: Pediatric resuscitation pharmacology, *Ann Emerg Med* 22:445-455, 1993.
13. Goetting MG, Paradis NA: High-dose epinephrine improves outcome from pediatric cardiac arrest, *Ann Emerg Med* 20:104-105, 1991.
14. Kirk CR, Gibbs JL, Thomas JL: Cardiovascular collapse after verapamil in supraventricular tachycardia, *Arch Dis Child* 62:1265-1266, 1987.
15. Camm AJ, Garrat CJ: Adenosine and supraventricular tachycardia, *N Engl J Med* 325:1621-1629, 1991.

16. Weiss ME, Adkinson NF, Hirshman CA: Evaluation of allergic drug reactions in the postoperative period, *Anesthesiology* 71:483-486, 1989.

17. American Diabetes Association: Report of the Expert Committee on the Diagnosis and Classification of Diabetes Mellitus, *Diabetes Care* 20:1183-1197, 1997.

18. Gunning RR, Garber AJ: Bioactivity of instant glucose: failure of absorption through oral mucosa, JAMA 240:1611-1612, 1978.

19. Lowenstein DH, Alldredge BK: Status epilepticus, N Engl J Med 338:970-976, 1998.

20. Goodson JL, Moore PA: Life-threatening reactions after pedodontic sedation: an assessment of narcotic, local anesthetic and antiemetic drug interaction, J *Am Dent Assoc* 107:239-245, 1983.

21. Kulick RM: Pulse oximetry, *Pediatr Emerg Care* 3:127-135, 1987.

Geriatric Considerations

Noah A. Sandler
James Q. Swift

The average life span in the United States has increased from 47 years in 1900 to 75 years at the end of the twentieth century.[1] As the patient population ages and advances in dental care benefit the older adult, dentists are more likely to be treating older patients. With this comes a responsibility to prepare for potential complications and medical emergencies in the dental office setting.

The aging process can significantly limit a person's physiologic reserves. Symptoms of a disease process that are insignificant in young persons may be serious in older individuals. This chapter reviews major physiologic alterations that occur with aging. Subsequent chapters present specific examples of the management of emergency situations in older patients.

PHYSIOLOGY AND IMPACT OF PROGRESSIVE DISEASE IN THE OLDER ADULT

All age groups view visits to the dentist as high-stress events. Physiologic and pathologic organ changes can predispose older adults to medical emergencies during times of physiologic and psychologic stress. Recent research suggests that advanced age itself only minimally increases the risk for medical and dental procedures.[2] Systemic diseases, such as atherosclerosis, hypertension, and congestive heart failure, are more prevalent in older adults.[3,4] Progressively debilitating medical conditions likely play the greatest role in the risk of developing an acute medical emergency during an office visit.[3,4] The aging process, however, affects all organ systems. Aging can negatively impact patients' response to stress because of their diminished reserve.[2] Of greatest concern are the effects of aging and the insufficient response to stress within the cardiovascular, pulmonary, renal, he-

patic, and neurologic systems. Older adults also are more likely to be taking pharmacologic agents than younger adults. Additional concerns relate to the effects of aging on the ability to metabolize drugs.

Cardiovascular System

Decreased elasticity of the aorta and large vessels occurs with aging. Changes in elasticity are related to decreased elastin in the layers of the vessel wall (intima, media, and adventitia). Eventually, fragmentation of the elastic lamina occurs, with decreased elastic recoil of the vessel. These changes in elasticity partially account for an increased systolic blood pressure present in the elderly; the decreased distensibility of these vessels results in greater pressure needed to maintain adequate flow.[2]

Hypertension means that the heart must pump against an increased pressure load. *Atherosclerosis*, characterized by the deposition of fatty deposits on blood vessel walls, is typically more advanced in older individuals. Atherosclerosis contributes to narrowing of blood vessels with concomitant hypertension. Vasculature changes with higher pressures result in compensatory hypertrophy of the heart muscle.[2,5] Baseline cardiac output is maintained, but the heart responds less to catecholamine (epinephrine, norepinephrine) stimulation during stress.[6] The hypertrophied heart muscle has a decreased force of contraction and a decreased maximal heart rate in response to stress.[7] There is more dependence on the volume of blood returning to the heart to regulate the strength of contraction.[8] These individuals are therefore more susceptible to dehydration and volume depletion.[2,8]

When atherosclerosis occurs in the coronary arteries, decreased blood flow, or *ischemia*, may result. Patients with coronary ischemia may present acutely with angina pectoris (chest pain), which can lead to myocardial infarction (MI, heart tissue death). Atherosclerosis and aging can affect the heart valve leaflets, producing degeneration and calcification. The aortic valve is especially susceptible to these changes. Clinical signs of significant valvular stenosis include syncope (fainting), angina pectoris (chest pain), and dyspnea (labored breathing).[9]

Cardiac conditions, such as infarction or cardiomyopathy (dilated heart), are more common in the older adult. These conditions may ultimately lead to congestive heart failure (pump failure) and resultant pulmonary edema (fluid in the lung) or pleural effusion (fluid in the pleural space surrounding the lung). *Dyspnea*, or shortness of breath, is the most common initial presentation in most patients with heart failure. This symptom typically progresses to orthopnea (difficulty assuming a supine position), as well as paroxysmal nocturnal dyspnea (shortness of breath at night when a supine position is assumed). In severe cases, pulmonary edema may present with shortness of breath accompanied by a pink, frothy sputum in the mouth or gurgling, noisy breathing.[10]

Cardiac dysrhythmias (abnormal electrical conduction of the heart beat) are more common in persons 60 to 85 years old. The dysrhythmias result from cardiac disease in the atria or ventricles. Typically, patients are asymptomatic.[11] A common dysrhythmia in elderly patients is *atrial fibrillation*, found in 4% of people older than 60 in the Framingham Study. Patients with chronic atrial fibrillation had almost twice the mortality as patients without atrial fibrillation.[12] The primary concern in patients with atrial fibrillation is the risk of systemic *embolization* (a circulating blood clot formation) with resultant stroke. Thyroid disease, alcohol intoxication, hypoxia, drugs, acute MI, or acute stresses, such as a visit to the dental office, may precipitate atrial fibrillation. Treatment of acute atrial fibrillation consists of cardioversion by either direct-current countershock or medication.[13]

Sick sinus syndrome is a cardiac dysrhythmia characterized by abnormal sinus node pulse formation and abnormal conduction from the sinus node, primarily affecting older individuals.[14] The sinus node is located in the right atrium and is the normal initiation point of the electrical signal controlling contraction of the heart. Patients with sick sinus syndrome may have a slow heartbeat (bradycardia), an alternating fast and slow heartbeat (tachycardia-bradycardia), or pauses in their heartbeat (sinus arrest). Patients may

complain of fatigue, palpitations, lightheadedness, or syncope (50% of patients with sick sinus syndrome). Sick sinus syndrome may also result in sudden death.[14] Often these patients require medical therapy or cardiac pacing.

Ventricular dysrhythmias are also more common in elderly patients, but most are asymptomatic *premature ventricular complexes* (PVCs). In the presence of heart disease, two or more PVCs are associated with an increased mortality, as are complex ventricular dysrhythmias.[13] Other irregular heart rhythms in the older adult include atrioventricular node conduction disturbances and heart block (block of normal electrical conduction).[13,15]

Pulmonary System

Age-related changes in pulmonary function in older patients result from changes in the lung itself and surrounding structures associated with proper ventilation. The elasticity of the lung decreases with advancing age. Increased distensibility of the alveoli and small airways may result in the partial collapse of these structures. This results in a loss of alveolar surface area and uneven distribution of air exchange in the lungs.[7,16] Changes in associated ventilatory structures include alterations in the chest wall (e.g., calcification of costal cartilages), increased anteroposterior chest diameter, and reduced rib excursions secondary to decreased intervertebral spaces.[2,16] These factors place the older patient at an increased risk for hypoxia, especially during sedation procedures.

Pneumonia is a common pulmonary condition found in older patients. Difficulty with coughing, chronic aspiration, and immunocompromise predispose patients to developing secondary infection and pneumonia. High fevers, tachycardia (fast heart rate), hypotension (low blood pressure), tachypnea (rapid rate of respiration), dehydration, or mental status changes may indicate a more serious systemic infection. Immediate stabilization and referral to an emergency department is warranted for fluid resuscitation and antibiotics.[10]

Asthma and chronic obstructive pulmonary disease (COPD, or emphysema) are conditions that affect the terminal bronchi and bronchioles. Because of its chronic, progressive nature, COPD is a common diagnosis in elderly patients. A long-standing history of tobacco use increases the risk for COPD. Asthma is an increasingly recognized diagnosis and affects an estimated 6% to 8% of older individuals. Wheezing is the most common symptom, although difficulty breathing or coughing may be presenting symptoms. Asthma in the newly diagnosed older patient may be more severe than in younger patients, with marked ventilatory impairment, greater steroid dependency, and high mortality. [17] Asthma is often underdiagnosed since older individuals often do not report respiratory disability.

Precipitants of asthma in older individuals include the common environmental sources seen in younger patients, such as upper respiratory tract infection, tobacco smoke, changes in temperature or humidity, or esophageal reflux. In addition, aspirin, nonsteroidal antiinflammatory drugs (NSAIDs), and beta-adrenergic blockers (including topical ophthalmologic solutions) can induce attacks. [17]

Pulmonary embolism is characterized by infarction or death of a region of lung tissue caused by blockage of the blood supply due to the presence of a thrombus (a blood clot). Typically this blood clot forms in the deep veins of the legs as a *deep venous thrombosis* (DVT). The clot dislodges, then becomes trapped in the lungs. Older persons, particularly those who lead a sedentary lifestyle, are particularly susceptible to DVTs and subsequent pulmonary embolism. [10]

Additional organ changes that can affect pulmonary function related to dental treatment in older adults include esophageal motor dysfunction, which can result in abnormal motility and increased risk of aspiration. [18] The risk of aspiration is greater in older individuals because of decreased gastric emptying time and diminished protective reflexes. [7]

Renal System

Kidney mass diminishes with advanced age and may compromise normal kidney function. [2] This affects the kidney's ability to retain sodium and water during dehydration. The clearance of medications excreted primarily by the kidneys is also diminished. [19] Commonly prescribed drugs in dentistry, including antibiotics, local anesthetics, and analgesics, may therefore require dose modifications in elderly patients. The long-term effects of chronic progressive disease (e.g., hypertension, diabetes mellitus) can affect kidney function, also requiring dose alteration of medications primarily excreted by the kidneys.

Hepatic System

Blood flow to the liver and liver mass decrease with aging, and changes occur in microsomal en-

zymes. These factors result in altered drug metabolism in older individuals. [20,21] Long-standing alcohol abuse or chronic hepatitis can cause liver damage which may not be detected until later in life. Most drugs are metabolized in the liver, so all elderly patients should be questioned about previous potential hepatotoxic exposures. Referral for further work-up is indicated with possible liver function compromise.

Neurologic System

Some brain atrophy occurs with aging, but significant atrophy with cognitive dysfunction may be secondary to dementia caused by Alzheimer's disease, stroke, or multiple brain infarcts, frequently related to long-standing hypertension. It is important to distinguish gradual changes in cognition associated with progressive dementia from the more acute causes of mental decline characteristic of delirium. [22]

Dementia is defined as a chronic organic brain syndrome usually lasting more than 1 year. It is characterized by memory loss and impaired cognitive function. *Delirium*, in contrast, is an acute mental syndrome caused by an identifiable medical factor. It is characterized by an attention deficit, rambling or incoherent speech, a fluctuating course, and impaired cognition. [22]

Delirious patients typically exhibit attention deficits, disorganized cognition, delusions, perceptual abnormalities, and hyperactivity. Some patients with delirium, however, will exhibit hypoactivity with slowed behavior and speech. Initial consideration should be given to serious cardiac and pulmonary disease, including MI, dysrhythmias, and pulmonary embolism. Common, easily correctable causes of delirium include hypoglycemia, urinary tract infection, and dehydration with fluid and electrolyte abnormalities. [22,23]

PHARMACOLOGIC EFFECTS

Older patients are more likely to be using multiple medications. [1,24-26] In one study, drug use increased fourfold in patients over 80 compared with those 18 to 33 years of age. Older persons are more likely to take multiple medications, including one or more cardiovascular drugs. The potential for significant drug interactions and side effects is increased. Consideration of drug interactions among medications commonly used in dentistry is essential. [26]

Orthostatic hypotension occurs when the body is unable to adjust to changes to a more upright

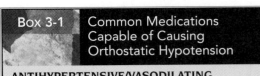

Box 3-1 Common Medications Capable of Causing Orthostatic Hypotension

ANTIHYPERTENSIVE/VASODILATING AGENTS
ACE inhibitors
Calcium channel blockers
Nitroglycerin-based products
Other vasodilating antihypertensives (e.g., hydralazine)

DRUGS AFFECTING AUTONOMIC FUNCTION
Sympatholytic antihypertensives (e.g., β-blockers)
Antianxiety drugs (e.g., benzodiazepines)
Tricyclic antidepressants
MAO inhibitors
Levodopa (drug used to treat Parkinson's disease)
Cholinergic agents

ACE, Angiotensin-converting enzyme.

position. With hypotension, patients experience lightheadedness, weakness, nausea, or syncope with postural changes. The incidence is 5% to 20% in older patients. Orthostatic hypotension may be idiopathic or secondary to a variety of medications (Box 3-1). Medication use is the most frequent cause of orthostatic hypotension in elderly patients and can occur even with therapeutic doses.[27]

Older adults demonstrate an increased sensitivity to drugs with central nervous system actions, including local anesthetics. Dosages of all local anesthetics should be carefully monitored to avoid toxicity.[21]

Pharmacokinetics

Drug metabolism relates to the dose administered and the concentration at the site of action,[21,28] which depends on the drug's absorption, distribution, metabolism, and elimination of the drug.

Absorption from the gastrointestinal tract is usually not affected by aging. Changes in body weight, total body water, muscle mass, and body fat affect drug distribution and ultimately the dose and drug effects. Body weight increases in both men and women as they age, and muscle mass decreases. Plasma volume is often also reduced, resulting in a contracted blood volume. These factors result in higher concentrations and exaggerated actions of many medications. The increased relative body fat in elderly patients re-

sults in a reservoir for lipid-soluble drugs, with slow elimination and prolonged effects.[21]

Aging is also associated with a decrease in plasma proteins. These proteins bind most drugs to varying degrees. The dosages of many medications need to be adjusted in older patients secondary to decreased protein binding.[21]

Pharmacodynamics

Changes in receptors may decrease drug effects in older patients, but most effects are pharmacokinetic rather than pharmacodynamic in older patients.[21,28]

PSYCHOLOGY OF AGING

Many physical diseases associated with aging can be more difficult to manage because of psychosocial issues. Some conditions, such as nutritional disturbances, may be a direct consequence of psychologic conditions (e.g., depression or dementia) seen more often in older patients.[24] Mental diseases will likely increase as people live longer. It is important to consider the effects of these disease processes and the side effects of medications administered for these conditions to prevent medical mishaps in the dental office.

SUMMARY

Changes that accompany aging diminish the physiologic reserve.[29] Although older persons may cope with activities of daily living, the increased stress of a dental appointment may cause them to decompensate. The result may be an emergency situation in the office setting. These problems can be managed best by not placing the patient in compromised situations. Optimal care of the aging patient requires careful review of the medical history and modification of dental management in consultation with the patient's primary physician.

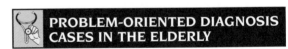

PROBLEM-ORIENTED DIAGNOSIS CASES IN THE ELDERLY

SYNCOPE
Situation

An 83-year-old patient in your waiting room suddenly stands, states she is dizzy, then falls to the ground unconscious. Review of her past medical history reveals hypertension. She is presently taking a calcium channel blocker, nifedipine and a diuretic, hydrochlorothiazide.

On examination, she is unresponsive to your voice or vigorous shaking; she is breathing spontaneously at a rate of 16 breaths per minute, she has a regular heart rate of 72 beats per minute, but her blood pressure is somewhat low at 98/65.

Recognition and Assessment

Patients experiencing syncope will be unconscious and unresponsive to external stimuli for seconds to minutes. During this time the victim should be breathing unlabored and spontaneously.

Initial Intervention

The degree of responsiveness should be assessed by gently shaking the person. Tight clothing should be loosened, and the patient should be placed in a supine position (laying on the back). In some cases it may be beneficial to raise the legs of the individual, especially for vasovagal syncope (see following discussion). Evaluating the "ABCs" (Airway, Breathing and Circulation) should routinely be performed on any patient experiencing a syncopal episode, especially older patients. Frequent blood pressure, pulse, and respiration should be checked as additional help is requested. Oxygen should be administered through a nasal hood, nasal cannula, or face mask. Local emergency personnel (i.e., paramedic unit, fire department, or ambulance) should be contacted in all cases of syncope in elderly patients.

Differential Diagnosis

Syncope (or fainting) represents a symptom of underlying pathology of the cardiac, neurologic, and pulmonary systems. Despite comprehensive evaluation, the source of syncope remains obscure in 30% to 50% of cases.[27] The etiology of syncope in the older patient is different than in younger patients. Vasovagal syncope is the most common cause of syncope in younger patients, especially in stressful situations such as a visit to the dental office. In the elderly, this form of syncope accounts for only 1% to 5% of the cases of syncope.[30,31]

Cardiac causes of syncope in elderly patients include acute with MI pump failure, valvular disease (especially progressive aortic stenosis), and symptomatic dysrhythmias (e.g.,

atrial fibrillation, sick sinus syndrome, or ventricular dysrhythmias).[9] Less common cardiac causes of syncope include congestive heart failure or the side effects of cardiac medications.[27] Because conditions can have severe consequences, all episodes of syncope in the elderly patient should be treated as cardiac related until proven otherwise.

Since this elderly patient experienced syncope after changing to a more upright position, orthostatic hypotension is high in the differential diagnosis. She was also taking two medications that could cause vascular or intravascular volume changes contributing to orthostatic hypotension (see earlier discussion). Medication use is the most frequent cause of orthostatic hypotension in the elderly, even if the dose of medication is in the therapeutic range.[27]

Patients with COPD and a sustained cough can develop syncope secondary to increased intrathoracic pressure with diminished venous return and reflex vasodilation.[27] Other causes of syncope more common in the older individual are often related to urination, defecation, and ingestion of a meal (postprandial syncope), which are related to parasympathetic nerve discharge.[27]

Secondary Intervention

Older patient experiencing syncope should be treated as if they are having a significant cardiac event, specifically an acute MI until tests can rule this out.

The pharmacologic management of MI in older patients is similar to that for younger patients, with nitroglycerin given early. If the patient takes sublingual nitroglycerin, the usual dose may be administered in the prehospital period. Older individuals and especially those patients with a recent episode of syncope should be carefully monitored for hypotension, since excessive reduction in arterial pressure may result in larger infarcts.[13,32] Aspirin is beneficial in the acute phase of MI by inhibiting platelet aggregation, and baby aspirin should be considered in patients with suspected MI.[33]

Thrombolytic agents help dissolve the blockage that causes MI. In the past, these agents were withheld in elderly persons because of their increased risk of stroke. Recent studies, however, suggest a reduction in mortality when thrombolytic agents were used, with greater benefit in older than younger patients without a significant risk of strokes.[13,34] These agents should be considered early in the management of patients with acute MI.

Reassessment

Potential causes for syncope should be ruled out, including MI, heart failure, dysrhythmias, or COPD with a chronic cough, and medications that may cause orthostatic hypotension. Future syncope episodes may be prevented by eliminating predisposing factors in older patients.

Disposition

The older patient should be referred for further evaluation even if the episode is short-lived or the patient demonstrates complete recovery.

CONFUSED PATIENT

Situation

A 78-year-old man in a nursing home appears agitated when you approach him. On further questioning, he says it is 1963, he is mayor of New York City, and he is trying to get back to his office. You question his primary nurse, who is surprised because the patient appeared normal earlier that morning.

Recognition and Assessment

You note that this patient has been oriented to self and surroundings on previous visits with no signs of cognitive impairment.

Initial Intervention

For acute onset of altered mental status, therapy should be directed at identifying life-threatening or easily treatable conditions. Emergency medical services or the nursing home physician should be contacted. Vital signs are monitored and ABCs are maintained until the arrival of support personnel. Oxygen should be administered because hypoxia is a potential cause of confusion.

Differential Diagnosis

As discussed earlier, the time course of impaired mental capacity is important in assessing older patients. For patients who may have cognitive impairments, relatives or close acquaintances should be questioned to determine the present mental status of the patient. Any questions regarding recent mental status changes should be referred to the patient's primary physician, who can assess for possible delirium and coordinate any nursing home treatment.

Secondary Intervention

The responding team should obtain an electrocardiogram (ECG) and treat the patient empirically if signs of an acute MI are present. A finger-stick (glucose) reading, blood chemistry, and complete blood count can identify common, easily treatable causes of delirium (i.e., hypoglycemia, dehydration, electrolyte disturbances). Any electrolyte disturbance or hypoglycemia should be corrected. Antibiotic therapy and fluids should be administered to treat underlying infection with dehydration.

Disposition

The nursing home patient with changes in mental status should be considered for transfer to a more acute setting for evaluation and treatment.

DYSPNEA

Situation

A 76-year-old man having a routine scaling procedure states that he is having difficulty "catching his breath" as you place him in a flat position in the dental chair. In the last week he has experienced this same problem at home and has used an extra pillow at night to sleep. His breathing difficulty continues, and toward the end of the appointment, he sits forward to "get enough air." He is breathing very fast (tachypnea) at a rate of 23 breaths per minute. He has had three heart attacks and underwent heart surgery 6 years earlier.

Initial Intervention

Ensure that the patient is maintaining a patent airway and that no foreign bodies remain in the mouth or pharynx. All tight clothing (e.g., neckties, collar buttons) should be loosened or removed. Allow the patient to posture in a position where breathing is most comfortable. Administration of oxygen via a face mask, if available, or nasal hood is warranted. Emergency services should be contacted early and preparations made if the patient requires rescue breathing, as per basic life support protocols.

Differential Diagnosis

Dyspnea is "disordered breathing," typically associated with uncomfortable, difficult, or labored breathing. Dyspnea describes a physical finding, not a diagnosis. It is not a normal consequence of aging; dyspnea usually results from respiratory or cardiovascular disease. Many medical conditions may present with dyspnea and may be identified by the history and physical examination.[35]

Cardiac conditions, such as MI or cardiomyopathy, may lead to pump failure and fluid in the lung or pleural space, which can cause difficulties with oxygen exchange, especially when the patient assumes a supine position.[10] Pulmonary embolism, pneumonia, and bronchitis secondary to COPD also may cause dyspnea. Audible wheezing should suggest asthma.

Secondary Intervention

Since this patient has signs of pulmonary edema, therapy is directed at reducing the fluid load to the failing heart (preload) so that less fluid is pumped more efficiently. Pharmacologic therapy would include the diuretic furosemide (Lasix), nitroglycerin, and morphine. Some medications given to the patient with acute pulmonary edema or pleural effusions also reduce the force that the heart must pump against (afterload) by causing peripheral blood vessels to vasodilate. Recommended agents include nitroprusside and hydralazine.[10]

If symptoms do not resolve or improve, further work-up includes ruling out pulmonary embolism (ventilation/perfusion scan of lungs, angiography of pulmonary vasculature), pneumonia (decreased breath sounds in lung on physical examination, chest x-ray film), or asthma (wheezing on expiration, response to bronchodilators).

Reassessment

The patient's respiratory rate, breathing effort, heart rate, and blood pressure are monitored. If signs of respiratory failure develop, rescue breathing should be initiated or an airway established.

Disposition

Any patient with labored breathing should be immediately taken to an emergency department for further evaluation.

CHRONIC OBSTRUCTIVE PULMONARY DISEASE

Situation

A 62-year-old man with a history of COPD and cigarette smoking suddenly becomes short of breath in your waiting room. He cannot "catch his breath" and is breathing very fast.

Initial Intervention

A common question is whether oxygen can be administered safely to the patient with COPD, who frequently has a high resting level of carbon dioxide (CO_2) in the bloodstream. The chemoreceptors that regulate respiration do not respond to changes in the CO_2 concentration, however, but to the level of oxygen in the blood (oxygen-dependent drive). Administration of oxygen may increase the oxygen level in the blood and theoretically decrease the rate and depth of respiration, possibly leading to hypoxia. Supplemental oxygen should *never* be withheld in the patient with COPD because hypoxia can predispose the patient to cardiac decompensation. Oxygen should be administered cautiously, however, at low flow rates (1 to 2 L/min by nasal hood or nasal cannula), and the patient should be monitored for worsening of COPD.[10]

Differential Diagnosis

In addition to the conditions listed previously for dyspnea, the differential diagnosis includes spontaneous pneumothorax. A *pneumothorax* is caused by the introduction of air into the pleural space, which can result in total or partial collapse of the adjacent lung. Patients with COPD are particularly at risk for the development of a pneumothorax, since emphysematous changes in the lung may result in the formation of "blebs" in the lung surface that may rupture spontaneously.

Secondary Intervention

Bronchodilators are typically administered to reduce the muscle spasm of the small airways. Theophylline and beta2-selective agents are also often used. A chest x-ray film may rule out pneumothorax with resultant lung collapse. Antibiotics may be initiated as well, since dyspnea in a patient with COPD is frequently related to bronchitis or infection of the small airways.[10]

Reassessment

Respiratory rate and "work of breathing" are monitored. If the patient has labored breathing, consideration should be given to possibly assisting the patient through assisted ventilation. Endotracheal tube placement should be considered.

Disposition

Even patients with brief attacks treated by bronchodilators should be referred to their physician for further evaluation.

REFERENCES

1. Levy SM, Baker KA, Semla TP, et al: Use of medications with dental significance by a non-institutionalized elderly population, *Gerodontics* 4:119-125, 1988.
2. Evers MB, Townsend CM Jr, Thompson JC: Organ physiology of aging, *Surg Clin North Am* 74(1): 23-39, 1994.
3. Goldman L, Caldera D, Southwick F, et al: Cardiac risk, factors and complications in non-cardiac surgery, *Medicine* 57: 357-370, 1978.
4. Linn B, Linn M, Wallen N: Evaluation of results of surgical procedures in the elderly, *Ann Surg* 195:90-96, 1982.
5. Arora RR, Machac J, Goldman ME, et al.: Atrial kinetics and left ventricular diastolic filling in the healthy elderly. *J Am Coll Cardiol* 9: 1255-1260, 1987.
6. Guarnieri T, Filburn CR, Zitnik G, et al: Contractile and biochemical correlates of beta-adrenergic stimulation of the aged heart, *Am J Physiol* 239: H501-508, 1980.
7. Katz SM, Fagraeus L: Anesthetic considerations in geriatric patients, *Clin Geriatr Med* 6(3):499-510, 1990.
8. Josephson RA, Lakatta EG: Cardiovascular changes in the elderly. In Kattic MR, editor: *Geriatric surgery*, Baltimore, 1990, Urban and Schwarzenberg.
9. Bayer AJ, Chadha JS, Faring RR, et al: Changing presentation of myocardial infarction with increasing old age, *J Am Geriatr Soc* 34(4):263-266, 1986.
10. Runge JW, Schafermeyer RW: Respiratory emergencies, *Prim Care* 13(1):177-192, 1986.
11. Fleg JL, Kennedy HL: Cardiac arrhythmias in a healthy elderly population: detection by 24-hour ambulatory electrocardiology, *Chest* 81: 302-307, 1982.
12. Kannel WB, Abbott RD, Savage DP, et al: Epidemiologic features of chronic atrial fibrillation: the Framingham Study, *N Engl J Med* 306:1018-1022, 1982.

13. Duncan AK, Vittone J, Fleming KC, et al: Cardiovascular disease in elderly patients, *Mayo Clin Proceed* 71(2):184-196, 1996.
14. Rodriguez RD, Schoken DP: Update on sick sinus syndrome, a cardiac disorder of aging, *Geriatrics* 45:26-30, 33-36, 1990.
15. Olsky M, Murray J: Dizziness and fainting in the elderly, *Emerg Med Clin North Am* 8(2):295-307, 1990.
16. Tockman MS: Aging of the respiratory system. In Kattic MR, editor: *Geriatric surgery*, Baltimore, 1990, Urban and Schwarzenburg.
17. Luce PJ: Asthma in the elderly, *Br J Hosp Med* 55(3):118-120, 1996.
18. Pelemans W, Vantrappen G: Oesophageal disease in the elderly, *Clin Gastroenerol* 14:635-656, 1985.
19. Epstein M: Effects of aging on the kidney, *J Pathol* 38:168-172, 1979.
20. Koruda MJ, Sheldon GF: Surgery in the aged, *Adv Surg* 24:293-331, 1991.
21. Muravchick S: Anesthesia for the elderly. In Miller RD, editor: *Anesthesia*, ed 5, Philadelphia, 2000, Churchill Livingstone.
22. Pousada L: Common neurologic emergencies in the elderly population, *Clin Ger Med* 9(3):577-590, 1993.
23. Johnson JC: Delirium in the elderly, *Emerg Med Clin North Am* 8(2):255-265, 1990.
24. Jeste DV: Psychiatry of old age is coming of age, *Am J Psych* 154(10):1356-1358, 1997.
25. Baker KA, Levy SM, Chrischilles EA: Medications with dental significance: usage in a nursing home population, *Spec Care Dentist* 11:19-25, 1991.
26. Miller CS, Kaplan AL, Guest GF, et al: Documenting medication use in adult dental patients: 1987-1991, *J Am Dent Assoc* 123:41-48, 1992.
27. Bonema JD, Maddens ME: Syncope in elderly patients: why their risk is higher, *Postgrad Med* 91(1):129-144, 1992.
28. McLeskey CH: Anesthesia for the geriatric patient. In Barash PG, Cullen BF, Stoetling RK, editors: *Clinical anesthesia*, ed 2, Philadelphia, 1992, Lippincott.
29. Buxbaum JL, Schwartz AJ: Perianesthetic considerations for the elderly patient, *Surg Clin North Am* 74(1):41-58, 1994.
30. Lipsitz LA, Wei JY, Rowe JW: Syncope in an elderly, institutionalized population: prevalence, incidence and associated risk, *Q J Med* 55:45-54, 1985.
31. Kapoor W, Snustad D, Peterson J, et al: Syncope in the elderly, *Am J Med* 80(3):419-428, 1986.
32. Jugdutt BI: Myocardial salvage by intravenous nitroglycerin in conscious dogs: loss of beneficial effect with marked nitroglycerin induced hypotension, *Circulation* 68:673-684, 1983.
33. Collins R, Peto R, Baisent C, et al: Drug therapy: aspirin, heparin, and fibrinolytic therapy in suspected acute myocardial infarction, *N Eng J Med* 366(12):847-860, 1997.
34. Forman DE, Bernal JL, Wei JY: Management of acute myocardial infarction in the very elderly, *Am J Med* 93:315-326, 1992.
35. Silvestri GA, Mahler DA: Evaluation of dyspnea in the elderly patient, *Clin Chest Med* 14(3):393-404, 1993.

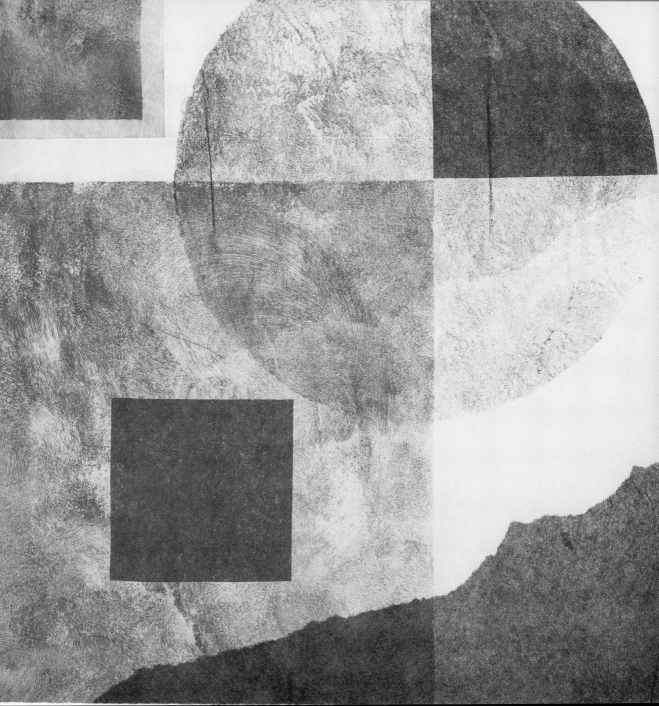

II

Problem-Based Assessment

Wheezing

Daniel McNally

Wheezes are high-pitched, continuous sounds. Because they are not part of the normal breath sounds heard on the chest examination, wheezes are termed *adventitious sounds*. These adventitious sounds also include *rhonchi*, which are low-pitched, continuous sounds, and *crackles*, which are discontinuous bursts of sound. Rhonchi are associated with secretions and crackles with alveolar filling. Wheezes are strongly associated with decreased airflow, however, and the examiner usually concludes that an obstruction is present.

Wheezes are both an objective finding and a subjective report. Many patients will describe high-pitched noisy breathing, especially when it is a response to the common environmental triggers of their disease. A description by a patient (or a parent) of wheezing that "comes and goes" in response to certain triggers can be accepted as *asthma*, at least as a starting point.

AIRWAY PHYSIOLOGY

Understanding why wheezes occur requires a review of how and where resistance occurs in the airways. The airways can be divided into intrathoracic and extrathoracic. The *intrathoracic airways* are within the chest space and are surrounded by the interstitium or the mediastinum. The pressure surrounding the intrathoracic airways is that of the pleural space. The *extrathoracic airways* are in the neck and are surrounded by tissues that are at ambient or room pressure. This difference in airways explains why most wheezing is in expiration and involves the intrathoracic airways, whereas high-pitched sounds in inspiration typically involve obstruction to flow in the extrathoracic airways.

Airways are not perfect cylinders. They contain varying amounts of cartilage so that the largest airways have the greatest amount of structural support, and the smaller airways have lesser amounts of structural support. The airways become smaller moving toward the periphery of the lung, but because the number of airways increases, the total cross-sectional area increases as well. Airways are held open by the pressure differences across their walls and by the structural support provided by the cartilage and surrounding lung. Thus the size of an airway is a function of (1) the lung volume at that point in inspiration and (2) the amount of intrathoracic pressure present around that airway compared with the pressure within the airway itself.

During a moderate or forceful exhalation, a person creates positive intrathoracic pressure by using the abdominal muscles to force the diaphragm upward. This creates pressure in the alveoli, and this gradient of pressure from the alveoli through the bronchi to the mouth creates the flow of air in exhalation. Depending on the pressures involved and the size of the airways, however, there is usually a point where the intrathoracic pressure surrounding an airway equals the pressure within the airway. At this *equal-pressure point* the airway itself may be narrowed by compression, made possible by the lack of full support from surrounding cartilage. For breaths of moderate or greater effort, this is the point of resistance that limits airflow in expiration. Any effort to increase the force generated by the abdominal muscles in order to increase airflow from alveoli is unsuccessful because that force is also applied to the airways at the equal-pressure points. This added resistance continues to narrow the airways and limits airflow.

PATHOPHYSIOLOGY OF AIRWAY OBSTRUCTION

Equal-pressure points and airway resistance are part of normal physiology. However, when a pathologic process narrows an airway or causes the loss of a supporting structure that helps to keep the airway open, resistance may be increased and airflow limited. Decreased airflow is accompanied by vibrations in the bronchial wall, which is either narrowed or inadequately supported. These vibrations give rise to wheezing.

In *decreased inspiratory flow* the site of obstruction usually changes to the extrathoracic airways. On inspiration, when the intrathoracic pressure surrounding the airways within the chest is negative, the airways are held open and flow is generally less limited. This may not be true in more severe cases where airway edema or secretions have narrowed the airway consistently in both inspiration and expiration; these patients may have both inspiratory and expiratory wheezing. Severe inspiratory wheezing alone, however, called *stridor*, usually reflects narrowing or loss of a supporting structure around the extrathoracic airways. During inspiration the negative pressure within the extrathoracic airways is surrounded by ambient room pressure outside. Coupled with a loss of support or marked intrinsic narrowing, this pressure can cause enough added resistance to create airflow obstruction.

In the more common process of intrathoracic airway obstruction, with relatively unimpaired inspiration, *decreased expiratory flow* leads to trapping of air. Air trapping causes overexpansion of some lung units and leads to ventilation/perfusion ($\dot{V}/\dot{Q}$) mismatch. These events are often seen as a secondary process compared with the high work of breathing of an obstructive airway. The hypoxemia resulting from air trapping and $\dot{V}/\dot{Q}$ mismatch may be very important, however, especially when coupled with inflammatory processes (e.g., poor secretion clearing, increased mucus formation) that also alter regional lung ventilation.

The bronchial tubes are surrounded by smooth muscle, with innervation from the parasympathetic and sympathetic pathways. The parasympathetic system, which predominates in number of nerve endings, causes *bronchoconstriction*, whereas the sympathetic system produces *bronchodilation* by relaxing the smooth muscle. This nerve supply is usually seen as causing disease and/or providing therapeutic options. The ability to adjust airflow to lung regions by changes in bronchial smooth motor tone, however, is part of the lung's natural autoregulating ability and is necessary for optimum gas transfer.

Defense Mechanisms

The mechanism for increased airway obstruction in disease states results largely from the body's efforts at airway defense. The most peripheral portions of the bronchial system and the alveolar gas exchanging surfaces beyond are largely defended by *alveolar macrophages*. These nonspecific phagocytes can clear foreign or unwanted materials and can signal specific immune defenses to activate both cell-mediated defenses through lymphocytes and humoral defenses through antibody production. In turn, these specific immune defenses release other cytokines, which serve to attract and activate alveolar macrophages and amplify the alveolar and the most distal airway defense.

This two-part defense mechanism, however, has a price. Many cytokines produced by or directed at cells in the bronchial system also produce other inflammatory changes, such as airway edema or increased smooth muscle constriction, leading to more airway obstruction. The inflammatory mediators also change airway permeability; inhaled substances that normally do not elicit a response can now reach the smooth muscle underlying the mucosal surfaces and cause bronchoconstriction.

Mucus

For much of the medium-sized bronchial tree the mucociliary escalator is the principal defense. Mucus is produced both in glands and by individual mucus-producing cells at the bronchial surface. Mucus lies in small islands on top of a more fluid phase that coats the bronchial surfaces. *Cilia*, with a primitive locomotor system of dynein-based microtubules that allows coordinated movement, lie in this fluid phase just below the islands of mucus. In a pattern described as a "field of wheat moving in the wind," the cilia extend upward and move the islands of mucus proximally, back toward the throat, then relax and retreat through the fluid phase until they begin another movement cycle. This repetitive movement brings the islands of mucus up through the tracheobronchial tree. Material inspired and caught on the mucus or debris from airway inflammation will gradually rise in the tracheobronchial escalator. The velocity of mucus flow varies in different airways, ranging from less than 1 millimeter per minute (mm/min) up to 12 mm/min, with the greater velocities in the larger airways.[1]

Cough

When mucus reaches the most proximal and largest airways, the mechanism of cough takes over. At this point the advantage of a flexible and incompletely supported airway becomes clearer.

The lack of cartilage in the posterior quarter of the large airways allows that portion to bulge inward, narrowing the airway and thus increasing the velocity of flow at that point. A cough requires (1) an inspiratory effort, (2) closure of the glottic mechanism, (3) creation of positive intraabdominal pressure, and (4) upward force on the diaphragm causing positive intrathoracic pressure. This is followed by an explosive opening of the glottic mechanism, allowing abrupt and forceful flow of air through narrowed airways, raising and clearing the confluent islands of mucus brought up by the mucociliary escalator.

An individual's cough may fail for a number of reasons, including inability to generate increased abdominal pressure, lack of coordination in inspiratory effort and abdominal forces, and poor closure of the glottic mechanism while increased intrathoracic pressure is generated. Although these mechanisms can occur, ordinary airflow limitation from edematous or narrowed airways can produce the same result with decreased flow and an ineffective cough.

Hyperreactivity Response

In addition to the narrowing of airways through edema, secretions, and smooth muscle constriction, most mechanisms that cause airflow obstruction also bring a dynamic quality of hyperreactivity to these airways. This increased reactivity has many possible triggers but is most easily viewed in terms of a nonspecific stimulus, such as cold air. Almost all individuals with asthma and many with airflow-obstructing diseases have a response to breathing very cold air, measurable in terms of bronchial smooth muscle constriction and airflow limitation, that is not seen in normal individuals. This increased responsiveness does not depend on an *allergic* mechanism, even though it often occurs in individuals who have asthma on an allergic basis. The reaction is also not purely an *irritant* phenomenon; although they can trigger it in susceptible individuals, irritants are not necessary to the reaction's cause or demonstration. An inflammatory response in the airways and hyperreactivity of those airways to both *specific* immune triggers (e.g., irritants) and *nonspecific* triggers (e.g., cold air, exercise) are the hallmarks of asthma.

Mild hyperreactivity occurs much more often than might be expected. After a typical upper airway viral infection, many individuals will show reactivity if rigorously tested for several weeks. They may even have symptoms of mild cough or wheezing brought about by normally inoffensive stimuli.

The cause of hyperreactivity is probably multifactorial. Changes in the number of smooth muscle sympathetic and parasympathetic receptors may be a factor, although asthma is now known to have many causes. The ability to examine the airway during asthma attacks and to note the changes in cell-to-cell junctions and wholesale sloughing of ciliated epithelial cells clearly demonstrates the altered permeability and defenses of this surface. Coupled with the presence of many more inflammatory mediators in the submucosal region, it is clear that the inflammatory response is both a result of the airflow obstruction and one of its causes. Determination of the molecular biology of asthma continues, but leukotrienes, histamine, proteins from eosinophils, and other cytokines all may play a role in changing both the responsiveness and the defenses of the bronchial system.

Decreased Oxygenation

Airflow obstruction that manifests as wheezing will increase the work of breathing. In the most severe cases, obstruction will lead to an inability to clear carbon dioxide, with an increase in partial pressure of arterial carbon dioxide ($Paco_2$) and eventually respiratory failure. Even without respiratory failure, however, the potential for problems from decreased oxygenation may be significant. Oxygen transfer in the lungs requires good regional $\dot{V}/\dot{Q}$ matching. Mucous plugging in areas of narrowed airways, aggravated by damage to the mucociliary escalator and by $\dot{V}/\dot{Q}$ mismatch and air trapping (obstructive mechanism), can cause significant hypoxia, even while an individual successfully increases work of breathing to maintain normal carbon dioxide transfer.

DIFFERENTIAL DIAGNOSIS
Upper Airway Obstruction

Upper airway obstruction may result from (1) damage to the supporting cartilage of the extrathoracic airways or larynx, (2) inflammatory or malignant growths impinging on the airway, or (3) neurologic disorders causing failure of the abductors of the vocal cords. These obstructions unique to the upper airway cause wheezing on inspiration, often accompanied by a harsh, strained quality, or stridor. Inspiratory wheezing that greatly exceeds expiratory wheeze in quantity or intensity strongly suggests the diagnosis of an upper airway obstruction. However, sufficiently severe obstruction, even in the lower intrathoracic airways, often causes both inspiratory and expiratory wheezing, although the expiratory component usually predominates. Obstruction that is mechanical or "fixed," such as a metallic foreign body or rigid tumor, may produce wheezing throughout the respiratory cycle. Such mechanical obstructions may be deceptive, however, and the distinction between intrathoracic and extrathoracic obstruction is usually helpful but not always completely accurate.

Chronic Obstructive Pulmonary Disease

Wheezing occurs most often in the family of diseases known as *chronic obstructive pulmonary disease* (COPD). Grouping these diseases is useful as shorthand, but each has a different definition, pathophysiology, and timing for therapeutic interventions. They share the pathophysiology of airflow obstruction and the capacity to cause wheezing.

Asthma

Asthma is defined as reversible airway obstruction. In this functional definition, *reversibility* means that between episodes, even with severe asthma, airflow can normalize and symptoms resolve. Asthma is a common disorder of younger patients and may be associated with allergies or elevated blood eosinophil counts. Allergic reactions are no longer seen as central to the definition, however, and are only one source of the hyperreactivity response and one trigger of the asthmatic attacks.

Chronic Bronchitis

Chronic bronchitis is defined historically as chronic sputum production on most days during 3 months of each of the last 2 years. Clinically, however, the difficulty is usually not the duration of symptoms but rather the recognition by patients that morning "smoker's cough" or raising and swallowing mucus may be a significant symptom. Many patients with chronic bronchitis do not consider these common symptoms as worthy of reporting. Many older patients who use the term "asthma" actually have *asthmatic bronchitis*, or chronic sputum production coupled with variable amounts of obstruction. Unlike patients with pure asthma, those with asthmatic bronchitis have persistent if mild symptoms, even on "good days," and a more chronic course with less dramatic attacks.

Emphysema

Emphysema is best defined morphologically as dilation and destruction of the distal air spaces. Although not immediately obvious as such, the importance of supporting structure to functioning of the bronchial system makes emphysema an obstructive lung disorder. It is typically caused by smoking; neutrophils filled with proteolytic enzymes are attracted to the lungs, are activated, and release their proteases while the normal protective antiprotease system has been inhibited by substances in cigarette smoke. Because there is scant sputum production and often no history of repeated infections, individuals with emphysema may have a subtle course. Loss of the distal air space leads to loss of supporting structures around the bronchial system, which in turn causes increased resistance, airflow obstruction, and greater work of breathing. These individuals may use a significant percentage of their caloric requirements doing their daily work of breathing, and they are often surprisingly thin.

Because plugging and secretions are not a large part of the clinical picture, especially early in the course, hypoxemia and right-sided heart failure are uncommon until late in the natural history of this disease. Individuals with emphysema lose their ventilatory reserves over many years, which may be inapparent to them if they are inactive. They may think their illness has appeared over only a couple years or even months. In contrast, individuals with chronic bronchitis usually know they have a chronic respiratory impairment, often waxing and waning depending on the frequency and severity of infections.

Uncommon Problems

Individuals with acute allergic reactions, especially when immunoglobulin E bound to mast cells is a predominant factor, may have *anaphylactic reactions* to stimuli. Wheezing may result from bronchoconstriction with vasomotor collapse. With laryngeal spasm an inspiratory component predominates, and the acuteness of the presentation and the proximity of a triggering event are important.

Individuals with *pulmonary edema* from heart failure may also have wheezing. The interstitial space surrounding the small bronchi becomes filled with pulmonary edema fluid, causing narrowing of the bronchi. Some individuals may also show an increase in airway reactivity, suggesting a change in airway permeability as well. A careful examination of the event triggering the wheezing episode can be helpful, as can a search for the secondary signs of congestive heart failure, such as orthopnea, nocturia, and repeated episodes of nocturnal awakening.

Occasionally when sleeping, some individuals produce wheezing sounds that are upper airway in origin and analogous to *snoring* events. These snoring sounds may be sufficiently high pitched to suggest a wheeze, but unlike wheezing, they usually resolve on awakening. More severe snoring episodes are typically accompanied by a history of traditional snoring during sleep and sometimes by daytime sleepiness. Antianxiety, analgesic, and anesthetic medications may produce this effect, with variable airflow obstruction previously noted only by a spouse during the sleeping hours.

Stridor

Some individuals have severe upper airway wheezing, or stridor, that is often equally prominent on inspiration and expiration, with a variable pattern suggesting asthma. This symptom may improve by simply talking to the patient, however, and the repetitive nature or triggering circumstances of these events may suggest psychogenic factors. These individuals may have *vocal cord dysfunction*; on a volitional or psychogenic basis or as a maladaptive of response to more traditional airflow obstruction (e.g., asthma), they have "learned" to adduct their vocal cords during inspiration. They often report extensive evaluation in the past and care for asthma, thought to be remarkably refractory to therapy. They may have had invasive care such as intubation, only to recover and be free of wheezing as soon as an endotracheal tube was placed. Identifying these patients usually requires noticing an episode and visualizing the cords with this abnormal movement. Vocal cord dysfunction can be suspected, however, in a patient who has asthma symptoms inappropriately timed to the therapeutic interventions or who has asthma refractory to aggressive therapy but still shows extreme symptom variability daily or hourly.

PATIENT ASSESSMENT

Assessment of a patient with wheezing should include pertinent historical information. Wheezing episodes in the past and possible triggers provide information about the frequency of the disease and help to identify predictable precipitants that can be avoided. A childhood history of asthma is of limited value, but the severity of the episodes and their duration into childhood may be helpful. Patients with very strong allergic backgrounds, those who received corticosteroids, and those who needed hospitalization for asthma require extra caution. In adults the markers of significant disease include daily doses of bronchodilators or previous treatment with systemic corticosteroids for asthma. Other groups who require special care include (1) patients who are currently receiving corticosteroids, which suggests an active and unresolved process; (2) those who required hospitalization and intubation in the past; and (3) those who report extremely labile disease.

In this third respect, many individuals with asthma describe their exacerbations as beginning over the course of a few days, often with initial nocturnal symptoms, or in response to a viral upper respiratory infection. However, some go from asymptomatic to severely obstructed over 1 or 2 hours, given the right triggering circumstances. In these patients the reappearance of wheezing requires special care because they may move quickly to severe impairment.

Respiratory Evaluation

Assessment of the patient should include an evaluation of respiratory distress. Respiratory rates above 20 breaths per minute should suggest some degree of distress. The pattern of breathing may be important, especially if noteworthy for a prolonged expiratory phase or for audible wheezing heard without a stethoscope, which usually reflects at least moderately severe airflow obstruction. Increased work of breathing may be evaluated by examining the patient's use of accessory muscles (e.g., neck, shoulder girdle, arm) to assist in the respiratory effort or intercostal muscles to assist in more forceful expiration. Accessory muscle use suggests increased work of breathing. The chest and abdomen should expand together during inspiration. Rocking motion of the chest and abdomen, with inward movement of the lower chest segments during inspiration, suggests the intercostal muscles in the lower ribs have fatigued and are no longer able to stabilize the rib cage so that the diaphragm may work on it to full mechanical advantage. This suggests greatly increased work of breathing and impending respiratory failure.

In respiratory distress, other systems attempt to compensate for the increased work of breathing. The sympathetic nervous system output increases, and individuals typically have increased heart rate, increased blood pressure, and diaphoresis. In addition, if oxygenation is failing and cardiac output is inadequate for the peripheral requirements, especially with high energy expenditure for breathing, tissue hypoxia may become evident. Hypoxia may appear as classic cyanosis, but cyanosis requires 5 grams of unoxygenated hemoglobin to be visible and thus is not seen in many patients until the hypoxemia is quite severe. Hypoxia may manifest sooner in some patients as central nervous system (CNS) dysfunction, with confusion, agitation, or more subtle mental status changes. Patients in respiratory distress who are "not themselves" should be considered hypoxic until more data are available.

Chest Auscultation

Chest auscultation is the definitive way to identify wheezing. Good auscultation utilizes the natural symmetry of the body to compare one region of the lung with its corresponding area on the other side. Wheezing will present as a continuous high-pitched sound, but its absence should not lead to the conclusion that no obstruction is present. In normal patients without obstruction, durations of inspiration and expiration are about equal. Some individuals will have a prolonged expiratory phase, without wheezing, which may suggest obstruction. In addition, some with normal breath sounds, when taking tidal-size breaths, will have wheezing or prolonged expiration when asked to take a larger inspiration and then make a forced expiratory effort. This is a worthwhile addition to a basic lung examination and may be helpful even if the dentist does not use a stethoscope and auscultate patients. Individuals with significant intrathoracic airway obstruction will have better breath sounds on inspiration than expiration, and they may even have a "silent" expiration without wheeze if obstruction is severe.

A comparison of audible sounds and those heard with the stethoscope may be useful. Individuals with upper airway obstruction or those making volitional sounds during a forced expiration may have significant wheezing heard audibly, whereas the chest reveals good air movement and no wheezing in expiration. Listening directly over the trachea may also be helpful in identifying obstruction at that level, particularly when it clarifies that inspiratory wheezing is the predominant sound.

Pulse Oximetry and Arterial Blood Gases

Since the lungs function to transfer oxygen into and remove carbon dioxide from the blood, measurement of these values is helpful when available. Oxygenation shows much greater variability and may be affected not only by bronchospasm but also by plugging with secretions and airway edema. Definitive measurement of oxygen content in the blood requires an arterial sample, which must be collected anaerobically, conveyed to the laboratory on ice, and promptly analyzed. However, pulse oximetry now provides additional insight into oxygenation that is of great benefit despite its shortcomings. Pulse oximetry measures oxygen saturation. The flattening of the oxyhemoglobin saturation curve at high oxygen partial pressure values makes saturation less sensitive in distinguishing a small drop in oxygenation at the mid-90% saturation range in normal patients. Since many factors (e.g., pH, temperature) can affect oxygen saturation, pulse oximetry can identify individuals at risk because their oxygen saturation is less than 90%.

The major obstacle to their use is that current pulse oximeters measure carboxyhemoglobin (carbon monoxide combined with hemoglobin) as oxygenated hemoglobin. Thus a smoker with 7% carboxyhemoglobin in the bloodstream may be significantly hypoxemic even while giving a reassuring saturation reading of 92%. When possible, pulse oximetry measurements should be complemented by direct arterial blood gas measurement in significantly ill patients, at least until it is clear from the initial analysis that carboxyhemoglobin is not an issue.

Ventilation and Pa_{CO_2} are inversely linked. As net alveolar ventilation decreases, Pa_{CO_2} rises. This indicator represents the definitive tool for determining whether respiratory failure is imminent on the basis of work of breathing, or when muscle fatigue leads to decreased ventilation and increased Pa_{CO_2}. Measurement of the arterial pH or even the carbon dioxide representing mainly bicarbonate in venous blood may be helpful to predict a chronic elevation of Pa_{CO_2}. Even with chronic elevation, however, an elevated Pa_{CO_2} in the context of wheezing and respiratory distress is a worrisome finding. Even a normal Pa_{CO_2} in an individual with respiratory distress should be regarded with concern, since most individuals with early airflow obstruction have a Pa_{CO_2} lower than normal as they attempt to compensate with hyperventilation.

Spirometry and Peak Flow Measurement

In a hospital or multispecialty clinic setting, direct measurement of airflow may be helpful. Spirometry can measure both the inspiratory and the expiratory flow rates, as well as maximal vital capacity. These values can be compared to predicted values based on age, height, and gender. The comparison of flow in inspiration and expiration may help in identifying extrathoracic versus intrathoracic obstruction, and it provides the most accurate assessment of the degree of impairment. However, good data from spirometry requires a cooperative patient who can perform the necessary maneuvers, which is often impossible for individuals with significant respiratory distress.

Peak flow measurement is often used as an alternative in assessing degree of airflow obstruction. These measurement devices are relatively simple, and many patients use them at home to track the natural history of their disease and to identify exacerbations and triggering factors earlier than the clinical symptoms alone might allow.[2] Many different standards for peak flow measurement exist, but knowing the patient's personal-best values is very helpful. Patients who are at less than 50% of their personal-best values are likely symptomatic and at risk for additional problems and should be seen by their care providers. Having a peak flow measurement of less than 100 liters per minute (L/min) in raw numbers or less than 40% of the predicted value[3] is usually associated with a high risk of worsening if sent home and indicates the need for hospital care. A failure to achieve 200 to 300 L/min after treatment in an emergency department (ED) is often an indication to keep the patient in the hospital or under observation for a longer period.[4] Predicted values for peak flow also depend on the patient's height, age, and gender, but in general, values greater than 300 L/min are normal.

With no smoking in health care facilities and the proliferation of smoke detectors, asking a patient to blow out a match to assess flow rate is now no longer viable. However, the forced expiration mentioned earlier as a tool to supplement lung auscultation can be used in a semiquantitative manner as a substitute. The patient can perform a mouth-open full inspiration and forced expiration and count the seconds required to complete the maneuver. Normal values for this maneuver are 3 to 4 seconds, but severely obstructed patients may take 7 seconds or more.

TREATMENT

Bronchodilator therapy has been the mainstay for treatment of wheezing for many years. Bronchial smooth muscle has both sympathetic and parasympathetic innervation. *Sympathetic innervation causes bronchodilation.* Activation of the sympathetic receptors causes generation of second-messenger cyclic adenosine monophosphate (cAMP) within the cell, causing calcium flux and smooth muscle dilation. In this way the sympathetic nervous system prepares the organism for stressful events. Increases in heart rate and contractility and blood pressure result in dilation of the airways, allowing greater ventilation. *Parasympathetic innervation causes bronchoconstriction.* The parasympathetic side of the autonomic nervous system focuses on "housekeeping" functions, such as digestion and secretory processes. Most therapies for wheezing focus on augmenting the sympathetic side rather than blocking the parasympathetic pathways.

Sympathomimetic Drugs

A wide range of sympathomimetic drugs has been used to treat wheezing. Epinephrine, although a good bronchodilator with quick onset of action, also increases heart rate and blood pressure. This broad range of activity makes epinephrine the drug of choice when an allergic or anaphylactic reaction includes wheezing as well as hypotension or laryngospasm. Epinephrine is often used when bronchospasm is of short duration and more responsible for wheezing than any inflammatory component. Young patients are more tolerant of β-agonist drugs than older patients, who may have coronary artery disease compromised by tachycardia. A nonselective drug such as epinephrine will activate other β-adrenergic receptors in addition to the β$_2$-adrenoreceptors on the bronchial smooth muscle. In addition to possible tachycardia and hypertension, patients treated with epinephrine for wheezing may have tremor in other skeletal muscles as well as an anxious feeling.

Much effort in the development of new pharmaceuticals for bronchodilation has centered on seeking more selectivity, so that bronchial smooth muscle relaxes without increases in heart rate or other muscle tremors (Table 4-1). Other efforts have been to prolong the duration of effect so that less frequent doses of medication are needed.

Aerosol Therapy

A major advance in the delivery of bronchodilators has been the use of aerosol therapy. Drugs given as aerosols can produce very good effects while minimizing the dose delivered to organs outside the bronchial tree. This adds to the

Table 4-1	Common Asthma and Wheezing Medications			
Generic (Trade)	Mechanism of Action	Benefits	Adverse Effects	Typical Dose
Albuterol (Proventil, Ventolin) Metaproterenol (Alupent) Pirbuterol (Maxair)	Inhaled sympathomimetics Bronchial smooth muscle relaxation	Rapid onset Minimal systemic effects Easily accessible	Tachycardia Tremor Potential for overuse	2 puffs every 4-6 hours, with more frequent dosing up to every 2 hours if needed for short periods
Salmeterol (Serevent)	Inhaled long-acting sympathomimetic Bronchial smooth muscle relaxation	Sustained effect lasting 12 hours, avoiding need for repeated dosing	Potential for prolonged side effects	2 puffs every 12 hours
Ipratropium (Atrovent)	Inhaled anticholinergic Bronchial smooth muscle relaxation	In addition to bronchodilation, may reduce secretions Tremor unlikely	Tachycardia	2-4 puffs every 4-6 hours
Theophylline	Phosphodiesterase inhibitor Increases cAMP Smooth muscle dilation	Oral medication available in sustained-release form Intravenous forms also available	Nausea and vomiting Tachycardia Highly variable dosage adjustments	100-300 mg two to four times daily
Epinephrine	Direct-acting sympathomimetic bronchodilator	Available in inhaled, oral, and injectable forms Rapid onset and potent effect	Tachycardia, hypertension	0.01 ml/kg up to 0.5 ml/kg subcutaneously of 1:1000 solution (not 1:10,000 solution used for CPR)
Beclomethasone (Beclovent, Vanceril) Triamcinolone (Azmacort) Flunisolide (AeroBid) Fluticasone (Flovent)	Inhaled corticosteroid, antiinflammatory agents	Reduce airway inflammation and hyperreactivity	Oral candidiasis Hoarseness With high doses of potent steroids, growth changes in children may occur	2-12 puffs twice daily Dose depends on potency of corticosteroid.
Prednisone Methylpred-nisolone	Corticosteroid, antiinflammatory agents	Reduce airway inflammation and hyperreactivity	Sodium retention Elevated blood glucose Increased appetite Reduced defenses against infection Calcium loss from bone	Tapering doses from 40-60 mg daily to 5-10 mg every other day
Montelukast (Singulair) Zafirlukast (Accolate)	Oral medications Leukotriene inhibitors	Reduces airway inflammation and hyperreactivity	None significant	Montelukast: once daily Zafirlukast: twice daily
Cromolyn (Intal) Nedocromil (Tilade)	Inhaled anti-inflammatory mast cell stabilizers	Reduces airway inflammation and hyperreactivity	None significant	2 puffs 4 times a day

reduction in side effects achieved by more selective agents.

Aerosol therapy is often delivered in outpatients through the *metered-dose inhaler* (MDI). This compact device contains medication, a pressurized propellant, and a small valve that allows a specific dose to be released for inhalation with each actuation. The amount of drug delivered to the bronchial tree may be surprisingly small, often about 15%, even with patients who are well coached in proper technique. The remaining drug may escape into the room or be deposited in the oropharyngeal space, where some will be systemically absorbed. Even with these limitations, an effective dose of medication can be delivered, with a significantly reduced side effect profile.

Patients require training in proper use of the MDI. The traditional methodology places the barrel of the device between the lips, with the mouth sealed around it. Studies on deposition of radionuclide aerosols have shown that a technique in which the mouth is held open and the inhaler held a few inches from the mouth may allow better mixing of the aerosol with the inspired airflow and better deposition. For other patients, spacing devices (*spacers*) achieve the same separation and contain chambers where air for inspiration and medication may be mixed before delivering the aerosol. With the recent concern about ozone depletion by fluorocarbons, a number of companies have produced agents that are only dry powders and that do not require propellant spray for delivery. These devices have the same benefits as other aerosol units in terms of delivery and should become more common in the future.

β-Agonist Medications

Common selective β-agonists include *albuterol*, with a 4- to 6-hour duration of effect, and *salmeterol*, with a 12-hour duration of effect. Albuterol is also available in liquid and oral preparations, but these routes lack the advantages of aerosol therapy and are probably appropriate only in children. Children in general are quite tolerant of the nonspecific aspects of β-adrenergic stimulation in other organ systems and often receive doses of β-agonist systemically that adults would not tolerate.

Inhalants

In recent years there has been controversy about the risks of some of the potent β-agonist inhaled medications. Some argued that increased mortality might reflect only the use of more medication in patients with severe asthma, which also can be life threatening. However, subsequent studies carefully controlled for severity of disease and found that the added risk remains. This risk may relate to cardiac stimulation from drugs or other side effects but more likely reflects inability of bronchodilators to change the underlying natural history of inflammation and hyperreactivity. Asthmatic patients with airway reactivity and inflammatory response may have increasing symptoms that are controlled by a β-agonist for a time but that ultimately worsen and put the patient at significant risk for sudden death.

This observation underscores the importance of *balanced therapy* for asthma. Patients with significant disease should be treated not only with a bronchodilator to control symptoms but also with therapy to reduce airway inflammation. The amount and frequency of a patient's β-agonist dosage are also important factors.

Over-the-counter (OTC) β-agonist medications are still in common use. These include medications containing ephedrine, sometimes sold as nutritional supplements or herbal extracts, and MDI epinephrine (e.g., Primatene Mist). OTC drugs can cause the same side effects as other β-agonists and are more likely to produce adverse effects such as tachycardia because they are less selective. They have remained as OTC drugs because they are their own deterrent to overuse; the side effects are *more* likely to occur with these drugs than with the prescription β-agonists. If a more selective β-agonist is not available, the use of OTC drugs in response to an episode of wheezing in the dental office is reasonable, but they would not be the first choice.

Parasympathetic Inhibitors

Parasympathetic inhibitors include atropine and ipratropium. A*tropine* has been in infrequent use for many years; it has the disadvantage of crossing the blood-brain barrier and producing agitation and confusion in some patients. I*pratropium* is a charged quaternary ammonium derivative of atropine and does not produce CNS effects. As with the β-agonists, these medications also are best delivered as an aerosol and can increase heart rate, but they generally do not produce tremor. Many patients, especially those with increased secretions and chronic bronchitis, may respond well to ipratropium or MDI combinations of albuterol and ipratropium. These anticholinergic medications are effective bronchodilators and may have additive effects to β-agonists. Anticholinergics have a slower onset of action, however, and are not as useful as immediate therapy for an acute event.

Theophylline

Another bronchodilator with a long history of use but relatively uncommon in recent years is theophylline, a methylxanthine related to caffeine that acts as a phosphodiesterase inhibitor. Theophylline blocks the degradation of cAMP and thus perpetuates the level of the second messenger within smooth muscle cells, causing additional bronchodilation. Besides bronchodilation, theophylline may improve the efficiency of the diaphragm and its resistance to fatigue. Theophylline also changes the timing of the ventilatory drive, possibly improving inspiratory flow and allowing more time for a prolonged expiratory phase. It is available in both intravenous and oral forms.

The major drawback of theophylline therapy is a poor toxic/therapeutic ratio, so many individuals have side effects (e.g., tremor, nausea and vomiting, palpitations) at doses within the therapeutic range. Metabolism also varies greatly; factors such as common medications (e.g., antacid H_2 blockers) and diet can cause wide fluctuations in theophylline metabolism. Drug monitoring by serum level may be important because serious toxicity can occur with elevations of less than 25% above the therapeutic window.

Corticosteroids

The cornerstone of antiinflammatory therapy for wheezing is corticosteroids. These medications are the prototypes of the antiinflammatory agents; they stabilize cell membranes and reduce release of mediators from mast cells and other immune cells. They reduce the number and function of lymphocytes, reduce the response of polymorphonuclear leukocytes, and even serve to upregulate β-adrenergic receptors, which may help to increase sensitivity to both endogenous and pharmacologic bronchodilators.

Side effects of corticosteroids, especially when used systemically, are significant. Most effects relate to the duration of treatment, not the dosage used. Adverse effects include elevation of blood glucose levels, diabetic complications, reduction in bone strength and osteoporosis, increased capillary fragility and easy bruising, retention of salt and fluid, mood shifts and sleeplessness, and increased appetite and frequent weight gain. Again, using an aerosol in this setting to deliver medication to the airway improves drug selectivity and avoids systemic effects.

Patients treated with corticosteroids need clear instructions to understand the potential for adrenal suppression. Patients treated with corticosteroids above the baseline level of about 7.5 mg/day naturally produced as cortisol may fail to resume cortisol production when corticosteroid therapy is stopped. This process probably takes about 3 weeks, and although uncommon, it can be life threatening. Patients treated with corticosteroids should have clear description of the intended dosage and the duration of therapy. Ideally, patients taking oral steroids should have a calendar defining the dose intended for each day of the tapering schedule.

Typical doses of *prednisone* used to treat an outpatient exacerbation of asthma with wheezing are about 40 mg/day, whereas a hospitalized patient may receive doses of 160 to 500 mg/day. The onset of action of corticosteroids is usually reported as 6 to 8 hours, although some studies suggest a faster response. Even a patient responsive to corticosteroids will not respond immediately and will need adequate therapy with quicker-acting bronchodilators to provide symptomatic relief and to stabilize them while the corticosteroid takes effect.

Nonsteroidal Antiinflammatory Drugs

Cromolyn and *nedocromil* stabilize mast cells, inhibiting the release of preformed mediators and reducing the inflammatory response. Other nonsteroidal antiinflammatory drugs include inhibitors of the leukotrienes, prostaglandin derivatives that are potent inflammatory mediators. Both the mast cell stabilizers and the leukotriene inhibitors may be helpful in patients with mild disease, especially when used early before a significant inflammatory cascade. As with corticosteroids, leukotriene inhibitors can alter the natural history of the disease and reduce the inflammatory state, so they make a significant contribution to reversing the underlying problem in asthma and wheezing. They are also generally well tolerated with relatively few side effects. However, none of the leukotriene inhibitors has a sufficiently rapid onset of action to be useful in acute episodes.

Oxygen

Although it is often neglected as a "medication," oxygen can be very important in the treatment of asthma and wheezing. $\dot{V}/\dot{Q}$ mismatch may result in significant hypoxemia, even without cyanosis or altered mental status.

Stridor

Patients who have stridor rather than classic wheezing may require a different approach that focuses on the upper airway. Procedures to lift and extend the jaw are clearly helpful in securing the airway of unconscious patients, but they also may be useful in conscious patients with noisy breathing. Patients may be asked to protrude their jaw or tongue to determine if the stridor can be eliminated by changing position or to visualize oropharyngeal structures, providing clues about stridor's origin. It is often useful to compare the intensity of wheezing using a stethoscope over the chest with the stethoscope held in front of the mouth or over the neck. Patients with upper airway obstruction in the subglottic but extrathoracic region often have localizable wheezing, whereas those with vocal cord dysfunction may have louder wheezing audibly or with the stethoscope in front of the mouth rather than over the chest.

Severe Wheezing

Patients with severe wheezing and increased work of breathing may reach the point of respiratory muscle fatigue and respiratory failure with elevated $Paco_2$. These patients need the basics of basic life support to assist in doing part of their work of breathing until more definitive therapy can correct the problem or provide long-term support. In general, these patients can be handled well using *bag-valve-mask* (BVM) assistive equipment. Their lungs are not unusually stiff, and it is usually easy to ventilate them with the BVM device. They are at risk for air trapping, which may make it difficult to appreciate the amount of airflow occurring. An adequately high inspiratory flow rate may improve air trapping, with sufficient time for expiration to prevent additional air trapping.

The choice of a BVM device using good airway management technique, a laryngeal mask, or traditional intubation with laryngoscopy depends on training and experience. In general, the clinician should directly observe that the chest is rising and falling with each ventilation and use auscultation to assist and to assess air movement at the same time. More sophisticated devices that detect carbon dioxide from the lungs, not the stomach, are becoming more common and may be more reassuring in some settings. All these methods can do an effective job, but all require some experience and practice.

In the hospital setting, instead of providing full support of the work of breathing with mechanical ventilation, partial support is frequently provided using a nasal *continuous positive airway pressure* (CPAP) *mask.* The positive pressure delivered through this mask holds the nasopharyngeal airway in an open position. Bilevel CPAP devices can do a significant amount of the patient's work of breathing. They are generally used as "bridging" devices to support a patient long enough for bronchodilator therapy to control the wheezing. Often, however, patients may be inadequately supported and may still require intubation and mechanical ventilation.

MANAGEMENT APPROACH IN THE DENTAL OFFICE
Recognition and Assessment

Assess the patient to determine if respiratory failure is imminent (Box 4-1). Assess the patient's alertness and responsiveness, determine any use of accessory muscles or increase in respiratory rate, and auscultate for breath sounds and air movement. Use a pulse oximeter if available; significant hypoxemia with oxygen saturations less than 90% on room air should raise concerns. If no oximeter is available, cyanosis is not very reliable, and the patient's alertness and degree of anxiety may be the only useful markers of hypoxemia. In deciding the overall severity, ask the patient to speak and cough. The cough requires a forced expiratory effort and helps assess any obstruction and the patient's ability to raise secretions. Ability to speak indicates that the wheezing is not caused by vocal cord edema, and an upper airway obstruction or foreign body is less likely.

Listen to assess severity of the bronchospasm and to determine if the wheezing is localized. Upper airway obstruction or focal wheezing limited to one area of the chest may suggest aspiration of food or dental hardware. Look for symmetry between the right and left sides of the chest, and watch the chest for uniform and well-coordinated respiratory movements.

Elicit the patient history. Identify the patient's current position in the natural history of

---

Box 4-1	Management Approach to the Wheezing Patient

STEPS	PATIENT FACTORS
1. Assess for catastrophe. Is respiratory failure imminent?	Alertness, responsiveness Respiratory rate Accessory muscle use Pulse oximetry, peak flow measurement
2. Evaluate bronchospasm. How much wheezing or "tightness" is present? Can patient speak and cough?	Listen for air movement first, then wheezing. Note "silent" chest.
3. Review history. At what point is patient in natural history of wheezing or asthmatic episode? Are there risk factors for lability? What is nature of similar episodes in the past? Is another disease process at work?	Rate of change in symptoms Past intubations or hospitalizations Inhaled or oral steroids, past or current Concurrent cardiovascular disease Evidence of upper airway obstruction (e.g., stridor)
4. Administer β-agonist aerosol as diagnostic tool and as therapy.	1 or 2 puffs of albuterol with spacer
5. Reassess at 20 minutes.	Peak flow measurements should double. Forced expiratory volume is improved. Air movement has improved. β-Agonist has caused no adverse effects. For anaphylaxis, subcutaneous epinephrine is useful in some younger patients.
6. Provide antiinflammatory therapy for all except mildest cases.	Inhaled steroids are primary therapy for milder cases. Oral or intravenous steroids are used for more severe cases. Steroids can be stopped later if indicated by new data.
7. Arrange disposition of patient. Is improvement sustained?	Repeat peak flow measurement and examination 4 hours after β-agonist use. Follow-up plans should consider response to past episodes.

---

the wheezing episode. Determine duration and tempo of symptoms; the patient with progressive symptoms over a long period may have accumulated a significant inflammatory burden that is not easily reversible. The patient with a short duration of symptoms may respond quickly. Past events are reviewed for any intubation or hospitalization to determine severity of disease and time to onset of effective therapy.

Determine if the patient has received or is taking corticosteroids. Patients who have required steroids frequently in the past probably have more severe disease and will require them again. Patients currently being treated with corticosteroids for an exacerbation are at significant risk, since they have worsened to the point of symptoms despite therapy. They more likely will require transfer to a setting appropriate for a longer period of observation. Inquire about

the frequency of β-agonist bronchodilator therapy; overusers may be at greater risk for sudden death and probably had a longer course of more severe disease.

Differential Diagnosis

Patients with a cardiovascular history or those taking cardiac medications (e.g., antihypertensives, digoxin, diuretics, β-blockers) may have wheezing related to a cardiac cause. Congestive heart failure, even at the early stages when only increased interstitial fluid is present, may present as wheezing. These patients often show a greater tachypnea than the typical asthmatic patient, may have a cardiac gallop rhythm, and may want to sit in an upright position to relieve their dyspnea, but the clinical examination without chest radiographs can be deceptive. Most patients with dyspnea are more comfortable sitting, even if diaphragmatic function and abdominal excursion are issues rather than lung congestion from ischemic disease. Also, sitting is typically the best position to treat and evaluate them. Strong suspicion of a concurrent cardiac problem causing the wheezing mandates transfer to facility with radiographic ability and adequate follow-up.

Initial Intervention

Almost all patients with wheezing will benefit from a trial of a β-agonist. The toxic/therapeutic ratio of MDI medications, especially with a spacer to reduce oropharyngeal deposition, is excellent. In a whezing patient, only specific information about an adverse reaction to a β-agonist in the past would contraindicate its use. A typical dose is 2 puffs of albuterol a few minutes apart, with 1 or 2 additional puffs in 10 to 30 minutes if needed. Onset of action is about 5 minutes and duration of effect about 4 hours. The β-agonist provides diagnostic benefit as well, since few other problems that mimic wheezing (e.g., heart failure, aspiration) are likely to improve with bronchodilator therapy. A long-acting β-agonist is not appropriate because of slower onset of action.

In general, relative to the endogenous catecholamine release through the distressed breathing, inhaled β-agonists are not a source of added cardiac stimulation in patients who may have concurrent cardiac disease. Control of the bronchospasm will reduce cardiac demand. Unless the patient has a specific history of intolerance to the current β-agonists, they should be given by inhalation for wheezing, even if the patient has cardiac concerns.

Reassessment

Reassess the patient about 20 minutes after administering the β-agonist. The patient's subjective response is often useful, as is a repeat of the assessment of air movement by auscultation and observation of the patient for signs of improved or worsening respiratory symptoms. When available, peak flow measurements are helpful. The peak flow measurement taken before administration of the β-agonist typically will double in a good response. Consider the expected duration of effect of any therapy. Even in the patient who subjectively feels much better, repeat the objective assessment when the duration of effect should begin to decrease.

Second Intervention

Anticholinergic medications such as ipratropium are usually too slow in onset to be a good initial therapy for acute wheezing but may be useful as a combined albuterol-ipratropium inhalation (Combivent MDI).

If the patient has worsened despite the β-agonist, consider activating the emergency medical services (EMS) system and preparing to transfer the patient to a facility for more support and observation. If the patient has improved, observe and repeat the β-agonist dose in about 2 hours. Improvement probably will be slow, however, and longer observation is necessary.

Administer epinephrine (0.01 ml/kg, up to 0.3 to 0.5 ml/kg, of a 1:1000 solution subcutaneously) for suspected anaphylaxis or for hypotension that accompanies the wheezing in a nonselective allergic context. Epinephrine is better tolerated by younger patients and those without ischemic cardiac disease. The drug has a rapid onset of action and short duration of action. Sustained-release forms are available but may give false reassurance analogous to the "responsiveness" of patients to overuse of inhaled β-agonists. Use epinephrine only when the problem is well understood and adequate time is available to observe the stability of response, typically several hours.

Even patients responding well to β-agonists may need antiinflammatory therapy, especially with prior corticosteroid use or recent noncompliance with a regimen of inhaled steroids. In general, if patients require treatment for a flare-up of symptoms, include a plan to increase their current antiinflammatory therapy, not just symptom-relieving bronchodilators.

Disposition

Patients who do not have a sustained improvement at the end of the expected duration of therapy may be re-treated with additional medication, but this natural history suggests a longer period of hospital observation. Patients who are not currently taking corticosteroids and have a good response to β-agonists may be released as long as their history does not suggest marked lability, late worsening, or need for intubation. These latter patients are at greater risk and require more observation. If patients taking corticosteroids improve but are given an increased dose, they should be seen by their attending physician within 24 to 48 hours. The increased dose of steroid should not be reduced until the patient has seen the primary physician.

All patients with wheezing who are treated and sent home, even if wheezing improves completely, should be reminded that symptoms may recur. Because asthma and wheezing can be life threatening, seeking care at the ED is appropriate.

REFERENCES

1. Sleigh MA: The nature and action of respiratory tract cilia. In *Respiratory defense mechanisms*, New York, 1977, Dekker.
2. Kendrick AH, Higgs CM, Whitfield MJ, et al: Accuracy of perception of severity of asthma: patients treated in general practice, BMJ 307:422-424, 1993.
3. Emerman CL, Effron D, Lukens TW: Spirometric criteria for hospital admission of patients with acute exacerbation of COPD, Chest 99:595-599, 1991.
4. Nowak RM, Pensler MI, Sankar DD, et al: Comparison of peak expiratory flow and FEV$_1$ admission criteria for acute bronchial asthma, Ann Emerg Med 11:64-69, 1982.

Dyspnea

O. Ross Beirne

Dyspnea is the sensation of difficult, uncomfortable, and labored breathing. Although unpleasant and disturbing, dyspnea is not painful. As with pain, dyspnea is a subjective sensation that elicits different reactions in different patients and is described by many different terms. No specific terms accurately describe the sensation.[1]

The language used to describe dyspnea can be helpful in understanding the cause of the labored breathing.[1,2] Air hunger is reported as "cannot get enough air," "need to breathe," and "out of breath." An increased desire to breathe may be associated connected with exercise, congestive heart failure, pregnancy, and chronic obstructive pulmonary disease (COPD). No term or phrase describing dyspnea can be used to diagnose a specific disease.

PHYSIOLOGY OF BREATHING

Breathing is controlled by a complex interaction between the brain, lung, and chest muscles. The automatic and voluntary control of breathing resides in the brain.[3-5] The brainstem controls automatic breathing, whereas voluntary breathing is controlled by the cerebral cortex. Central and peripheral respiratory sensory receptors signal the respiratory control system. The central chemoreceptors respond to carbon dioxide (CO_2), and the peripheral chemoreceptors respond to oxygen. Peripheral sensory receptors are present in the chest wall, airways, and lungs. The respiratory muscles have sensory receptors that respond to stretching. The lung receptors are irritant receptors, which respond to physical or chemical stimulation; pulmonary stretch receptors, which respond to increases in lung volume; and C-fiber receptors, which respond to vascular engorgement and congestion.

The control centers in the brain stimulate the respiratory muscles (diaphragm; intercostal, scalene, and accessory muscles) and air is moved in and out of the lungs. Oxygen is trans-ported into the lungs, and CO_2 is exhaled. The changes in oxygen and CO_2 are fed back to the brain by the respiratory central and peripheral sensory receptors.

The phrenic nerves are the only motor neurons to the diaphragm and arise from the third, fourth, and fifth cervical segments. The phrenic nerve is also the major sensory nerve for the diaphragm. The intercostal nerves arising from the first to the twelfth thoracic segments are the motor and sensory innervation for the intercostal muscles. The cervical segments of the fourth to the eight segments supply motor innervation to the scalene muscles. The sternocleidomastoid and trapezius muscles are the major accessory muscles of respiration and are innervated by the spinal accessory nerve and the second to the fourth cervical segments.

The muscle spindles and tendon organs are the two major sensory receptors in the respiratory muscles. The muscle spindles are abundant in the intercostal muscles and scarce in the diaphragm. Tendon organs are found in both the intercostal muscles and the diaphragm. The muscle spindles help coordinate breathing during speech and assist with changes in posture. The tendon organs inhibit inspiration based on the force of muscle contraction.

The sensory receptors send information to the brain through the vagus nerve. Information from the sensory chemoreceptors of the carotid bodies travels in a branch of the carotid sinus nerve, reaching the brainstem via the glossopharyngeal nerve (Figure 5-1).

PATHOPHYSIOLOGY OF DYSPNEA

The sensation of dyspnea occurs when there is inadequate oxygenation, ventilation, or control of acid-base balance. Normal respiration depends on a balance between ventilatory demand and capacity. The chemoreceptors and mechanoreceptors signal the brain generating the sensation of dyspnea.[3-5]

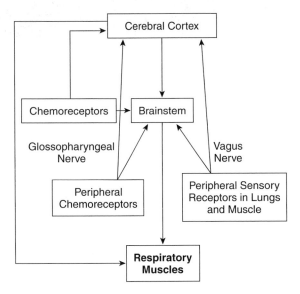

Figure 5-1. Normal regulation of respiration. *Arrows* show (1) afferent input to the brainstem and cerebral cortex from the central and peripheral sensory receptors and (2) efferent output from the brain to the respiratory muscles.

The effort of breathing associated with an increased work of breathing is observed with increased resistance in the airway. The sensation of effort may arise because the motor cortex sends impulses directly to the sensory cortex at the same moment that the outgoing motor signal is sent to the respiratory muscles. An alternative theory is that the receptors in the respiratory muscles provide direct feedback to the central nervous system (CNS) that is identified as increased work to breathe. As the effort of breathing increases, patients reach a point that the sensation is unpleasant or uncomfortable. However, effort is only one of the factors that contribute to the sensation of breathlessness. Even rapid breathing can become uncomfortable after strenuous exercise; because the sensation is uncomfortable, it is included in the definition of dyspnea.

Acute hypercapnia (increased CO_2 levels) can also produce the sensation of dyspnea. Although some studies suggest that respiratory muscle activity is needed to signal the CNS rather than CO_2 having a direct effect on the brain, recent studies support the theory that respiratory muscle contraction is not needed and that CO_2 directly triggers the sensation of dyspnea.[3] This CO_2-induced dyspnea is probably mediated by changes in pH at the central chemoreceptors. Patients with chronically elevated levels of CO_2, such as those with COPD or neuromuscular diseases, have developed a metabolic compensation for the chronic pH changes. These patients become less responsive to central chemoreceptors that react to CO_2, and their respiratory drive becomes dependent on the peripheral oxygen chemoreceptors.

Hypoxia (low arterial oxygen) can also be associated with dyspnea. As the oxygen level drops in normal patients breathing gas mixtures with low concentrations of oxygen, the patients experience greater breathlessness as the oxygen concentration decreases. However, dyspnea in patients with COPD does not always correlate with the level of hypoxia. Hypoxia probably exerts its effect on the sensation of dyspnea by increasing ventilation and directly stimulating the CNS.

Mechanoreceptors play a role in the pathogenesis of dyspnea. Upper airway receptors can alter the sensation of breathlessness.[3] Patients with COPD report relief of dyspnea when sitting by a fan or open window or when cold air is directed against the face. Stimulation of receptors in the trigeminal nerve distribution influences the intensity of breathlessness.

Lung receptors send impulses to the brain via the vagus nerves. Stretch receptors respond to increases in lung volume, irritant receptors respond to chemical and mechanical stimulation; and C fibers respond to pulmonary vascular congestion. The discomfort associated with bronchospasm is probably mediated by the irritant receptors. The C fibers respond to pulmonary congestion and cause breathing changes in patients with pulmonary edema.

Chemoreceptors and mechanoreceptors have different inputs to the brain. No single receptor causes the sensation of dyspnea. Under normal conditions the brain receives a balanced input from all the receptors that is recognized as a normal pattern. When there is deviation from the normal balance, patients will develop or observe an increase in the sensation of dyspnea.

DIFFERENTIAL DIAGNOSIS

Respiratory, cardiac, and neuromuscular diseases and anxiety can cause dyspnea (Box 5-1).[5-9] The onset of dyspnea can be acute or chronic. Patients with chronic dyspnea rarely present for emergency care. However, normal patients with acute onset of dyspnea or patients with chronic dyspnea who have greater difficulty breathing than usual require immediate management.

Box 5-1	Differential Diagnosis of Dyspnea

PULMONARY
Chronic obstructive pulmonary disease
Asthma
Upper airway obstruction
Aspiration
Pulmonary embolism
Pneumothorax
Laryngospasm
Laryngeal edema
Pulmonary edema

CARDIAC
Congestive heart failure
Myocardial infarction
Valvular heart disease

NEUROMUSCULAR
Myasthenia gravis
Guillain-Barré syndrome
Amyotrophic lateral sclerosis

Chronic Obstructive Pulmonary Disease

COPD affects millions of Americans, and the majority of cases are linked to cigarette smoking.[2,7] Patients are classically described as "blue bloaters" or "pink puffers." These individuals have chronic dyspnea with frequent episodes of decompensation and respiratory failure. An acute episode of dyspnea can be triggered by any stimulus that increases the need for oxygen. Anxiety, infection, administration of CNS depressants, and exhaustion can induce respiratory failure requiring emergency management.

The blue bloater has chronic bronchitis, which is associated with a chronic cough and significant sputum production. They are usually obese and cyanotic. They may retain CO_2 and become dependent on a hypoxic drive for normal respiration. Many of these patients have right-sided heart failure.

The pink puffer has emphysema with distention of the pulmonary alveoli and destruction of the alveolar walls. The airways lose their support and collapse with inspiration. These patients have to expend significant effort to breath. They are usually thin because of the work needed to breathe, and their lungs are hyperinflated, resulting in a barrel-chest appearance. They develop significant dyspnea, which can severely limit their activity. They do not have a productive cough, are not usually cyanotic, and do not usu-

ally retain CO_2. They frequently purse their lips when they exhale to maintain pressure on the alveoli to prevent them from collapsing.

The pink puffer and blue bloater represent two extremes of COPD. Most patients with COPD are between these two extremes. Patients with COPD have very little respiratory reserve; any increase in respiratory demand can result in significant dyspnea. When these patients develop acute respiratory distress, their hypoxemia can become extreme. Patients who retain CO_2 may be unable to eliminate it and the increasing serum CO_2 levels will cause lethargy and drowsiness. Because these patients develop severe airway obstruction, they have a prolonged expiratory phase.

The severity of the dyspnea cannot be used as an objective measure of obstruction.[1-3] Some patients report severe dyspnea with less obstruction than other patients, who report only minor dyspnea.[2,6] Spirometry and arterial blood gases are the most accurate objective measures of obstruction. The forced expiratory volume in 1 second, peak expiratory flow rate, and arterial CO_2 and oxygen tensions are especially useful measures of obstruction. A patient complaining of dyspnea must be treated for severe respiratory obstruction until proven otherwise.

Asthma

Asthma is a reversible obstructive disease. Unlike COPD, respiratory function is relatively normal between acute asthmatic attacks. The airways are hyperactive, and a variety of stimuli trigger reversible narrowing of these airways (bronchospasm). The acute asthmatic attack involves bronchospasm, swelling of the mucous membranes in the bronchial walls, and mucous plugging of the bronchi, all of which increase resistance to airflow. The effort or work of the respiratory muscles increases to overcome the resistance, and the lungs usually become hyperinflated to increase airway pressure and permit airflow. The increased respiratory motor output and muscle stretching from hyperinflation contribute to the sensation of dyspnea. Wheezing is associated with asthma (see Chapter 4).

Upper Airway Obstruction

Upper airway obstruction due to blockage by a foreign body is characterized by a distressed patient who may be grasping the throat area while attempting to breathe. If the obstruction is complete, the patient will be unable to exchange any air, and there will be no airflow. The chest will retract instead of expand with each attempt to inhale, and speech will be impossible. If there is partial obstruction, stridor will be heard as a *crowing* sound as the air passes the narrowed upper airway. Acute upper airway obstruction occurs with aspiration of a large foreign body, angioedema, and swelling of the neck and oral cavity associated with infection.

Pulmonary Embolism

Pulmonary embolism is the sudden blocking of a pulmonary artery. It can be life threatening but is uncommon in the dental setting. Dyspnea and chest pain are typical symptoms.[2,5,9] The increased pressure in the pulmonary vessels is sensed by the pulmonary C fibers, which signal the sensation of dyspnea.

Blood clots are a common cause of pulmonary embolism. The clots form in the veins of the legs or pelvis and break loose and become trapped in the progressively narrowing pulmonary vessels. Heart disease, advanced age, prolonged immobilization (e.g., a long airplane trip), malignancy, thrombophlebitis, and certain drugs (e.g., oral contraceptives) favor the development of blood clots in the legs and pelvis. Fat particles released from fractured bone, amniotic fluid released during delivery, and air entering the circulation from a wound or intravenous catheter can also obstruct a pulmonary artery.

The signs and symptoms of pulmonary embolism depend on the size of the obstruction. If a major pulmonary vessel is blocked, gas exchange will be impaired, and the patient will have severe respiratory distress. In addition, the right ventricle will have to move blood against greater pressure, and signs of right-sided heart failure can develop. With small obstruction, only dyspnea and chest pain may occur without major impairment of gas exchange.

Pneumothorax

A pneumothorax results in air leaking into the pleural cavity between the lung and pleura; it can be spontaneous or traumatic.[2,5,7,8] The lung collapses, causing dyspnea and chest pain. Spontaneous pneumothorax results from rupture of a bleb or bulla in patients with or without underlying lung disease. Primary spontaneous pneumothorax occurs most frequently in tall, thin, and young adult males. The clinical examination of the chest may be normal if the pneumothorax is small. If a tension pneumothorax develops,

however, the patient will have rapid deterioration with increasing dyspnea, absent breath sounds on the side of the pneumothorax, tracheal deviation to the opposite side of the chest, and impaired venous return and cardiac output. The rapidly declining patient needs immediate emergency management to reexpand the lung. This is a rare medical emergency in the dental office.

Allergic Reactions

Allergic reactions can cause dyspnea by two mechanisms.[8] Laryngeal edema may occur as an isolated allergic reaction or as part of an anaphylactic reaction. Laryngeal swelling results in upper airway obstruction. Dyspnea can also result from allergic bronchospasm. Bronchospasm is associated with severe dyspnea and wheezing and resembles an acute asthma attack.

Acute Pulmonary Edema

Acute pulmonary edema, another rare medical emergency in dental practice, occurs with increased intravascular hydrostatic pressure or increased permeability of the vascular endothelium.[2,5,8,9] The edema reduces lung volume and dyspnea is caused by hypoxemia and stimulation of receptors in the lung parenchyma and pulmonary vasculature. Pulmonary edema is usually the result of aspiration, hypotensive shock, drug overdose, trauma, or malignancy.

Aspiration

Aspiration of gastric contents can result in dyspnea. This unusual complication is most frequently associated with management of the sedated patient. The severity of the dyspnea depends on the amount of liquid aspirated and the pH of the material. The acidic gastric material causes a chemical pneumonitis. Because of the anatomy of the trachea, the material usually enters the right rather than the left lung. The constellation of symptoms associated with aspiration of gastric contents has been termed *Mendelson's syndrome*. Patients who aspirate liquid gastric contents develop wheezing, dyspnea, arrhythmias, cyanosis, and tachycardia. The onset of dyspnea may be a delayed rather than an immediate response.[7,10]

Respiratory Depression

Respiratory depression associated with narcotic overdose may be managed with naloxone, a reversal agent for narcotics. Naloxone can cause pulmonary edema because of increases in hydrostatic pressure, pulmonary capillary permeability, and possibly pulmonary vascular resistance.[11] Pulmonary edema usually occurs in critically ill patients but has also been reported in healthy patients who received naloxone.

The cardiac causes for dyspnea can be difficult to diagnose because the signs and symptoms are similar to dyspnea caused by pulmonary disease.[2,4,5,7-9] Congestive heart failure, myocardial infarction, and valvular heart disease are the most common cardiac causes of acute dyspnea. Dyspnea caused by pulmonary edema is the most common symptom of congestive heart failure. Heart failure patients may have orthopnea (shortness of breath when lying down) and paroxysmal nocturnal dyspnea (shortness of breath that awakens the patient at night). An acute increase in pulmonary edema as a result of heart failure may mimic an asthma attack.

A patient having a myocardial infarction can present with dyspnea. Infarction may result from congestive heart failure caused by damage to the cardiac muscle, with reduced cardiac output and pulmonary edema, or by decreased cardiac output from an abnormal rhythm that causes significant left-sided heart failure. In addition to dyspnea, the patient may present with substernal chest pain that radiates to the arms. Unlike pleuritic chest pain, the cardiac pain does not increase or decrease in relationship to breathing.

Although most valvular heart disease results in a gradual onset of chronic dyspnea, acute dyspnea is associated with acute aortic insufficiency and mitral regurgitation. Acute mitral regurgitation may result from papillary muscle dysfunction or rupture and can lead to pulmonary edema with acute onset of dyspnea.

Neuromuscular Diseases

Guillain-Barré syndrome, myasthenia gravis, and amyotrophic lateral sclerosis can cause acute dyspnea.[2,5,7] The contraction of the respiratory muscles is reduced because of these neuromuscular diseases. The muscles become weak, and more neuromotor output is required to breathe. This increase in output is the principal mechanism for breathlessness in these patients, who may develop significant hypoxia and hypercapnia, which contribute to the dyspnea.

Hyperventilation

A more common medical emergency in dentistry is the hyperventilation syndrome that presents as acute dyspnea.[2,4,7-9] The hyperventilating patient is usually a teenager or young adult with no underlying pulmonary disease. The syndrome occurs more frequently in women than in men. Rapid ventilation results in a decrease in the partial pressure of arterial CO_2, which decreases cerebral blood flow and alters serum electrolytes. The patients may experience lightheadedness; faintness; numbness or tingling of the mouth, hands, and feet; and sharp, stabbing chest pain. Patients with severe hyperventilation may develop carpopedal spasm, with the hands taking a flexed position and thumbs curved toward the palm. Hyperventilation syndrome is diagnosed by excluding organic causes of dyspnea aided by the health history.

PATIENT ASSESSMENT

The first step in evaluating a patient with acute dyspnea is to determine the urgency of the situation (Box 5-2).[4,5,7-9] Initially, the patient's position, level of consciousness, respiration rate, pulse rate, blood pressure, and airflow are assessed. Patients with severe dyspnea will be sitting upright and leaning forward to breathe. As hypoxia increases, the patient will become disoriented, confused, restless, and unable to answer questions. This requires immediate intervention to raise the level of oxygen and prevent the patient from losing consciousness. The effort of breathing is assessed by determining the respiratory rate, which normally is 14 to 16 breaths per minute, as well as the depth of respiration. If the rate is more than 20 breaths per minute, the patient has significant dyspnea. Severe airway obstruction will result in an inability to exhale air, and the patient may not be able to talk or may only be able to whisper. The urgency of the condition is established very quickly. The immediate concerns are to ensure that the airway and oxygenation are adequate.

After stabilizing the patient, the cause of the dyspnea must be established. A focused history can be helpful in formulating the differential diagnosis of the dyspnea. The history must focus on the cardiac, pulmonary, and neuromuscular systems. The medical history can help establish if the patient has underlying medical problems. Heart and lung disease, hypertension, and neuromuscular disease may be related to the acute episode of dyspnea. A patient with a history of asthma, congestive heart failure, or cardiac valvular disease may have poor control of the disease with inadequate functional reserve. A patient with a history of thrombophlebitis may

Box 5-2 Management of Dyspnea in the Dental Office

1. Evaluate the patient's position, level of consciousness, respiration rate, use of respiratory muscles, blood pressure, pulse rate, and chest movement.
2. Manage upper airway obstruction. If patient is conscious, repeat the Heimlich maneuver until the object is dislodged. If the patient loses consciousness, initiate the emergency medical system, and continue to attempt to dislodge the object with abdominal thrusts, followed by finger sweeps and positive-pressure ventilation with a bag-valve-mask attached to oxygen.
3. When the upper airway is open and air is moving, the patient should be given supplemental oxygen. Even before the diagnosis is established, oxygen should be administered using nasal prongs, nasal hood, or full-face mask. The patient should be allowed to sit up and find the most comfortable breathing position.
4. If the patient is unconscious, ventilatory support is required. Bag-valve-mask ventilation with oxygen is preferred over mouth-to-mouth resuscitation.
5. Once the upper airway is established, oxygen delivered, and ventilation supported, the diagnosis of the cause for the dyspnea must be determined. While the dentist does this, the emergency medical service is called to move the patient to the emergency room (ER) for definitive management of the problem.
6. Oxygen is administered and maintained until the patient can be transported to the ER. If hypoxia is so severe that the patient's level of consciousness is compromised, it may be necessary to expand the collapsed lung temporarily by inserting a large bore needle into the second intercostal space at the midclavicular line before transport to the ER.
7. If the patient has a history of asthma or COPD and the patient's usual management of bronchospasm reversed the acute episode, the patient can be discharged home. If the attack is difficult to reverse or is more severe than usual, however, the patient should be transported to the ER for evaluation.
8. If the patient has bronchospasm or laryngeal edema that is severe and possibly allergic in origin, subcutaneous epinephrine should be administered.
9. If vomiting occurs, the patient should be placed in a head-down position and suction used to remove the material from the mouth. Oxygen is administered and the patient transported to the ER for treatment.
10. Patients with pulmonary edema should receive oxygen and are transported to the hospital.
11. Patients with acute pulmonary embolism should receive oxygen and are transported to the hospital to receive anticoagulant therapy and supportive respiratory treatment.
12. If dyspnea and nonpleuritic chest pain are present, the patient may be having a myocardial infarction.
13. If all organic causes have been eliminated, hyperventilation syndrome or psychogenic hyperventilation should be suspected.

have dyspnea from pulmonary embolism. A patient with a history of allergies may be having an acute allergic reaction. The medications the patient takes or a recent need to increase dosage will help determine the severity of the disease and possible origin of the dyspnea.

A history of orthopnea or paroxysmal nocturnal dyspnea indicates that congestive heart failure may be contributing to an acute episode of dyspnea. A history of neuromuscular weakness may indicate underlying neuromuscular disease.[2,5,7] Past history of myocardial infarction may suggest a cardiac cause for the dyspnea.

The patient should describe the dyspnea to help identify the underlying cause of the breathlessness.[1] Asthmatic patients describe their dyspnea as "chest tightness" or "constriction."

Patients with emphysema often use "air hunger" and "gasping" to describe their dyspnea and do not report chest tightness. Patients with congestive heart failure report rapid breathing, a feeling of suffocation, and "air hunger." These descriptions are not diagnostic but can help guide the differential diagnosis.

The patients must be questioned about associated symptoms. Is chest pain associated with the dyspnea? If the pain is substernal and not altered by breathing, it is probably cardiac in origin. If the pain is pleuritic and increases with inspiration, it is probably pulmonary in origin and may be caused by a pulmonary embolism or pneumothorax.

A careful physical examination is done as the history is obtained.[8,9] General mental status provides information about the level of oxygenation. The respiratory rate is a useful indicator of the patient's distress and the efficacy of treatment. The examination is usually focused on the head, neck, and chest. The position of the trachea is determined, and the neck veins are examined for jugular venous distention in the semisitting position, which will show elevated right ventricular pressure. The chest and neck are examined for signs of respiratory distress. Inward movement of the soft tissue above the sternal notch with inhalation, retraction of the intercostal muscles on inhalation, and use of the accessory respiratory muscles indicate significant respiratory difficulty. The skin is examined for cyanosis, and the patient's body habitus is evaluated for obesity, thinness, and a barrel chest.

The chest is examined with a stethoscope for wheezing, decreased breath sounds, and crackles. Wheezing is heard with bronchoconstriction, decreased breath sounds are present with pneumothorax, and crackles are associated with increased fluid in the lungs. The respiratory cycle is carefully evaluated. Normally, inhalation occupies about two thirds of the cycle and exhalation one third of the cycle. A prolonged inhalation phase suggests upper airway obstruction and a prolonged exhalation phase is observed with lower airway obstruction in COPD and asthma.

The history and physical examination usually focus on the differential diagnosis but are not diagnostic of the cause for the dyspnea. If cardiac disease is suspected, the electrocardiogram (ECG), chest radiograph, and echocardiogram help make the final diagnosis after emergency medical personnel transport the patient to the hospital. The ECG reveals ischemia and dysrhythmia. The chest radiograph demonstrates dilated pulmonary veins and enlargement of the left atrium and ventricle associated with congestive heart failure. The echocardiogram shows valvular heart disease.

Pulmonary embolism, pneumothorax, and pulmonary edema can be difficult to diagnose with the history and physical examination. When pulmonary embolism is suspected, a ventilation/perfusion scan is done. A normal scan will rule out pulmonary embolism. If the scan is abnormal, a noninvasive lower extremity ultrasound is done. If the ultrasound is positive for thrombophlebitis, it is likely that that patient has pulmonary embolism. A chest radiograph is use to detect a pneumothorax. No definitive test exists for pulmonary edema, and the diagnosis depends on the clinical information and chest radiographic findings.

TREATMENT

The primary treatment for dyspnea is aimed at establishing and maintaining an airway and assisting ventilation as necessary.[6-11,12] This is accomplished in the dental office by airway management dictated by the algorithms of basic cardiopulmonary resuscitation.

The treatment of decompensated COPD is aimed at relieving the hypoxia. Therefore it is essential that these patients receive supplemental oxygen. Controversy surrounds the use of oxygen in patients who chronically retain CO_2. These patients presumably receive their respiratory drive from hypoxia, and if the hypoxia is corrected, they might stop breathing. It is not clear whether this actually occurs, and even so, these patients should be given supplemental oxygen when their condition is deteriorating.[9] If the oxygen suppresses their respirations, they can be given manual bag-valve-mask ventilation. Lifesaving oxygen should not be denied the patient in need.

After stabilizing the airway and achieving adequate ventilation, the underlying disease must be identified and treated. Treatments for pulmonary and cardiac causes of dyspnea are discussed in the appropriate chapters. The emergency treatment of dyspnea involves either (1) administering supplemental oxygen and stabilizing the patients with the medications they use to manage their disease or (2) transporting the unstable patient to the emergency room.

Patients with bronchospasm should receive oxygen and bronchodilators. Patients with upper airway obstruction must have the obstruction removed or have an airway surgically established. Patients who aspirate gastric content should be transported to the hospital for monitoring and treatment. A pneumothorax requires surgical management to reexpand the lung. Inadequate oxygenation mandates immediate surgical treatment. Emergency medical personnel can place a needle in the pleural cavity at the midclavicular line in the second intercostal space to expand the lung temporarily if immediate treatment is needed to correct severe hypoxia. Pulmonary embolism requires anticoagulant therapy and supportive respiratory therapy to maintain oxygenation. Pulmonary edema must be managed by treating the underlying cause.

Allergic reactions causing laryngeal edema or bronchospasm must be treated similar to any allergic reaction. β-Sympathetic agonists are used to manage the allergic reaction and bronchospasm. If the laryngeal edema causes severe upper airway obstruction, the patient may require endotracheal intubation or cricothyrotomy to establish a patent airway.

If the dyspnea is caused by cardiac disease, the underlying congestive heart failure, myocardial infarction, or valvular disease must be stabilized.[6-9] In the emergency situation, oxygen can be administered to correct hypoxemia. An intravenous catheter is placed to administer the medications needed to manage the complications associated with a myocardial infarction.

SUMMARY

The differential diagnosis of dyspnea includes cardiac, pulmonary, neurologic, and psychological causes.[5-9] When a patient develops dyspnea in the office, the dentist first must establish the severity of the problem and urgency for treatment. Upper airway obstruction must be eliminated and oxygen administered. If the patient is not breathing, ventilatory support is needed using a bag-mask system or endotracheal tube. The medical history and clinical examination are used to make a preliminary diagnosis; more specific treatments can then be instituted. As with any acute medical emergency, the key to successful management and outcome is early diagnosis and treatment. Dyspnea is a warning of an impending respiratory emergency that cannot be ignored without severe consequences.

REFERENCES

1. Schwartzstein RM: The language of dyspnea. In Mahler DA, editor: *Dyspnea*, New York, 1998, Dekker.
2. Mahler DA: Diagnosis of dyspnea. In Mahler DA, editor: *Dyspnea*, New York, 1998, Dekker.
3. Manning HL, Schwartzstein RM: Mechanism of dyspnea. In Mahler DA, editor: *Dyspnea*, New York, 1998, Dekker.
4. Tobin MJ: Dyspnea: pathophysiologic basis, clinical presentation, and management. *Arch Intern Med* 150:1604, 1990.
5. Ferrin MS, Tino G: Acute dyspnea, AACN *Clin Issues* 8:398, 1997.
6. Dailey RH: Evaluation of dyspnea. In Schwartz GR, editor: *Principles and practice of emergency medicine*, ed 4, Baltimore, 1999, Williams & Wilkins.
7. Spears KL, Williams JA, Hutson HR: Dyspnea. In Rosen P, Barkin R, editors: *Emergency medicine: concepts and clinical practice*, ed 4, St Louis, 1998, Mosby.
8. Mills J, Luce JM: Dyspnea, respiratory distress, and respiratory failure. In Saunder CE, Ho MT, editors: *Current emergency diagnosis and treatment*, ed 4, East Norwalk, Conn, 1992, Appleton & Lange.
9. Caroline NL: Respiratory emergencies. In *Emergency care in the streets*, ed 5, Boston, 1995, Little, Brown.
10. James CF: Pulmonary aspiration of gastric contents. In Gravenstein N, Kirby RR, editors: *Complication in anesthesiology*, ed 2, Philadelphia, 1996, Lippincott.
11. Johnson C, Mayer P, Grosz D: Pulmonary edema following naloxone administration in a healthy orthopedic patient, *J Clin Anesth* 7:356, 1995.
12. Trayner Jr. EM, Celli Br: Strategies in the treatment of dyspnea. In Mahler DA, editor: *Dyspnea*, New York, 1998, Dekker.

Hyperventilation

Brent B. Ward
Stephen E. Feinberg

Hyperventilation is a pathologic state in which alveolar ventilation is increased above the requirements of normal metabolism. It results from an increase in respiratory rate, tidal volume, or both, causing a decrease in the partial pressure of arterial carbon dioxide ($Paco_2$). Stress-induced (psychological) hyperventilation is known as *hyperventilation syndrome*, which occurs in 6% to 11% of the population.[1] It is estimated that hyperventilation syndrome accounts for more than 9% of all emergencies in the dental office.[2] Although anxiety is the most likely etiology of hyperventilation in the dental setting, it is important to consider and rule out other causes that may mimic the clinical presentation of hyperventilation.[3,4] This chapter focuses on the pathophysiology, clinical manifestations, and management of the differential diagnosis of hyperventilation, with a focus on the most common cause of acute hyperventilation, hyperventilation syndrome.

UNIVERSAL MEASURES

Regardless of the ultimate diagnosis, respiratory abnormalities are frequently associated with anxiety. Stress reduction is always appropriate even if it is not the primary etiologic factor. Stress may exacerbate and perpetuate episodes of respiratory distress and many of its symptoms. The release of adrenaline and activation of the sympathetic nervous system may also aggravate the situation. A vicious cycle ensues. To break this cycle, all stress-inducing procedures should be terminated when hyperventilation is first noticed. Initial positioning of the hyperventilating patient is dictated primarily by patient comfort. The vast majority of patients prefer an upright seated position. Supine patients tend to have increased difficulty in breathing due to pressure on the diaphragm from the abdominal contents. Additionally, increased difficulty of breathing has a high propensity to increase the stress associated with hyperventilation and therefore potentially increase and prolong the symptoms.

Active measures to calm the patient with verbal intervention by the dentist are the most important means to reduce the patient's stress levels. This approach may be curative for some etiologies of hyperventilation and should therefore be the first and a continued intervention during any episode. The personal patient contact and reassurance can also reduce the symptoms of those etiologies that are not cured by decreasing the patient's stress response. With all procedures stopped and the patient appropriately positioned and reassured, an "ABC" (airway-breathing-circulation) approach should then be used (Box 6-1).

ACID-BASE BALANCE

The primary function of the respiratory system is to ensure an adequate exchange of oxygen and carbon dioxide (CO_2) between the blood and the atmosphere. Oxygen is essential for aerobic metabolism. An increased requirement for oxygen or a decreased ability to deliver such oxygen to the peripheral tissues will result in increased alveolar ventilation. CO_2 is an end product of aerobic metabolism. When combined with water, CO_2 forms carbonic acid, which dissociates into free hydrogen ions (H^+) and bicarbonate (HCO_3^-). The equilibration between these compounds forms the carbonic acid–bicarbonate buffer system, as follows:

$$HCO_3^- + H^+ \leftrightarrow H_2CO_3 \leftrightarrow CO_2 + H_2O$$

The body has four major buffer systems. The carbonic acid–bicarbonate buffer system is the primary buffer of the extracellular space. The buffer systems function by absorbing H^+, which would otherwise cause significant changes in the body's hydrogen ion concentration (pH). Buffer systems maintain the body within a narrow pH range that allows proper cellular function.

Box 6-1   The "ABC" Approach

A: AIRWAY
What is the integrity of the patient's airway? An evaluation determines whether the airway is sufficient or is compromised by blockage (e.g., foreign object, gastric contents aspiration, laryngospasm) or constriction (e.g., asthma, chronic obstructive pulmonary disease, anaphylaxis, epiglottitis).

B: BREATHING
What is the quality of the patient's breathing? The rate, depth, and pattern of breathing are important. The *rate* can be easily calculated by counting the number of respirations over 15 seconds. However, a longer interval may be necessary to observe for irregularities in the *pattern* of breathing. The *depth* is a clinical assessment of the amount of air being exchanged. Useful tools in assessing depth include visualization of chest excursions and accessory muscles. Often, placing of the back of the dentist's hand in front of the patient's mouth without obstruction allows a subjective assessment of the flow being produced by the patient. Auscultation of lung fields to listen for air exchange will identify abnormal sounds consistent with specific diagnoses. Pulse

oximetry, if available, will identify abnormalities in oxygenation (not ventilation) and may assist in arriving at a suspected or definitive diagnosis depending on the condition. *Cyanosis* is the desaturation of at least 5 g of hemoglobin. Examining the tongue, lips, tip of the nose and ears will detect central cyanosis, which represents a lack of oxygenation. Detection of cyanosis on the peripheral skin may suggest a circulatory abnormality rather than a respiratory abnormality.

C: CIRCULATION
Hemodynamic stability of the patient should be assessed. Rate and regularity of pulse should be evaluated. Tachycardia should be anticipated. Cardiac arrhythmias, such as atrial fibrillation, may indicate an underlying cardiac abnormality. A blood pressure reading should also be obtained. These parameters should be repeated at appropriate intervals. The neck should be examined for jugular venous distention. However, labored breathing causes continuous fluctuations in intrathoracic pressure, which makes a diagnosis of increased central venous pressure more difficult.

Of the acidic byproducts of metabolism, CO_2 is unique in that the lungs can eliminate it. Increases in CO_2 result in an increase in free hydrogen ion and are synonymous with *respiratory acidosis*. Decreases in CO_2 result in a decrease in H^+ and are synonymous with *respiratory alkalosis*. The kidneys eliminate all other acid byproducts of metabolism. An increase in these acidic byproducts is referred to as *metabolic acidosis*. The numerous causes for metabolic acidosis and metabolic alkalosis are not significant to this discussion.

The body strives to maintain a physiologic pH by continuously balancing the respiratory and metabolic components. Changes in ventilation can result in rapid changes in $Paco_2$. Increases or decreases in alveolar ventilation can rapidly and predictably cause a respiratory alkalosis or respiratory acidosis, respectively. This allows prompt compensation for metabolic disturbances. Metabolic compensation for primary respiratory acid-base disturbances requires significant time.

DIFFERENTIAL DIAGNOSIS

Hyperventilation is an increase in respiratory rate and depth beyond that required for normal me-

tabolism. Various disease states may cause an increase in respiratory rate and depth, which may represent either hyperventilation or hyperpnea. In *hyperpnea*, respirations are deeper and more rapid than normal, which may reflect a metabolic abnormality, such as lack of oxygenation or need to compensate for a metabolic acidosis. Some of the complexity associated with hyperventilation is demonstrated in Figure 6-1.

The differential diagnosis of hyperventilation requires the retrieval of a complete medical history and its correlation to the history of the present illness, the patient's vital signs, and the physical findings (Box 6-2). The medical history may be obtained from the patient, a friend or relative, or past records. Observers may be able to provide necessary information pertaining to the development of the episode, if necessary. For a patient who is actively hyperventilating, the history of present illness should elucidate the length of time the patient has been hyperventilating, as well as the precipitating, alleviating, and exacerbating factors. The clinician should also elucidate the symptoms, and, if they have occurred previously, the treatment regimens used and their effect. Depending on the severity of the situation, taking the history may have to be delayed until initial therapy has been provided.

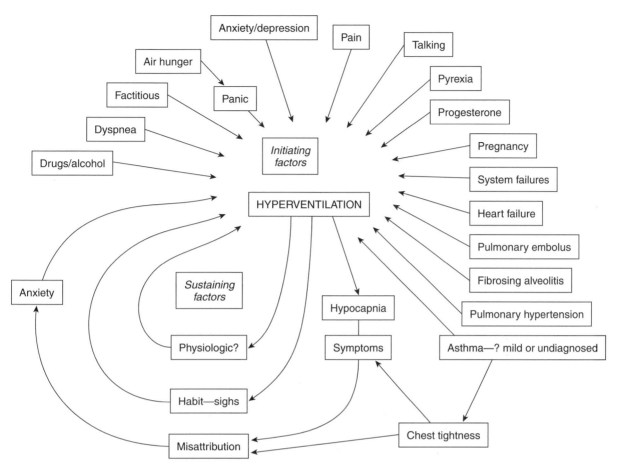

Figure 6-1. Interaction of factors initiating (*top* and *right*) and sustaining *(bottom left)* acute and subacute hyperventilation. *From Gardner W: Chest 109:516-534, 1996.*

Box 6-2	Differential Diagnosis of Hyperventilation

METABOLIC DISORDERS
Lactic acidosis
Diabetic ketoacidosis*
Biotin-dependent multicarboxylase deficiency
Malignant hyperthermia
Dehydrogenase deficiency
Liver failure
Sepsis*

CARDIOPULMONARY
Asthma*
Pulmonary embolus
Pulmonary hypertension
Congestive heart failure*

CHEMICAL-INDUCED CONDITIONS
Progesterone
Aspirin*

Drugs of abuse
Alcohol
Dinitrophenol
Nicotine
Tricyclic antidepressants

NEUROLOGIC DISORDERS
Central hyperventilation
Cerebral lymphomas

PSYCHIATRIC DISORDERS
Panic disorder
Hyperventilation syndrome

OTHER CONDITIONS
Pregnancy
Heat exhaustion
Stroke

*Diagnoses are discussed in this chapter.

Although it may be readily apparent that the diagnosis is hyperventilation, the clinician should perform a gross inspection and assess the respiratory rate. The normal respiratory rate for an adult patient is 14 to 20 breaths/minute. The clinician should also assess the respiratory depth and pattern, looking for differences in inspiration and expiration, paradoxical chest movements, signs of obstruction, wheezing, coughing, aphonia, pallor, cyanosis, and jugular venous distention. The clinician should inquire about dyspnea, even though this may not help confirm a diagnosis of hyperventilation syndrome, which may occur with or without dyspnea.

HYPERVENTILATION SYNDROME

Hyperventilation syndrome (*stress-induced hyperventilation*) is the type of hyperventilation most often seen in the dental setting, although it only accounts for 1% of all episodes of hyperventilation.[5] In arriving at the diagnosis of hyperventilation syndrome, the dentist must recognize the clinical signs associated with this disorder to separate it from other disorders in the differential diagnosis. The overall medical history of the patient should be carefully considered so as not to overlook a more serious condition. Recognition of this syndrome's acute onset in association with stress-inducing factors is the most helpful indicator in its delineation. Importantly, hyperventilation syndrome is normally self-limiting and is most often rapidly treated to resolution. The persistence of symptoms in the face of appropriate treatment should raise significant concerns about a more serious diagnosis.

Historical Perspective

In 1937 Kerr and others introduced the term *hyperventilation syndrome.*[6] Descriptions date back to 1871, when Da Costa published his observations of soldiers in the Civil War in "On Irritable Heart: a Clinical Study of a Functional Cardiac Disorder and Its Consequences." *Soldiers heart* was used to describe these symptoms during World War I. Not until the early 1900s was a clinical study undertaken to elucidate the causes and effects of hyperventilation syndrome. Even today, debate continues over the exact etiology and the many symptoms.

Pathophysiology and Clinical Course

The period after injection of a local anesthetic is the most common time for initiation of hyper-

ventilation, with subsequent cascading of signs and symptoms (Box 6-3). However, the situation may also occur at any time during the course of treatment. Some patients show obvious signs of increased respiration in association with a "panic attack." Others have more subtle signs, which may even go unnoticed by the patient and the practitioner. Usually, the patient initially complains of lightheadedness, dizziness, chest discomfort, dysphagia, and nausea. Symptoms such as palpitations, trembling, and sweating are nonspecific and associated with the adrenergic stimulation secondary to anxiety. These sensations increase the patient's anxiety and elicit a positive-feedback perpetuation of symptoms.

Respiratory changes in the acute setting include an increased ventilatory response in depth and rate of respiration. Minimal respiratory elevation may be present, but patients often gasp for breath at a rate that approaches the mid-60s. Ultimately, this can result in exhaustion of respiratory musculature and chest pain.

The increase in minute ventilation (tidal volume × respiratory rate) results in a decrease in $Paco_2$ (normal, 35 to 45 mm Hg). This results in an increase in the blood pH above the normal physiologic pH of 7.40 (range 7.35 to 7.45). *Respiratory alkalosis* shifts the oxyhemoglobin dissociation curve to the left, increasing the affinity of oxygen for hemoglobin and decreasing the delivery of oxygen to tissues. Alterations in pH also result in changes in the balance of both ionized and bound electrolytes, as well as intracellular and extracellular electrolytes.

Several adverse consequences occur in the cardiovascular system. *Hypocapnia* (low $Paco_2$) induces coronary artery vasoconstriction. The release of adrenaline and activation of the sympathetic nervous system secondary to anxiety are associated with an increase in heart rate. Myocardial oxygen demand increases as the ability to satisfy that demand decreases. The shift in the oxyhemoglobin dissociation curve further compromises the oxygen supply to the myocardium. The net effect is a potential imbalance between oxygen supply and demand. *Chest pain* in the hyperventilating patient is most often caused by the exhausted respiratory musculature and is compounded by the palpitations associated with anxiety and adrenergic stimulation. Chest pain may be difficult to distinguish from anginal pain, although in select patients the pain may be of myocardial etiology and either secondary to or aggravated by the oxygen imbalance. This is not significant for all patients, but it creates a diagnostic dilemma for the patient with atheroscle-

| Box 6-3 | Clinical Manifestations of Acute Hyperventilation |

NEUROLOGIC
Lightheadedness
Headache
Visual disturbances (blurred or tunnel vision)
Paresthesias of face, chest extremities, or trunk
Dizziness, faintness, vertigo, seizures

CARDIOVASCULAR
Palpitations
Precordial pain
Tachycardia

RESPIRATORY
Shortness of breath
Tachypnea, hyperpnea
Painful breathing

MUSCULOSKELETAL
Muscle cramps or pains
Tremors
Tetany

GASTROINTESTINAL
Epigastric pain
Xerostomia
Dysphagia
Nausea and vomiting

PSYCHOLOGICAL
Anxiety
Apprehension
Panic
Disorientation

rotic heart disease, who may be more susceptible to the potential oxygen imbalances (see Chapter 7).

Neurologic symptoms include headaches, visual disturbances, dizziness, tinnitus, ataxia, altered consciousness, and syncope. These are produced by the decreased cerebral perfusion associated with the hypocapnia-induced cerebral vasoconstriction.[7] Symptoms worsen because of the increased affinity of oxygen for hemoglobin, which decreases the availability of oxygen to the tissues. *Paresthesias*, occurring either unilaterally or bilaterally on the face, chest, and extremities, are one of the most frequent complaints of patients. *Tetany* is the most common sign in the musculoskeletal system and can lead to carpopedal spasms. This state of altered sensation may be associated with central causes or a reduced concentration of ionized calcium, which may increase peripheral nerve excitability.[8] This state has more recently been associated with the cellular influx of phosphorus secondary to increases in glycolysis.[9]

Prevention

Prevention of acute hyperventilation begins with the identification of patients at risk for episodes. Patients with previous attacks are especially prone to recurrence. Furthermore, patients whose medical histories are positive for anxiety disorders or other psychological disturbances are more prone to events in the dental setting. Signs of anxiety include increased perspiration, mild tachycardia, elevations in blood pressure, and a mild increase in the respiratory rate. Initial vital signs should be taken in a "nonstress-

ful" environment so that a baseline is established for comparison. Anxious patients may be very talkative or difficult to engage in conversation. They usually appear uncomfortable and untrusting. Procedures that reduce stress are preventive in patients at risk for hyperventilation syndrome. Pharmacologic or verbal sedative techniques can assist in allaying the fears of the apprehensive patient. The effective administration and appropriate use of local anesthetics is of paramount importance, and failure to do so is associated with the majority of events.

 Rapid Assessment of Acute Hyperventilation

PMH: Previous history of hyperventilation, psychiatric disorders (panic disorder, phobias, etc.)
MEDS: Medications of psychiatric disorders
All: Noncontributory
HPI: Acute onset associated with stressful stimuli, generally rapidly treated successfully
Key Vital Signs and Physical Findings: Tachypnea, sighing, shortness of breath, pain on respiration, nonradiating chest pain, tachycardia, mild hypertension, lungs clear to auscultation, normal oxygen saturation, dizziness, faintness, altered consciousness, peripheral paresthesias, muscle cramps, tremor, myalgia

TREATMENT

Patients who clinically begin to hyperventilate should be reassured and encouraged to slow the rate and decrease the depth of their breathing. Procedures should be terminated and all objects removed from the oral cavity. The patient should be positioned in the most comfortable position, usually seated upright in this situation. Restrictive clothing about the neck should be loosened. Universal measures should ensue. A physical examination should include an assessment of respiratory rate, dyspnea, auscultation of the lungs, skin and mucosal color, oxygen saturation (if available), and heart rate and rhythm. Vital signs and physical examination are likely to reveal tachypnea with or without dyspnea, lungs clear to auscultation, mucosa without signs of cyanosis, a normal oxygen saturation, tachycardia, and mild hypertension.

Once a definitive diagnosis of hyperventilation syndrome is reached, forced nasal breathing has been reported to be successful as an initial treatment.[10] Individuals who do not resolve with this approach may be directed to slow their breathing. Several methods may be employed. The dentist may rhythmically count, instructing the patient to take a breath at specific intervals. Instructing the patient to breath-hold after each exhalation is also advantageous. It is important to reassure the patient continuously.

In the event that they are unable to control their hyperventilation, patients may be instructed to cup their hands over their mouth and nose (Figure 6-2). This method is useful in the initial stages to elevate the $Paco_2$ minimally and, more importantly, to calm patients who will feel the warmth of their breath on their hands and face. Use of a noncollapsible paper bag over the mouth and nose is more effective in severe cases and allows a much fuller rebreathing of air rich in CO_2 (Figure 6-3). Patients should continually be reassured that all is well and encouraged to slow their respiration.

If these measures are not effective, pharmacologic anxiolytic therapy is indicated. Intramuscular, intravenous, or nasal administration of a benzodiazepine is usually effective but is rarely required. Individuals should not administer a parenteral benzodiazepine for the management of hyperventilation unless they are appropriately trained in sedative measures. Oxygen therapy is contraindicated in the routine management of hyperventilation syndrome. The oxygen flow tends

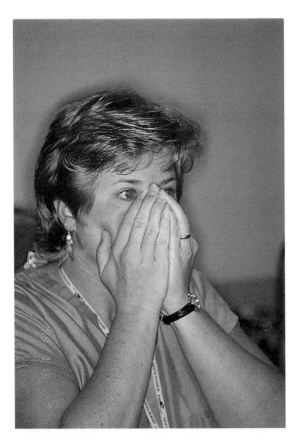

Figure 6-2. Initial treatment for episode of acute hyperventilation.

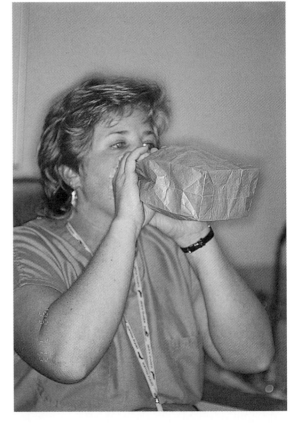

Figure 6-3. Active correction of decreased $Paco_2$ through full rebreathing in a paper bag.

to dilute the expired gases and decrease the amount of CO_2 available to be rebreathed. Excessive flow can exacerbate the symptoms. More likely, oxygen flow will diminish the rise in $Paco_2$ and slow the course of recovery. In select patients at risk for myocardial ischemia, low-flow oxygen may be indicated. A nasal cannula with an oxygen flow of 2 liters per minute may be attached to the patient. The patient then breathes through the paper bag. The low flow minimizes the CO_2 "washout" effect and provides supplemental oxygen to counter the adverse effects of peripheral oxygen release.

The symptoms of hyperventilation syndrome can resolve within minutes of effective treatment. Resolution is inversely proportional to the severity of symptoms (Box 6-4).

Disposition

After resolution of symptoms, the dentist should engage the patient in conversation regarding the onset and causes of the episode. If a direct psychological factor cannot be identified, a medical work-up to rule out other causes is appropriate, and further dental treatment should be delayed. In the absence of other medical concerns, the physician and patient should decide whether to continue treatment for that day. Factors to consider include severity and length of the episode, whether the patient is past the stress-inducing portion of the procedure (i.e., the patient now has adequate anesthesia), and most importantly the patient's feelings regarding continuing the procedure.

Regardless of whether the procedure is completed, plans regarding definitive stress reduction at future visits should be discussed with the patient. Pharmacologic agents often help reduce anxiety for patients and prevent attacks. Generally, benzodiazepines at standard doses given the previous evening and 1 hour before (perioperative) the appointment are effective. Patients need an escort if a perioperative sedative agent is used. Additionally, patients may opt for intravenous sedation as a

---

| **Box 6-4** | **Case Study: Hyperventilation Syndrome** |

A 32-year-old male presents on an emergency basis for evaluation and treatment of tooth no. 29, which has been bothersome for some time. His past medical history is negative, and his blood pressure is 112/80, heart rate 78 and regular, and respirations 14. On oral examination you find evidence of a generalized lack of dental care. The patient requires simple extraction of tooth no. 29 today and multiple restorative procedures in the future. When questioned regarding previous dental care, the patient responds that he has not been to a dentist in a long time.

On administration of the local anesthetic, the patient forcefully grabs the arms of the chair and takes multiple deep, rapid breaths, which are discontinued as the administration of local anesthesia ends. The patient initially seems to return to his baseline recordings but on careful evaluation has a respiratory rate of 20 with a minor increase in depth that continues over the next 30 seconds. Attempts to reassure the patent are unsuccessful, and universal measures begin. Vital signs and physical examination reveal an increased blood pressure of 135/88, a heart rate of 100, and an increase in respiratory rate to 24 with a significant increase in depth. The patient's mucosal membranes are of normal coloration. The patient begins to complain of chest pains associated with numbness and tingling of the arms and face. The patient is encouraged only to use nasal breathing into cupped hands while a staff member is sent for a paper bag in the office emergency kit. By the time the bag arrives, the patient has had some resolution of symptoms.

The patient is allowed to continue to breathe into the paper bag until all his symptoms have resolved.

Questioning of the patient after the episode reveals that 5 years earlier he had a similar attack associated with "the shot" that he was too embarrassed to report and that had kept him from routine dental care. The patient now has complete anesthesia and would like to proceed with the procedure. The patient's vital signs have returned to normal, and tooth no. 29 is extracted uneventfully.

On discharge, both the patient and doctor are comfortable with the patient's ability to leave unaccompanied. Definitive plans for stress prevention in future visits are made with the patient. In this case the plan includes oral pharmacologic presedation with triazolam (halcion) 0.25 mg the night before and 1 hour before the appointment, and nitrous oxide sedation during the administration of local anesthesia.

The patient understands that he will need an escort to and from the office for the next visit, due to the administration of an oral sedative. Furthermore, the patient is referred to a psychologist to discuss stress-coping strategies because of the recurrent nature of the episodes.

means of coping with the stresses of future dental care. Psychological evaluation should be considered for prevention of future episodes and is especially indicated in individuals with recurrent attacks. Regardless of the ultimate decision, the patient should participate in this planning process and feel comfortable with its result. After formulating the plan, the patient may be discharged without an escort.

METABOLIC ACIDOSIS SECONDARY TO DIABETIC KETOACIDOSIS

Metabolic acidosis secondary to diabetes is precipitated by a deficiency in insulin in conjunction with a relative or absolute increase in glucagon. This complication of diabetes may lead to diabetic ketoacidosis (DKA), which is usually associated with type I diabetes mellitus patients who discontinue their insulin regimen. Occasionally, DKA may be seen in "well-controlled" type I diabetics who undergo a physically or emotionally stressful procedure. A decrease in circulating insulin results in impaired peripheral utilization of glucose and a relative increase in glucagon. The shift in the balance of the insulin/glucagon ratio in favor of glucagon ultimately results in a decrease in peripheral glucose transport and is associated with a massive gluconeogenesis, leading to severe hyperglycemia, osmotic diuresis, and volume depletion. Relative increases in glucagon also activate ketone body production, which results in ketosis for energy and a ketoacidotic state.

The body attempts to correct its pH by a variety of compensatory mechanisms, initially by lowering serum CO_2 levels through hyperventilation. *Kussmaul breathing*, classically described as "air hunger," is associated with prolonged rapid and deep breathing. Accessory muscles of respiration are used in this process. The breathing is unrelenting until either the underlying metabolic acidosis is corrected or the exhausted patient can no longer tolerate the respiratory demand. Cramping and direct or referred pain from the diaphragm and accessory muscles accompany later stages of the process.

HEART FAILURE

Heart failure is the result of decreased cardiac function that leads to blood flow inadequate to meet the metabolic needs of the body. Its causes include primary myocardial failure and myocardial failure secondary to other abnor-

 Rapid Assessment of Diabetic Ketoacidosis

PMH: Disease occurs almost exclusively in type I diabetes; rarely, reported in type 2 diabetes
MEDS: Insulin, oral hypoglycemic agents
All: Noncontributory
HPI: Noncompliance with medications, may be precipitated by stressful event (e.g., sepsis, myocardial infarction)
Key Vital Signs and Physical Findings: Kussmaul breathing, acetone (fruity) breath, tachycardia, hypotension, thirst associated with increased urination and signs of volume depletion, clear lungs to auscultation, normal oxygen saturation, nausea and vomiting, abdominal pain, increased blood glucose levels, lethargy, fatigue, altered consciousness and coma.

malities, such as in valves or vessels. *Congestive heart failure* results when the failure leads to the retention of fluid in excess of normal body water.

Specific predisposing events include infection, arrhythmia, myocardial infarction, pulmonary embolism, and emotional or physical stress. Most important to the dental professional, emotional stress may precipitate events in individuals with or without previous history if they were previously marginally compensated.

Dyspnea is a common manifestation in heart failure. It results from increased pulmonary venous pressure with fluid shifts into the pulmonary interstitium, resulting in compression of the alveoli and impaired gas exchange. Clinical symptoms include anxiety, restlessness, and air hunger. *Cheyne-Stokes respiration*, a cyclic respiratory pattern that alternates between periods of hyperventilation and apnea, is also characteristic of the heart failure patient. This phenomena is the product of a decrease in the respiratory centers sensitivity to $Paco_2$ and an increase in blood circulation time. Due to the increase in circulation time the respiratory center does not synchronize respiratory drive with $Paco_2$ and partial pressure of arterial oxygen ($Paco_2$). The result is hypoventilation leading to an increase in $Paco_2$ and decrease in $Paco_2$. As the respiratory center senses these changes late, the patient compensates with hyperventilation, resulting in hyperoxygenation and hypocapnia. The resulting compensation is a prolonged period of apnea. The more impaired the circulation, the longer are the periods of hyperventilation and apnea. Cheynes-Stokes

Rapid Assessment of Heart Failure

PMH: Hypertension, valvular dysfunction, idiopathic or acquired cardiomyopathy, anemia, arrhythmia
MEDS: Antihypertensives, vasodilators, inotropes, diuretics
All: Noncontributory
HPI: Acute decompensation of a previously well or well-compensated cardiac patient
Key Vital Signs and Physical Findings: Tachycardia, pulsus paradoxus, dyspnea, moderate-to-severe hyperventilation with Cheyne-Stokes respiration, lung auscultation with rales, pink frothy fluid, cyanosis, decreased oxygen saturation

breathing is exacerbated by hypertension and cerebrovascular disease.

ASTHMA

Asthma is a disease of increased airway reactivity caused by a variety of stimuli and resulting in significant narrowing of the respiratory complex. An estimated 4% of the population have a component of asthma. Attacks tend to be episodic in nature and may occur frequently or rarely, depending on the severity of disease and the adequacy of treatment. Attacks are usually brief and self-limited, especially when bronchodilator "rescue therapy" is utilized. The most severe complication is associated with *status asthmaticus*, in which obstruction remains for days or weeks. Under extremely rare circumstances, acute episodes may result in death.

A variety of stimuli have been hypothesized, including environmental allergens, medications (e.g., aspirin, nonsteroidal antiinflammatory drugs [NSAIDS], β-blockers), infections, exercise, and emotional stress. In the dental setting, stress undoubtedly plays the most significant role in induction.

The key difference between other differential diagnoses and asthma is the physical findings of wheezing and cough in association with a decrease in air movement due to airway constriction. These physical changes lead to hyperventilation to compensate for the low amounts of oxygen delivered to the lungs with each breath. Ultimately, asthma may result in hypoxia as well. Additional physical signs of acute attack include the patient's use of accessory breathing muscles and a visualized, palpated, or auscultated paradoxical pulse.

Patients with a history of asthma should bring their bronchodilator inhalers with them to appointments in the event an attack occurs.

Rapid Assessment of Asthma

PMH: Severity elucidated by questions regarding hospitalizations, emergency department visits, use of systemic steroids, most recent attack, and frequency of attacks
MEDS: Inhaled corticosteroids and ß-agonists, methylxanthines (theophylline), anticholinergics, mast cell stabilizers (cromolyn)
All: Multiple environmental factors; intolerance to aspirin, NSAIDS, or ß-blockers
HPI: Acute onset with increased difficulty in breathing from known etiologic agent or associated with stress induction, wheezing, dyspnea, and hyperventilation associated from increased rate with decreased airflow
Key Vital Signs and Physical Findings: Tachycardia, pulsus paradoxus, mild hypertension, moderate-to-severe hyperventilation demonstrated by increase rate with decreased volumes, lung wheezing to auscultation, normal to decreased oxygen saturation.

PULMONARY EMBOLISM

Pulmonary embolism (PE) is estimated to cause more than 50,000 deaths per year. It generally results from migration of deep venous thrombosis (DVT) from the lower extremity. Classically the pathophysiology of the disease process was described by Virchow, who defined its risks as being a triad of vessel wall changes, stasis, and thrombogenic changes in the blood.

The many risk factors for PE are beyond the scope of this review. Specific associations likely to be encountered in the dental office include (but are not limited to) male gender, age over 40, obesity, malignancy, pregnancy, recent surgical procedure or period of inactivity, and previous history of DVT or PE. Medications that alert the dentist to increased risk include oral contraceptive use and anticoagulant therapy.

Rapid Assessment of Pulmonary Embolism

PMH: Obesity, recent surgery, malignancy, need for anticoagulation, current pregnancy
MEDS: Oral contraceptives, coumadin
All: Noncontributory
HPI: Acute onset dyspnea associated with cough, pleuritic pain, and hemoptysis
Key Vital Signs and Physical Findings: Tachycardia, systemic hypotension, moderate to severe hyperventilation, lung auscultation positive for rales, decreased oxygen saturation

Hyperventilation in the patient with PE is the result of hypoxia due to ventilation/perfusion mismatch, which deprives an area of the lung from perfusion. Its severity is determined by the size of the affected area and the health of the residual lung tissue.

SEPSIS

Gram-negative sepsis is a bacterial disease that may be associated with significant hyperventilation secondary to acidosis and hypoxia. Sepsis affects both normal and immunocompromised hosts and is lethal in up to 30% of patients. Predisposing factors can include underlying host diseases (e.g., malignancy, diabetes, congestive heart failure, immunocompromising condition), malnutrition, or previous or current antibiotic therapy.

The pathophysiology associated with sepsis involves the release of host defense mediators in response to the lipopolysaccharide (LPS) endotoxin of the gram-negative bacteria. The LPS is capable of activating factors such as complement, tumor necrosis factor, interleukins, and lysosomal enzymes. These activated factors, which normally contain and localize infections, can lead to widespread injuries with septic shock and multiorgan system failure.

Hyperventilation associated with sepsis is the result of two contributing factors. *Hypoxemia* (low Pao_2) results from a ventilation/perfusion mismatch due to an increase in pulmonary capillary permeability, leading to an increase in pulmonary water content. Severe *hypotension* can cause a decrease in tissue perfusion, resulting in a metabolic (lactic) acidosis. As described with

 Rapid Assessment of Sepsis

PMH: Immunocompromised status, diabetes, congestive heart failure, malignancy, parotitis, sinusitis, significant facial space infection, recent surgical procedure requiring intubation or bladder catheterization
MEDS: Recent or current antibiotic therapy
All: Noncontributory
HPI: Recent fevers, hyperventilation; history of infection, hospitalization, or surgical procedures; process not consistent with acute decompensation of a previously normal dental patient
Key Vital Signs and Physical Findings: Tachycardia, hypotension, moderate to severe hyperventilation, lung auscultation positive for rales, decreased oxygen saturation

diabetes, metabolic acidosis is immediately compensated by the respiratory system through hyperventilation. This situation is exacerbated because the respiratory system is compromised due to the ventilation/perfusion mismatch.

SALICYLATE (ASPIRIN) OVERDOSE

Drug overdose reactions may lead to medical emergencies in the dental office. This section focuses on reactions that lead to hyperventilation, but overdose in general may lead to hyperventilation or hypoventilation, depending on the causative agent. Hyperventilation as a result of drug overdose is associated with a variety of medications, including aspirin (most common), dinitrophenol, nicotine, and xanthines.

Aspirin is prescribed or taken as an over-the-counter (OTC) medication by a large percentage of adult patients. Its primary prescriptive indications include the treatment of pain and inflammation; it is especially useful in rheumatoid arthritis and osteoarthritis, systemic lupus erythematosus, ankylosing spondylitis, and Reiter's syndrome. Aspirin is also useful as an antiplatelet agent for prevention of myocardial infarction and transient ischemic attacks. The OTC maximal dose, 4 g every 24 hours, may be increased under the care of a physician. Aspirin-induced hyperventilation is associated with immediate and late responses that are modulated by independent mechanisms. The immediate response results from direct stimulation of carotid chemoreceptors by salicylate, which uncouples oxidative phosphorylation. Experiments have shown this reaction in humans occurs at doses below the 24-hour OTC maximum (3.9 g).[4] Accordingly, most patients on high-dose aspirin therapy present with respiratory rates slightly above the norm and above their baseline (if baseline taken before aspirin therapy). Late-response aspirin toxicity is seen only at significantly higher levels of aspirin ingestion, 150 to 300 mg/kg of body weight (10.5 to 21 g in a 70-kg individual) or greater. Toxicity is associated with severe metabolic acidosis, vomiting, diaphoresis, dehydration, and tinnitus. Hyperventilation is a result of the severe metabolic acidosis associated with this type of overdose.

Treatment

Immediate-response aspirin-induced hyperventilation is of little consequence in the dental setting. Patients do not require treatment for this

Rapid Assessment of Aspirin Overdose

PMH: Rheumatoid arthritis, osteoarthritis, systemic lupus erythematosus, ankylosing spondylitis, Reiter's syndrome, myocardial infarction, transient ischemic attacks, chronic pain
MEDS: Acetylsalicylic acid (ASA)
All: Noncontributory
HPI: Immediate response: noncontributory; late response: history of acute ingestion of large quantities of aspirin
Key Vital Signs and Physical Findings: Mild tachycardia and hypertension, moderate-to-severe hyperventilation, lungs clear to auscultation, normal oxygen saturation

condition, other than ruling out possible late-response conditions, as well as other conditions in the differential diagnosis.

Late-response salicylate toxicity is associated with acute (one-time dose) and chronic (excessive therapeutic administration over 12 hours) overdoses. The treatment of either of these conditions requires evaluation of the patient in a hospital emergency department (ED). Cathartics are not beneficial in non-enteric-coated salicylate poisoning but may be of minimal value in enteric-coated overdose, depending on the proximity to ingestion.

ED treatment consists of activated charcoal administration (1 g/kg) and repeated serum salicylate levels. Intravenous hydration with close monitoring of electrolytes, coagulation, glucose, and renal function is indicated. Urine alkalinization is often performed to enhance the excretion of salicylate. Hemodialysis is indicated in patients who deteriorate in the face of appropriate medical management.

SUMMARY

Anxiety-induced hyperventilation is one of the most common medical emergencies in the dental office. A complete medical history, including psychological history and previous dental experiences, is important in identifying individuals at higher risk. Stress reduction procedures, either pharmacologic or nonpharmacologic, are indicated for all patients and can be preventive for episodes of stress-induced hyperventilation. When hyperventilation occurs, its clinical manifestations should be recognized and diseases in the differential diagnosis ruled out. Until the diagnosis is confirmed, universal intervention principles are followed.

Treatment of hyperventilation syndrome requires both physiologic and psychological support for rapid resolution of symptoms. This disorder is rarely life threatening if other medical causes have been eliminated. Open dialogue with the patient after an episode is important to identify a causative factor and to make definitive plans for future prevention. Recurrent episodes of hyperventilation syndrome should be rare if the practitioner uses stress-reduction procedures. Recurrence mandates referral to a psychologist for counseling and coping strategies for stress.

REFERENCES

1. Brasher RE: Hyperventilation syndrome, *Lung* 161:257-73, 1983.
2. Malamed SF: Managing medical emergencies, *J Am Dent Assoc* 124:40-53, 1993.
3. Garssen B, Rijken H: Hyperventilation syndrome. In Kaptein AA, Vander Ploeg HM, Schreurs PJG, et al, editors: *Behavioural medicine*, New York, 1990, Wiley & Sons.
4. Riley DJ, Legawiec BA, Santiago TV, et al: Ventilatory responses to hypercapnia and hypoxia during continuous aspirin ingestion, *J Appl Physiol* 43:971-976, 1977.
5. Lum LC: Hyperventilation: the tip and the iceberg, *J Psychosom Res* 19:375-384, 1975.
6. Kerr WJ, Dalton JW, Gliebe PA: Some physical phenomena associated with the anxiety states and their relation to hyperventilation, *Ann Intern Med* 11:961-991, 1937.
7. Jibiki I, Kurokawa K, Matsuda H, et al: Widespread reduction of regional cerebral blood flow during hyperventilatoin-induced EEG slowing ('buildup'), *Neuropsychobiology* 26:120-124, 1992.
8. Kugelberg E: Activation of human nerves by hyperventilation and hypocalcemia: neurologic mechanism of symptoms of irritation in tetany, *Arch Neurol Psych* 60:153-164, 1948.
9. Brautbar N, Leibovici H, Finander P, et al: Mechanisms of hypophosphatemia during acute hyperventilation, *Clin Res* 28:387A, 1980.
10. Backon J: Nasal breathing as a treatment of hyperventilation: relevance of hemispheric activation, *Br J Clin Pract* 43:161-162, 1989.
11. Gardner W: The pathophysiology of hyperventilation disorders, *Chest* 109:516-534, 1996.

Acute Chest Pain

Remy H. Blanchaert, Jr.

Chest pain is the presenting symptom for a multitude of clinical conditions, from minor dyspepsia to life-threatening aortic dissection. Chest pain is such a common complaint that the practitioner should anticipate its occurrence during otherwise routine dental health care delivery. As with all medical emergencies, preparation by the dentist and the staff is instrumental in prompt implementation of potentially lifesaving measures. This chapter provides the clinician with a useful algorithm for the management of chest pain.

RECOGNITION AND ASSESSMENT

Early recognition of alterations in a patient's physiology distinguishes the astute clinician. Often, only subtle clues are present, and the clinician must elicit a complaint through appropriate patient questioning. At other times, clinical signs such as diaphoresis, cyanosis, and pallor are evident. Whenever a clinician suspects such alterations in physiology, the primary tools available remain the verbal history and the physical examination. Patient denial of the potential severity of acute chest pain is the most common factor leading to a delay in appropriate therapy.

When faced with a patient reporting chest pain, the dentist must ask relevant questions about specific factors (Box 7-1). Patient descriptions of pain tend to be stated in rather vague terms and need further specification. This is especially true for patients with acute chest pain. Assessment should specify *onset* by time and association with what event or activity. The *location* of the pain is identified by having the patient point to the specific site. The *character* of pain is important in the formulation of a relevant differential diagnosis. In regard to chest pain the most useful divisions of character of pain are deep visceral, superficial, and pleuritic. *Deep visceral pain* is a constant, central discomfort most often associated with angina, myocardial infarction, or esophageal disease. *Superficial* (musculoskeletal)

pain is easily aggravated or reproduced by palpation of the chest wall, especially the costochondral junctions. P*leuritic pain* is sharp, exaggerated by inspiration, and most closely associated with pneumonia, pericarditis, pneumothorax, and pulmonary embolism. The presence or absence of *radiation* and the site to which the pain radiates should be identified. Associated abdominal or back pain may indicate duodenal ulcer, cholecystitis, pancreatitis, gastritis, or aortic dissection. Exacerbating and alleviating factors have particular relevance to the diagnosis of chest pain.

Assessment of vital signs and a directed physical examination should take place at the identification of any medical emergency. The examination should initially determine the patient's mental status. Evaluation of a patient with chest pain involves an assessment of perfusion and the presence or absence of central plethora; skin assessment, cardiovascular examination (jugular venous distention), palpation and auscultation of the precordium, and auscultation of the lung fields are the primary means used. An altered sensorium in the patient with acute chest pain is a clear indication of inadequate perfusion. Palpation of the skin may reveal *diaphoresis*, a cool clammy finding indicative of hypoperfusion. Palpation of the pulse provides assessment of heart rate (bradycardia, tachycardia), rhythm (irregular, regular), and character of the pulse (thready, strong, absent). Blood pressure measurement further indicates the effectiveness of the myocardium as a pump. Blood pressure measurement in both seated and standing positions is particularly relevant to the determination of hypovolemia (e.g., peptic ulcer disease with hemorrhage, aortic dissection) or inadequate venous return (e.g., tension pneumothorax).

Box 7-2 lists a useful differential diagnosis for acute chest pain in clinical dentistry. Pneumonia and pericarditis are excluded because they have a more insidious onset and are unlikely to confront the dental practitioner in the office setting.

| Box 7-1 | Relevant Factors in the Diagnosis of Pain |

Onset: time, association with event
Location
Radiation: absence or site
Character: deep visceral, superficial, pleuritic
Exacerbating or alleviating factors

| Box 7-2 | Differential Diagnosis of Acute Chest Pain |

Angina
Myocardial infarction
Dyspepsia, gastroesophageal reflux disease
Musculoskeletal chest pain
Pulmonary embolus
Spontaneous pneumothorax
Aortic dissection, cardiac tamponade
Esophageal rupture
Panic disorder

| Box 7-3 | Initial Interventions for Acute Chest Pain |

- Initiate office emergency protocol using appropriate assistance and materials.
- Supply supplemental oxygen.
- Position patient.
- Evaluate and record vital signs.
- Ensure continuous cardiac monitoring.
- Complete initial assessment.
- Review medical history.

INITIAL INTERVENTION

The purpose of the initial interventions in the patient with acute chest pain is to ensure adequate oxygenation, optimize venous return, and ensure that the physician has sufficient assistance to complete the patient assessment and provide necessary secondary interventions (Box 7-3). Supplemental oxygen is delivered to ensure adequate oxygenation. The patient is placed in a semirecumbent position to optimize venous return.

The dentist must activate the office emergency protocol promptly at the earliest sign of any medical emergency to mobilize the team created to deal with such emergencies. Ancillary staff must be summoned immediately at any sign of trouble to perform the necessary tasks so that the dentist can assess the patient and initiate appropriate interventions. The dentist must assign specific persons to obtain the emergency drugs and equipment, oxygen, monitors, and defibrillator if available. Two persons should be with the patient at all times to provide cardiopulmonary resuscitation (CPR) if necessary. One assistant should transcribe events (time of onset of symptoms, interventions taken, time of drug administration, continuous recording of vital signs), and another person should be assigned to notify emergency medical services (EMS) if necessary.

Frequent practice and review of procedures for medical emergencies in the dental practice should be standard office protocol. Such review reinforces necessary skills and allows the dentist to focus on the emergency and not the functions of the office staff. Assigning roles to personnel within the office helps maintain a calm atmosphere throughout the emergency and ensures that the dentist will have adequate assistance to intervene appropriately.

All patients should receive supplemental oxygen immediately at the recognition of chest pain. The administration of oxygen is most appropriately done in an emergency setting through the use of a face mask with a reservoir (10 liters per minute). If such a device is unavailable, a nasal cannula (4 liters per minute) or nasal hood (4 to 6 liters per minute) can be used. The patient should be placed in a semirecumbent position to prevent peripheral venous pooling and to encourage venous return. The flexed knees should approximate the level of the heart. Vital signs should be taken and recorded. If available, an automatic blood pressure monitoring device should be set to cycle frequently (every 3 to 5 minutes). A continuous electrocardiogram (ECG) monitor (a defibrillator can be used in a monitoring mode) and a pulse oximeter should be used if available. Equipping the dental office with a defibrillator (automatic or conventional) and providing instruction with periodic review are encouraged.

These initial interventions should be made while maintaining continuous dialogue with the patient. The patient should be reassured frequently and reassessed often for alteration in mental status or symptoms. The medical history is quickly reviewed. The dentist must then proceed rapidly into a diagnostic mode, reviewing the most common and most devastating disease processes first. Early in the evaluation the dentist should decide if EMS should be contacted. When in doubt, the physician should establish contact and arrange for hospital transfer. In a patient with known stable angina, it may not be necessary to use EMS, and it is appropriate to wait 15 minutes for resolution of symptoms and response to topical nitrates. Any sign of hemodynamic instability (hypotension), however, requires prompt EMS notification.

DIFFERENTIAL DIAGNOSIS
Angina

The presenting symptoms of angina and acute myocardial infarction (MI) are similar. The patient describes the chest pain of angina and MI as heaviness or a squeezing, smothering, or choking sensation, often while holding a clenched fist to the chest wall at the precordium. Pain is perceived to originate deeply and is often substernal. It can also be perceived to originate or radiate to the left shoulder, either arm, jaw, back, or epigastrium. Anginal pain generally exhibits a crescendo-decrescendo pattern. The major difference in the presenting symptom differentiating angina from MI is duration. Pain from angina is usually relieved 5 to 15 minutes after cessation of the initiating event.

The pathophysiology of myocardial ischemia has been well described. Critical narrowing of the major cardiac vessels by atherosclerosis is a major factor. Such narrowing must be in the range of 70% before becoming evident. The resultant diminution of coronary blood flow results in local vasodilation of arterioles within the myocardium even at rest (autoregulation). Cold, stress, increased heart rate, and increased contractility cause increased myocardial oxygen demand. Increased demands for oxygen delivery cannot be met through the normal mechanism because it is already maximized. The perfusion of coronary vessels is directly proportional to the pressure gradient established between the aorta and the ventricular myocardium during systole or between the aorta and the ventricular cavity pressure during diastole. Therefore myocardial perfusion occurs primarily during diastole. Elevations in heart rate shorten diastolic time and therefore decrease myocardial perfusion.

Angina is the clinical expression of ongoing imbalance between myocardial oxygen delivery and oxygen demand (Box 7-4). Cessation of the ischemic event results in rapid resolution and explains why angina is of short duration. This is similar to the mechanism for claudication seen in arterial insufficiency of peripheral vascular disease. Angina can therefore be considered *myocardial claudication*. Persons with stable angina

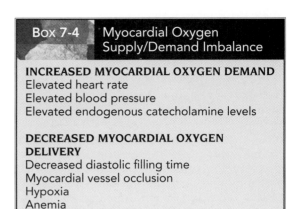

Box 7-4   Myocardial Oxygen Supply/Demand Imbalance

INCREASED MYOCARDIAL OXYGEN DEMAND
Elevated heart rate
Elevated blood pressure
Elevated endogenous catecholamine levels

DECREASED MYOCARDIAL OXYGEN DELIVERY
Decreased diastolic filling time
Myocardial vessel occlusion
Hypoxia
Anemia

often find that their tolerance for increased workloads is greater in the midday than the morning hours. This may be related to the circulating levels of endogenous catecholamines, which are at their highest unstimulated level in the morning. Stress and emotional disturbances also increase the catecholamine levels and result in lower thresholds for ischemia.

An additional mechanism for angina is present in *Prinzmetal's angina*; vasospasm of the coronary circulation results in the decreased flow state. The vasospasm is most evident at the site of an existing atheroma in the major coronary vessels and within the arterioles of the myocardium.

Nitrates

Angina responds to the administration of nitrates because of two mechanisms. First, nitrates reduce the preload of the ventricle, greatly decreasing the heart's work and oxygen demands. Second, the vasodilation mediated by nitrates improves cardiac blood flow and thus myocardial oxygen delivery. Routes of administration for nitrates include sublingual rapidly dissolving tablets, sublingual spray, long-acting tablets, and transdermal patch. The long-acting tablet and patch are used most often for patients with severe cardiac ischemia who are not candidates for revascularization (e.g., percutaneous transluminal coronary angioplasty, coronary artery bypass grafting). Tolerance is a significant issue in long-term use of nitrates. Patients using the long-acting forms require daily breaks from the drugs.

In the dental office, patients with known angina should be treated with their own supply of nitrates, if available. Clinicians should check expiration dates because nitrates lose their effectiveness rapidly.

Myocardial Infarction

MI is a common cause of acute chest pain. Ischemic heart disease remains the number-one cause of death among adults in the United States, annually with about 1 million deaths. Two thirds of deaths from coronary artery disease occur outside the hospital environment, and most of these deaths occur within 2 hours of the onset of symptoms.[1] Thus prompt diagnosis and appropriate intervention are extremely important for patients with acute MI.

Symptoms of acute MI mimic those of angina. The World Health Organization requires that a patient meet two of three criteria to justify a diagnosis of acute MI: (1) chest pain for at least 20 minutes, (2) evidence of ischemia, and (3) increased levels of cardiac enzymes. Although neither the patient nor the dentist can know if the event is an acute MI, initial interventions outlined earlier and short-term observation are appropriate. Failure to respond to these interventions should result in urgent transfer to a hospital emergency department (ED) for diagnosis and potential thrombolytic therapy.

The formation of a thrombus within a coronary artery results from disruption (fissure, rupture, ulceration) of an atherosclerotic plaque, with exposed collagen, platelet aggregation, and vessel obstruction. Clinical characteristics of the event depend on the area perfused by the occluded vessel, the presence of collateral circulation, and whether the induced ischemia affects a critical area of cardiac conduction or impulse initiation.[2]

Time to the initiation of thrombolytic therapy is the most important variable in determining benefit from intervention in acute MI. The largest improvements in outcomes are seen in those receiving thrombolytic therapy within the 2 hours after onset of symptoms.[3] Outcome, however, is still improved when thrombolytic therapy is initiated 6 to 12 hours later.[4]

Atypical presentations of acute MI occur in specific groups. Patients over 85 years of age and those with diabetes mellitus are most likely to have acute MI without the typical complaints of chest pain, diaphoresis, nausea, and vomiting. Patients with such "silent" MI are also more likely to be nonsmokers and to have no history of angina.[5,6] Dentists should recognize that alterations in the physiology of elderly or diabetic patients (e.g., syncope, weakness, confusion) may be silent MIs but are often interpreted as strokes or hypoglycemic events.

Dyspepsia and Gastroesophageal Reflux Disease

Epigastric pain can be the presenting sign for a number of clinical conditions. In patients with dyspepsia or gastroesophageal reflux disease (GERD) the typical chair position used in dentistry can aggravate the condition and produce epigastric pain. Clinicians should consider such processes in their patients before initiation of dental therapy but must be careful not to rush to such a diagnosis in the acute setting. The symptomatology is similar to many life-threatening conditions described in this chapter. The absence of diaphoresis, a feeling of doom, abnormalities in vital signs, and a strong clinical history of dyspepsia or GERD help to rule out more severe conditions. A thorough history before dental treatment should alert the clinician to this disorder. Questioning the patient about GERD and dyspepsia after the development of symptoms may mislead the clinician. Patients who develop acute chest pain often delay treatment because they believe the discomfort is related to dyspepsia or GERD.

Musculoskeletal Chest Pain

Complaints related to musculoskeletal chest pain are rather easy to diagnose, typically occurring after a fall, motor vehicle accident, and other causes of chest trauma; prolonged coughing episodes; or periods of emesis. The typical mechanisms are (1) disruption of the junction between the bone of the rib and the cartilaginous insertion into the sternum, (2) stretch of intercostal muscles, and (3) rib fracture. Patients show no evidence of physiologic disturbance, such as tachypnea, tachycardia, dyspnea, and diaphoresis. The patient reports that pain is increased by maximal inspiration, or the clinician may observe shallow breaths. The pain is reliably reproduced by direct palpation of the costocartilaginous junction or by pressure on the rib cage.

Patients with musculoskeletal chest pain do not require urgent evaluation. They should notify their physician, who will determine if they require evaluation and nonsteroidal antiinflammatory drugs (NSAIDs).

Pulmonary Embolus

The obstruction of a pulmonary artery by an embolus results in the failure to perfuse the portion of the lung that receives its blood supply through that artery. The most common cause is the embolization of clots from the deep veins of the lower extremity. Obstructing emboli can arise from other venous locations or rarely involve other substances (e.g., fat, air, amniotic fluid). Well-defined risk factors for the development of pulmonary emboli include immobility, heart disease, cancer (particularly nonsolid malignancies), estrogen therapy, hypercoagulability, abnormal thrombolysis, and previous deep venous thrombosis or pulmonary embolus.

Patients that develop a pulmonary embolus complain of chest pain and dyspnea. The chest pain increases with inspiration (pleuritic). A cough (nonproductive or with hemoptysis) may be present. Syncope occurs in severe cases. Tachypnea, hypoxemia, diaphoresis, and tachycardia are common. Hypotension occurs in cases of massive embolism. Clinical examination may demonstrate pathologic splitting of the second heart sound, rales, and a friction rub. Patients with mild disease may demonstrate only tachycardia, mild hypoxemia (decreased oxygen saturation on pulse oximetry), and tachypnea.

Urgent diagnosis and prompt referral to an ED for the initiation of anticoagulation, thrombolytic therapy, or surgical intervention are warranted because the clinical condition can deteriorate rapidly, with further emboli. The vast majority of patients require anticoagulation only. Thrombolytic therapy and surgical embolectomy are reserved for severe cases.

Spontaneous Pneumothorax

Spontaneous pneumothorax is an uncommon cause of acute chest pain. An abnormality in the lung ruptures, causing air to accumulate between the pleural spaces within the thorax, without any antecedent event. In an otherwise normal lung the event is called a *primary* spontaneous pneumothorax. In a patient with known lung disease (e.g., bullous emphysema) the term *secondary* spontaneous pneumothorax is more appropriate.

Primary spontaneous pneumothorax most often occurs in young adults (20 to 40 years of age), usually associated with high levels of physical activity and less likely with rest. A disproportionately high percentage of patients with spontaneous pneumothorax are tall, thin smokers. Pleuritic chest pain is generally observed, but because of the high degree of pulmonary reserve, no overt signs of hypoxemia or air hunger may be seen if the pneumothorax is small. Pneumothorax can be difficult to diagnose if the col-

lection of air is small. A larger pneumothorax causes the patient to feel short of breath. Anxiety, a rapid respiratory rate, cyanosis, and hypoxemia may be observed.

A serious form of pneumothorax occurs when a large volume of air enters the intrapleural space and develops higher pressures than the underlying lung and central vasculature. This *tension pneumothorax* results from the development of a valvelike mechanism that allows air entry during periods of high airway pressure, and air cannot escape. The rising pressure overcomes the inflation pressure of the lung parenchyma and results in its collapse. Complete collapse of an entire lung causes hypoxemia and elevated levels of carbon dioxide because of diminished area for diffusion of gas. Likewise, the intrapleural pressure elevation can overwhelm the intravascular pressure of the central venous system and therefore decrease cardiac return. The decreased cardiac return results from both vascular collapse and kinking of the vessels as the pneumothorax "shifts" structures to the opposite side of the chest.

Nitrous oxide sedation is contraindicated in persons with a recent pneumothorax because the gas can dissipate easily into the cavity and increase the size of the pneumothorax. Inhalation sedation should be used cautiously in persons with recent chest trauma or a history of pneumothorax.

Aortic Dissection

Acute aortic dissection is a clinical condition that manifests as severe, catastrophic chest pain. The pain may radiate to the back or extremities. Aortic dissection occurs approximately 60,000 times per year in the United States. Men are three times more likely to be affected than women, with persons 45 to 70 years of age most often affected. Marfan syndrome, Ehlers-Danlos syndrome type IV, congenital disease of the aorta (coarctation) or aortic valve, hypertension, atherosclerosis, and trauma are common historical findings.[7] The underlying disease process is necrosis of the media (cystic medial necrosis) of the aorta, which contains the elastic fibers that allow the vessel to withstand 40 to 50 million pulsations per year.

Common clinical findings in aortic dissection are catastrophic chest, back, and abdominal pain; diminished peripheral pulsation; differential differences in blood pressure between upper and lower extremities or right and left sides; dyspnea secondary to pulmonary edema; neurologic deficit; and nausea and vomiting. The pain is usually severe enough for patients to seek immediate medical attention. Pain may radiate to the extremities. Diminished peripheral pulses are evident because of decreased cardiac outflow (cardiac tamponade), aortic valve incompetence (proximal dissection), or collapse of a vessel lumen by the pressure within the surrounding dissection. Blood pressure differences occur in the upper and lower extremities with descending aortic dissection and in the right and left sides of the body with ascending (proximal) aortic dissection. Pulmonary edema results from inadequate forward flow of blood and subsequent pulmonary hypertension, as in cardiac tamponade. Neurologic deficits are related to the degree of the dissection and the involvement of branches of the aortic arch.

Patient outcome in aortic dissection is poor; 20% of patients die within the first 15 minutes, 40% by 24 hours, and 50% by 48 hours with treatment.[8]

Esophageal Rupture

The clinical presentation of esophageal rupture usually involves severe chest pain. The site of the pain correlates well with the location of the esophageal injury. Neck pain results from injuries occurring in the cervical esophagus. Epigastric pain often radiates to the back in lower esophageal injury and is often severe. Excruciating pain after straining is seen in most cases of postemetic rupture. Tachycardia and tachypnea are common. Hypotension and shock are seen with the development of sepsis. Subcutaneous emphysema may occur in patients with cervical esophageal injury. A "crunch" may be heard on auscultation of the precordium in patients with a pneumomediastinum caused by rupture of the thoracic esophagus.

Esophageal perforation or rupture results from iatrogenic causes (endoscopy; esophageal dilation, biopsy, or intubation), surgery (anterior approach to cervical spine, mediastinoscopy, tracheostomy, thoracic procedures), trauma (penetrating, foreign body, blunt, pneumatic rupture), and esophageal disease (carcinoma, Barrett's esophagus, infectious esophagitis). These causes are unlikely to occur during a visit to the dental office. A more likely cause in this setting is the syndrome named for Boerhaave, who first described spontaneous esophageal rupture secondary to excessive vomiting.

Spontaneous esophageal rupture (Boerhaave's syndrome) can occur with acute rises in in-

traabdominal pressure against a closed glottis. Spontaneous rupture accounts for approximately 20% of all cases of esophageal rupture. The tear usually occurs just above the diaphragm at the left lateral wall.[9] Typical precipitating situations are emesis, childbirth, defecation, and lifting heavy objects. The symptoms are often not apparent immediately, and the delayed presentation means that signs must be correlated with clinical suspicion for an accurate diagnosis. The most common disease processes confused with esophageal rupture are MI and gastric perforation.

Of patients with cervical esophageal perforation, 85% will survive, as do 90% with abdominal perforations. However, only 65% to 75% of those with thoracic disruptions survive their injury. Survival is strongly correlated with time elapsed before treatment.

Panic Disorder

Up to 20% of all patients presenting to an ED with a complaint of chest pain are eventually diagnosed with panic disorder.[10] This clinical situation is too complex for ED diagnosis in the majority of cases. Many patients with panic disorders have existing coronary artery disease. Fear of an MI is a significant factor, especially in patients with previous angina or infarction. Clinical signs and symptoms of panic disorder mimic acute MI. The dentist should manage all such cases, even with suspected panic disorder, as if they are an acute MI. These cases typically require diagnostic laboratory testing and serial electrocardiography to rule out MI.

SECONDARY INTERVENTION

After the initial interventions allow the time and the means to consider the differential diagnosis, the clinician considers the secondary management of a patient with acute chest pain (Box 7-5). Most patients with chest pain in the dental office will subsequently require transfer to an emergency medical facility. The physician should direct a member of the emergency response team to contact 911.

The diagnosis most often managed in the dental office and associated with chest pain is stable angina, with prompt resolution of symptoms after administration of nitroglycerine in tablet or spray form to the sublingual area in normotensive or hypertensive patients. Time of administration and response are carefully observed and recorded. Nitroglycerin administra-

Box 7-5	Secondary Interventions for Acute Chest Pain

HYPOTENSION
Arrange transport.
Provide intravenous access.
Administer crystalloid solutions (normal saline, lactated Ringer's).
Consider pulmonary embolus, aortic dissection, massive myocardial infarction (cardiogenic shock), and pneumothorax.

NO HYPOTENSION
Administer sublingual nitroglycerin.

PAIN
Arrange transport.
Provide intravenous access.
Administer morphine sulfate.
Consider myocardial infarction and unstable angina.

NO PAIN
Observe patient.

ALL CASES
Prepare for arrival of EMS.

tion can be repeated up to three times in 5 minutes. Continued support of all patients with chest pain with supplemental oxygen is required. Dentists comfortable with initiating an intravenous line should do so promptly. If the patient is normotensive, a slow infusion of 5% dextrose in water is ideal to maintain patency of the line and allow the administration of medications. In the patient with significant hypotension, normal saline and lactated Ringer's solution are appropriate choices. When the normotensive patient does not respond to nitrates, intravenous morphine sulfate may be administered to decrease the pain. Typical doses are 2 to 5 mg every 15 to 30 minutes (as long as the blood pressure remains stable) to effect until the desired pain relief is achieved.

Without intravenous access it is difficult to provide effective narcotic analgesia, and instead the physician should continue nitrate therapy and patient reassurance. Intramuscular or subcutaneous injections should be avoided because of the likely need to anticoagulate the patient, which could result in hematoma formation. Nitrous oxide analgesia might be appropriate if the clinician cannot administer morphine. When the diagnosis is clearly MI, aspirin is effective in de-

creasing platelets to aggregation and further clotting. A child's dose of aspirin is adequate, although administering a typical 325-mg tablet is also appropriate; the clinician should communicate this to the EMS on their arrival.

The clinician performs serial examination and initiates interventions according to level of training and comfort. The training and equipment for the administration of advanced cardiac life support (ACLS, e.g., *defibrillation*) is not currently the standard in general dental practice. However, dental specialties that provide anesthesia services in their office should have ACLS capacity and should employ it when necessary.

REASSESSMENT

The supervising dentist should ensure that the patient's vital signs and condition are monitored at least every 5 minutes. Accurate recording of the time of drug administration or initiation of other therapies (e.g., supplemental oxygen, establishment of intravenous line) is required. Such data are critical to the ongoing reassessment and evaluation of therapeutic effectiveness. The dentist should state the working diagnosis and any changes to team members. The dentist's statements should be recorded, photocopied, and given to the EMS on arrival.

DISPOSITION

Since most patients with acute chest pain in the dental office require transport to an emergency medical facility, the office emergency response team prepares for the arrival of the EMS personnel and facilitates the transfer. A team member should greet the ambulance and direct personnel to the location of the emergency. Typically, one EMS responder evaluates the patient while the other obtains demographic data, medical history, and a description of the event. The dentist should provide a copy of the recorded events (with the dentist's name and office number) to the EMS team (Box 7-6).

After the patient's transfer the dentist should conduct a debriefing of the office response team. All relevant recollections of the events should be recorded. The physician should then write a narrative summary of the event in the patient's office record and affix the recordings of the emergency and debriefing. The dentist should contact the patient's spouse or relatives, using plain language to describe the event and providing the name and telephone number of the hospital where the patient was transferred. The dentist

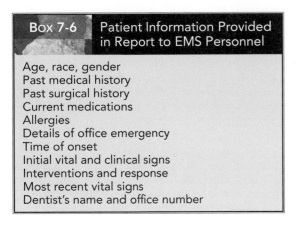

| Box 7-6 | Patient Information Provided in Report to EMS Personnel |

Age, race, gender
Past medical history
Past surgical history
Current medications
Allergies
Details of office emergency
Time of onset
Initial vital and clinical signs
Interventions and response
Most recent vital signs
Dentist's name and office number

should remain available for questions from the ED staff and follow up with them in 2 to 24 hours.

DEFINITIVE DIAGNOSIS AND MANAGEMENT
Myocardial Infarction

The clinical management of MI is well studied because of the large volume of cases, the relative ease of standardization of assessment (ECG changes, cardiac enzyme elevation, echocardiogram, radionucleotide perfusion studies, angiogram), and the standardization of outcome measures (cardiac failure, in-hospital death, left ventricular function, continued ischemia). Revascularization involves thrombolytic therapy and percutaneous transluminal coronary angioplasty (PTCA). On arrival at the ED, patients with chest pain receive immediate screening for thrombolytic therapy. The most important exclusions to intervention with thrombolytic agents are (1) delay in presentation (beyond 6 hours), (2) recent major surgery, and (3) prior hemorrhagic cerebrovascular accident (stroke). Current emphasis on the use of "accelerated" or "front-loaded" thrombolytic protocols has decreased the differences in outcome between thrombolytic therapy and primary PTCA.[11] This is extremely important because of the special facilities, increased cost, and expertise required for PTCA.

In the absence of specific contraindications, well-controlled studies have demonstrated improved survival in patients with acute MI who receive aspirin and beta-blockers. The most valuable interventions by the dentist for acute MI in the office are (1) recognition, (2) nitrate administration, and (3) prompt transfer to a medical facility.

Dyspepsia and Gastroesophageal Reflux Disease

Dyspepsia and GERD are best prevented in patients with existing disease through changes in positioning and avoidance of large meals before dental therapy. Antacids, histamine blockers, and proton pump inhibitors are helpful. These two disease processes are the most common diagnoses when MI has been ruled out in the patient with acute chest pain.

Musculoskeletal Chest Pain

The physical examination and history readily distinguish musculoskeletal chest pain from the other entities discussed in this chapter. Confirmation of the diagnosis may include chest radiograph, normal cardiac enzyme values, and a normal ECG tracing. Most patients will be managed with NSAIDs or mild narcotics.

Pulmonary Embolus

Although it is the definitive test for pulmonary embolus, the angiogram is seldom necessary because ventilation/perfusion ($\dot{V}/\dot{Q}$) nucleotide scans are readily available and accurate in the majority of cases. The combination of $\dot{V}/\dot{Q}$ scans and Doppler ultrasonography of the legs (identification of deep venous thrombosis) is the typical mechanism utilized to confirm the diagnosis of pulmonary embolus. Therapy consists of anticoagulation in the absence of contraindications.

Spontaneous Pneumothorax

The diagnosis of spontaneous pneumothorax is made by the history, physical examination, and chest radiograph. A large pneumothorax is easily diagnosed and treated with closed-thoracostomy (chest tube) drainage. Often the thoracostomy tube causes sufficient scarring between the pleura to prevent recurrence. In the event of recurrence, thoracoscopy for resection of blebs and pleurodesis (mechanical or chemical abrasion of the pleura) are necessary.

Aortic Dissection

Chest radiograph, aortogram, and echocardiogram are useful in the definitive diagnosis of aortic dissection. Definitive management depends on the patient's ability to tolerate surgical correction and on extent and location of the dissection. Medical management is directed at the normalization of blood pressure (avoidance of hypertension) and is reserved for patients with stable dissection of the ascending aorta and nonsurgical patients. Cases of proximal dissection with aortic valve incompetence or cardiac tamponade are surgical emergencies. Descending aortic dissection, although stabilized medically, requires surgical correction.

Esophageal Rupture

Definitive diagnosis of esophageal rupture is based on radiographic features. Chest x-ray films may show pneumomediastinum. Barium swallow may demonstrate extravasation of contrast material. Computed tomography can demonstrate pneumomediastinum and mediastinitis. Most patients with spontaneous esophageal rupture undergo conservative management of the rupture with aggressive antibiotic therapy and nutritional support.

Panic Disorder

The exclusion of all other diagnoses may lead to the diagnosis of panic disorder. Therapy of the underlying depression and anxiety is necessary.

SUMMARY

Chest pain is a common complaint on presentation to an ED. For many disease processes with chest pain as the presenting symptom, the time between onset of symptoms and initiation of therapy is critical. Initial interventions include prompt recognition of a problem, attempts to alleviate the symptom or ameliorate the disease process, and rapid transport to an ED. Patients may deteriorate rapidly, illustrating the importance of supportive measures and transfer of care.

Ischemic heart disease may be the most likely cause of acute chest pain during routine dental practice and even in the waiting area. Dentists should organize the staff and practice the management of medical emergencies. Prompt recognition of signs and symptoms of chest pain should activate the office response team. Initial interventions are then made as the dentist assesses the situation and considers the differential diagnosis and disposition of the patient.

REFERENCES

1. Emergency Cardiac Care Committee and Subcommittees, American Heart Association: Guidelines for cardiopulmonary resuscitation and emergency cardiac care, JAMA 268(16):2174, 1992.
2. Fuster V, Badimon L, Badimon JJ, et al: The pathogenesis of coronary artery disease and acute coronary syndromes. Part I, N Engl J Med 326:242, 1992.
3. Weaver WD et al: Prehospital-initiated vs hospital initiated thrombolytic therapy: the Myocardial Infarction Triage and Intervention Trial, JAMA 270(10):1211, 1993.
4. Late assessment of thrombolytic efficacy (LATE) study with alteplase 6-24 hours after onset of acute myocardial infarction, Lancet 343:759, 1993.
5. Uretsky BF, Farquhar DS, Berezin AF, et al: Symptomatic myocardial infarction without chest pain: prevalence and clinical action, Am J Cardiol 40:498, 1977.
6. Bayer AJ, Chadha JS, Farag RR, et al: Changing presentation of myocardial infarction with increasing age, J Am Geriatr Soc 34:263, 1986.
7. Wolfe WG: Dissecting aneurysms of the aorta. In Sabiston DC, Lyerly HK, editors: Textbook of surgery: the biological basis of modern surgical practice, ed 15, Philadelphia, 1997, WB Saunders.
8. Hirst AE, Johns VL, Kime SW: Dissecting aneurysm of the aorta: a review of 505 cases, Medicine 37:217, 1958.
9. Tidman MK, John HT: Spontaneous rupture of the oesophagus, Br J Surg 54:286, 1967.
10. Carter SC, Servan-Schreiber D, Perlstein WM: Anxiety disorders and the syndrome of chest pain with normal coronary arteries: prevalence and pathophysiology, J Clin Psychiatry 58(suppl 3):70, 1997.
11. Verheugt FW: Primary angioplasty for acute myocardial infarction: is the balloon half empty? Lancet 347:1276, 1996.

Palpitations and Arrhythmias

David M. Shafer

- Does it ever feel like your heart skips a beat?
- Are you ever aware of feeling your heartbeat?
- Do you have a history of an irregular heartbeat?

A dentist often asks these or similar questions when taking a medical history, and patients may answer such questions when filling out a health questionnaire. Unfortunately, a positive patient response to any of these questions frequently is dismissed with little thought or is ignored. If these warning signs of potentially severe underlying heart disease are recognized and investigated further, a serious medical emergency may be prevented.

Sudden cardiac death is a leading cause of mortality in adults, and arrhythmias are often the precipitating factor initiating sudden cardiac death. Although many palpitations may be benign from a functional cardiac standpoint, they may also be one of the few clinical clues to underlying cardiac disease. Therefore an understanding of the pathophysiology and significance of palpitations is crucial not only to the treatment and prevention of medical emergencies, but also to the overall medical evaluation of patients presenting for dental treatment.

CLINICAL PRESENTATION

Palpitations are defined as any conscious sensation of cardiac activity. Typically the sensation is unpleasant and may be very provoking for patients. Patients may report that they feel a skipping, fluttering, flopping, pounding, or a racing sensation in the pericardium. After ruling out any immediate cardiac emergency, it is important to calm these patients because the associated feeling of anxiety and sense of impending doom may worsen the situation. Patients may experience palpitations even with a normal heartbeat. Any alteration in cardiac rate, rhythm, stroke volume, or contractility can cause a patient to experience palpitations.

PATHOPHYSIOLOGY

Palpitations are a nonspecific patient complaint because they can have many different underlying causes. Therefore consideration of the pathophysiology of palpitations may involve diverse disease processes. Palpitations can be separated into two broad categories: palpitations without discernible change in cardiac function and those with changes in cardiac function. Palpitations associated with changes in cardiac function can be subdivided into those with and without cardiac arrhythmia. Palpitations not associated with an arrhythmia can be further subdivided into those of cardiac origin and those not of cardiac origin.

The term *arrhythmia* can have several definitions depending on its usage. The classic definition of arrhythmia is the complete absence of rhythm, as in ventricular fibrillation, or asystole; however, it is rarely used only in such a narrow way. Typically, arrhythmia is used to refer to any abnormal alteration in heart rate (increase or decrease) or rhythm (regular or irregular). In this context, arrhythmias, or *dysrhythmias*, also include ventricular tachycardia, bradycardia, and supraventricular tachycardias.

Palpitations experienced with no change in heart rate, rhythm, or function are most likely precipitated by anxiety. Palpitations without changes in cardiac function are least likely to represent a true medical emergency but may still be stressful to the patient. The patient may be simply describing normal cardiac function. *Neurocirculatory asthenia*, also referred to as *cardiac neurosis*, is a psychosomatic disorder in which patients describe shortness of breath, palpitations, lightheadedness, and precordial pain. These patients may indeed have some underlying cardiac disease, but the magnitude of the complaints is out of proportion to the problem. Other patients may become aware of completely normal cardiac activity in the nighttime as they are falling asleep, particularly those who sleep on their left side. More often, however, palpitations are the result of some change in function caused by altered heart rate or rhythm.

It is important not to dismiss palpitations as minor psychogenic complaints that require no further investigation or intervention. They may be the harbinger of a serious underlying cardiac condition, or they may represent an existing cardiac neurosis so severe that it may cause significant disability. In one study describing the natural history of patients presenting for evaluation of palpitations, 84% had recurrent palpitations at 6-month follow-up.[1] Patients with recurrent palpitations scored significantly higher than control patients on measures of cardiac symptoms and had more physician visits in the preceding 6 months. Interestingly, these patients also had a higher prevalence of panic disorders and more psychopathologic symptoms, somatized more, and were more hypochondriacal than the control group. Therefore palpitations may represent more complex psychological problems.

Palpitations perceived as a sudden abnormal change in heart rate or rhythm may result from normal physiologic changes in cardiac function. A normal increase in stroke volume or cardiac contractility, as occurs during strenuous physical activity, may be perceived as palpitations. Similarly, a sudden change in cardiac rate or rhythm caused by adrenergic stimulation may also result in a sensation of palpitations. Pathologic stressors, such as fever, hyperparathyroidism, anemia, and pheochromocytoma, increase adrenergic stimulation. Any increase in catecholamines is a common pathway in many different causes of palpitations (Box 8-1).

In conditions that result in an abnormally increased stroke volume, patients may experience forceful, regular palpitations. Such conditions include aortic and mitral regurgitation, ventricular septal defects, and hyperkinetic circulatory states such as anemia and thyrotoxicosis. Patients with these conditions typically complain of forceful, regular palpitations, generally at night while lying on their left side (Box 8-2).

Palpitations that occur with arrhythmias are the least common encountered but potentially the most life threatening. Therefore understanding their cause is extremely important. Emergency therapy is directed toward the arrhythmia and its cause. Intermittent rapid, slow heart rhythms or premature atrial and ventricular contractions may cause palpitations by erratic alterations in heart motion. Patients become most aware of palpitations during either the beginning

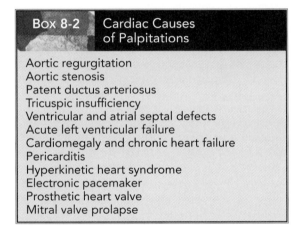

Box 8-2	Cardiac Causes of Palpitations

Aortic regurgitation
Aortic stenosis
Patent ductus arteriosus
Tricuspic insufficiency
Ventricular and atrial septal defects
Acute left ventricular failure
Cardiomegaly and chronic heart failure
Pericarditis
Hyperkinetic heart syndrome
Electronic pacemaker
Prosthetic heart valve
Mitral valve prolapse

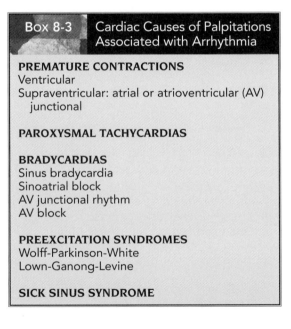

Box 8-3	Cardiac Causes of Palpitations Associated with Arrhythmia

PREMATURE CONTRACTIONS
Ventricular
Supraventricular: atrial or atrioventricular (AV) junctional

PAROXYSMAL TACHYCARDIAS

BRADYCARDIAS
Sinus bradycardia
Sinoatrial block
AV junctional rhythm
AV block

PREEXCITATION SYNDROMES
Wolff-Parkinson-White
Lown-Ganong-Levine

SICK SINUS SYNDROME

Box 8-1	Noncardiac Causes of Palpitations

Anxiety
Iatrogenic administration of sympathomimetic agent
Anemia
Fever
Thyrotoxicosis
Hypoglycemia
Migraine
Arteriovenous fistula
Drugs (e.g., vasodilators, (β-agonists, vasopressors)
Pheochromocytoma
Diaphragmatic flutter

or end of an arrhythmia. With premature contractions the patient often identifies the post-extrasystolic beat as a palpitation. This beat generally is accompanied by an increase in stroke volume. Patients whose palpitations are due to atrioventicular nodal reentrant tachycardia (Wolff-Parkinson-White syndrome or Lown-Ganong-Levine syndrome) may have simultaneous atrial and ventricular contraction, elevated right atrial pressure, and retrograde flow in the great veins, leading to a pounding sensation in the neck (Box 8-3).

PATIENT EVALUATION

The basic principles of patient evaluation apply to the assessment of a patient presenting with palpitations. Every attempt should be made to determine the underlying pathophysiology, severity of signs and symptoms, whether the palpitations are the result of a cardiac or noncardiac abnormality, and whether the palpitations correlate with a cardiac arrhythmia.

History

Questions in the history should determine the patient's use of prescription and nonprescription medications and substances. Prescription medications, such as β-blockers and antiarrhythmics (e.g., digitalis, calcium channel blockers), may cause palpitations. Over-the-counter medications, such as cold remedies with decongestants (e.g., pseudoephedrine) or stimulants (e.g., caffeine) are frequent causes of palpitations. Patients should be questioned about what (if anything) initiates or resolves the palpitations. It is extremely important to determine whether the patient is experiencing other symptoms (e.g., concurrent chest pain, changes in neurologic function) that may indicate either a

direct or an indirect consequence of the palpitations (Box 8-4).

Physical Examination

A focused physical examination should be performed, including assessment of the patient's peripheral pulses. The simple act of taking the pulse can reveal a tachycardia or bradycardia. The character of the pulse, whether regular or irregular, can distinguish between a sinus tachycardia and atrial fibrillation. A more advanced examination consists of precordial palpation and heart and carotid auscultation. Auscultation, whether during or between episodes of palpitations, may uncover the characteristic murmur associated with a valvular defect.

Laboratory Studies

Laboratory evaluation should be conducted to aid in diagnosis. For example, a blood glucose level can be done to rule out hypoglycemia. Thyroid function tests, including T_3, T_4, and thyroid-stimulating hormone (TSH) levels, may be indicated if hyperthyroidism is suspected. A toxicology screen is indicated if illicit drug use or overdose is suspected. Serum digoxin levels should be checked in patients taking cardiac glycosides.

Pheochromocytoma is a rare condition that may be considered in patients who have palpitations in conjunction with labile hypertension. The preferred screening test is the analysis of a 24-hour urine collection for catecholamines and either vanillylmandelic acid or metanephrines. Two normal 24-hour urinalyses essentially rule out the diagnosis of pheochromocytoma. If the patient's 24-hour urine collection is positive, a plasma catecholamine assay and computed tomography (CT) of the adrenal glands should be performed.

Box 8-4	Patient Descriptions of Palpation and Probable Causes
DESCRIPTION	**CAUSE**
Sudden onset, rapid and regular	Supraventricular tachycardia
Sudden onset, rapid and irregular	Paroxysmal atrial fibrillation
Gradual onset, regular with exercise	Sinus tachycardia
Occasional skipped beats, "flip-flops"	Premature contractions
Occurs with noncardiogenic chest pain or hyperventilation	Anxiety related
Associated with medications or substance ingestion	Caffeine, tobacco, coffee, tea, xanthines, catecholamines, thyroid hormone

The potential for arrhythmias should be evaluated using a 12-lead electrocardiogram (ECG); however, an ECG will only detect an arrhythmia while it is occurring. If a routine 12-lead ECG does not confirm the diagnosis but an arrhythmia is still suspected, a 24-hour ambulatory ECG (Holter monitor) can be performed. In rare instances a 24-hour examination will be inadequate, and even longer monitoring will be used if an arrhythmia is still suspected. If an exercise-induced arrhythmia or underlying coronary artery disease is suspected, treadmill testing may be appropriate. Echocardiography may be necessary to evaluate subtle valvular and flow abnormalities.

ETIOLOGY AND DIFFERENTIAL DIAGNOSIS
Noncardiac Causes

In responding to an emergency situation, it is important to differentiate palpitations that are secondary to a noncardiac cause from those that are cardiac in origin, particularly palpitations that represent an arrhythmia.

Psychiatric Disorders

Palpitation is a common symptom in patients with certain psychiatric illnesses, including panic disorders, anxiety reaction, depression, and somatization. In one study, nearly 50% of outpatients referred for ambulatory ECG monitoring for a complaint of palpitations had a psychiatric disorder.[2]

A history of a gradual onset of a palpitation during routine, typically nonstressful activities is characteristic in patients with anxiety disorders. These patients may even describe chest pain, which is not cardiac in origin. The patient may simply become acutely aware of normal heart activity, particularly during quiet times, such as before falling asleep or during periods of deep thought. Occasionally this may be associated with premature ventricular contractions. These contractions can also be perceived as palpitations as a reaction to stress in otherwise healthy individuals.

Neurocirculatory asthenia. In a subgroup of patients, palpitations can become part of a chronic anxiety neurosis associated with chronic autonomic nervous system hyperactivity. Neurocirculatory asthenia (cardiac neurosis, Da Costa's syndrome, soldier's heart, functional cardiovascular disease) is often confused with true organic heart disease, compounding the patient's anxiety and exacerbating the problem. Correctly identifying these patients is therefore extremely important. They often have physical findings consistent with a hyperkinetic state, including excessive perspiration, resting sinus tachycardia, widened pulse pressure, and a functional systolic flow murmur. Frequently these patients have nonspecific ST changes on a resting ECG, and combined with chest pain, this can lead to an incorrect diagnosis of coronary artery disease. Hyperventilation alone during stress ECG testing can lead to ST-segment depression (a sign of cardiac ischemia), making the incorrect diagnosis of coronary artery disease more likely. Hyperthyroidism can cause many of the same signs and also must be ruled out in these patients before establishing the diagnosis of neurocirculatory asthenia.

Medical Disorders

Conditions such as anemia, electrolyte abnormalities, thyrotoxicosis, hypoglycemia, migraine, and pheochromocytoma must be ruled out by a detailed medical history, focused physical examination, and appropriate laboratory tests. The patient history often reveals the potential for these conditons. For example, patients taking loop or thiazide diuretics are at risk of hypokalemia. Patients at risk for an acute episode of hyperthyroidism will likely have a history consistent with thyroid disease. The most common arrhythmia in patients with noncardiac medically induced palpitations is a sinus tachycardia with a gradual onset.

Cardiac Causes

Cardiac causes of palpitations may include either congenital (e.g., patent ductus arteriosis, ventricular and atrial septal defects) or acquired functional disturbances of the heart such as valvular disease (e.g., aortic regurgitation, aortic stenosis, tricuspid insufficiency, mitral valve prolapse), heart failure, or pericarditis. Corrective surgical procedures, such as prosthetic heart valves and coronary artery bypass grafts, and devices to regulate electrical cardiac activity, such as pacemakers and automatic implantable cardiodefibrillators, may also result in palpitations.

Mitral Valve Prolapse

A cohort of patients with mitral valve prolapse (MVP) has been identified who have a psychological profile and signs of autonomic dysfunction similar to that seen in neurocirculatory asthenia. The patient may also exhibit premature ventricular contractions, paroxysmal tachycardias, and atypical chest pain. These patients may have significant valvular compromise and often undergo stress testing and an echocardiogram to rule out pathology other than the typical click and murmur of MVP. Therefore, although it is important to identify patients with MVP who have a regurgitant murmur so that they can receive antibiotic prophylaxis, realization of this diagnosis can also be of benefit in an emergency when palpitations may be present.

Arrhythmias

There are multiple cardiac arrhythmias during which a patient may describe an unpleasant awareness of their heartbeat. Arrhythmias can be rapid (tachycardia) or slow (bradycardia) and can arise in the atria, ventricles, sinoatrial (SA) node,

atrioventricular (AV) node, or any location along the conduction pathway. Arrhythmias can result from antegrade conduction, retrograde conduction, or reentrant conduction. Table 8-1 summarizes characteristics of common and clinically relevant arrhythmias associated with palpitations.

Premature Ventricular and Atrial Contractions

Premature contractions are among the most common causes of palpitations and can occur in otherwise healthy individuals. They may occur with or without organic heart disease and can be supraventricular or ventricular in origin. Most episodes of premature contractions are benign, but rarely they may signify a serious clinical condition (see Table 8-1). As with all arrhythmias, definitive diagnosis requires an ECG.

Table 8-1   Clinical Presentation of Common Arrhythmias with Palpitations

Arrhythmia	History	Physical Findings
Sinus tachycardia	Gradual onset, anxiety, drug use, underlying medical problem	Regular rhythm, rate 100-170 beats/min; transiently slows with vagal maneuvers then returns to rapid rate
Premature atrial and ventricular contractions	Brief sensation of a skipped beat or pause with increased intensity after pause	Premature beat followed by compensatory or non-compensatory pause; may have diminished or absent pulse
Atrial fibrillation	Sudden onset; usually a history of heart disease, hypertension, diabetes, or thyroid disease	Irregular rhythm with variable rate; peripheral pulse dropout because of variable diastolic filling; variable ventricular response; gradually slows with vagal maneuver, with return to previous rate
Atrial flutter	Sudden onset and termination; coexistent cardiovascular or lung disease	Regular pulse, rate 150 beats/min because of 2:1 conduction; without block, rate up 350 beats/min; conduction block variable
Ventricular tachycardia	Sudden onset; elderly patients with history of coronary artery disease	Rapid, regular rhythm; variable first heart sound and jugular venous cannon A waves due to atrioventricular dissociation; no effect from vagal maneuvers
Paroxysmal reentrant supraventricular tachycardia	Sudden onset and termination; long history of recurrent symptoms	Rapid regular rhythm, rate 140-200 beats/min; may terminate with vagal maneuvers or may have no effect; normal or cannon A waves
Complete heart block	Extreme fatigue, syncope, dyspnea on exertion; complaint of pounding in neck	Rate slow, 40-60 beats/min; rhythm generally regular; jugular venous cannon A waves with variable amplitude; variable intensity of first heart sound

Premature ventricular contractions (PVCs) are generally benign if less than one contraction occurs per minute. However, organic heart disease should be suspected if more than six PVCs occur per minute or if they are in pairs or groups, are multifocal, are closely coupled to the preceding beat, or have a very wide QRS complex (>0.16 second). If PVCs occur with chest pain, myocardial ischemia and infarction should be considered. When they occur during infarction, PVCs may lead to ventricular fibrillation. The risk of ventricular fibrillation is increased if the PVC falls on the preceding T wave, representing ventricular repolarization ("R on T phenomenon").

A common cause of PVCs during dentistry is hypoxia, when sedative drugs are administered without adequate monitoring, leading to cardiac ischemia.

Premature atrial contractions (PACs) occur in normal individuals but may be associated with febrile states, mitral valve disease, pericarditis, chronic obstructive pulmonary diseases, or digitalis overdose. PACs can also be precursors to ominous arrhythmias, such as atrial tachycardia, flutter, or fibrillation. Therefore underlying causes should be eliminated, and the presence of PACs should not be simply dismissed.

Bradycardia

Bradycardia is a heart rate below 60 beats per minute. The patient may perceive bradycardia as palpitations because of the associated increased stroke volume with a slow heart rate. Patients may initially describe palpitations without other functional problems. However, if they start to decompensate, with decreased cardiac output and a resulting decrease in cerebral blood flow, patients may experience syncope or lightheadedness. In patients with bradycardia, it is particularly important to differentiate between those with and those without symptoms. Patients who are symptomatic need to be treated as true emergencies, and basic life support (BLS) or advanced cardiac life support (ACLS) may need to be initiated.

The most common causes of a slow pulse rate are sinus bradycardia, SA block, AV block, AV junctional rhythms, and extrasystolic bigeminy. In patients with a history of cardiac disorders, medication-related bradycardia must be considered. Medications that can cause bradycardia include: β-blockers, calcium channel blockers, digitalis, and antiarrhythmics (e.g., amiodarone). Also, bradycardia may be normal in certain patients. It is not unusual for well-conditioned athletes to have resting pulse rates of 50 beats/min or rarely as low as 40 beats/min.

Paroxysmal Tachycardias

Paroxysmal tachycardias may occur with and without underlying heart disease. Similar to bradycardia, tachycardias may also be drug induced. Digitalis and class I antiarrhythmics (e.g., quinidine, procainamide, disopyramide, lidocaine, tocainide, mexiletine, phenytoin, flecainide, propafenone) are among the most common medications causing tachycardia. Paroxysmal tachycardias may last from less than a minute to several days and may recur, with frequent "stops and starts." Similar to the origins of premature contractions, *paroxysmal supraventricular tachycardia* (PSVT) or *paroxysmal ventricular tachycarida* (PVT) can occur.

As with any arrhythmia, the presence of paroxysmal tachycardia is most significant if the patient develops symptoms of cardiac insufficiency or ischemia. This is most likely to occur if the course of the tachycardia is prolonged for more than several minutes or if the patient is elderly or has diminished cardiac function.

An episode of paroxysmal tachycardia is associated with lightheadedness, faintness, syncope, dyspnea, and angina, with signs of congestive heart failure (see Table 8-2). Vagal maneuvers such as carotid massage or ocular pressure can diagnose and in some cases treat tachycardias. However, these maneuvers should be used with extreme caution. Carotid massage can dislodge plaques in the carotid artery, leading to cerebral ischemia and stroke. Pressure over the globes can cause intraocular damage. Vagal maneuvers can lead to asystole, especially in patients with PSVT and heart block.

Preexcitation Syndromes

Preexcitation occurs when there is an accessory conduction pathway between the atria and ventricles bypassing the AV node. Preexcitation appears as a shortened PR interval on an ECG. Both atrial and ventricular tachycardias can occur. These arrhythmias are rarely life threatening. *Wolff-Parkinson-White* (WPW) *syndrome* is the most common form of an accessory conduction path leading to preexcitation. In this variant there is a bypass of the AV node leading to direct connection between the atria and ventricles. Another preexcitation syndrome is *Lown-Ganong-Levine* (LGL) *syndrome*, in which a direct, rapid connection occurs between the atria and His-Purkinje system.

Diagnosis of preexcitation syndromes is important because of the increased risk of fatal arrhythmias, such as ventricular fibrillation. Treatment is different for PSVT with or without pre-excitation. Conventional forms of antiarrhythmic treatment may be ineffective. Chronic medical therapy for PSVT includes digoxin and procainamide. Digoxin is contraindicated in WPW because it may paradoxically accelerate the ventricular response. *Radiofrequency catheter ablation* of the accessory pathway is successful treatment in removing the aberrant accessory pathway. This treatment appears to have a success rate in excess of 95%, with very low morbidity and mortality. In fact, because it may eliminate the longterm administration of medication, radiofrequency ablation may result in lower overall costs.[3,4]

Sick Sinus Syndrome (Tachycardia-Bradycardia Syndrome)

Sick sinus syndrome is a common cause of palpitations associated with dizziness and syncope. It can occur in patients of all ages but is more common in patients over 60. Sick sinus syndrome actually refers to a constellation of arrhythmias. Presenting dysrhythmias include (1) persistent sinus bradycardia, (2) sinus pauses, (3) intraatrial and AV node conduction abnormalities, (4) PSVTs alternating with periods of bradycardia, and (5) a lack of extranodal escape pacemakers that respond to the bradycardia. Patients may complain of symptoms during periods of bradycardia, tachycardia, or both. Degen-

erative changes within the sinus node or chronic use of cardiac medications, such as β-blockers, calcium channel blockers, or class III antiarrhythmics (e.g., amiodarone), may initiate the syndrome. Atrial fibrillation may also be present. These patients may require placement of a permanent pacemaker because treatment of their tachycardia with medications results in symptomatic bradycardia.

MANAGEMENT
Medical Management

The medical management of patients with palpitations is summarized in Figure 8-1.[5] Many cardiac diseases may be associated with arrhythmias and palpitations. If the patient is being treated and the palpitations continue, chronic stress reduction techniques are useful. Patients who are syncopal will need electrophysiologic studies (EPS). Dental treatment should be deferred until a definitive diagnosis is made and the patient is considered to be in optimal condition.

General Emergency Treatment

Palpitations may precede or be part of a true medical emergency. An emergency results when an arrhythmia is associated with instability or cardiac insufficiency (Figure 8-2). Recognition and treatment of these emergencies are outlined in the ACLS guidelines published by the American Heart Association.[6]

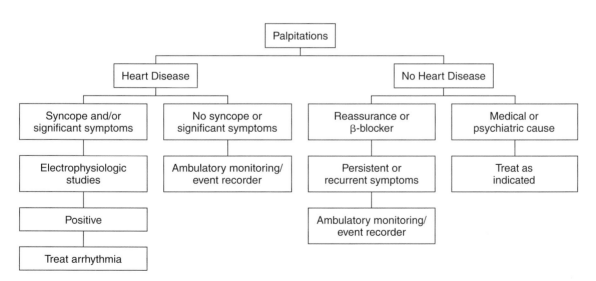

Figure 8-1. Medical management of the patient with palpitations. The first step is the determination of cardiac disease. *Modified from De Lurgio DB, Barbour A: Palpitations and tachycardia. In Branch WT, Alexander RW, Schlant RC, Hurst JW, editors:* Cardiology in primary care, *New York, 2000, McGraw-Hill.*

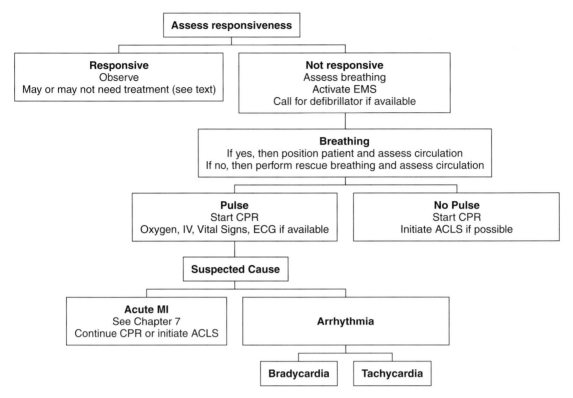

Figure 8-2. Emergency treatment of tachycardia. *VT,* Ventricular tachycardia; *SVT,* supraventricular tachycardia; *WPW,* Wolff-Parkinson-White syndrome; *ECG,* electrocardiogram.

Generally, when approaching the emergency management of a patient undergoing dental treatment with a significant arrhythmia, the first action is to suspend all dental treatment and remove all objects that may obstruct the airway or that may be dislodged into the airway. The patient's responsiveness should then be assessed. The patient who remains responsive and has stable neurologic status and blood pressure can be referred for routine medical work-up and treatment (see earlier). If the patient is unresponsive, the emergency medical services (EMS) system should be activated. The emergency medical plan should be implemented and a manual defibrillator or an automatic external defibrillator (AED) procured. Evaluation of the airway, breathing, and circulation (ABCs) follows, as described in BLS protocols. At this point, if an ECG and defibrillator are not available, the patient should have vital signs continually monitored and should be transferred to an emergency facility for evaluation. If the patient becomes pulseless or stops breathing, BLS is initiated.

If the practitioner has an AED, the pads are appropriately applied to the patient's chest wall, the device is turned on and allowed to assess the rhythm, and a shock is delivered, if indicated. Health care providers trained in ACLS and with an ECG can initiate advanced therapies.

Bradycardia

If detected, it is important to remember that bradycardia may represent a normal condition. The presence of accompanying lightheadedness, loss of consciousness, chest pain, or heart failure (e.g., low blood pressure, pulmonary edema) dictates immediate intervention (Figure 8-3). If the patient is unstable, EMS should be notified, oxygen administered, and intravenous (IV) access established for administration of emergency medications. The patient must be monitored continually. If bradycardia or any other arrhythmia is associated with chest pain, the chest pain may need to be treated (see Chapter 7).

A patient with bradycardia who is not symptomatic can then be observed and referred to a

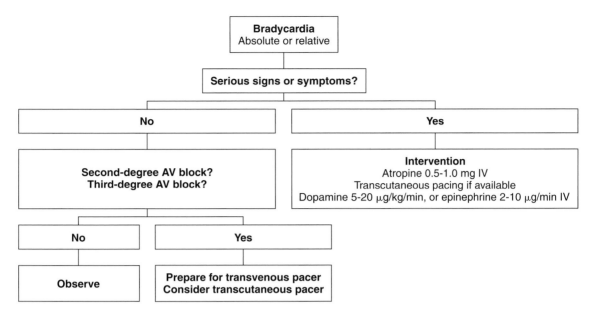

Figure 8-3. General emergency treatment of arrhythmias. *EMS,* Emergency medical system; *CPR,* cardiopulmonary resuscitation; *IV,* intravenous line; *ECG,* electrocardiogram; *ACLS,* advanced cardiac life support.

medical colleague for assessment and treatment. The work-up should not be delayed because bradycardia can quickly become an emergency, including atypical myocardial infarction (MI) without chest pain and type II (second-degree) or type III (third-degree) AV block.

Tachycardia

Initial treatment of tachycardia is the same as for bradycardia. If the patient does have an abnormally rapid heart rate and accompanying signs of lightheadedness, loss of consciousness, chest pain, or heart failure (e.g., low blood pressure, pulmonary edema), EMS should be immediately notified, oxygen administered, and IV access established for medications (Figure 8-4). Continual patient monitoring is important because tachycardia could progress to an acute MI or ventricular fibrillation, especially in the elderly patient with undiagnosed ischemic heart disease.

If stable with no serious signs or symptoms, the patient is first treated with vagal maneuvers and medications. This is most effective if the medication is directed toward a specific arrhythmia, so an ECG is required. If the heart rate is greater than 150 beats/min and the patient is unstable, immediate cardioversion may

be necessary. An attempt can be made to control the arrhythmia and stabilize the patient first with vagal maneuvers and then with medications, but the universal recommendation in the most recent ACLS protocol is immediate cardioversion for unstable patients with a tachycardia.[7]

Based on ECG results, tachycardias can be divided into four categories for treatment purposes: (1) atrial fibrillation and flutter, (2) narrow-complex tachycardia (e.g., PSVT), (3) stable wide-complex tachycardia (e.g., PVC), and (4) stable monomorphic or polymorphic ventricular tachycardia.

Atrial Fibrillation and Flutter

When treating patients with tachycardia secondary to atrial fibrillation or atrial flutter, the patient must be evaluated for four clinical factors: (1) clinical stability, (2) impaired cardiac function, (3) WPW syndrome, and (4) duration of tachycardia greater than 48 hours. Symptomatic tachycardia secondary to atrial fibrillation or flutter can be treated effectively with synchronized cardioversion. Although digoxin is often used for the chronic treatment of atrial fibrillation, it is not recommended for emergency treatment. For emergency control of ventricular rate in patients

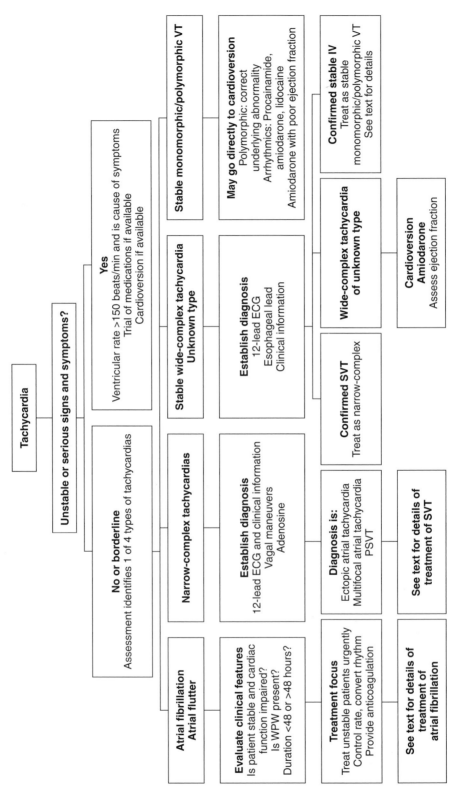

Figure 8-4. Emergency treatment of bradycardia. AV, Atrioventricular; IV, intravenously.

with well-preserved cardiac function, a calcium channel blocker (e.g., diltiazem, verapamil) or a β-blocker (e.g., esmolol, metoprolol, atenolol, propranolol) is recommended. Many consider *diltiazem* to be the first-line drug.[8]

Narrow-Complex Tachycardia

Narrow-complex tachycardias producing symptomatic PSVT can be treated initially by vagal maneuvers. Patients with a history of PSVT usually are familiar with the treatment modalities that are successful for them. Sympathomimetic agents should be avoided in the local anesthetic in patients with suspected PSVT.

The drug of choice for PSVT in a patient with a well-preserved cardiac output is IV *adenosine*. The next medications to consider are a calcium channel blocker, a β-blocker, and digoxin. If these are ineffective, cardioversion can be performed and IV procainamide or amiodarone considered. In patients with poor cardiac output, digoxin, amiodarone and diltiazem can be considered.

Stable Wide-Complex Tachycardia (PVCs)

PVCs typically do not represent an emergency condition. PVCs do not require treatment if they occur less often than six per minute, do not occur in couplets, or are multifocal in nature (requires ECG evaluation). Frequent or multifocal PVCs or couplets may require treatment because they could degrade to a more serious arrhythmia, such as ventricular tachycardia, or because cardiac output may be altered, as evidenced by hypotension. PVCs are best treated with IV infusion of lidocaine, 1.0 to 1.5 mg/kg. PACs alone do not require emergency treatment. If they are associated with significant tachycardia or bradycardia, however, these arrhythmias will need to be treated.

Ventricular Tachycardia

Ventricular tachycardia (VT) is treated whether it is monomorphic or polymorphic and depending on the presence or absence of a prolonged QT interval on ECG. An IV bolus of lidocaine, 1.0 to 1.5 mg/kg repeated at 5- to 10-minute intervals, up to a maximum dose of 3 mg/kg, has been recommended for the treatment of most VTs. ACLS guidelines now include other medications as well, based on the criteria discussed.

Amiodarone is now recommended not only as a secondary medication but also as a replacement for lidocaine in the first-line treatment for some VTs. Amiodarone should be considered a

first-line drug particularly in elderly patients and those with poor cardiac output. Amiodarone is administered in three phases: (1) rapid infusion of 150 mg over 10 minutes, (2) early maintenance infusion of 1mg/min for 6 hours, and (3) late maintenance infusion of 0.5 mg/min, if needed. The maximum daily dose is 2 g. The primary complication is hypotension, and therefore a patient's blood pressure should be carefully monitored when amiodarone is administered. The incidence of hypotension with amiodarone appears to be less than that seen with bretylium, and therefore IV bretylium is no longer recommended as a second-line medication.[9] In patients with well-preserved cardiac output, *procainamide* should be considered a first-line medication before lidocaine (see Figure 8-4).

If VT is present without significant physical findings, care is suspended, vital signs (heart rate and blood pressure) monitored, and oxygen administered via a nasal cannula. *The most common cause of palpitations in dentistry is anxiety or iatrogenic injection of a local anesthetic agent containing epinephrine.* VT secondary to the accidental administration of an IV sympathomimetic is of relatively short duration.

OUTCOMES

Generally, for patients with a history of chronic atrial fibrillation, if they are not showing signs of cardiac ischemia or heart failure, they will spontaneously revert to slower rhythm and can then be discharged for a routine evaluation by their physician. Patients with a PSVT can also be monitored and will likely return to a slower rhythm. In those with a history of PSVT, patients generally can be referred for routine evaluation. In those with new-onset PSVT, patients should be evaluated more emergently for some underlying acute change, such as acute MI.

As with other arrhythmias, VT may be self-limiting. However, VT should never be allowed to persist for more than several seconds treated (even in a hemodynamically stable patient) because of the high likelihood that it could degrade to ventricular fibrillation. Elderly patients and those with ischemic heart disease are at high risk for MI because of increased myocardial oxygen demand.

SUMMARY

Figures 8-2 to 8-4 summarize the algorithms for treatment of arrhythmias. Table 8-2 provides an overview of antiarrhythmic medications.

Table 8-2	Medications for Treatment of Arrhythmias			
Drug	**Common Use**	**Typical Dose**	**Drug Class/Action**	**Precautions**
Epinephrine	Symptomatic bradycardia	1 mg IV push; 10 ml of 1:10,000 solution; can be given via endotracheal tube (2-2.5 mg)	Catecholamine, (α/β-adrenergic agonist	Can exacerbate myocardial ischemia or ventricular ectopy
Atropine	Symptomatic bradycardia	0.5-1.0 mg IV push; can be given via endotracheal tube (1-2 mg)	Parasympatholytic	Can induce tachycardia; anticholinergic syndrome with delirium
Lidocaine	Ventricular tachycardia and fibrillation, symptomatic ectopy	1.0-1.5 mg/kg IV push; can be given via endotracheal tube	Antiarrhythmic (class IB), local anesthetic	Neurologic depression with large dose; seizure induction; can lead to heart block
Procainamide	Ventricular fibrillation and tachycardia, PVCs not controlled by lidocaine	20 mg/min until arrhythmia suppressed, hypotension controlled, or QRS complex widened by 50%; maximum of 17 mg/kg	Antiarrhythmic (class IA), ganglionic blocker	Can cause hypotension with rapid infusion; can induce arrhythmia, including heart block; may be worsened by hypokalemia and hypomagnesemia
Amiodarone	Ventricular tachycardia, supraventricular tachycardia, ventricular fibrillation	IV bolus, 150 mg over 10 minutes, then 1 mg/min IV for 6 hours, then 0.5 mg/min; maximum 24-hour dose of 2 g	Antiarrhythmic; affects sodium, potassium, and calcium channels; (α/β-adrenergic antagonist	Can cause hypotension and bradycardia
Verapamil	PSVT; control of rapid ventricular response in atrial fibrillation and flutter	2.5-5.0 mg IV push over 1-2 minutes; 5-10 mg repeated in 15 to 30 minutes; slower in elderly patients	Calcium channel blocker; slows conduction and prolongs refractoriness at AV node	Transient decrease in blood pressure; can be prevented by pretreatment with calcium chloride

Drug	Indication	Dose	Mechanism	Comments
Diltiazem	PSVT; control of rapid ventricular response in atrial fibrillation and flutter	0.25 mg/kg (20 mg for average patient); IV bolus over 2 minutes; second bolus of 0.35 mg/kg can be administered in 15 minutes if first not effective.	Calcium channel blocker; slows conduction and prolongs refractoriness at AV node	Transient decrease in blood pressure; can be prevented by pretreatment with calcium chloride
Propranolol	Acute myocardial infarction; reduces risk of ventricular fibrillation and mortality	Total dose of 0.1 mg/kg by slow IV push divided into 2-3 doses 2-3 minutes apart; oral maintenance of 180-320 mg/day in divided doses	Nonselective β-adrenergic blocker	See esmolol; use with caution in patients with bronchospasm
Esmolol	Acute treatment of tachycardias, including PSVT and sinus tachycardia; rate control in atrial fibrillation	0.5 mg/kg IV loading dose over 1 minute, then infusion of 50 μg/kg/min for 4 minutes; may repeat cycle every 4 minutes and increase infusion to maximum of 300 μg/kg/min; may continue for up to 48 hours	Selective β_1-adrenergic blocker	Bradycardia, AV conduction delay, hypotension; heart failure: use with caution in severe heart failure, especially with calcium channel blocker; contraindicated in second- or third-degree heart block
Adenosine	PSVT	6-mg rapid bolus over 1-3 seconds, followed by a 20-ml saline flush; may administer 12-mg repeat dose in 1-2 minutes if no response	Endogenous purine nucleoside; slows conduction at AV node; half-life <10 seconds	Transient flushing, dyspnea, chest pain; effect potentiated in patients taking dipyridamole; effect decreased in patients taking methylxanthines (e.g., theophylline)

PVCs, Premature ventricular contractions; PSVT, paroxysmal supraventricular tachycardia; AV, atrioventricular.

Although palpitations may represent a benign process, the risk of potentially life-threatening arrhythmia must always be considered when a patient reports their presence in their medical history. The dentist or other practitioner must have a realistic appreciation of the potential severity of a patient complaint of palpitations and a basic understanding of both the general management and the emergency treatment of patients with cardiac arrhythmias.

REFERENCES

1. Barsky AJ, Cleary PD, Coeytaux RR, Ruskin JN: The clinical course of palpitations in medical outpatients, *Arch Intern Med* 155:1782-1788, 1995.
2. Barsky AJ, Cleary PD, Coeytaux RR, Ruskin JN: Psychiatric disorders in medical outpatients complaining of palpitations, *J Gen Intern Med* 9:306-313, 1994.
3. Jackman WM, Wang XZ, Friday KJ, et al: Catheter ablation of accessory atrioventricular pathways (Wolff-Parkinson-White syndrome) by radiofrequency current, *N Engl J Med* 324:1605-1611, 1991.
4. Kalbfleisch SJ, Calkin H, Langberg JJ, et al: Comparison of the cost of radiofrequency catheter modification of the atrioventricular node and medical therapy for drug refractory atrioventricular nodal reentrant tachycardia, *J Am Coll Cardiol* 19:1583-1587, 1992.
5. De Lurgio DB, Barbour A: Palpitations and tachycardia. In Branch WT, Alexander RW, Schlant RC, Hurst JW, editors: *Cardiology in primary care*, New York, 2000, McGraw-Hill.
6. American Heart Association: Guidelines 2000 for cardiopulmonary resuscitation and emergency cardiovascular care: advanced cardiovascular life support, *Circulation* 102(suppl I):86-171, 2000.
7. American Heart Association: Guidelines 2000 for cardiopulmonary resuscitation and emergency cardiovascular care: the tachycardia algorithms, *Circulation* 102 (suppl I):158-165, 2000.
8. Salemo DM, Dias VC, Kleiger RE, et al: Efficacy and safety of intravenous diltiazem for treatment of atrial fibrillation and atrial flutter, *Am J Cardiol* 63:1046-1051, 1989.
9. Kowey PR, Levine JH, Herre JM, et al: Randomized, double-blind comparison of intravenous amiodarone and bretylium in the treatment of patients with recurrent, hemodynamically destabilizing ventricular tachycardia or fibrillation: the Intravenous Amiodarone Multicenter Investigators Group, *Circulation* 92:3255-3263, 1995.

Hypertension

John A. Yagiela
Reuben N. Turner

Hypertension is a condition in which the systolic blood pressure is 140 mm Hg or greater, the diastolic blood pressure is 90 mm Hg or greater, or the patient is taking medication to control blood pressure.[1] Hypertension is a "modern" disorder in that (1) humans living in primitive cultures rarely have it, and (2) it was only recognized in the twentieth century as posing a significant health risk. Even the term *essential hypertension*, now used to indicate hypertension of unknown etiology (i.e., idiopathic or primary hypertension), originated from the mistaken belief that some people needed blood pressures higher than normal for adequate perfusion of tissues. Table 9-1 lists the various categories of hypertension.[1]

Approximately 70% of the American population with hypertension are aware of their condition. However, only two fifths of these individuals are adequately controlled, leaving almost 75% of the more than 50 million Americans with hypertension at increased risk of cardiovascular disorders, cerebrovascular accidents (CVAs, strokes), peripheral vascular disease, renal problems, and progressive retinopathy.

Hypertensive crises ensue when the blood pressure becomes so high that acute organ damage occurs or threatens. True emergencies include hypertension accompanied by acute encephalopathy, intracranial hemorrhage, retinal hemorrhage and papilledema, dissecting aortic aneurysm, microangiopathic hemolytic anemia, myocardial ischemia, acute pulmonary edema, acute renal insufficiency, or severe preeclampsia.

Hypertension manifesting as a medical emergency in the dental office is a rare but potentially catastrophic event. The dentist must be able to recognize a hypertensive emergency and ensure that the patient receives immediate and appropriate care. Identifying the undiagnosed hypertensive patient and assessing the adequacy of antihypertensive therapy in patients with known high blood pressure are also essential responsibilities. Finally, the dentist must be able to modify the dental treatment plan as appropriate in response to the patient's medical status.[2]

PATHOPHYSIOLOGY

The arterial blood pressure is a dynamic product of the *cardiac output* and *peripheral vascular resistance* (PVR). It is one of the most highly regulated physiologic parameters, dependent on local factors governing the microcirculation and on the integrated actions of the cardiovascular, autonomic, renal, and endocrine systems. Because the delivery of nutrients to and removal of waste products from the various tissues of the body are essential requirements for life, the blood pressure, which powers this transport in complex animals, is highly controlled.

Cardiovascular Risk

Hypertension occurs when the resting blood pressure reaches a certain value, whether the 95th percentile for a given age in childhood or a 140 mm Hg systolic or 90 mm Hg diastolic measurement for adults. This definition is necessarily arbitrary because hypertension is usually without symptoms for decades but is clearly a major risk factor for two leading causes of death, heart attack and stroke. The relationship between blood pressure and cardiovascular risk has been described as "strong, continuous, graded, consistent, independent, predictive, and etiologically significant."[1] Recent findings suggest that systolic blood pressure higher than a certain threshold (e.g., above 160 mm Hg in men ages 65 to 74) and increased pulse width (difference between systolic and diastolic blood pressures) are especially important predictors of cardiovascular risk.[3,4] Compared with their normotensive counterparts, hypertensive individuals (ages 55 to 64) experience three times as much occlusive peripheral arterial disease and

Table 9-1	Classification of Blood Pressure for Adults and Dental Recommendations			
Category	**Systolic (mm Hg)**		**Diastolic (mm Hg)**	**Recommendation**
Optimal	<120	and	<80	Regular dental care.
Normal	<130	and	<85	Regular dental care.
High-normal	130-139	or	85-89	Regular dental care; advise patient of blood pressure status.
HYPERTENSION				
Stage 1	140-159	or	90-99	Regular dental care; recommend physician consultation.
Stage 2	160-179	or	100-109	Noninvasive elective care or definitive emergency care; refer to physician for evaluation and treatment.
Stage 3	≥180	or	≥110	Noninvasive emergency care only; refer to physician for immediate follow-up.
Hypertensive crisis	>220	or	>120	Hospitalization and immediate blood pressure reduction if signs and symptoms of organ damage; otherwise refer to physician for immediate follow-up.

Modified from National Heart, Lung, and Blood Institute, National High Blood Pressure Education Program: *The sixth report of the Joint Committee on Prevention, Detection, Evaluation, and Treatment of High Blood Pressure*, NIH Pub No 98-4080, Bethesda, Md, National Institutes of Health.

coronary heart disease, more than seven times as many strokes, and a fourfold increase in the incidence of congestive heart failure.[5]

Many substances in the body influence cardiac output and PVR (Figure 9-1). In cases of *secondary hypertension* a single definite factor can be identified that is causing the increased blood pressure. Rectifying the underlying problem in these patients (10% or less of all hypertensive individuals) can normalize the blood pressure.

Primary (Essential) Hypertension

Primary hypertension, which is diagnosed by excluding secondary forms of the disorder, has not been attributed to any particular etiology. Rather, it is the consequence of a homeostatic system whose "set point" is inappropriately high for the relatively sedentary nature and animal-rich, high-calorie diet of Western civilization.

In most cases of primary hypertension, PVR is increased throughout the body.[6] Enhanced smooth muscle contraction in the resistance arterioles accounts for much of this increase. Flow resistance in arterioles is also influenced by fluid dynamics. Resistance is inversely correlated with blood volume and changes in osmolarity and temperature. Local tissue edema and overhydra-

tion of the arteriolar wall, along with increased blood viscosity, tend to increase resistance to flow. Venules are responsive to these same influences and react similarly to their arteriolar counterparts.

Most patients with primary hypertension have a normal cardiac output despite the increased PVR. Compensatory mechanisms, including venular contraction and increased venous return to the heart, activation of the renin-angiotensin system, and maintenance of sympathetic tone, increase myocardial work to overcome the elevated afterload associated with increased PVR.

Enhanced sympathetic nervous system activity plays a prominent role in promoting vasoconstriction in essential hypertension. The complexity of this system makes it difficult to isolate a particular component for study, let alone assign causation, in this disease.

Signals from baroreceptors in the carotid sinus and aortic arch are carried by afferent autonomic nerve fibers to the nucleus tractus solitarius (NTS) in the medulla. Stretch receptors located in the lungs and heart (both atria and ventricles) provide additional stimuli to the NTS. These signals activate the NTS in response to increased blood pressure and volume; they inhibit the NTS when there is hypotension and hypo-

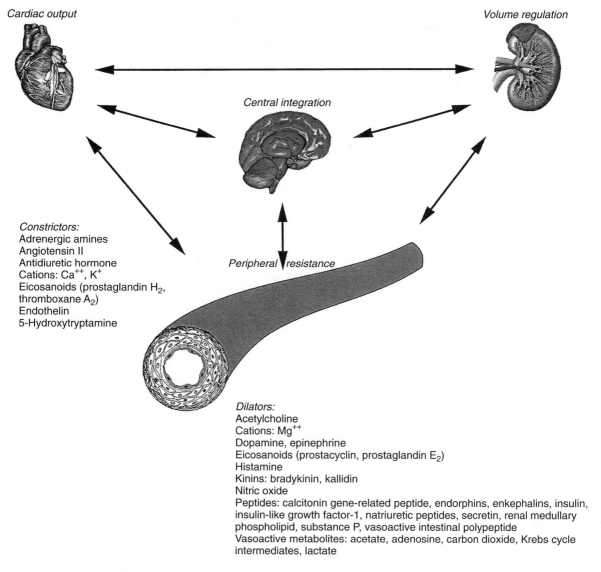

Cardiac output

Volume regulation

Central integration

Constrictors:
Adrenergic amines
Angiotensin II
Antidiuretic hormone
Cations: Ca^{++}, K^+
Eicosanoids (prostaglandin H_2,
thromboxane A_2)
Endothelin
5-Hydroxytryptamine

Peripheral resistance

Dilators:
Acetylcholine
Cations: Mg^{++}
Dopamine, epinephrine
Eicosanoids (prostacyclin, prostaglandin E_2)
Histamine
Kinins: bradykinin, kallidin
Nitric oxide
Peptides: calcitonin gene-related peptide, endorphins, enkephalins, insulin,
insulin-like growth factor-1, natriuretic peptides, secretin, renal medullary
phospholipid, substance P, vasoactive intestinal polypeptide
Vasoactive metabolites: acetate, adenosine, carbon dioxide, Krebs cycle
intermediates, lactate

Figure 9-1. Regulation of blood pressure, with specific endogenous modifiers of vascular tone.

volemia. Afferent fibers from skeletal muscle and the kidneys are inhibitory to the NTS. The NTS also integrates inhibitory and stimulatory inputs from the cerebral cortex, basal ganglia, and brainstem.

The NTS provides inhibitory tone to the rostral ventrolateral nucleus, also known as the *vasomotor control center*. The hypothalamus is another primary source of information to the vasomotor center, helping to mediate acute responses to physical and emotional stress while integrating homeostatic inputs dealing with thermoregulation and salt and water balance.

Impulses arising from activation of sympathetic neurons in the vasomotor center are carried by axons that emerge from the thoracolumbar spinal cord to synapse with postganglionic neurons in the sympathetic ganglia and the adrenal medulla. In turn, these neurons release norepinephrine, along with adenosine triphosphate (ATP) and other vasoactive substances, onto receptors located on target cells (e.g., vascular myocytes, myocardial cells). In the adrenal medulla, specialized postganglionic cells release catecholamines, principally epinephrine but also norepinephrine, directly into the circulation. A pronounced axonal arborization of sympathetic neurons and the release of catecholamines by the adrenal medulla support a generalized response to sympathetic nervous system activation.

In addition to causing vasoconstriction (both in resistance and capacitance vessels) and stimulating myocardial function (increasing cardiac output), sympathetic stimulation raises blood pressure less directly by invoking other systems, especially the renin-angiotensin system, that regulate blood volume, PVR, and cardiac output. Stimulation of β_1-adrenergic receptors by norepinephrine and epinephrine promotes the release of renin from the juxtaglomerular cells of the kidney. Renin, a glycoprotein protease, cleaves the decapeptide angiotensin I from the circulating α_2-globulin angiotensinogen. In turn, angiotensin I is converted to the octapeptide angiotensin II by angiotensin-converting enzyme (ACE, also known as kininase II because of its ability to degrade bradykinin).

Angiotensin II is a powerful vasoconstrictor. It stimulates angiotensin I receptors to constrict arterioles directly; it also amplifies the action of norepinephrine on vascular α-adrenergic receptors. In addition, angiotensin II promotes sympathetic function by (1) increasing norepinephrine synthesis, (2) promoting norepinephrine release from postganglionic nerve terminals, and (3) preventing norepinephrine reuptake. Centrally, angiotensin II stimulates the vasomotor center by binding to receptors in the area postrema of the medulla. These actions, almost immediate in onset, are supported by other actions that result in delayed and even long-term changes in cardiovascular function. Angiotensin II stimulates the release of aldosterone from the adrenal cortex, a hormone that promotes sodium-potassium exchange and water retention in the distal convoluted tubules of the kidney. Over time this action, with complementary enhancement of antidiuretic hormone (ADH) secretion from the pituitary gland, increases blood volume. Long-term changes over years are associated with the role of angiotensin II in cardiovascular cell growth and hypertrophy.

An increased hemodynamic load, whether caused by angiotensin II, norepinephrine, or another inciter, eventually results in tissue remodeling to accommodate the load. The muscle walls of both the vasculature and the ventricles become thicker and less compliant. Reduced compliance in turn blunts the ability of mechanoreceptors to respond to increased arterial pressure and blood volume. Angiotensin II alone and in association with cate-

cholamines also stimulates vascular and cardiac muscle cells to grow independently of its hemodynamic effects. Trophic factors are released in these tissues, causing activation of intracellular mediators of cellular division and hypertrophy. The net result of these long-term changes is anatomic reinforcement of the hypertension and development of other diseases associated with high blood pressure, or essential hypertension.

Hypertensive Crisis

A hypertensive crisis is an acute increase in blood pressure to a value, usually considered to be greater than 220 mm Hg systolic and/or 120 mm Hg diastolic, where target organ damage is occurring or impending. Such crises generally develop in persons with preexisting hypertension; they may also arise in late pregnancy (preeclampsia-eclampsia) and result from management errors such as acute vasoconstrictor overdosage.

When systemic vascular resistance is greatly increased (e.g., with cessation of antihypertensive medication, acute renal impairment, or excessive stimulation of the sympathetic nervous system), arteriolar fibrinoid necrosis may ensue from the endothelial damage, platelet aggregation, and fibrin deposition secondary to the extreme blood pressure. Loss of the local blood supply causes ischemia in the target tissue. Ischemia then triggers the release of additional vasoactive substances. Unchecked, this vicious cycle results in infarction and irreversible damage to the affected organ. Death is the ultimate outcome.

DIFFERENTIAL DIAGNOSIS
Chronic Hypertension

Although most patients with chronic hypertension are simply classified as having "primary hypertension," this designation belies the diversity of abnormalities expressed in this group. For example, patients with primary hypertension can be differentiated by their (1) plasma renin activity; (2) sensitivity to dietary sodium, chloride, and calcium; and (3) resistance to insulin. Future research likely will uncover distinct causes of high blood pressure in these patients.

More than half of all cases of secondary hypertension are related to *renal disease*, such as pyelonephritis, glomerulonephritis, polycystic renal disease, and renovascular disease. Especially in renovascular disease, activation of the renin-angiotensin system in response to impaired renal perfusion is a common finding. Sodium retention and increased blood volume are prominent in patients with parenchymal renal disease.

Additional causes of secondary hypertension include primary hyperaldosteronism, Cushing's syndrome, thyroid disease, hypercalcemic disorders, pheochromocytoma, acromegaly, central nervous system tumors, and coarctation of the aorta. Drug use (e.g., alcohol, adrenergic drugs, cocaine, corticosteroids, cyclosporine, erythropoietin, oral contraceptives) constitutes another form of secondary hypertension.

Acute Hypertension

Significantly elevated blood pressure in anticipation of dental procedures is uncommon in healthy adults but more likely to occur in the hypertensive patient.[7] In the highly anxious patient without underlying hypertension, however, "white-coat syndrome" may result in spuriously high recordings, particularly systolic blood pressure, whenever measurements are taken in the office setting. Labile blood pressures are also encountered in individuals who go on to develop sustained hypertension.

Acute increases in blood pressure are frequently observed in stressful situations. Hypertensive responses during dental procedures and similar interventions may be linked to a variety of causes. For example, a noticeable increase in blood pressure and heart rate often occurs when patients are subjected to extractions under local anesthesia.[8] Hypertensive patients show a greater increase in blood pressure under these circumstances than do normotensive patients. Activation of the sympathetic nervous system response may be associated with fear and anxiety, pain, or the vasoconstrictor in the local anesthetic solution. Patients who have received general anesthesia or deep sedation may also become hypertensive because of hypoxia, hypercarbia, a full urinary bladder, overhydration, gastric distention, or delirium (e.g., during emergence from anesthesia). Acute hypertension during general anesthesia is more likely to occur in the chronically hypertensive patient, especially with a history of inadequate blood pressure control.[9]

Many of the drugs listed previously as causes of secondary hypertension also play a role in acute increases in blood pressure. Cocaine, amphetamines, certain dietary suppressants, and other sympathomimetics typically cause rapid elevations in blood pressure when taken in toxic amounts. Patients receiving monoamine oxidase inhibitors (e.g., pargyline) are likely to experience pressor crises when ingesting foods rich in tyramine (aged meats, cheeses, fermented beverages) or when given indirect-acting adrenergic agents (e.g., amphetamine) and certain other drugs (e.g., meperidine). The sudden cessation of adrenolytic antihypertensive therapy may result in *rebound hypertension*. Adrenolytic agents comprise the α- and β-adrenergic blockers, centrally acting antihypertensives, and adrenergic neuron blockers.

True hypertensive emergencies are diagnosed according to the organ affected. *Hypertensive encephalopathy* is characterized by severe headache, vomiting, confusion, visual and motor disturbances, convulsions, and coma. In this emergency, excessive cerebral blood flow from a loss of autoregulation is superimposed on arteriolar fibrinoid necrosis. Ocular damage in the form of swelling of the optic disc (papilledema) and hemorrhagic edema of the retina often occurs in conjunction with hypertensive encephalopathy, but eye injury is also itself a true emergency.

Hypertension often accompanies stroke, both as a risk factor for stroke and as a consequence of the disrupted cerebral circulation. Strokes are caused by thrombotic or embolic occlusion of a cerebral artery resulting in brain tissue infarction or by spontaneous rupture of a vessel resulting in intracerebral or subarachnoid hemorrhage. Common manifestations of CVA include sudden alterations in vision, paralysis or numbness (both usually unilateral), and language disturbances. Abnormal sensations, vertigo, and ataxia are other indicators. Sudden severe headache, nausea and vomiting, and decreased consciousness suggest hemorrhagic stroke.

Myocardial ischemia is often a complication of severe hypertension. The increased workload of the heart causes the oxygen demand to exceed the available supply in persons with coronary artery disease. Sympathetic nervous system arousal may also follow an acute myocardial infarction. Retrosternal chest pain or pressure is the most common symptom of myocardial ischemia. The pain may be localized or spread to the shoulders, neck, arms, jaw, or back. Other indicators include a feeling of anxiety or impending doom, lightheadedness or fainting, nausea, excessive perspiration, and shortness of breath. The 12-lead electrocardiogram (ECG) is the most important evaluative tool for diagnosing the acute coronary syndrome and determining early therapy.[10]

Aortic dissection as a consequence of high blood pressure may produce pain similar to that of a myocardial infarction. If blood forced through a tear in the aortic intima involves the ascending aorta, it may block a coronary artery and even cause a heart attack. Rupture of a dissecting aneurysm rapidly leads to hypovolemic shock. Aortic dissection is usually diagnosed by computed tomography.

Acute *pulmonary edema* and other signs of congestive heart failure may be associated with severe hypertension when the heart is unable to pump blood sufficiently against the elevated PVR. Inadequate perfusion of tissues may lead to fatigue or weakness; pulmonary congestion results in rapid labored breathing, rales, frothy sputum, and cyanosis. These manifestations of acute heart failure also may be associated with profound hypotension. Jugular venous distention, peripheral edema, and hepatomegaly are signs of right ventricular failure.

Acute *renal failure* is both a cause and result of severe hypertension. As renal vasoconstriction contributes to the increased PVR, the decreased blood flow activates the renin-angiotensin system. Interference with urine production, elevated urinary protein, decreased creatinine clearance, and plasma electrolyte disturbances are indicative of this condition.

Preeclampsia is a systemic disorder of pregnancy in which greatly increased PVR results from heightened responsiveness to angiotensin II and other vasoactive peptides. Proteinuria, liver abnormalities, thrombocytopenia, rapid weight gain, and peripheral edema are common manifestations of the disorder. Upper abdominal pain, mental confusion, blood pressures above 160/110 mm Hg, and rapid declines in kidney function predict an impending emergency. When convulsions ensue, the full-blown syndrome of eclampsia is evident.

Microangiopathic hemolytic anemia may develop when red blood cells are disrupted and platelets are trapped by fibrin deposits in damaged blood vessels. Because it is unlikely for clinical signs and symptoms to develop quickly as a consequence of this disorder, diagnosis is usually made by detecting red cell fragments in peripheral blood.

PATIENT ASSESSMENT

Hypertension is diagnosed and monitored by measuring the blood pressure at repeated intervals. A standard approach is necessary to obtain accurate recordings that can be compared over time. As an initial requirement, the patient should be free of drugs that increase blood pressure. For example, the patient should not smoke or ingest caffeine-containing substances for at least 30 minutes before the blood pressure is recorded. The patient should also rest for 5 minutes before measurement.

With the patient seated in a chair supporting the back and the arm at heart level, a blood pressure cuff that encircles at least 80% of the upper arm is placed snugly. The systolic and diastolic blood pressures are then taken with a mercury sphygmomanometer or a recently calibrated manual or automatic device in a manner recommended by the American Heart Association[11] or the manufacturer. A second reading is taken 2 minutes later, and the measurements are then averaged. Additional recordings—using the opposite arm, with the patient standing, or by the patient at home—may be necessary for specific diagnostic purposes. Repeated measurements, at 1-week to 2-month intervals depending on the clinical situation, are regularly taken to confirm the diagnosis of hypertension.

Initial evaluation of the hypertensive patient includes a detailed medical history, physical examination, and laboratory studies. The goals of this investigation are (1) to identify correctable causes of the high blood pressure; (2) to determine the extent, if any, of hypertension-associated organ damage; and (3) to identify risk or health factors that may modify antihypertensive therapy.

To supplement information obtained with a typical medical history form, the physician should inquire about the patient's personal and family history of hypertension and closely related ailments (heart disease, vascular disease, dyslipidemia, renal disease, diabetes mellitus). The patient should also be asked about recent changes in lifestyle, body weight, dietary habits, drug use (including prescription drugs as well as over-the-counter remedies, alcohol, tobacco products, and illicit substances), or physical activity and exercise tolerance.

The physical examination begins with an assessment of the patient's general appearance, including skin color and fat and muscle distribution. The neck should be evaluated for carotid bruits (abnormal sounds caused by blood rushing through a stenotic artery), distended jugular veins, and thyroid gland hypertrophy. Auscultation of the heart and lungs is performed to detect abnormal cardiac rhythms or sounds or evidence of congestive heart failure. The abdomen is examined for enlarged organs or abnormal blood flow, and the extremities are checked for peripheral pulses, bruits, edema, and loss of function. Finally, a funduscopic examination is necessary to detect the presence and degree of retinopathy.

Basic laboratory studies in all newly identified hypertensive patients generally include a urinalysis, complete blood count, blood chemistry (glucose, creatinine, uric acid, electrolytes, lipid profile), 12-lead ECG, and chest radiograph. Additional tests may be ordered depending on the results of the initial investigation. For example, an abdominal bruit suggests renovascular hypertension, and the physician might order a renal angiogram and renal vein renin determination to confirm the diagnosis.

Once the diagnosis is established and treatment initiated, continued monitoring of the hypertensive patient is required to assess the effectiveness of therapy and make any necessary adjustments to treatment. Periodic evaluations also help maintain patient compliance and detect progression of the disorder or presence of a comorbid disease (e.g., atherosclerosis, congestive heart disease).

Because many individuals schedule dental appointments on a regular basis but seek medical care infrequently, the dentist is strategically positioned to detect hypertension and related disorders. It is a standard of care for the dentist to take a medical history and record the patient's blood pressure before initiating treatment. The dentist should also be observant for evidence of disease states that may involve hypertension as an integral component, such as chest pain, shortness of breath, exercise intolerance, and dizzy spells. Referring the patient for medical evaluation and follow-up consultation with the patient's physician are indicated for every patient who may have undiagnosed hypertension.

TREATMENT
Chronic Hypertension

The goal of therapy in patients with primary hypertension is to reduce the blood pressure to the normal range (e.g., below 140/90 mm Hg). In the case of secondary hypertension, there is the additional goal of correcting, if possible, the underlying cause of the elevated blood pressure. Even small decreases in blood pressure can prove highly beneficial. Long-term reduction of the diastolic pressure by 5 to 6 mm Hg may be associated with 35% to 40% fewer strokes and 20% to 25% less coronary heart disease.[12]

Lifestyle modifications are a key to both prevention and successful management of hypertension in all patients. Weight reduction in the obese patient is a crucial if challenging aim. Caloric restriction and regular aerobic exercise provide benefits of reduced blood pressure and decreased risk of comorbid diseases such as diabetes mellitus and atherosclerotic heart disease. Specific dietary modifications useful in hypertensive patients include modest restriction of sodium (to no more than 6 g sodium chloride per day) and alcohol (daily maximum of 1 oz for males, 0.5 oz for females), and adequate intake of potassium (at least 90 mmol per day). Although cessation of smoking and avoidance of foods high in cholesterol and saturated fat have little effect on blood pressure itself, they are vital to minimizing the risk of atherosclerosis.

Initiation of drug therapy is based on the stage of hypertension (see Table 9-1), the presence of major risk factors for cardiovascular disease (age over 60 years, diabetes mellitus, dyslipidemia, male gender, postmenopausal women, smoking, significant family history of cardiovascular disease), and the existence of cardiovascular disease or other target organ damage. All patients with stage 2 or stage 3 hypertension are started on pharmacotherapy without delay, but patients with stage 1 high blood pressure and no evidence of existing disease may be managed from 6 to 12 months with lifestyle modifications only.

Drug therapy generally should begin with a diuretic or a β-adrenergic blocker (Table 9-2).[1] This recommendation is based on accumulated information that these drugs reduce mortality and morbidity associated with hypertension. Specific situations may dictate the choice of one group over the other or even the selection of a different agent as initial therapy. For example, diuretics are more effective than β-blockers in the African-American population, but a β-blocker would be preferred in a patient with a history of angina pectoris, myocardial infarction, or hyperthyroidism because its ability to minimize myocardial ischemia and prevent cardiac dysrhythmias. Alternative agents used as first-line drugs include ACE inhibitors in patients with heart failure, renal insufficiency, or diabetes mellitus; α_1-adrenergic blockers with coexisting dyslipidemia or prostatism; and calcium channel blockers in patients with isolated systolic hypertension. Occasionally, preexisting medical conditions contraindicate the use of a first-choice drug. Thus β-blockers are not an initial agent of choice in the patient with asthma or congestive heart failure, and other drugs are preferred over the diuretics in the patient with gout. Finally, many practitioners use an ACE inhibitor or a calcium channel blocker as initial therapy. The most

Table 9-2	Antihypertensive Drugs	
Drug Class	**Mechanism of Action**	**Adverse Effects**
FIRST-CHOICE DRUGS*		
Diuretics (e.g., hydrochloro-thiazide)	Decreased extracellular fluid volume and cardiac output initially, followed by decreased total peripheral resistance with normalization of cardiac output	Increased cholesterol and uric acid concentrations, potassium and other electrolyte disturbances, orthostatic hypotension, renal insufficiency
β-Adrenergic blockers (e.g., metoprolol)	Decreased cardiac output, plasma renin activity, peripheral vascular resistance (delayed effect except for labetalol and carvedilol), and pressor responses to sympathetic nervous system activation	Bronchospasm, bradycardia, decreased exercise tolerance, fatigue, heart failure, insomnia, rebound hypertension and cardiac disturbances from sudden termination; may mask signs of insulin-induced hypoglycemia
ALTERNATIVE FIRST-CHOICE DRUGS*		
ACE inhibitors (e.g., enalapril)	Decreased angiotensin II formation initially, bradykinin inactivation with persistent vasodilation, decreased aldosterone production and adrenergic tone, improved vascular compliance	Angioedema, cough, dysgeusia, fetal toxicity, hyperkalemia, leukopenia, rash, renal insufficiency
α_1-Adrenergic blockers (e.g., terazosin)	Blockade of α_1-adrenergic receptors, decreased vascular resistance	Orthostatic hypotension, tachycardia, fluid retention, dizziness, headache
Angiotensin II receptor blockers (e.g., losartan)	Blockade of angiotensin I receptors, leading to vasodilation, decreased aldosterone production and adrenergic activity, and improved vascular compliance	Similar to ACE inhibitors, but no cough and angioedema less likely
Calcium channel blockers (e.g., nicardipine)	Blocked inward movement of calcium ions across cell membranes, reducing vascular smooth muscle contraction; cardioactive blockers (e.g., verapamil) also decrease heart rate and cardiac output	Headache, edema, flushing, gingival hyperplasia; bradycardia, heart block, and heart failure with verapamil and diltiazem; nifedipine-like drugs may cause tachycardia and anginal pain
OTHER DRUGS*		
Adrenergic neuronal blockers (e.g., guanethidine)	Decreased adrenergic tone by interference with catecholamine storage and/or catecholamine release	Bradycardia, diarrhea, fluid retention, muscle weakness, orthostatic hypotension (strong), impotence, renal insufficiency, bronchospasm
Centrally acting α_2-adrenergic agonists (e.g., clonidine)	Stimulation of central α_2-adrenergic receptors that inhibit efferent sympathetic activity	Fluid retention, orthostatic hypotension, somnolence, xerostomia; rebound hypertension from sudden termination; autoimmune reactions with methyldopa
Direct-acting vasodilators (e.g., minoxidil)	Relaxation of vascular smooth muscle, decreased peripheral vascular resistance	Fluid retention, headache, muscle weakness, orthostatic hypotension, tachycardia; hirsutism with minoxidil, lupuslike syndrome with hydralazine

Modified from National Heart, Lung, and Blood Institute, National High Blood Pressure Education Program: *The sixth report of the Joint National Committee on Prevention, Detection, Evaluation, and Treatment of High Blood Pressure,* NIH Pub No 98-4080, Bethesda, Md, 1997, National Institutes of Health.

**First-choice drugs* are indicated for uncomplicated hypertension. *Alternative first-choice drugs* may be preferred if there is a compelling indication for their selection or if they may have favorable effects on comorbid conditions, such as diabetes mellitus or prostatism. *Other drugs* may be tried in combination with one or more first-choice drugs for refractory hypertension.

common justification given is that compliance is better with these drugs because of fewer adverse effects.

The selected drug is started at a low dose, which is then increased in stepwise fashion over the next few months until the blood pressure is controlled, adverse effects intervene, or the maximum recommended dose is reached. If full or tolerated doses of the initial drug prove insufficient to normalize the blood pressure, alternative agents are selected or added to the therapeutic regimen. Diuretics are often used in combination with other first-line drugs because diuretics often potentiate the effects and reduce adverse effects of these drugs. Refractory cases of hypertension may require the addition or substitution of one or more additional agents. The physician must also seek out possible reasons for therapeutic failure, such as patient noncompliance, excessive sodium or alcohol intake, or drug interactions.

Dental Considerations

The dentist plays an important supportive role in the medical management of patients with chronic hypertension. Blood pressure recordings of known hypertensive individuals should be taken during regular checkups and at every appointment when an invasive procedure is planned. These measurements help determine the effectiveness of the antihypertensive therapy and provide a baseline for the dentist should an untoward event occur during a planned procedure. Recommended responses by the dentist to specific blood pressure measurements are listed in Table 9-1.

Important drug interactions occur between common antihypertensive agents and drugs used for pain and anxiety control in dentistry (Table 9-3). Interactions involving the vasoconstrictors epinephrine and levonordefrin are quick in onset and short-lived because of their rapid absorption and metabolism after intraoral injection. Rarely, life-threatening responses have occurred with vasoconstrictor dosages used in dentistry. Interactions involving nonsteroidal antiinflammatory analgesics are slower to develop but likely to continue for as long as the analgesic is taken. Recommendations to minimize problems associated with these and related drug interactions are given in Table 9-3.

Postural hypotension or *orthostatic hypotension* may develop as the hypertensive patient rises from

Table 9-3	Drug Interactions Between Antihypertensives and Dental Agents		
Antihypertensive	**Dental Agent**	**Possible Effect**	**Recommendation**
Diuretics (e.g., furosemide, hydrochlorothiazide)	NSAIDs (e.g., ibuprofen)	Decreased renal blood flow, loss of antihypertensive effect	Warn patient about possible interaction; consult physician regarding use in stage 3 hypertension.
	Epinephrine, levonordefrin	Transient hypokalemia	Consult physician; avoid use if patient is hypokalemic.
β-Adrenergic blockers (e.g., metoprolol)	NSAIDs (e.g., ibuprofen)	Decreased renal blood flow, loss of antihypertensive effect	Warn patient about possible interaction; consult physician regarding use in stage 3 hypertension.
Nonselective β-blockers (e.g., propranolol)	Epinephrine, levonordefrin	Hypertension, bradycardia	Use cautiously; monitor blood pressure.
ACE inhibitors (e.g., captopril)	NSAIDs (e.g., ibuprofen)	Decreased renal blood flow, loss of antihypertensive effect	Warn patient about possible interaction; consult physician regarding use in stage 3 hypertension.
Centrally acting α_2-adrenergic receptor agonists (e.g., clonidine)	CNS depressants, opioid analgesics	Increased CNS depression	Use cautiously.
Peripheral adrenergic neuron blockers (e.g., guanethidine	Epinephrine, levonordefrin	Increased cardiovascular responses to vasoconstrictor	Use cautiously; monitor blood pressure.

NSAIDs, Nonsteroidal antiinflammatory drugs; *CNS*, central nervous system.

the dental chair after a treatment session (see Chapter 10). Particularly with such secondary agents as the adrenergic neuronal blockers, postural hypotension may cause the patient to transiently lose balance or even consciousness and fall down. Extensive injuries, including facial trauma and broken hips, have resulted. As a general rule, patients receiving antihypertensive medication should be slowly raised from a reclining to a fully upright position with constant observation to ensure safety.

Hypertensive Crisis

Medical management of a hypertensive crisis depends on the presence or likelihood of target organ damage. In the true emergency, therapy must be instituted to reduce the blood pressure, by no more than 25% initially (several minutes to 2 hours), then toward 160/100 mm Hg over the next 2 to 4 hours while avoiding complications of inadequate tissue perfusion. Intravenous therapy with vasodilators is standard treatment (Table 9-4).

A possible exception to immediate blood pressure control is hypertension in association with an ischemic stroke. Although occlusion of a cerebral artery frequently results in extreme elevations of blood pressure, stroke patients often exhibit heightened responses to antihypertensive medication, and a reduction in cerebral perfusion pressure may increase tissue ischemia. Therefore, in patients who are not candidates for thrombolytic therapy, pressures below 220/120 mm Hg are generally not treated unless there is evidence of concomitant cardiovascular decompensation or hypertensive encephalopathy.[10] Hypertension in thrombolytic candidates and in patients with hemorrhagic stroke is generally treated if the pressure is above 185/105 mm Hg.

Hypertensive urgencies do not require immediate reduction in blood pressure. In fact, oral or sublingual administration of nifedipine has led to uncontrolled, precipitous falls in blood pressure and sudden death. Oral agents with relatively rapid onsets of action and more predictable effects are preferred in the management of hypertensive urgencies, so that dosages can be adjusted over the course of a few days to weeks in the outpatient setting to elicit the desired response.

Dental Management

If a hypertensive crisis occurs in the dental office, the dental team must respond quickly and appropriately. If the patient experiences some difficulty, as for any emergency the initial response includes (1) ceasing treatment, (2) positioning the patient (supine for most emergencies, sitting upright for acute breathing problems in the conscious patient), and (3) assessing the airway, breathing, and circulation (ABCs). If an excessive blood pressure is discovered in this process, the treatment protocol outlined in Figure 9-2 should be followed. The same algorithm should also be used if an excessive blood pressure is recorded during routine monitoring of the patient with no obvious signs or symptoms of a medical emergency.

Once the abnormal blood pressure is verified as described previously, the patient should be examined for any manifestations of target organ damage or dysfunction that might presage such damage. If a true hypertensive emergency is suspected, the dentist should immediately request emergency medical services (EMS). Continuous monitoring of the patient and recording of vital signs at 5-minute intervals until EMS personnel arrive is necessary to ensure optimal safety of the potentially decompensating patient. Oxygen supplementation by mask or nasal prongs may help ameliorate tissue ischemia. Drug therapy by the dentist is usually indicated only when the hypertension is accompanied by signs of myocardial ischemia. Nitroglycerin in the form of sublingual tablets or spray is administered to reduce the blood pressure and lessen myocardial workload. Acute anginal pain may dissipate as the oxygen supply to the heart becomes more in line with the oxygen demand of the myocardium.

If there is no evidence of target organ damage and the blood pressure is stabilized or decreasing, the dentist can then discharge the patient to the primary physician for immediate follow-up. Consultation with the physician while the patient is being monitored is advised. If the patient does not have medical support, the dentist should arrange a referral.

Dentists who provide deep sedation or general anesthesia services for patients assume additional responsibilities in the management of perioperative high blood pressure. Hypertensive responses to surgical stimuli, inadequate oxygenation or ventilation, and other inducers of sympathetic nervous system activity must be treated to minimize myocardial ischemia and other hypertension-related problems. If specific interventions, such as the administration of opioids and local anesthetics for pain relief, fail to ameliorate the cardiovascular stimulation, antihypertensive medications may be used (see

Table 9-4 Antihypertensive Drugs for Intraoperative Hypertension and Hypertensive Emergencies

Drug Dose	Onset of Action Time	Duration	Adverse Effects	Comments
Sodium nitroprusside (Nitropress): 0.3-10 µg/kg/min IV infusion (10 min only at high infusion rate)	0.5-2 min	1-2 min	Cyanide and thiocyanate toxicity, fluid retention, flushing, methemoglobinemia, nausea	Direct-acting vasodilator; usually drug of choice; requires continuous blood pressure monitoring; tolerance with volume expansion
Nitroglycerin (Nitro-Bid IV, Tridil): 5-100 µg/min IV infusion	2-5 min	2-5 min	Dizziness, headache, methemoglobinemia, nausea, rash, tachycardia	Direct vasodilator; indicated with myocardial ischemia; tolerance with prolonged use
Trimethaphan camsylate (Arfonad): 0.3-6 mg/min IV infusion	1-2 min	10-30 min	Histamine release, paralytic ileus, respiratory arrest, urinary retention	Ganglionic blocker; indicated for short-term control of blood pressure; tolerance with prolonged use
Esmolol (Brevibloc): 500 µg/kg/min IV for 1 min, then 50 µg/kg/min for 4 min; if inadequate, repeat loading dose and increase infusion by 50 µg/kg/min (up to 300 µg/kg/min)	1-2 min	10-20 min	Nausea, bradycardia; venous irritation with concentrations >10 mg/ml	β₁-Adrenergic receptor blocker; indicated for perioperative hypertension, aortic dissection (with vasodilator)
Fenoldopam mesylate (Corlopam): 0.1-0.3 µg/kg/min IV infusion initially, adjusting by 0.05-0.1 µg/kg/min every 15 min as needed	<5 min	30 min	Headache, hypokalemia, nausea, myocardial ischemia, tachycardia	Dopamine (D1) receptor blocker; indicated for most hypertensive emergencies
Phentolamine (Regitine): 5-10 mg IV every 5-15 min	1-2 min	3-10 min	Dysrhythmias, myocardial ischemia, nausea, stroke, tachycardia	α-Adrenergic receptor blocker; indicated for catecholamine excess (e.g., pheochromocytoma)
Labetalol (Normodyne, Trandate): 10-80 mg IV bolus repeated every 10 min to 300 mg or 0.5-2 mg/min IV infusion (to 300 mg) until desired response	5-10 min	3-6 hr	Bronchospasm, bradycardia, dizziness, flushing, heart block, heart failure, nausea, tingling	α/β-Adrenergic receptor blocker; indicated for most hypertensive emergencies except with heart failure
Diazoxide (Hyperstat IV): 5-15 mg/hr IV infusion (0.1 mg/mL) until desired response, then 3 mg/hr	2-4 min	6-12 hr	Chest pain, dizziness, fluid retention, flushing, hyperglycemia, nausea, tachycardia	Direct-acting vasodilator; used only if continuous monitoring unavailable
Nicardipine (Cardene IV): 5-15 mg/hr IV infusion (0.1 mg/mL) until desired response, then 3 mg/hr	5-10 min	1-4 hr	Flushing, headache, myocardial ischemia, tachycardia, venous irritation	Calcium channel blocker; contraindicated in acute heart failure, myocardial ischemia
Hydralazine (Apresoline): 5-10 mg IV every 20 min to 20 mg	10-30 min	2-8 hr	Flushing, headache, myocardial ischemia, nausea, tachycardia, tartrazine sensitivity	Direct-acting vasodilator; indicated in eclampsia

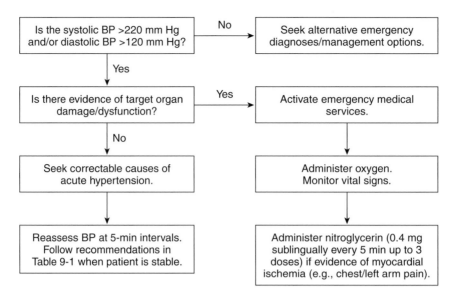

Figure 9-2. Hypertensive crisis algorithm. *BP,* Blood pressure.

Table 9-4). Agents that do not require continuous monitoring of blood pressure are generally preferred in the office setting. *Labetalol,* 5 to 10 mg every 5 to 10 minutes, is a common choice. Because hypertension often develops in the first 1/2-hour after emergence from general anesthesia, regular blood pressure monitoring of the hypertensive patient is strongly advised during the recovery period.[13]

REFERENCES

1. National Heart, Lung, and Blood Institute, National High Blood Pressure Education Program: *The sixth report of the Joint National Committee on Prevention, Detection, Evaluation, and Treatment of High Blood Pressure,* NIH Pub No 98-4080, Bethesda, Md, 1997, National Institutes of Health.
2. Kaplan EL, editor: *Cardiovascular disease in dental practice,* Dallas, 1986, American Heart Association.
3. Port S, Demer L, Jennrich R, et al: Systolic blood pressure and mortality, *Lancet* 355(9199):175-180, 2000.
4. Benetos A, Zureik M, Morcet, J, et al: A decrease in diastolic blood pressure combined with an increase in systolic blood pressure is associated with a higher cardiovascular mortality in men, *J Am Coll Cardiol* 35(3):673-680, 2000.
5. Kannel WB: Role of blood pressure in cardiovascular disease: the Framingham study, *Angiology* 26(1):1-14, 1975.
6. Frohlich ED: *Hypertension: evaluation and treatment,* Baltimore, 1998, Williams & Wilkins.
7. Beck FM, Weaver JM II: Blood pressure and heart rate responses to anticipated high-stress dental treatment, *J Dent Res* 60(1):26-29, 1981.
8. Abraham-Inpijn L, Borgmeijer-Hoelen A, Gortzak RA: Changes in blood pressure, heart rate, and electrocardiogram during dental treatment with use of local anesthesia, *J Am Dent Assoc* 116(4):531-536, 1988.
9. Stoelting RK, Dierdorf SF, McCammon RL, editors: *Anesthesia and co-existing disease,* ed 2, New York, 1988, Churchill Livingstone.
10. Commins RO, editor: *Advanced cardiac life support,* Dallas, 1997, American Heart Association.
11. Perloff D, Grim C, Flack J, et al: Human blood pressure determination by sphygmomanometry, *Circulation* 88(5):2460-2470, 1993.
12. MacMahon S, Peto R, Cutter J, et al: Blood pressure, stroke, and coronary heart disease. Part 1. Prolonged differences in blood pressure: prospective observational studies corrected for the regression dilution bias, *Lancet* 335(8692):765-774, 1990.
13. Feeley TW, Macario A: The postanesthesia care unit. In Miller RD, editor: *Anesthesia,* ed 5, Philadelphia, 2000, Churchill Livingstone.

Hypotension

Vincent B. Ziccardi
Eric M. Alltucker

Any condition that interferes with the tissue perfusion of oxygenated blood to major organ systems will result in an acute medical emergency and lead to unconsciousness and/or cardiac ischemia. If this condition persists, other organ systems will become involved, and the emergency will deteriorate to cardiac arrest. Adequate perfusion depends on maintenance of an adequate mean arterial pressure, which is essentially the average of systolic and diastolic pressures. Hypotension is a relative term that is difficult to define numerically from patient to patient, but decreases in systolic or diastolic pressure of 15 to 20 mm Hg from baseline warrant immediate assessment and possible treatment to prevent escalation into shock. Proper assessment of blood pressure readings across the population requires an understanding that normal variations in many cohorts (e.g., individuals, age groups) are the rule rather than the exception (Table 10-1). Understanding fundamental physiologic and pathologic concepts will greatly aid the diagnosis and treatment of patients with emergency hypotensive conditions.

PHYSIOLOGY AND PATHOPHYSIOLOGY

Systolic blood pressure is determined by *cardiac output*, which is the volume of blood ejected by the left ventricle each minute. Cardiac output is the product of heart rate and stroke volume. *Stroke volume*, or amount of blood pumped with each contraction is influenced by myocardial contractility, which in turn depends on sympathetic stimulation and the intrinsic ability of cardiac muscle to contract more forcefully when it is stretched. This explains why venous return to the heart (*preload*) is such an important determinant in maintaining stroke volume and why heart failure occurs when the myocardium is overstretched.

Peripheral vascular resistance (PVR), on the other hand, largely maintains diastolic blood pressure. During ventricular systole, PVR (*afterload*) op-

poses ventricular ejection and is instrumental in providing the backflow pressure required for coronary artery perfusion. Blood pressure is the product of cardiac output and total PVR. Any direct or indirect changes in one or more of these physiologic parameters will result in changes in blood pressure[1] (Figure 10-1).

An understanding of the physiology of the cardiovascular system elucidates the mechanisms of antihypertensive medications, the changes seen in athletes conditioned by training, the pathophysiology of heart failure, and the management of acute cardiovascular emergencies (Box 10-1).

PATIENT ASSESSMENT

The determination of baseline blood pressure should be an integral part of the physical examination and should be done at every dental examination. This baseline establishes "normal" values for an individual because it is difficult to give an absolute value at which hypotension begins. Blood pressure determination may be inaccurate because of improper patient positioning; incorrect cuff width, position, rate of cuff deflation; or misinterpretation of Kortokoff sounds.

Table 10-1	Normal Variations in Blood Pressure	
Age	**Systolic (mm Hg)**	**Diastolic (mm Hg)**
Infant (2 years)	95-105	53-66
Adolescent (15 years)*	112-128	66-88
Adult*	90-130†	60-90

*With athletes, note that blood pressure may be at the lower end of the scale, depending on age and level of conditioning.

†With elderly patients, note that systolic pressure tends to increase with age.

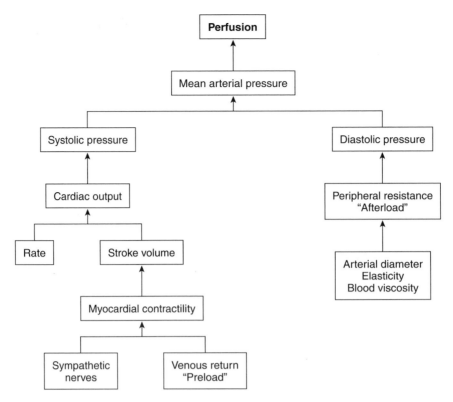

Figure 10-1. Physiologic regulation of arterial pressure.

Box 10-1   **Physiologic Changes in Athletes**

A well-conditioned athlete (e.g., marathon runner) may clinically demonstrate bradycardia and hypotension by conventional measures. Because of rigorous physical conditioning, however, this state may be normal for the athlete and requires no medical treatment. In the athlete the heart pumps more efficiently with each contraction, and stroke volume is greater than in the unconditioned person. In athletes, for a given cardiac output, the heart rate will be lower because of the greater stroke volume. At rest, a lower heart rate will provide the same cardiac output because the stroke volume is greater.

Conversely, a patient who tends to be hypertensive and experiences a sudden drop in blood pressure to the level of the marathon runner would constitute a medical emergency requiring prompt action. In this patient the compensatory mechanism would be to increase the stroke volume and heart rate to maintain the cardiac output. If unable to compensate, a state of hypoperfusion and eventual cardiac arrest would develop.

Pulse pressure and mean arterial pressure (MAP) are calculated as follows:

Pulse pressure = Systolic pressure − Diastolic pressure

MAP = Diastolic pressure + (1/3 × Pulse pressure)

MAP is classically defined as 100 mm Hg, but variations from baseline and the patient's clinical condition are still the best guide in any emergency situation. Generally, a systolic pressure of 90 to 100 mm Hg for patients in a supine position will generate an MAP sufficient for tissue perfusion.

In emergency situations, rapid determination of peripheral and central perfusion will often dictate treatment and outcome. *Peripheral perfusion* is assessed by simply applying finger pressure to the nail beds or oral mucosa and observing for return of normal color. *Central perfusion* is assessed by the patient's response to verbal, and if necessary, painful, stimuli. In unconscious patients, pupillary reflexes can also be an important sign of adequate cerebral perfusion. Hypotensive patients may feel dizzy; may be flushed, weak, or nauseous; or may develop cardiac palpitations. They may have cold extremities, tachycardia or bradycardia, nausea, or confusion and may lose consciousness if the situation is not diagnosed and corrected.

The most common causes of hypotension in dental practice are vasovagal syncope and orthostatic hypotension. These minor, predictable medical emergencies can gravitate to a more serious situation if not immediately diagnosed and treated. Uncommon causes of hypotension include dialysis-associated hypotensive episodes, hemorrhagic shock, cardiogenic shock, and congestive heart failure (CHF). Supine hypotensive syndrome, encountered during the last trimester of pregnancy, may be a particular concern to the practitioner.

INITIAL INTERVENTION

The initial treatment of hypotension, regardless of its etiology, is the traditional "syncope" protocol that consists of placing the patient in a semisupine position with the feet slightly elevated and applying an oxygen mask (Figure 10-2). As with any medical emergency, airway, breathing, and circulation (ABCs) are immediately assessed. Treatment is instituted depending on the patient's medical history, drugs administered during dental treatment, and most important the patient's state of consciousness. If repositioning does not elevate the blood pressure to acceptable levels, establishment of an intravenous (IV) line and the rapid infusion of 500 ml of a physiologic solution should be considered. If an IV line cannot be established or a fluid challenge is unsuccessful, the heart rate should be immediately assessed and further therapy contemplated.

If the heart rate is less than 60 beats per minute (bradycardia), atropine should be considered. However, if the heart rate is normal or elevated and the blood pressure is low, increasing the heart rate will not elevate systolic pressure.[2] A this time, injection of a vasopressor to increase PVR, stroke volume, or both is suggested. *Ephedrine*, a vasopressor that acts directly on both α- and β-adrenergic receptors, is a good choice to treat hypotension in emergency situations. Ephedrine will increase both cardiac out-

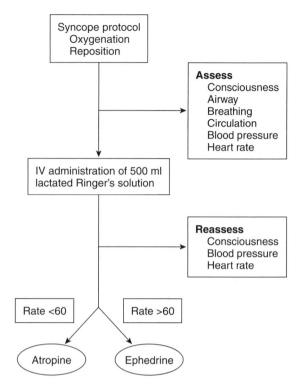

Figure 10-2. Routine treatment approach for patient with hypotension and inadequate perfusion.

put and PVR for 60 to 90 minutes but should be used judiciously in the patient with ischemic heart disease.

VASOVAGAL SYNCOPE

The most common cause of hypotension and associated unconsciousness encountered during routine dental treatment in healthy individuals is vasovagal syncope. Vasovagal syncope is usually initiated by stressful physical, psychological, or surgical stimuli. A variant of vasovagal syncope, termed *situational* or *visceral* vasovagal syncope, is mediated by autonomic reflexes (e.g., gagging, acute pain, coughing) and is usually initiated by a Valsalva response to stressful stimuli.[3] A prodromal phase usually precedes the vagal event and may consist of nausea, vomiting, weakness, diaphoresis, tachycardia, tachypnea, confusion, blurred vision, and possibly abdominal pain.

The pathogenesis of vasovagal syncope involves activation of efferent vasodepressor and cardioinhibitory reflexes.[4] The afferent signal that initiates neurally mediated syncope may originate within the central nervous system or from associated peripheral receptors that respond to chemical, mechanical, pain, or temperature stimuli. These impulses are transmitted directly to the nucleus solitarius in the medulla, closely related to the dorsal and ambiguous nuclei of the vagus nerve. The characteristic bradycardia associated with vasovagal syncope results from the enhanced parasympathetic tone of the vagus nerve. Vasodilation is primarily caused by diminished sympathetic vasoconstrictor tone. Together these factors are responsible for the resulting hypotension.[5]

Clinically, there is a marked decrease in MAP and PVR. Cardiac output may be unchanged but cannot adequately compensate for the decreased arterial pressure. Since it is vagally mediated, bradycardia can be corrected by the administration of atropine. Since the hypotension itself is not vagally mediated, it may be resistant to increases in heart rate. If the syndrome progresses, unconsciousness results from temporary reductions in cerebral blood flow caused by either vasomotor instability or a sudden reduction in systemic vascular resistance and cardiac output.[5]

Vasovagal syncope is usually reversible when diagnosed early. Treatment consists of removing the initiating stimuli, repositioning the patient in the Trendelenburg position in the dental chair, and ensuring adequate ventilation and oxygenation. Vasovagal syncope in healthy patients should resolve rapidly with proper treatment. If a return of consciousness does not occur quickly, attention must be directed to other, more serious causes of unconsciousness, such as major cerebrovascular or cardiac, metabolic, or drug-related emergencies.[7]

ORTHOSTATIC HYPOTENSION

Orthostatic hypotension is a sudden and dramatic fall in systolic blood pressure associated with changes in body position (e.g., supine to upright, sitting to standing). Homeostatic maintenance of blood pressure is primarily regulated by the autonomic nervous system, thus any autonomic interference can result in hypotension. With PVR dependent on sympathetic control, any condition or medication that disrupts normal sympathetic input also can result in orthostatic hypotension.[8]

Orthostatic hypotension can be divided into neurogenic and nonneurogenic causes. Neurogenic causes of orthostatic hypotension result from primary[9] or secondary[10] failure of the auto-

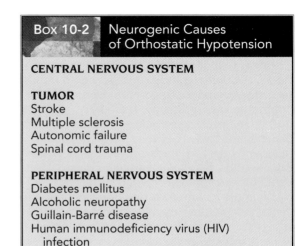

Box 10-2 Neurogenic Causes of Orthostatic Hypotension

CENTRAL NERVOUS SYSTEM

TUMOR
Stroke
Multiple sclerosis
Autonomic failure
Spinal cord trauma

PERIPHERAL NERVOUS SYSTEM
Diabetes mellitus
Alcoholic neuropathy
Guillain-Barré disease
Human immunodeficiency virus (HIV) infection

nomic system (Box 10-2). Nonneurogenic causes of orthostatic hypotension result from cardiac failure, reduced intravascular volume, venous pooling, and drug side effects and interactions (Box 10-3).

Patients at risk for orthostatic hypotension may also report episodes of hypoperfusion, manifesting as dimming of vision, decreased hearing, and lightheadedness.[11] To increase circulating blood volume and reduce the incidence of hypotensive events, these patients may receive salt supplementation, fluid therapy, and support stockings. They are advised to perform regular exercise, sleep with their head elevated, and arise slowly from a supine or seated position.[12]

A determination of risk factors for orthostatic hypotension during the preoperative evaluation and review of the medical history help to prevent the acute medical emergency of patient injury on standing after a prolonged dental procedure. Patients at risk should have their blood pressure monitored throughout the perioperative period and before discharge. Slow, careful changes in patient position are mandatory. When it does occur, orthostatic hypotension should be treated with the routine syncope protocol.

Neurogenic-Mediated Hypotension

Primary autonomic system failure is exceedingly rare and includes pure autonomic failure, multisystem atrophy, and subacute dysautonomia. Pure autonomic failure is of unknown etiology and is not associated with a peripheral neuropathy.[9] This syndrome usually begins in middle age and results in

---

Box 10-3 Nonneurogenic Causes of Orthostatic Hypotension

CARDIAC PUMP FAILURE
Myocardial infarction
Aortic stenosis
Arrhythmias

REDUCED INTRAVASCULAR VOLUME
Dehydration
Diarrhea
Vomiting
Burns

VENOUS POOLING
Alcohol
Vigorous exercise
Sepsis
Extremes of heat

MEDICATION SIDE EFFECTS
Antihypertensives
Diuretics
Vasodilators (nitrates)
Central nervous system sedatives

Box 10-4 Medications Associated with Hypotension

VASODILATING DRUGS
Angiotensin-converting enzyme (ACE) inhibitors
Calcium channel blockers
Nitroglycerine preparations
Antihypertensives

DRUGS AFFECTING AUTONOMIC FUNCTION
Sympatholytic antihypertensives
Neuroleptics, antipsychotics
Tricyclics, monoamine oxidase (MAO) inhibitors
Levodopa
Cholinergic agents

CENTRAL NERVOUS SYSTEM DRUGS
Benzodiazepines
Barbiturates
Narcotics

---

the loss of postganglionic sympathetic neurons and decreased levels of plasma norepinephrine when the affected patient is supine. The resultant orthostatic hypotension can be disabling. Multisystem atrophy (Shy-Drager syndrome) involves several overlapping disorders, including striatonigral degeneration and olivopontocerebral atrophy. These patients have orthostatic hypotension accompanied by parkinsonian features, cerebellar dysfunction, or pyramidal signs.[11]

Secondary failure of the autonomic system is the more common cause of neurogenic orthostatic hypotension and is related to diseases of the peripheral and central nervous systems. Lesions can occur in the brain, brainstem, spinal cord, or peripheral nervous system. The autonomic dysfunction occurs most often in conditions that affect small fibers, such as diabetes, alcohol neuropathy, and amyloidosis. It also affects diseases that cause acute demyelination of small myelinated fibers, such as Guillain-Barré syndrome or multiple sclerosis. The postural maintenance of blood pressure depends on sympathetic-induced reflex vasoconstriction in the splanchnic vascular bed and peripheral blood vessels. The loss of normal sympathetic efferents to these vascular systems results in hypotension.[10]

Patients with spinal cord injuries are also prone to orthostatic hypotensive episodes. Be-

cause of the interruption in the efferent pathways from the brainstem vasomotor center to the sympathetic nerves involved in vasoconstriction, blood pressure responses to position changes are abnormal.[13]

Medication-Induced Hypotension

In the dental setting, hypotensive events may occur in patients taking certain classes of medications, including antihypertensives and psychotropics (Box 10-4). These drugs usually cause orthostatic hypotension, which may be exacerbated by positional changes in the dental chair required for common dental procedures.

Although orthostatic hypotension secondary to medications can occur at any age, a higher incidence is seen in the elderly population. Aging and coronary artery disease are associated with impaired blood pressure regulation, which may further increase the risk of hypotension in response to positional changes. For example, aging is associated with a decrease in the baroreflex mechanism, which may impair the cardioacceleratory response to preload reduction during upright posture. To prevent orthostatic hypotension, elderly people must compensate for an abnormal chronotropic or rate response through systemic vasoconstriction. Vasodilator therapy may further exacerbate the risk of orthostatic hypotension in these susceptible patients.[14] Orthostatic hypotension has been reported to occur in 27% of elderly hypertensive patients.[15]

The risk of orthostatic hypotension is also associated with drug interactions. In one study, orthostatic hypotension accounted for more than 20% of the total number of side effects from drug interactions in an elderly population.[16]

SUPINE HYPOTENSIVE SYNDROME

Some pregnant women in the third trimester experience compression of the inferior vena cava by the gravid uterus when lying supine. The resulting hypotension causes unconsciousness, and lack of oxygenated blood, which can impair the patient and fetus. Simply turning the patient on her left side will alleviate this condition. Placing a pillow under the right buttock of pregnant women prone to this condition on being seated in the dental chair may prevent this cause of hypotension.[17]

DIFFERENTIAL DIAGNOSIS
Hemorrhagic Shock

Acute and severe hemorrhage is rarely encountered in routine dental practice but can be associated with epistaxis, scalp lacerations, and maxillofacial trauma.[18,19] The circulatory responses to blood loss are compensatory and progressive, with vasoconstriction of cutaneous, visceral, and muscular circulation to maintain blood flow to vital organs, including the heart, brain, and kidneys. An increase in the heart rate is usually the first compensatory response. However, after a blood loss of 15% to 30% of blood volume, the pulse pressure decreases; after a blood loss greater than 30%, hypotension develops. The acute loss of circulating blood volume is a life-threatening situation that can be initially treated only with infusion of large volumes of lactated Ringer's solution. Plasma expanders and substitutes or blood and blood products may also be needed to optimize the perfusion and oxygenation of vital organs and maintain blood pressure.

Renal Failure and Dialysis

Hypotension associated with patients in chronic renal failure may by encountered during and after hemodialysis. Altered sympathetic regulation resulting from dialysis treatment and impaired ability to regulate peripheral and autonomic nervous function resulting from renal failure are responsible for the hypotensive episodes.[20,21]

Acute Congestive Heart Failure

Although rarely seen as an acute emergency in dental practice, acute congestive heart failure (CHF) must be considered in the differential diagnosis of the hypotensive elderly patient. Heart failure is defined as the state in which the heart is not able to pump blood at a rate to meet metabolic requirements, resulting in inadequate cellular perfusion and oxygen delivery. CHF causes more than 30,000 deaths, 700,000 hospitalizations, and 2 million outpatient visits each year in the United States at an estimated cost of $10 billion. As the population ages, CHF becomes an increasingly important clinical problem.[22] These patients have a systolic pressure of less than 90 mm Hg, or a decrease of greater than 80 mm Hg in those with a hypertensive history, and exhibit cool, clammy, and cyanotic skin. They have decreased urine output and develop an altered sensorium from decreased organ perfusion as the hypotensive state persists. Failure of the myocardium to pump efficiently and a profound decrease in peripheral vascular tone make treatment difficult and complex. Acute CHF is a major medical emergency, and emergency medical services (EMS) should be contacted immediately.

Cardiogenic Shock

Cardiogenic shock is also rarely seen as a dental emergency. Diagnosis of shock may be difficult, however, with the emergency state multifactorial and the treatment usually beyond the purview of most dental practitioners. Causes other than cardiogenic shock must be considered, including pulmonary embolism, sepsis, hypovolemia, anaphylactic shock, and neurogenic disorders. Hypovolemia, heart rate and rhythm, and ventricular contractility must be assessed to guide treatment. An advanced life support treatment algorithm for shock provides an overview to the treatment of clinically significant hypotension when routine measures (oxygenation, repositioning, fluid, atropine, or vasopressor) are ineffective[23] (Figure 10-3).

SUMMARY

Hypotension can precipitate major cardiac and cerebrovascular events leading to morbidity and mortality. An understanding of physiologic concepts helps to formulate a rational, cognitive approach to diagnosis and treatment (Box 10-5).

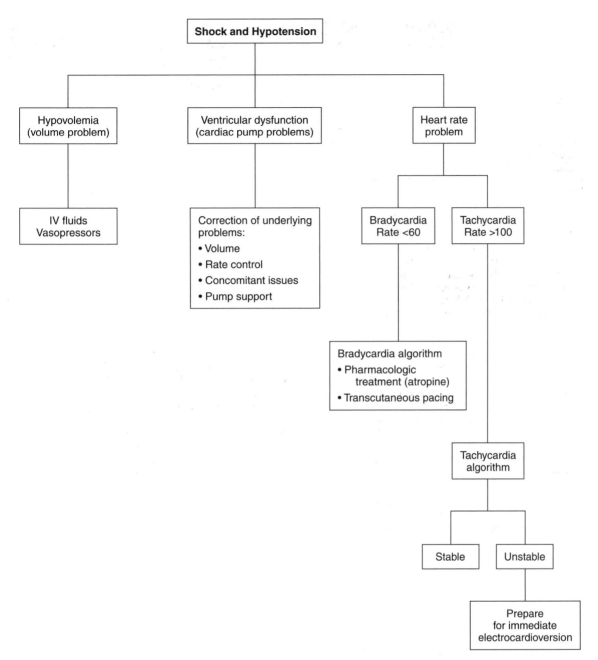

Figure 10-3. Management of hypotension associated with shock.

Box 10-5   Case Studies—Hypotension in the Dental Office

CASE SCENARIO 1

A 21-year-old female patient presents for dental treatment, including restoration of a carious mandibular first molar. The patient has never received a local anesthetic block and is apprehensive about the proposed treatment. When she sees the dental syringe, the patient becomes clammy and faints.

Questions: What do you suspect happened to this patient? What is the best management scenario for her?

Answers: Vasovagal response. The patient is best managed by discontinuing dental treatment and removing any objects from the oral cavity. Administer oxygen, and place the patient placed in Trendelenburg position to increase cerebral blood flow, with the head lowered to a level below the lower extremities. Maintain vigilance and monitor ABCs. Implement emergency procedures if patient does not quickly become alert and responsive.

CASE SCENARIO 2

A 74-year-old male presents for dental treatment that includes the restoration of a maxillary molar. His medical history is significant for hypertension and diabetes mellitus, for which he is taking insulin, a diuretic, and a calcium channel blocker. His diabetes and hypertension have been fairly well controlled on this regimen. In the office his pretreatment blood pressure is 165/85 mm Hg. The dental procedure is performed without difficulty or complications. When the patient is discharged, he abruptly attempts to stand up but complains that he feels weak and dizzy.

Questions: What has happened? What should be done for this patient?

Answers: Because the patient has been supine for a significant period, he has probably experienced an event of orthostatic hypotension. Causative factors may include age, sudden positional change, effects of hypertensive medications, and neurogenic effects of diabetes mellitus. Impaired cardioacceleration and sympathetic vasocontrol associated with age and disease can make older patients vulnerable to hypotensive episodes. Assist the patient back into the dental chair, monitor vital signs, and implement a more subtle positional change. Administer oxygen if the patient does not respond quickly to repositioning.

CASE SCENARIO 3

A 55-year-old male presents for the extraction of a maxillary bicuspid tooth. His past medical history is significant for quadriplegia after a motor vehicle accident about 10 years ago. He states that he has low blood pressure and that he passed out several years ago when he had a similar dental extraction. His current blood pressure is 85/47 mm Hg while sitting in his wheelchair.

Questions: Why is this patient hypotensive? How should he be managed?

Answers: The patient is hypotensive secondary to loss of autonomic control of his vascular system, a result of his previous spinal cord injury. Monitor blood pressure, and ensure that he does not make any rapid positional changes. He likely will have a large increase in blood pressure when placed supine for the extraction. If he is positioned upright too rapidly, he may experience an episode of orthostatic hypotension and lose consciousness.

REFERENCES

1. Stoelting RK: *Pharmacology and physiology in anesthetic practice,* Philadelphia, 1987, Lippincott.
2. Morilo CA, Eckberg DL, Ellenbogen KA, et al: Vagal and sympathetic mechanisms in patients with orthostatic vasovagal syncope, *Circulation* 96:2509-2513, 1997.
3. Kaufmann H: Neurally mediated syncope: pathogenesis, diagnosis, and treatment, *Neurology* 45(suppl 5):S12-S28, 1995.
4. Abboud FM: Neurocardiogenic syncope, *N Engl J Med* 328:1117-1120, 1993.
5. Benditt DG: Neurally mediated syncopal syndromes: pathophysiological concepts and clinical evaluation, PACE 20:572-584, 1997.
6. O'Rourke RA: Syncope: current diagnosis and treatment, Curr Probl Cardiol 22:242-296, 1997.
7. DeJong-DeVos, Van Steenwijk CCE, Wieling W, et al: Variability of near-fainting responses in healthy 6-16-year-old subjects, *Clin Sci* 93:205-211, 1997.
8. Grubb BP, Kosinski D: Dysautonomic and reflex syncope syndromes, *Cardiol Clin* 15:257-268, 1997.
9. Polinsky RJ, Martin JB: Disorders of the autonomic nervous system. In Isselbacher KJ, editor: *Harrison's principles of internal medicine,* ed 13, New York, 1994, McGraw-Hill.
10. McDougall AJ, McLeod JG. Autonomic neuropathy. I. Clinical features, investigation, pathophysiology, and treatment, *J Neurol Sci* 137:79-88, 1996.
11. Engstrom JW, Aminoff MJ: Evaluation and treatment of orthostatic hypotension, *Am Fam Physician* 56:1378-1384, 1997.
12. Bass EB, Lewis RF: Dizziness, vertigo, motion sickness, near syncope, syncope, and disequilibrium. In Barder LR, Burton JR, Zieve PD, editors: *Principles of ambulatory medicine,* ed 4, Baltimore, 1997, Williams & Wilkins.
13. Blackmer J: Orthostatic hypotension in spinal cord injured patients, *J Spinal Cord Med* 20:212-217, 1997.

14. Lipsitz LA, Connelly CM, Kelly-Gagnon M, et al: Cardiovascular adaptation to orthostatic stress during vasodilator therapy, *Clin Pharmacol Ther* 60:461-471, 1996.
15. Masuo K, Mikami H, Ogihasa T, et al: Changes in frequency of orthostatic hypotension in elderly hypertension patients under medications, *Am J Hypertension* 9:263-268, 1996.
16. Doucet J, Chassapne P, Trivalle C, et al: Drug-drug interactions related to hospital admissions in older adults: a prospective study of 1000 patients, *J Am Geriatr Soc* 44:944-948, 1996.
17. Ikeda T: Maternal cerebral hemodynamics in the supine hypotensive syndrome, *Obstet Gynecol* 79:27-31, 1992.
18. Committee on Trauma: Shock. In *Advanced trauma life support*, Chicago, 1989, American College of Surgeons.
19. Shoemaker WC, Peitzman AB, Bellamy R, et al: Resuscitation for severe hemorrhage *Crit Care Med* 24(suppl):S12-S23, 1996.
20. Nishimura M, Takahashi H, Maruyama K, et al: Enhanced production of nitric oxide may be involved in acute hypotension during maintenance hemodialysis, *Am J Kidney Dis* 31:809-817, 1998.
21. Shetty A, Afthentopoulos IE, Oreopoulos DG: Hypotension on continuous ambulatory peritoneal dialysis, *Clin Nephrol* 45:390-397, 1996.
22. Chin MH, Goldman L: Correlates of major complications or death in patients admitted to the hospital with congestive heart failure, *Arch Intern Med* 156:1814-1820, 1996.
23. Essentials of ACLS. In Cummins RO, editor: *Textbook of advanced cardiac life support*, Dallas, 1994, American Heart Association.

KVCC KALAMAZOO VALLEY COMMUNITY COLLEGE LIBRARY

Drug Allergy and Anaphylaxis

Martin R. Boorin

It is extremely difficult to prepare adequately for the frightening experience of a patient with laryngeal edema secondary to an allergic reaction. Severe or fatal drug reactions in the dental office are rare, and allergic reactions constitute only a small proportion of adverse drug reactions. However, allergic reactions may occur unpredictably whenever drugs are administered or materials with allergic potential are employed. Severe hypersensitivity reactions can lead to significant morbidity and mortality in any health care setting. The response to suspected allergic reactions by the clinician and office staff must be swift to impede if not prevent the progression of a potentially severe response. Dental clinicians and staff should regularly review the clinical signs and management of allergy and anaphylaxis.

IMMUNOGENESIS

Knowledge of the normal immune response facilitates an understanding of abnormal immune responses and clinical allergy syndromes. This discussion focuses on the primary immunologic components of the allergic response. The reader should refer to an immunology text for a complete discussion.

Lymphoid Cells

The bone marrow is the site of production and initial maturation for cells of the immune system. Pluripotential bone marrow stem cells receive signaling cues from the microenvironment to produce both lymphoid and myeloid cell lines. The lymphoid stem cell gives rise to T lymphocytes, B lymphocytes, and non-T, non-B large granular lymphocytes. Final differentiation of lymphocytes occurs in the periphery, specifically the thymus, lymph nodes, and spleen.

T *lymphocytes* are responsible for organization and direction of B lymphocytes and macrophage response, antigen-specific cell killing, and production of cytokines. T-lymphocyte maturation in the thymus involves T-cell receptors, major histocompatibility complex (MHC) molecules, and surface membrane molecules (CD nomenclature, e.g., CD4, CD8). The final peripheral T cell is specifically targeted toward recognition of antigen within the context of a host's MHC (avoidance of attack on host tissue). The principal stimulus of T cells by antigen occurs through interaction of antigen with receptors.[1]

B *lymphocytes* are responsible for antibody production. B cells interact with antigen through immunoglobulin at the cell surface. Early maturation of the B cell occurs in the bone marrow or in the fetal liver and is independent of antigen presence. Differentiation is completed after B cells migrate to the spleen and lymph nodes, where they may respond to specific antigen. Activated B cells may secrete immunoglobulin as plasma cells, and a small number of activated B cells may develop into memory cells, which are responsible for the secondary immune response that occurs after reexposure to antigen. The initial signal of B-cell activation is cross-linking of surface immunoglobulin by antigen and a series of signal transduction steps to activate the cytoplasm.

Myeloid Cells

Myeloid stem cells give rise to mononuclear phagocytes and granulocytes. Mononuclear cells reach full maturity in the soft tissues of the body, whereas granulocytes mature primarily in the bloodstream and are classified according to their specific cytoplasmic granules (polymorphonuclear neutrophils, eosinophils, basophils, mast cells). These cells primarily function to provide a controlled nonspecific inflammatory response to foreign stimuli. Unlike lymphocytes, myeloid cells are not predetermined for a specific immune response and do not have immune memory.

Mononuclear phagocytes exist in different locations within the body. On entering the bloodstream from the bone marrow, these cells traverse the endothelial lining of capillaries into the interstitial tissues, where they reside as macrophages. Their promotion of the general inflammatory response is by the production of cytokines and phagocytosis. They also interact with lymphocytes to process antigen for specific responses. Polymorphonuclear neutrophils are the most numerous peripheral leukocytes and the major cells in the acute inflammatory response. They contain surface receptors for complement and the Fc portion (see Figure 11-1) of immunoglobulin that enable them to phagocytose opsonized particles. Their characteristic lobules are filled with granules that contain acid hydrolase, lysozyme, and myeloperoxidase.[1]

Eosinophils primarily function through extracellular release of granules against large targets that are poorly phagocytosed. Eosinophils do not express high affinity for immunoglobulin E (IgE) but appear to be stimulated by the chemotactic effects of lymphocyte-released cytokines. In addition, eosinophils are primary inflammatory cells during late phase reactions.[2]

Basophils are inflammatory granulocytes recruited from the circulation to sites of local inflammation. *Mast cells* remain in interstitial tissues within many organs. Intracellular secretory granules of both cell types contain histamine that is complexed with proteoglycans and other inflammatory mediators. Cell activation occurs by allergen to IgE cross-linking on the cell surface. Intracellular fusion of granules is followed by degranulation, thus mediating many allergic symptoms. The basophils and mast cells (BMC) appear to differ in granule composition and localization within the body.

Other Factors

Immunoglobulin proteins are secreted by differentiated B cells and designed to respond to an extremely diverse group of organisms and molecules. Secreted or membrane-bound immunoglobulins exert their biologic influence by binding antigen. The immunoglobulin structure consists of a Y-shaped complex consisting of two pairs of light and heavy chains with significant structural diversity at one terminal (left arm of the Y). A hypervariable region of the variable end of the molecule functions as the antigen-binding region.

Of the five immunoglobulin classes, *IgE* is the antibody class that participates in immediate hypersensitivity. The biologic and clinical features of IgE are established by direct interaction with eosinophils, basophils, and mast cells. Both basophils and mast cells express Fc receptors for IgE with high affinity.

Cytokines represent a diverse group of soluble proteins that play an important role in mediation and regulation of the immune response. Both general and specific inflammatory responses are influenced by cytokines. Cytokines also function as stimulators for immune cell development.

Complement plays a vital role in natural immunity as an independent humoral immune system that primarily protects the host from infection. However, complement often acts in concert with the other humoral system of antibodies to facilitate clearance of pathogens and perpetuate nonspecific inflammation by marking or opsonization of allergen molecules. Complement activation often leads to vascular permeability changes, mast cell activation, release of inflammatory mediators and chemotactic agents, and influx of neutrophils.

IgE-MEDIATED HYPERSENSITIVITY REACTION
Step 1: Sensitization

Allergens are macromolecular compounds, usually proteins or glycoproteins, capable of inducing IgE antibody responses. *Haptens* are low-molecular-weight molecules that individually are incapable of stimulating an IgE response but, when combined with host proteins, can become immunogenic. This is the primary mechanism for penicillin sensitization, such as penicillin binding to albumin. Compounds that become allergenic must (1) gain access to the body's immune system by absorption or injection, (2) be soluble in body fluids, and (3) be recognized by the immune system as foreign.[3] As antigen presenting cells, macrophages process and then present the phagocytosed antigen to T lymphocytes through direct contact and cell surface molecules. In response to the antigen, these T-cell clones then produce large amounts of cytokine and induce B lymphocytes to produce IgE synthesis. The secreted IgE is then bound by high-affinity receptors on mast cells and basophils despite low serum concentrations. Thus, initial contact with allergen by the immune system leads to production of allergen-specific IgE (Figure 11-1).

Step 2: Early Phase Reaction (Immediate Hypersensitivity)

On reexposure to a multivalent allergen, rapid cross-linking of specific membrane-bound IgE on the BMC high-affinity binding sites triggers

Immediate Hypersensitivity Reaction

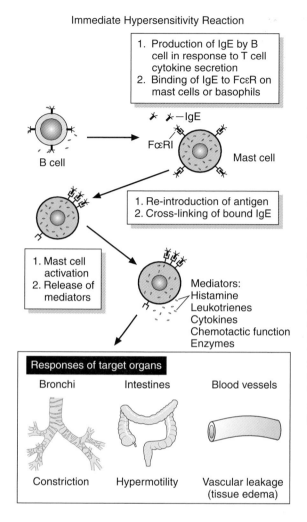

1. Production of IgE by B cell in response to T cell cytokine secretion
2. Binding of IgE to FcεR on mast cells or basophils

IgE

FcεRI

B cell

Mast cell

1. Re-introduction of antigen
2. Cross-linking of bound IgE

1. Mast cell activation
2. Release of mediators

Mediators:
Histamine
Leukotrienes
Cytokines
Chemotactic function
Enzymes

Responses of target organs

Bronchi — Constriction

Intestines — Hypermotility

Blood vessels — Vascular leakage (tissue edema)

Figure 11-1. Immediate IgE-mediated hypersensitivity reaction. The first two steps of an IgE-mediated allergic response are sensitization and the early phase reaction. *Sensitization* includes identification and processing of antigen by multiple lymphocytic cells, leading to B-lymphocyte production of allergen-specific IgE. The IgE molecule is then bound by a high-affinity receptor ($F_{C\epsilon}R1$, crystallizable epsilon fragment receptor) on circulating mast cells. The Fc portion of the IgE molecule is the nonvariable stalk region where cell binds IgE. The end of Y portion of IgE molecule, the region of variability, is the region of allergen-specific-binding to circulating allergen (macromolecules or haptens bound to protein). The *early phase, or immediate hypersensitivity, reaction* occurs on reexposure of circulating allergen to mast cells and cross-linking of allergen-specific IgE. Mast cell degranulation releases multiple preformed mediators, chemotactic agents, and enzymes, with formation of new mediators and amplification of the inflammatory response. *Redrawn from American Academy of Allergy, Asthma, and Immunology: The allergy report: overview of allergic diseases, Milwaukee, 2000, The Academy.*

acute degranulation. Plasma and interstitial histamine, mast cell–derived tryptase, other vasoactive preformed mediators, and leukocyte chemotactic factors are increased. These factors are responsible for the clinical manifestations of immediate hypersensitivity reactions. A second group of newly formed, BMC-derived, lipid breakdown products with proinflammatory effects includes the leukotrienes, prostaglandins, and platelet-activating factors. These preformed or newly formed mediators have potent effects on vascular bronchiolar tissue and stimulate interstitial cell chemotaxis (Table 11-1).[2]

The second step in the IgE-mediated allergic response occurs within minutes of subsequent exposure of the IgE antibody to the allergen. This reaction subsides in 30 to 90 minutes. The sustained response to environmental allergens characteristic in atopic individuals consists of an *IgE-dependent biphasic response* (Figure 11-2).

Step 3: Late Phase Reaction

The late phase response consists of an intense, localized infiltration of inflammatory cells that may play a key role in the pathogenesis of chronic allergic disease as well as prolonged allergic manifestations. Within 3 to 4 hours after a decline in the immediate reaction, allergen stimulates immune cells through IgE bound to low-affinity IgE receptors on lymphocytes, macrophages, and eosinophils. Over several hours this IgE-allergen cross-linking leads to synthesis and release of numerous cytokines, mediators, and other cell factors (e.g., tumor necrosis factor) from lymphocytes. Cytokines play a critical role in the induction of late phase allergic responses, stimulation and regulation of IgE synthesis, mast cell differentiation, and perpetuation of a chronic allergic inflammatory state.[2]

Numerous types of inflammatory cells, predominantly eosinophils, accumulate within the

Table 11-1 Inflammatory Mediators in Anaphylactic and Anaphylactoid Reactions

Mediator	Pathophysiologic, Cellular, and Biochemical Events	Proposed Clinical Effect
Histamine (actions by H_1/H_2 receptors)	Vascular permeability (H_1)	Urticaria, angioedema
	Vasodilation (H_1, H_2)	Hypotension, flushing, wheezing
	Smooth muscle contraction (H_1)	Abdominal cramping, diarrhea
	Exocrine gland secretion (H_2)	Rhinorrhea, bronchial secretions
ARACHIDONIC ACID METABOLITES		
Cyclooxygenase pathway (prostaglandins D_2 and F_2, thromboxane A_2)	Peripheral vasodilation	Hypotension, flushing
	Bronchiolar smooth muscle contraction	Bronchoconstriction
	Coronary vasoconstriction	Coronary vasospasm, ischemia
	Submucosal gland secretions	
Lipooxygenase pathway (leuko-trienes)	Chemotaxis	Possible late phase response
	Bronchiolar smooth muscle contraction	Bronchoconstriction
	Increased vascular permeability	Possible hypotension
	Submucosal gland secretions	
Platelet-activating factors	Bronchiolar smooth muscle contraction	Bronchoconstriction
	Increased vascular permeability	Hypotension
Chemotactic factors	Infiltration/activation of eosinophils and neutrophils	Lymphocyte infiltration
		Possible prolongation of inflammatory reaction and late phase reaction
Tryptase	May activate complement	Unclear; may recruit or amplify other inflammatory pathways
	Cleaves fibrinogen	
Heparin	Inhibits clotting, plasmin, and kallikrein	Possible antiinflammatory effect
	Anticomplement pathways	

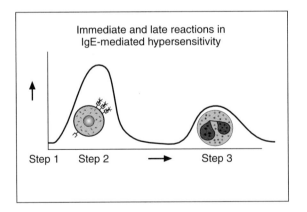

Figure 11-2. IgE-mediated hypersensitivity reaction over time. Immediate hypersensitivity reactions occur within minutes of exposure to allergen in sensitized individuals. With repeat exposure to allergen, multiple IgE-$F_{C\kappa}$R1 complexes are cross-linked, resulting in immediate hypersensitivity reactions (mast cell degranulation, release of mediators, e.g., histamine, leukotrienes, cytokines, proteases). Late reactions begin 2 to 4 hours after exposure to allergen and can last for 24 hours before subsiding. Inflammatory leukocytes (e.g., neutrophils, basophils, eosinophils) release cytokines and chemotactic mediators during the response. In atopic patients the late response is mediated primarily by eosinophils. *Redrawn from American Academy of Allergy, Asthma, and Immunology: The allergy report: overview of allergic diseases, Milwaukee, 2000, The Academy.*

local tissue within 6 to 8 hours. The intensity of the late phase reaction may correlate with the potential for chronic inflammation and respiratory injury found in asthma and other chronic allergic diseases.

ETIOLOGY AND CLASSIFICATION

Adverse drug reactions are common iatrogenic disorders, occurring in 1% to 15% of drug regimens. Most result from toxic mechanisms (overdosage), known side effects, impaired metabolism, or drug interactions, but 5% to 10% of adverse drug reactions may be caused by immunologic mechanisms.[4] The incidence of drug allergy is probably less than 2% overall, except for several common agents, including penicillin, cephalosporins, and trimethoprim-sulfamethoxazole (sulfa).

Allergic drug reactions are based on drug-specific immune mechanisms, are caused by a range of drug classes, and present in a wide array of clinical syndromes. The diagnosis of an immunologic drug reaction is often based on the clinical presentation, although identification of antibodies or sensitized T cells directed against the drug, serum mediator levels, and skin testing may help confirm the diagnosis.

Risk Factors

The risk for development of drug reactions may be influenced by route of administration, clinical features of the specific drug, or the host. Multiple intermittent exposures to a drug increase the risk of an IgE-mediated allergic reaction, usually in the early weeks of a drug course. The route of drug administration can alter the risk and presentation of an immunologic reaction. Parenteral administration increases the risk of sensitization, severe reaction, and anaphylaxis. When anaphylaxis develops after oral administration, the onset will often have a more delayed onset and a prolonged course.

The allergic potential of drugs depends in part on their chemical properties. Non-β-lactam antibiotics do not react directly with self-protein but develop reactive complexes after metabolism. Skin testing or in vitro testing of the parent compound may thus not identify allergenicity to a reactive intermediate product.

Several host factors may influence the risk of immunologic sensitization. Children may have a lower risk for developing allergic drug reactions than adults, presumably because of shorter periods of drug exposure. Women have an in-

creased incidence of cutaneous and anaphylactic reactions, thought to be associated with increased exposure to cosmetics and latex gloves. Individuals with multiple medical illnesses requiring polypharmacy and numerous medication trials develop allergic drug reactions more frequently. A multidrug allergy syndrome has been reported in patients with a history of penicillin reactions (anaphylaxis, urticaria, angioedema) who also have reactions to drugs that are antigenically unrelated to penicillins (e.g., erythromycin).[4] Clinical signs and symptoms of allergy to the nonpenicillin agents (e.g., rash) can significantly differ from reactions resulting from penicillin. The risk of unpredictable anaphylaxis is increased in patients with allergies to foods, insect venom, latex, and parenteral drugs, vaccines, or contrast media.

Classification
Temporal Course

The clinical course of all allergic drug reactions, regardless of immunologic mechanism, can be categorized into one of three time courses of clinical manifestations after drug administration. *Immediate reactions* evolve within the first hour of drug administration and include manifestations of immediate hypersensitivity (e.g., anaphylaxis, urticaria, pruritus, angioedema). *Accelerated reactions* occur from 1 to 72 hours and may present as urticaria, nonurticarial rashes, angioedema, or fever. *Delayed reactions* or *late reactions* occur 72 hours or more after administration and often present as benign skin eruptions, serum sickness–like reactions, fever, or systemic disorders (cardiovascular, hematopoietic, vasculitic, renal, hepatic).

Gell and Coombs

The Gell and Coombs classification defines four basic immunologic mechanisms responsible for the majority of allergic drug reactions. A combination of mechanisms may be operating simultaneously in a single patient. Type 1 (immediate hypersensitivity) and type 4 (delayed hypersensitivity) reactions are the primary areas of interest for this chapter.

Type 1 (IgE-mediated hypersensitivity) reactions pose the greatest threat to clinicians in office practice. Type 1 reactions usually occur within seconds to minutes, although oral drug administration may slow the onset to several hours. This can be significant in the dental office, where oral antibiotics are used as prophylaxis for subacute bacterial (infectious) endocarditis, as recommended by the American Heart Association. Anaphylactoid (non-IgE-mediated) reactions often have clinical presentations similar to the IgE-mediated type but are caused by BMC mediator release or complement activation without IgE antibody.

Type 2 (cytotoxic/cytolytic antibody-mediated) reactions occur when IgG or IgM antibodies recognize a drug antigen associated with cell membranes or a cross-reactive cell membrane antigen. Type 2 reactions to therapeutic agents generally involve blood elements (e.g., blood group, platelet membrane glycoprotein). The resultant interaction with complement causes cell destruction.

Type 3 (immune complex) reactions occur when a drug or drug metabolite combines with IgM or IgG antibodies in the circulation to form soluble immune complexes. Deposited within blood vessels and basement membranes, these complexes activate the complement cascade, promote platelet aggregation, and cause tissue damage. Circulating immune complexes cause serum sickness reactions that may present as fever, varied skin lesions (rash, angioedema, urticaria), lymphadenopathy, arthralgias, nephritis, or hepatitis. Serum sickness reactions are produced by several drugs, including penicillin. The onset of clinical illness is generally 1 to 4 weeks after onset of drug use or within days with previous drug exposure.

Type 4 (delayed hypersensitivity) reactions are mediated by specifically sensitized T-cell lymphocytes. Most reactions result from cutaneous contact and are characterized by infiltration of lymphocytes. Allergic contact dermatitis is the primary example of a type 4 reaction. Clinical onset of dermatitis is usually 24 to 72 hours after topical drug application but may develop up to 1 week later. Causative agents include local anesthetics, latex, and paraben preservatives.

PATHOPHYSIOLOGY
Urticaria and Angioedema

The most common manifestations of drug reactions involve the skin. Skin eruptions may present as maculopapular, morbilliform, or erythematous rashes; urticaria and angioedema; and erythema multiforme, bullous eruptions, and exfoliation. Skin reactions typically develop within days to weeks after initiation of a drug course, presenting with a symmetric distribution that initially involves the proximal trunk and then progresses to the extremities. Fever and pruritus often develop concurrently with urticaria. Urticaria and angioedema are extremely common, affecting about one fifth of the population. Approximately one half of patients experiencing urticaria also develop deeper subcutaneous tissue involvement, resulting in angioedema. Numerous forms of urticaria and angioedema exist, but the IgE-dependent, drug-related form is uniformly acute in onset and duration. Both disorders are associated with the release of various vasoactive mediators from activated cells or enzyme pathways. Inflammatory mediators (e.g., histamine, bradykinin, leukotrienes, prostaglandins) and cytokines cause itching, vasodilation, increased vascular permeability, and a neurologic axon reflex causing a more extensive reaction, possibly through substance P and other neuropeptides (see Table 11-1).

Acute urticaria, usually of viral infection or drug etiology, usually presents as a flat or raised wheal with an erythematous border (*flare*). It is associated with varying degrees of pruritus, from mild itching to a severe and unrelenting itch that interferes with work and sleep. The lesions are variably transient, usually waxing and waning over minutes to hours. They typically resolve within 48 hours. The wheal blanches with pressure, indicating the presence of dilated blood vessels and edema within the dermis. Early acute lesions are composed of subcutaneous edema and are modified by the onset of a perivascular lymphocyte infiltrate within hours (Box 11-1).

Drugs are a common and identifiable cause of urticaria. Almost any drug is capable of inducing urticaria. Antibiotics (e.g., penicillin) may pro-

Box 11-1	Signs and Symptoms of Minor Allergic Reactions
SIGN	**SYMPTOMS**
Urticaria (wheal and flare)	Trunk, face, and extremities affected
	Blanching, hives
Pruritus	Lesions specific or generalized
	Mild to severe itching
Angioedema (localized)	Face, lips, and periorbital areas affected
	Localized skin swelling, edema
	Puffiness
	Lesions painful or burning but nonpruritic
Erythema	Generalized or localized (hives)
	Flushing

duce urticaria through an IgE-mediated mechanism. Other medications (e.g., meperidine, codeine, vancomycin) and contrast agents can directly activate mast cells. A significant percentage of patients with a history of urticaria or angioedema experience exacerbations with aspirin or other nonsteroidal antiinflammatory drugs (NSAIDs) through an unknown mechanism. Angiotensin-converting enzyme (ACE) inhibitors may cause angioedema by interfering with the degradation of bradykinin or complement system components.[5]

Food-induced urticaria is generally temporally related to ingestion. Although gastrointestinal (GI) symptoms (e.g., abdominal cramping, diarrhea, nausea) are common, hypersensitivity-related reactions (e.g., bronchospasm, hypotension) may also occur. Dermatologic disorders must be differentiated from urticaria and include erythema multiforme and the autoimmune diseases of bullous pemphigoid and dermatitis herpetiformis. Physical urticaria is relatively common and includes numerous syndromes induced by application of physical stimuli. Hives usually develop within 30 minutes and may either be localized to the area of stimulus or distributed diffusely. Physical and emotional stressors have been associated with cholinergic and adrenergic urticaria syndromes. Contact urticaria is seen in extremely sensitive patients and has been described with latex, chemicals, medications, and cosmetics. Inhalant allergens, which cause acute respiratory symptoms, may in rare circumstances cause urticaria.[6] Papular urticaria from insect bites may mimic drug-induced urticaria.

Persistent urticaria and idiopathic pruritus should not be regarded as allergic manifestations but rather as symptoms of a systemic disorder that requires further medical evaluation for autoimmune, vasculitic, and dermatologic etiologies. Diagnosis often requires skin biopsy. Multidrug regimens may complicate the search for the cause of urticaria. For acute urticaria, unless the reaction is severe or recurs frequently, an extensive evaluation is neither useful nor cost-effective.

Allergic angioedema results from the same or similar edematous manifestations as urticaria but extends deeper into the dermis and the subcutaneous tissue, resulting in less circumscribed swelling. The face, eyelids, lips, tongue, and extremities are composed of loose connective tissue and are the primary sites affected. These tissues contain fewer mast cells, so the lesions are rarely pruritic, and the skin may appear normal. Frequently the affected tissues are painful, burn-

ing, or paresthetic. The time course is similar to that of urticaria, with rapid onset and peak effect often in less than 1 hour.

Progressive laryngeal edema leading to asphyxiation is a common cause of mortality after anaphylaxis and chronic angioedema syndromes. This is clinically recognized by hoarseness, dysphagia, stridor ("crowing"), and air gasping. Hereditary and acquired causes of angioedema (e.g., inherited angioneurotic edema, cellulitis, edema from cardiac/renal/hepatic disease, and acquired C1-esterase inhibitor deficiency associated with malignancy) must be sought to provide appropriate medical management.

Allergic Contact Stomatitis

Allergies in dentistry most often constitute delayed hypersensitivity reactions to specific dental restorative materials or oral hygiene products. The relative infrequency of contact allergic stomatitis may be attributable to the presence of saliva, increased mucosal vascularity, and decreased keratinization of the mucosa, which results in less keratin-derived protein for hapten formation.[7] The stomatitis reaction is often nonspecific histologically and clinically. The lesions are characterized by intracellular edema, vesiculation of the epithelium, and inflammatory lymphocyte-rich infiltrates.

The diagnosis of intraoral contact allergy generally requires recognition of a temporal relationship between exposure to a suspected dental allergen and the onset of clinical symptoms and signs. Intraoral contact allergies must be differentiated from sources of irritation by history and examination because the clinical picture may be nondescriptive. Mucosal irritation from toothpastes with pyrophosphates and zinc citrate, often a component in tartar control products, may present in a similar manner but is not a true allergy. The distribution of affected mucosa may suggest the source of allergen. Localized lichenoid lesions more often suggest direct mucosal contact, whereas a generalized erythema, edema, and desquamation suggest mouthwash or liquid dental materials.[8]

Contact allergies resulting from oral hygiene products and foods often present in a heterogenous manner. Clinical findings may include erythema, edema, tissue sloughing, burning, and pain.[9,10] The lesion localizes to areas of greatest concentrations where pooling may occur (e.g., labial and buccal mucosa, floor of mouth). Gingival symptoms are also common.[8] Delayed hypersensitivity has been reported with many dental materials, including gold, amalgam, acrylic, orthodontic wire, and prosthetic metals. Allergic reactions to orthodontic hardware (nickel), gold, amalgam, and prosthetic metals tend to arise directly adjacent to the fixed restorations. Contact allergies to acrylic are based on sensitivity to the free monomer, which has significant sensitization potential.[11] The liquid acrylic's ability to distribute throughout the mouth leads to more diffuse presentations. Hypersensitivities to the metal components of amalgam often present in a variety of mucosal lichenoid patterns.[12] In rare cases, oral hypersensitivity reactions can lead to complex systemic clinical presentations or anaphylaxis.[13,14]

Diagnostic skin or patch testing is often not necessary for a diagnosis. When oral lesions are adjacent to dental restorations, however, the decision to remove them may be greatly aided by referral to an allergist or dermatologist for definitive testing. Patch testing consists of placing test substances within metal cups that are applied to the skin. The patches are removed after 48 to 96 hours for examination. Standardized screening patch kits for dental materials are available.

Treatment of oral lesions that develop from a contact allergy should include palliative management of symptoms or removal of the identified material. Oral hygiene products may be easily withdrawn. In patients with lesions caused by restorative dental materials, removal and replacement with another material are often necessary. When desquamative or painful ulcerative lesions result from removal of the causative agent, potent topical corticosteroids will provide short-term relief.[8]

Anaphylaxis and Anaphylactoid Reactions

Anaphylaxis and anaphylactoid events are the result of the rapid activation of several inflammation pathways. These pathways may include the BMC degranulation syndromes, the kallikrein-kinin system, the complement system, and coagulation abnormalities. *Anaphylactic reactions* are defined as those mediated through IgE-antigen complex–induced BMC degranulation. Anaphylaxis may arise from drugs, foods, insect bites, and stings and possibly exercise. The term *anaphylaxis*, first used in 1902 by Portier and Richet to describe lethal consequences of anemone venom in sensitized dogs, literally means *against or without protection*.[15] Studies suggest an in-hospital incidence of anaphylaxis of 0.04%.[16,17]

The incidence of anaphylactic reactions may be greater in women, adults (versus children), and atopic individuals. Sensitization by exposure to cosmetics and latex gloves may explain the increase in women. The severity and incidence of anaphylaxis appear to be greatest after administration by injection. Frequency of exposure to a drug and reinstitution of a drug after cessation of therapy increase the potential for anaphylactic reactions.

Anaphylactoid reactions, also known as *pseudoallergic reactions*, mimic true IgE-mediated anaphylactic events but have a different and often more complex underlying pathophysiology without evidence of hypersensitivity. The most common mechanism of anaphylactoid reactions involves the direct (non-IgE) release of BMC mediators. In contrast to true allergic reactions, this idiosyncratic reaction occurs promptly on initial contact with various drugs, such as opiates (morphine, codeine, meperidine) and antibiotics (polymyxin B, vancomycin), as well as with contrast media and muscle relaxants used during general anesthesia. Other immunologic pathways (e.g., immune aggregate anaphylaxis, cytotoxic and complement-mediated reactions) also contribute or predominate in some anaphylactoid reactions (e.g., from radiographic media, protamine, and transfusions).[18]

Patients with combined histories of asthma, chronic rhinosinusitis, and nasal polyps who ingest NSAIDs or aspirin may develop nonimmunologic clinical syndromes of intolerance and respiratory distress. The reaction occurs in up to 40% of this subpopulation. The degree of intolerance varies widely, and most patients are adults with histories of atopic disease. Intolerance may develop in adolescents and older children. NSAIDs inhibit the enzyme cyclooxygenase and thus the generation of prostaglandin from arachidonic acid. Inhibition of cyclooxygenase may lead to greater arachidonic metabolism through the lipooxygenase pathway, thus increasing the levels of other inflammatory mediators (e.g., leukotrienes). Hyperreactive mast cells may also play a role. Some patients develop only mild reduction in pulmonary function and no clinical symptoms, whereas others have severe anaphylactoid reactions leading to shock and death.

Most anaphylactic and anaphylactoid events involve BMC degranulation, resulting in rapid elevation of tissue and serum levels of multiple inflammatory mediators. Mediators released from these cells include histamine, arachidonic acid metabolites (lipooxygenase and cyclooxygenase pathway), platelet-activating factors, and eosinophil/neutrophil chemotactic factors (see Table 11-1). The major pathophysiologic events caused by the release of these mediators include smooth muscle spasm (bronchus, coronary arteries, GI tract), increased vascular permeability, vasodilation, reflex vagal stimulation, and myocardial depression. The classic clinical picture consists of flushing, urticaria, and angioedema; wheezing; hypotension with possible shock; GI smooth muscle contraction with nausea, vomiting, and diarrhea; and myocardial ischemia. Many mediators can activate other inflammatory pathways, such as the kinin system, complement system, or clotting and clot lysis, and can prolong and intensify the overall reaction. A protracted anaphylactic syndrome may result from combined direct mediator effects.

Drug Fever

Fever may represent the only manifestation of a drug reaction or may present with other systemic manifestations. *Pyrogens*, which cause the febrile response, are released from macrophages after drug-IgG immune complexes are engulfed or cytokines released from sensitized T cells. Drug fevers generally occur 7 to 10 days after initiation of drug therapy. The fever usually recedes within 48 hours of drug discontinuation.[4] Penicillin is one of the many drugs that cause isolated drug fever.

Other Drug Reactions

Other adverse drug reactions involving hypersensitive or inflammatory mechanisms include dermatologic reactions, internal organ involvement, and febrile mucocutaneous syndromes, which may have a delayed onset over days to weeks.

SPECIFIC DRUG ALLERGIES
Local Anesthetics

The majority of adverse reactions from local anesthetic agents are toxic reactions caused by overdosage, rapid drug absorption, and inadvertent intravenous (IV) injection. Toxic reactions present with central nervous system (CNS) and cardiovascular manifestations and may include hypotension, altered consciousness, and convulsions. Epinephrine-induced vasoconstrictors are often responsible for the side effects reported by patients as allergic reactions (e.g., tachycardia, tremor, diaphoresis).

True allergic reactions (e.g., urticaria, angioedema, anaphylactoid reactions) to local anesthetics are extremely rare and should always be confirmed by allergist referral for skin testing. IgE-mediated anesthetic reactions are rare and limited to several case reports. Delayed-type lymphocytic reactivity is responsible for a contact stomatitis and for some localized reactions from local anesthetics. Immunologic cross-reactivity exists for the type 4 delayed hypersensitivity within the group 1 agents (esters of benzoic acid, e.g., benzocaine, procaine) but not from among the group 2 drugs (amides, e.g., lidocaine, mepivicaine, bupivacaine). A patient with an allergy to lidocaine would therefore not be expected to react adversely to bupivacaine.

A history of a severe reaction to local anesthetic before the 1970s would have suggested either a vasovagal reflex or an ester anesthetic or preservative as the cause. *Parabens*, which are structurally related to ester local anesthetics, are no longer contained within dental anesthesia cartridges but are used as a preservative in cosmetics and some topical anesthetic agents. They may cross-react with group 1 agents. Patients may also exhibit hypersensitivity to *sulfites* contained in many dental local anesthetics. Sodium metabisulfite continues to be used as an antioxidant in epinephrine vasoconstrictors. Most patients affected by sulfites are asthmatics with hyperreactive airways stimulated by sulfur dioxide, a metabolite of inhaled or ingested sulfites. Total avoidance is rarely necessary. A stepwise reintroduction of the local anesthetic from dental cartridges in aliquots of 1 to 2 ml (cc) can be used to assess patient sensitivity.[19,20]

Latex Allergy

In the context of allergy, *natural rubber latex* (NRL) has undergone a reversal of roles from lifesaving protection against hepatitis and human immunodeficiency virus (HIV) infection to a widespread and well-recognized medical and occupational health hazard. NRL is used not only in medical and dental practice, in the form of gloves and thousands of surgical, anesthetic, and medical supplies, but also by food handlers, housekeepers, law enforcement officers, and others. Factors that contribute to the risk of developing an allergy to latex include repeat exposure, frequent "wet work" with the hands, and increased exposure to residual allergen through universal precautions against blood-borne infections. Latex allergy may present as either a type 1 IgE-mediated reaction or a type IV delayed reaction.

Delayed hypersensitivity reactions to NRL manifest primarily as an allergic contact dermatitis, although contact urticaria has also been described. The primary sensitizing additives in NRL dermatitis are usually low-molecular-weight accelerators (thiurams and carbamates) and antioxidants added during latex processing. Dermatologic reactions generally begin to appear 4 to 6 hours after exposure and peak within 48 hours. The clinical picture is characterized by a subacute or chronic pruritic, eczematous dermatitis identified by vesicles, erythema, and induration. A sharp line of demarcation often develops between affected and uninvolved skin ("glove dermatitis"). In dental patients, delayed reactions have been reported after exposure to rubber dams, gloves, and orthodontic elastics. Although topical and oral steroids can be used to treat acute symptoms, the primary treatment of allergy to latex is the complete avoidance of all latex-containing products or use of alternative NRL products without allergen chemicals.[21]

Type 1 hypersensitivity reactions, unlike type 4 reactions, are mediated by IgE antibodies to water-extractable proteins of NRL. Immediate hypersensitivity to the natural protein allergen occurs much more often in women, in patients who have undergone multiple surgical procedures, in children with spina bifida, in patients with repeated catheterization (e.g., spinal cord injuries), in those with an atopic history, and in individuals with high occupational exposure (e.g., health care workers). Patients with these histories should be questioned for previous latex or rubber contact experiences (e.g., with balloons, tire stores, medical settings). The IgE specific for the natural proteins of latex can cross-react with several foods (e.g., avocado, bananas, chestnuts, kiwi). Thus dental patients may be easily screened for susceptibility, but some may not understand the cause of reported symptoms or provide information during the medical history interview without directed questions.

Type 1 reactions usually occur within 20 minutes after reexposure to antigen. Clinical reactions range from mild to severe depending on individual susceptibility to NRL and circumstances of exposure. Exposure of NRL to mucosal tissue is a common factor that increases the risk of anaphylaxis; this situation is intrinsic to dental practice.[22] Mild reactions tend to be cutaneous, including localized urticaria and or nonspecific pruritus. Symptoms may rapidly progress from severe generalized urticaria to anaphylaxis. Until otherwise identified, the cause of perioperative anaphylaxis is often assumed to be latex. Individuals at high risk for IgE-mediated hypersensitivity must avoid physical exposure to NRL or inhalation of airborne latex allergen.

The cornstarch powder used to improve glove placement can adsorb the NRL protein allergen migrating from latex gloves. After glove use, this protein-powder combination readily becomes airborne and is capable of sensitization if inhaled. The aerosolized antigen can induce the classic allergic respiratory symptoms of conjunctivitis, rhinitis, cough, and asthma. Patients with this syndrome must have dental treatment or examination early in the day before air contamination with latex particles or preferably in an air-conditioned environment latex free for 24 hours. Emergency resuscitative drugs and equipment must be readily available in case anaphylaxis develops despite all precautions.

CLINICAL MANIFESTATIONS OF ANAPHYLAXIS

Symptoms of anaphylaxis usually begin 5 to 30 minutes after antigen injection. The onset of symptoms after oral ingestion may be delayed up to 2 hours. A major allergic reaction often progresses rapidly toward anaphylaxis. Patients may be incoherent or unconscious and unable to aid in the diagnosis. In this circumstance a quick physical examination and check of vital signs are the only tools available. Immediacy of symptom onset may be associated with severity of an anaphylactic attack. Recovery from anaphylaxis is related to the rapidity of recognition and onset of effective treatment. The rapid onset of symptoms may lead to death within 30 minutes. The original clinical complex can withdraw and then redevelop several hours later in a biphasic manner. The cardiovascular and respiratory pathophysiologic changes may persist for more than 24 hours (Table 11-2).

Urticaria and angioedema are the most common reactions (90% of cases) and occur with remarkable consistency. Upper airway edema may be identified in a majority of patients. Cutaneous symptoms are not usually reported, but pruritus and a diffuse erythematous rash may often occur. Patients frequently report a "sense of impending doom" and a generalized warmth or flush. Tingling or pruritus of the palms, soles of the feet, lips, genitalia, axilla, and scalp may occur.

Airway complaints often include a lump in the throat or throat tightness, hoarseness or difficulty swallowing, and fear induced by developing stridor. A swelling of the lips, tongue, uvula, and eyes as well as an audible inspiratory stridor may be observed. Lower respiratory distress, including

System	Signs	Symptoms
Skin	Flush*	Generalized warmth
	Skin rashes	Pruritus*
	Diffuse urticaria	Tingling* (palms, soles, lips, scalp, axilla, groin)
	Angioedema	
Respiratory	Dyspnea	Shortness of breath*
	Laryngeal edema	Lump in throat,* hoarseness,* dysphagia,* drooling, dysphonia,* inspiratory stridor*
	Upper airway obstruction	Throat tightness,* nasal congestion, rhinorrhea
	Bronchospasm	Wheezing,* chest tightness,* cough
	Hypoxia	Cyanosis
	Hypercarbia	
Central nervous system	Altered consciousness	Sense of "impending doom"*
	Unconsciousness	
	Seizure	
Cardiovascular	Diaphoresis	Faintness
	Pallor	Dizziness
	Hypotension	
	Syncope	
	Tachycardia/bradycardia	Palpitations
	Vascular collapse	
	Cardiac arrest	
	Arrhythmia	
Gastrointestinal		Abdominal bloating, cramping, nausea, vomiting

Table 11-2   Signs and Symptoms of Anaphylactic and Anaphylactoid Reactions

*Common early symptom.

shortness of breath, dyspnea, or wheezing, is very common (nearly 50%), with decreased oxygen saturation expected in serious cases. Early arterial blood gas abnormalities are usually characterized by a low partial pressure of oxygen (cyanosis) and carbon dioxide (Pco_2). Subsequently, Pco_2 increases with severe respiratory distress and evolving metabolic acidosis. Dizziness, syncope, and hypotension are the next most common symptoms (33%), followed by GI symptoms of nausea, vomiting, diarrhea, and abdominal cramping.[23-25] Patients often complain of lightheadedness and faintness. Neurologic symptoms and signs are also common and include seizure, altered or loss of consciousness, and muscle spasm.

Cardiovascular abnormalities associated with severe immediate hypersensitivity are extensive and complex. The primary cardiovascular feature of anaphylaxis is an initial and rapid loss of intravascular fluid into the extravascular space through vascular endothelial permeability and vasodilation. Up to 50% of the intravascular volume can be lost within the first 15 minutes of the allergic reaction. Cardiac output and pulmonary artery pressure decrease, whereas pulmonary vascular resistance increases. Because of these changes, adult respiratory distress syndrome (ARDS) with pulmonary edema may develop. Anaphylaxis is often associated with a compensatory tachycardia in response to the hypovolemia. Coronary vasospasm with ischemia and myocardial depression may subsequently develop. Patients may complain of chest tightness and palpitations. Some patients may have bradycardia from increased autonomic vagal tone and a cardioinhibitory reflex associated with ischemia.[18] Intrinsic myocardial depression with decreased cardiac output may persist for days. Electrocardiographic (ECG) changes may include ST-segment and T-wave abnormalities.

The rapid loss of blood volume stimulates numerous compensatory cardiovascular and autonomic nervous system mechanisms to increase peripheral resistance, including catecholamine secretion and angiotensin pathway activation.

These intrinsic vasoconstrictor agents can yield variable results on total peripheral resistance and thus on blood pressure and cardiac output. As a result of high plasma levels of catecholamines and angiotensin II, patients in shock may be maximally vasoconstricted and therefore unresponsive to vasopressor agents. A critical requirement in clinical resuscitation is the aggressive and preferential use of fluid replacement and volume expanders rather than only vasoconstrictor agents to treat shock and hypotension.

MANAGEMENT
Initial Intervention

In all patients with suspected allergic reactions, initial management must include a standard evaluation of the patient's general condition and an activation of primary emergency treatment (Box 11-2). The treatment of anaphylaxis should never be restricted to the dental office. If anaphylaxis is suspected, emergency medical services (EMS) should be requested without delay. When hypotension is suspected, the patient should be positioned either supine in a dental chair or couch with feet above the level of the heart unless medically contraindicated. The patient should be positioned semisupine when signs and symptoms suggest only mild reactions. The patient's general physical state and vital signs should be taken with the standard airway, breathing, and circulation (ABC) assessment protocol of basic life support (BLS). Airway patency must be evaluated, confirmed, and if necessary maintained. Supplemental oxygen should be administered to all patients because progression of an allergic reaction is impossible to predict. Vital signs (blood pressure, carotid pulse, respiration) should be repeated every 5 minutes and documented. If not currently on record, the patient's weight should be estimated to help guide medication dosing decisions. The patient should never be left unmonitored.

On completion of these initial steps, the clinician must consider the severity of the observed reaction to establish a plan of clinical management. *Syncope* should always be considered in the differential diagnosis due to the high incidence of this syndrome in dental office settings. If clinical signs and symptoms progress in severity (hypotension or airway compromise), EMS must be requested. Definitive medical care should be instituted when possible and necessary, including IV fluids, medications, and cardiopulmonary resuscitation (CPR). Supportive care should be maintained until EMS personnel

Box 11-2	Primary Emergency Management for Major and Minor Allergic Reactions

1. Patient assessment
   a. General condition
   b. Level of consciousness
   c. Vital signs (every 5 minutes)
   d. Weight estimation
2. Emergency medical services activation
   a. Decision based on extent and progression of signs/symptoms
3. Patient positioning
   a. Semisupine
   b. Supine, feet elevated if hypotension
4. Basic life support monitoring
   a. Airway
   b. Breathing
   c. Circulation
5. Oxygen supplementation
   a. *No respiratory distress:* nasal cannula or nasal mask
   b. *Respiratory distress:* full-face mask with 100% oxygen

arrive. When the patient is stable and can be transported to a hospital emergency department, the clinician should accompany the patient and assist emergency personnel as needed.

Minor Allergic Reactions

Minor reactions involving nonpruritic, localized or generalized rash, fever, and limited urticaria may often be managed by stopping the use of a suspected drug or dental material to prevent further absorption (Figure 11-3). Latex should always be suspected and withdrawn if present in the immediate environment. The differential diagnosis of the cutaneous reaction should be considered. Scattered or mild hives are usually self-limited and require no treatment or only a mild antihistamine. Localized urticaria and other skin eruptions should be treated initially with oral H_1-receptor antihistaminic drugs, such as the first-generation diphenhydramine (Benadryl) or chlorpheniramine (Chlor-Trimeton); both have mild sedative side effects. Newer nonsedating oral H_1-blocking antihistamines, such as loratadine or cetirizine, could be considered as alternatives. The success of these medications may be limited by the magnitude of the ongoing release of histamine and other unblocked mediators. Also, some actions of histamine are mediated through H_2 as well as H_1 receptors.[26] Thus both histamine receptors

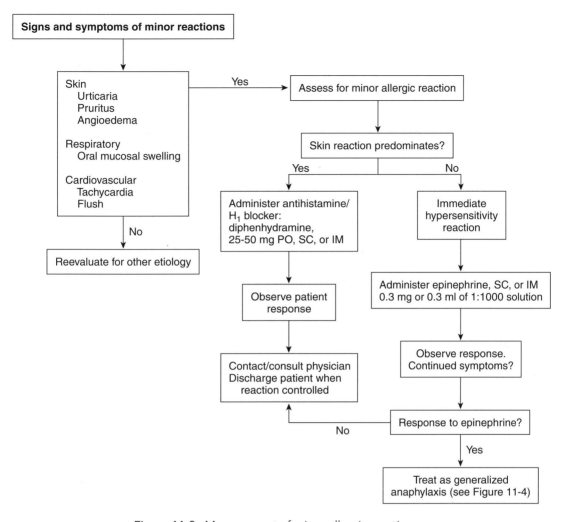

Figure 11-3. Management of minor allergic reactions.

must be blocked for maximal effect. The onset of acute and generalized urticaria or angioedema should be treated similar to anaphylactic reactions, using epinephrine in addition to the antihistamine (Table 11-3).

Anaphylactic and Anaphylactoid Reactions

Anaphylactic reactions may include cutaneous reactions, but these often are not early harbingers of the syndrome. The major features of anaphylactic reactions include the life-threatening pathophysiologic states of cardiovascular instability (hypotension) and airway compromise (bronchospasm and laryngeal edema), which are mediated not only by histamine but also by numerous potent inflammatory mediators that cannot be pharmacologically reversed by competitive receptor binding as can histamines. Rapid recognition and treatment of anaphylaxis are crucial to prevent a possible fatality (Figure 11-4).

The immediate goal is to maintain adequate airway and blood pressure support during this "hurricane" of mediator release. Together with instituting primary emergency care (see Box 11-2) and contacting EMS, subcutaneous (SQ) or intramuscular (IM) *epinephrine* must be administered as soon as possible. Epinephrine possesses sympathomimetic agonist activity at α-, β_1-, and β_2-adrenergic receptors, antagonizing the main cardiopulmonary pathophysiologic changes associated with anaphylaxis. Binding to receptors on mast cells, epinephrine inhibits continued mediator release and may reduce the extent of the late phase response. The dose and route of administration of epinephrine should be

Table 11-3	Primary Medications for Minor Allergy and Anaphylaxis	
Drug	**Dose/Route**	**Comments**
ANTIHISTAMINES		
Diphenhydramine	*Adult*: 25-50 mg PO q6-8h, *or* 10-50 mg IM/IV q2-4h *Child* (>10 kg): 12.5-25 mg PO q6-8h, *or* 1 mg/kg IM/IV q6-8h	Route of administration depends on severity of episode. Sedation will occur.
Ranitidine/famotidine (H_2-receptor blockers)	*Adult* Ranitidine: 150 mg PO q12h, *or* 50 mg IM q6h Famotidine: 20 mg PO q6h *Child* (>10 kg) Ranitidine: 1-2 mg/kg PO q12h, *or* 0.75 mg/kg IM q6h Famotidine: 1 mg/kg PO q6h	
Epinephrine	*Adult*: 1:1000, 0.3-0.5 ml SC/IM *Child*: 1:1000, 0.01 mg/kg SC/IM, *or* 0.1-0.3 ml SC/IM	Initial drug of choice for all allergic reactions involving laryngeal edema, bronchospasm, or hypotension.
Albuterol (β_2-agonist inhalant)	Initially as for asthma/bronchospasm: 2 or 3 metered doses (puffs)	Used for bronchospasm resistant to epinephrine. Additional puffs of inhaler may be used if bronchospasm persists or inhalation effort is poor.
Glucagon	*Adult*: 0.5-1 mg SC/IM q20min	Patients receiving β-blockers are resistant to β-adrenergic effects of epinephrine.
Oxygen	See Chapter 1.	Required for all patients except those with mild reactions.

PO, Orally; SC, subcutaneously; IM, intramuscularly; IV, intravenously; *q6-8h*, every 6 to 8 hours.

guided by the severity of the reaction. IM administration is more rapidly absorbed and should be used for severe reactions. SC administration results in slower absorption and is appropriate for the patient with generalized urticaria or cutaneous reactions who is unresponsive to antihistamines but without compromised cardiopulmonary function. The epinephrine dose is 0.3 to 0.5 mg (0.3 to 0.5 ml) of a 1:1000 concentration (1 mg/ml) for adults and 0.1 to 0.3 mg (0.1 to 0.3 ml) or 0.01 mg/kg in children. The dose may be repeated two or three times every 10 to 15 minutes in adults. Dosage adjustment down to one half of recommendations may be required for elderly patients or those with compromised cardiovascular status.

Vital signs must be retaken frequently to assess stabilization or progression of signs and symptoms. The patient's airway must be maintained, and oxygen should be administered using full-face oxygen masks. IM *diphenhydramine*

(or other H_1-receptor antihistamine) may be administered to conscious patients and may provide significant symptomatic relief.

Secondary Intervention and Emergency Medical Services

Once these primary steps have been taken, further therapy must be guided by the clinical course and the extent of the clinician's training. After an anaphylactic event, patients should be transported to the hospital, regardless of early resolution of signs and symptoms before or on EMS arrival, to ensure that a late response does not occur away from immediate medical care. Biphasic and "protracted" cases of anaphylaxis can lead to death even though the patient survives the first several hours after the initial event. Although most allergic reactions respond well to parenteral epinephrine and antihistamine, the three life-threatening components of anaphy-

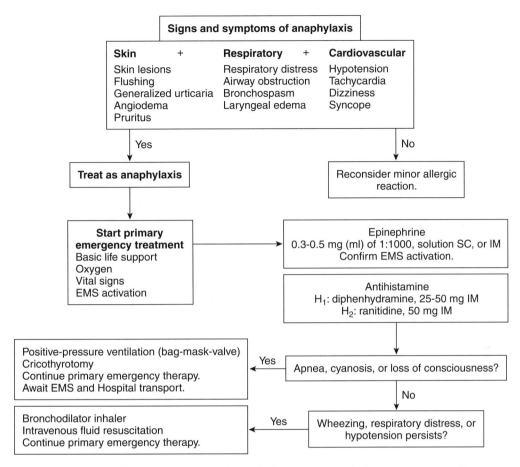

Figure 11-4. Office management of anaphylactic and anaphylactoid reactions. *EMS,* Emergency medical services.

laxis—hypotension, bronchospasm, and laryngeal edema—may be so severe as to be refractory to primary treatment. Advanced, rapid, and aggressive medical management is then necessary. Subsequent emergency management steps may be provided by the clinician experienced with advanced emergency procedures and parenteral drug administration as well as the arriving EMS team. EMS personnel will increase the level of monitoring by using ECG, pulse oximetry, and possibly automated blood pressure monitoring to better evaluate the patient's cardiopulmonary parameters affected by anaphylaxis as well as subsequent therapeutic interventions.

Airway closure or laryngeal edema that is largely unresponsive to epinephrine may develop into a complete airway obstruction. Apnea and unconsciousness must be recognized rapidly so that adequate ventilation can immediately replace the oxygen supplementation provided at the onset. The primary therapeutic goal must be to provide oxygenation and ventilation to prevent severe metabolic acidosis and hypoxia. Ventilation of the unconscious patient using the bag-valve-mask device (Ambu bag) for positive-pressure ventilation with 100% oxygen should begin immediately. Secretions in the patient's airway should be suctioned. If mask ventilation is unsuccessful, the trained clinician or EMS team will intubate the patient's trachea. If these airway maneuvers fail, lifesaving emergency airway access through a transtracheal catheter or surgical cricothyrotomy is necessary.

Bronchospasm (wheezing or diminished breath sounds when severe) may remain unresponsive or incompletely corrected by the epinephrine injections and must be treated with aerosolized and IM β_2-agonists (e.g., terbutaline), as in asthmatic patients. The management of bronchospasm may require multiple inhalation treatments due to limited or poor patient cooperation. Aggressive use of the metered-dose inhalers with approximately 10 to 20 inhalations may be necessary.

Except for acute upper airway obstruction, the manifestation of anaphylaxis that may be most difficult to treat and most threatening is profound and protracted *hypotension*. In severe cases, epinephrine may not correct intravascular volume contraction. The primary treatment must be intravascular volume expansion with rapid administration of IV crystalloid and colloid fluids. A rapid rate of fluid resuscitation requires large-bore IV needle access. Large volumes of crystalloid (lactated Ringer's solution or normal saline) may be required; 1 to 2 L is given to adults (up to 5 to 7 L), at an initial rate of 5 to 10 ml/kg in the first 5 minutes.[27] Children should receive up to 30 ml/kg of crystalloid solution within the first hour.[28] An IV epinephrine infusion (10 to 20 µg/min) titrated to clinical effect may be used while the patient is monitored for dysrhythmias.

Patients taking nonselective β-blockers (e.g., propranolol, nadolol) present a particular problem in the therapy of anaphylaxis and are associated with more severe reactions, including refractory hypotension, bradycardia, and bronchospasm.[29,30] These patients may be resistant to the β-adrenergic effects of epinephrine. High doses of epinephrine or alternative drugs are needed to reverse the negative chronotropic and inotropic effects of the β-blocker and counteract the allergy-induced bronchoconstriction. The administration of epinephrine in the presence of a preexisting blockade of peripheral β₂-adrenergic receptors on arterioles may lead to a severe α-receptor-mediated hypertensive event. *Glucagon*, a polypeptide hormone with positive inotropic and chronotropic effects on the heart independent of adrenergic receptors, should be administered in a 1- to 5-mg bolus intravenously, followed by IV infusion. IM glucagon can be given if IV access is not available. When glucagon is unavailable, hypotension may require treatment with reduced epinephrine doses combined with alternative vasopressors. Selective β₂-agonist inhalation (e.g., albuterol) is used in the management of bronchospasm.[26]

A combination of both both H₁- and H₂-receptor blockers appears to improve symptomatology better than H₁ antihistamines alone.[31,32] As such, antihistamine therapy should include IV diphenhydramine and ranitidine or famotidine.

The role of *corticosteroids* in the acute management of anaphylaxis has not been established. The onset of therapeutic effects, including inhibition of inflammatory mediator release and stabilization of mast cells, is delayed for several hours. Based on their known effects on chronic allergic disease, however, systemic corticosteroids should be considered, especially in patients with severe anaphylactic reactions involving laryngeal edema or recent glucocorticoid therapy. Corticosteroids should also be considered because of the potential for a late phase response or biphasic reaction and thus recurrence of the allergic reaction. Clear recommendations of the steroid form and dose, however, are empiric at best.

Hospital Emergency Care

After stabilization, patients experiencing anaphylaxis should be transported by EMS to a tertiary care medical center for advanced medical management and monitoring. Patients with severe reactions may redevelop earlier symptoms during late phase responses. Aggressive cardiopulmonary management of decompensated patients may require further administration of IV fluids and vasopressor infusions, based on invasive cardiovascular monitoring of central venous and pulmonary pressures, cardiac output, and oxygen consumption, as well as ECG analysis, urine output, and other physiologic parameters. Patients may require tracheal intubation for several days until fluid status and cardiovascular and respiratory function have normalized.

DIFFERENTIAL DIAGNOSIS

The differentiation between anaphylaxis and other acute-onset conditions follows primary emergency management protocols. The clinician must consider alternative diagnoses during the secondary and tertiary management phases. The most common syndrome masquerading as anaphylaxis is the *vasodepressor (syncope) reaction*, characterized by pallor, weakness, nausea, vomiting, diaphoresis, hypotension, and bradycardia. Syncope often arises from intense fear or emotional upset. Bradycardia occurs more frequently during syncope, but this cannot be used as the only factor to distinguish it from anaphylaxis. Normal heart rates or bradycardia may exist during anaphylaxis.[32] Vasodepressor reactions do not involve cutaneous reactions (urticaria, flush, angioedema) and usually improve rapidly with a recumbent position.

Symptoms of respiratory distress are consistent features of numerous alternative medical diagnoses that must be considered during emergency management. Several acute-onset emergencies with features similar to anaphylaxis include nonorganic syndromes, such as panic attacks, hyperventilation, and upper airway obstructions. *Foreign body aspiration* and *airway obstruction* often present with inspiratory stridor and diminished breath sounds, with acute or even violent onset of symptoms. Except for facial flush and tachycardia, cutaneous and cardiovascular signs and symptoms are not present. *Panic attacks* and *hyperventilation* may be accompanied by tachycardia, chest pain, flush, and shortness of breath.

Patients with the chronic diseases of asthma and congestive heart failure should be familiar to the dental clinician. Bronchospasm secondary to *asthma* or reactive airway disease might develop in response to inhaled fumes or to aspiration of water in the back of the mouth during dental therapy. However, hypotension and skin changes are absent. Patients developing *congestive heart failure* often have respiratory distress, dizziness, pallor, and weakness. Clinical signs include hypotension, wheezing, and syncope. Cyanosis is the only cutaneous sign usually present. This syndrome must be quickly distinguished from anaphylaxis because of the very different medical management required.

Disorders that produce flush reactions should be considered in the differential diagnosis. *Postmenopausal flush* involves flushing over the upper half of the body and lasts for 2 to 5 minutes without hypotension. This may occur several times a day and may be stimulated by alcohol or stress. *Thyroid medullary carcinoma* may present with an extended flush of the face and upper extremities. *Carcinoid syndrome* arises from tumors secreting histamine, prostaglandins, serotonins, and other inflammatory mediators. Patients also experience abdominal pain, cardiovascular instability, and bronchospasm. *Drug interactions* between ingested alcohol and sulfonylureas (e.g., chlorpropamide) can induce a flush associated with hypoglycemia, tachycardia, and diaphoresis, but not hypotension or GI symptoms.

Patients with postprandial syndromes may present with several features also common in anaphylaxis. Patients ingesting foods with high concentrations of *sulfites* (e.g., dried fruits, wine, fruit juices, shellfish) may experience flushing, hypotension, and bronchospasm. *Monosodium glutamate* (MSG) ingestion can cause chest pain, facial burning, flushing, sweating, dizziness, headaches, palpitations, or nausea and vomiting. Children may present with irritability, shivering, and chills. Symptoms usually begin within an hour after ingestion. *Scombroidosis* occurs after ingestion of spoiled fish, with symptoms of urticaria, itching, headache, nausea, and vomiting as well as flushing. The symptoms are experienced by all those who ate the fish, and cardiovascular signs are usually absent.[33]

PREVENTION

The first steps in reducing the risk of adverse drug reactions, including allergy, is to avoid using drugs or to reduce multidrug regimens except when absolutely indicated. Patient and occupational exposure to potentially allergenic materials (e.g., antibiotics, latex, chemical solvents, methylparaben preservatives) should be avoided or eliminated when possible.

A thorough history is the most important clinical tool to reduce the risk of allergic reactions. Previous drug reactions or allergies must be reviewed with patients during their initial office visit. Subsequent office visits should incorporate a regular history review, including new-onset drug allergies or recent illness that suggest allergic reactions. Over-the-counter drugs and herbal remedies should be included; these drugs are often forgotten by patients but often contain multiple medications that could aggravate chronic allergic or asthmatic states or even provoke anaphylaxis. When a drug allergy is reported, the clinician should seek a more complete description of the type and severity of symptoms as well as necessary medical management. Special care is necessary in selecting and prescribing *any* drug for the patient with a history of allergy to multiple medications. When the patient history suggests true drug allergy, an alternative, non-cross-reactive medication should be administered.

Inevitably, some patients will be labeled incorrectly or will state they are allergic to the medication. Thorough questioning is often sufficient to clarify the history. Symptoms of previous drug reactions that suggest a nonimmunologic etiology include nausea and vomiting, diarrhea, stomachache, headache, lethargy, and palpitations. Patients often give a history of penicillin allergy but on further questioning have received related drugs (e.g., ampicillin, cephalosporin) without reaction. Acute viral infections typically present with cutaneous manifestations, and sick children usually receive multiple medications in the course of these illnesses. Allergic reactions in children are relatively uncommon except with repeated courses of treatment.

DIAGNOSTIC ALLERGY TESTING

Allergy testing is recommended before dental treatment in certain situations. These circumstances include elective or urgent dental surgery with a risk of infection and a history of multiple antibiotic allergies and anaphylaxis, suspected latex or local anesthetic allergy, and mucocutaneous reactions after previous dental treatment that required medical management. When alternative, equally effective medications without cross-reactivity or increased toxicity can be used, allergy testing may be avoided. However, knowing that (1) no allergy exists, (2) a latex allergy is not present (considering the ubiquitous use of latex in dental practice), and (3) the most efficacious antibiotic or local anesthetic can be safely used is often worth the relative risk of diagnostic testing.

Skin Testing

Skin prick/puncture and intradermal testing are used for identifying type 1 IgE-mediated allergy. The *skin prick/puncture test* is the most convenient and specific screening method for detecting IgE antibodies. Skin testing involves stepwise cutaneous challenge to a diluted and later an undiluted test drug. Anaphylaxis during allergy testing is rare, but the setting for skin testing must include a clinician trained to treat anaphylactic reactions, all necessary basic and advanced emergency medications and equipment, and a fully monitored setting. A skin prick test with 1:1000 (prior allergic reaction) to 1:100,000 dilution (history of anaphylaxis) is followed by intracutaneous tests with negative and positive control injections. Anaphylactic reactions during testing are almost exclusively related to circumstances where intracutaneous testing occurred without a prior prick test and where an allergen caused anaphylaxis in the past. Intracutaneous tests should be considered when the prick test is negative to an allergen that is strongly suggested by patient history.[34] Skin testing is currently available for penicillin and local anesthetics.

The diagnostic test for type 4 allergens is the *patch test*, which is applied according to a standard methodology. Suspected allergens are mixed in petrolatum in appropriate concentrations and then applied to the patient's back underneath a small aluminum disk. The test sites are read at 48 hours, 96 hours, and if indicated, up to 1 week after application.

Serologic Testing

Serologic methods for measuring IgE antibodies, such as the radioallergosorbent test (RAST) and the enzyme-linked immunosorbent assay (ELISA), are available for testing some drugs but often provide no more information than skin testing; they are also less sensitive, and results take longer to obtain. However, serologic testing may be preferred in patients who cannot submit to skin testing, have severe dermatologic disease, are receiving nonwithdrawable antihistamines, or have a very high risk of anaphylaxis with skin testing. In vitro IgE immunoassay is the standard testing procedure for latex currently used in the United States. In vitro tests for IgE antibodies to penicillin lack negative predictive value and should not be used to evaluate penicillin allergy.[35]

Specific Drug Testing

Testing for penicillin (but not cephalosporin) has become well established as a screening mechanism for patients with strongly suggestive reactions to drugs of the penicillin class. Testing for penicillin allergy should ideally include both the major and the minor determinant reagents, which are composed of the principal and lesser metabolites (plus the drug penicillin G), respectively. These haptens form stable conjugates in vitro with protein or polypeptide carrier molecules. Inclusion of major and minor determinants during testing provides a reliable confirmation or exclusion of allergy and risk of anaphylaxis to penicillin. Some allergists administer the undiluted drug after testing, particularly when only the major determinant and penicillin G are tested.[34]

Identifying latex sensitization is important for its negative predictive value. Patients without latex sensitivity do not develop generalized anaphylaxis. Currently, however, no standard latex allergen extract is commercially available in the United States for skin testing. The skin prick test, which incorporates incubated NRL in saline, is controversial as a result of an increased risk of anaphylaxis. The latex RAST, an in vitro alternative test, is specific for latex allergen but has only moderate sensitivity, with detection in about 60% of true cases. A negative latex RAST does not exclude NRL type 4 reactions, such as contact dermatitis.[22] A series of standard NRL allergens is available for skin patch testing to confirm type 4 delayed hypersensitivity.

REFERENCES

1. Sandberg ET, Shearer WT: Normal immune response. In Bierman CW, Pearlman DS, Shapiro GG, et al, editors: *Allergy, asthma, and immunology from infancy to adulthood*, ed 3, Philadelphia, 1996, WB Saunders.

2. Leung DYM: Allergic immune response. In Bierman CW, Pearlman DS, Shapiro GG, et al, editors: *Allergy, asthma, and immunology from infancy to adulthood*, ed 3, Philadelphia, 1996, WB Saunders.
3. Holgate ST, Church MK: Allergens. In Holgate ST, Church MK, editors: *Allergy*, New York, 1993, Raven.
4. Dykewicz MS: Drug allergy. In Slavin RG, Reisman RE, editors: *Expert guide to allergy and immunology*, Philadelphia, 1999, American College of Physicians.
5. Israili ZH, Hall WD: Cough and angioneurotic edema associated with angiotensin-converting enzyme inhibitor therapy: a review of the literature and pathophysiology, *Ann Intern Med* 117:234, 1992.
6. Hobbs KF, Schocket A: Urticaria and angioedema. In Bierman CW, Pearlman DS, Shapiro GG, et al, editors: *Allergy, asthma, and immunology from infancy to adulthood*, ed 3, Philadelphia, 1996, WB Saunders.
7. Reitschel RL, Fowler JF: Contact stomatitis and cheilitis. In Fisher AA, editor: *Fischer's contact dermatitis*, ed 4, Baltimore, 1995, Williams & Wilkins.
8. De Rossi SS, Greenberg MS: Intraoral contact allergy: a literature review and case reports, *J Am Dent Assoc* 129:1435, 1998.
9. Lamey PJ, Lewis MA, Rees TD, et al: Sensitivity reaction to the cinnamonaldehyde component of toothpaste, *Br Dent J* 70:529, 1990.
10. Miller RL, Gould AR, Bernstein ML: Cinnamon-induced stomatitis venenata, *Oral Surg Oral Med Oral Pathol* 73:708, 1992.
11. Kanerva L, Estlander T, Jolanki R: Allergic contact dermatitis from dental composite resins due to aromatic epoxy acrylates and aliphatic acrylates, *Contact Dermatitis* 20:201, 1989.
12. Koch P, Bahmer FA: Oral lichenoid lesions, mercury hypersensitivity and combined hypersensitivity to mercury and other metals: histologically-proven reproduction of the reaction by patch testing with metal salts, *Contact Dermatitis* 33:323, 1995.
13. Hansen PA, West LA: Allergic reaction following insertion of a Pd-Cu-Au fixed partial denture: a clinical report, *J Prosthodont* 6:144, 1997.
14. Wantke F, Hemmer W, Haglmuller T, et al: Anaphylaxis after dental treatment with a formaldehyde-containing tooth-filling material, *Allergy* 50:274, 1995.
15. Portier P, Richet C: De l'action anaphylactique de certains venins, *CR Soc Biol* (Paris) 54:170, 1902.
16. Amornmarn L, Bernard L, Kumar N: Anaphylaxis admissions to a university hospital, *J Allergy Clin Immunol* 89(suppl):349, 1992.
17. Porter J, Jick H: Boston collaborative drug surveillance programs: drug-induced anaphylaxis, convulsions, deafness, and extrapyramidal symptoms, *Lancet* 1: 587, 1977.
18. Lieberman PL: Specific and idiopathic anaphylaxis: pathophysiology and treatment. In Bierman CW, Pearlman DS, Shapiro GG, et al, editors: *Allergy, asthma, and immunology from infancy to adulthood*, ed 3, Philadelphia, 1996, WB Saunders.
19. Simon RA: Sulfite sensitivity, *Ann Allergy* 56:281, 1986.
20. Yagiela JA: Local anesthetics. In Dionne RA, Phero JC: *Management of pain and anxiety in dental practice*, New York, 1991, Elsevier.
21. Virant FS: Radiocontrast, local anesthetic, and latex reactions. In Bierman CW, Pearlman DS, Shapiro GG, et al, editors: *Allergy, asthma, and immunology from infancy to adulthood*, ed 3, Philadelphia, 1996, WB Saunders.
22. Hamann B, Hamann C, Taylor JS: Managing latex allergies in the dental office, *Calif Dent J* 23:45, 1995.
23. Orfan NA, Stoloff RS, Harris KE, et al: Idiopathic anaphylaxis: total experience with 225 patients, *Allergy Proc* 13:35, 1992.
24. Kemp S, Lieberman P, Wolf B: A review of 267 cases of anaphylaxis in clinical practice, *J Allergy Clin Immunol* 91S:153, 1993.
25. Wiggins CA: Characteristics and etiology of 30 patients with anaphylaxis, *Immunol Allergy* Pract 13:313, 1991.
26. Becker DE: Management of immediate allergic reactions, *Dent Clin North Am* 39:582, 1995.
27. Eon B, Papazian L, Gouin F: Management of anaphylactic and anaphylactoid reactions during anesthesia, *Clin Rev Allergy* 9:415, 1991.
28. Saryan JA, O'Loughlin JM: Anaphylaxis in children, *Pediatr Ann* 21:590, 1992.
29. Toogood JH: Beta-blocker therapy and the risk of anaphylaxis, *Can Med Assoc J* 136:929, 1987.
30. De Soto H, Turk M: Cimetidine in anaphylactic shock refractory to standard therapy, *Anesth Analg* 69:260, 1989.
31. Vidovich RR, Heiselman DE, Hudock D: Treatment of urokinase-related anaphylactic reaction with intravenous famotidine, *Ann Pharmacother* 26:782, 1992.
32. Simon MR: Anaphylaxis associated with relative bradycardia, *Ann Allergy* 62:495, 1989.
33. Settipane GA: The restaurant syndromes, *Arch Intern Med* 146:2129, 1986.
34. Van Arsdel PP: Drug hypersensitivity. In Bierman CW, Pearlman DS, Shapiro GG, et al, editors: *Allergy, asthma, and immunology from infancy to adulthood*, ed 3, Philadelphia, 1996, WB Saunders.
35. Diagnostic testing. In American Academy of Allergy, Asthma, and Immunology: *The allergy report: overview of allergic diseases*, Milwaukee, 2000, The Academy.

Syncope

George Blakey III

Simple fainting, or *vasodepressor syncope*, is generally regarded as the most common medical emergency occurring in dentistry. In general, syncope describes a sudden, brief loss of consciousness caused by a reduction or interruption in cerebral blood flow, usually resulting from an abrupt loss of cardiac output. Thirty percent of the adult population will experience at least one syncopal episode, accounting for approximately 3% of emergency department visits.[1]

Causes of syncope range from benign vasovagal episodes to life-threatening cardiac dysrhythmias. The dental clinician must identify the cause of the episode, provide supportive care, and stabilize and treat the patient if necessary. The dentist must also identify patients who require activation of the emergency medical services (EMS) system and more comprehensive care in a hospital setting.

ETIOLOGY

Syncopal episodes can be grouped under four major headings: peripheral vascular or circulatory, central nervous system, metabolic, and cardiac (Table 12-1). A specific cause can be identified in about 50% of patients during the initial evaluation. The prognosis is relatively benign if accompanying cardiac or neurologic disease is absent. Syncope is more likely to occur in patients with known heart disease, young women, and older men. It is most often abrupt in onset, transient, and followed by prompt return to full consciousness.

Syncope may be caused by excessive vagal tone or impaired reflex control of the peripheral vascular circulation. Enhanced vagal tone is the cause of syncope in carotid sinus hypersensitivity and postmicturition syncope. Vagal-induced sinus bradycardia, atrioventricular blocks, and sinus arrest are common sequelae and may even be the cause of syncope.

Orthostatic hypotension is a common cause of syncope, especially in elderly, diabetic, hypovolemic, and other patients with autonomic neuropathy. Patients taking vasodilators, diuretics, and adrenergic blocking drugs may have orthostatic hypotension. The normal vasoconstrictive response to assuming an upright position, which compensates for the decrease in venous return, is impaired in the patient taking these medications. Blood pressure declines more than 20 mm Hg on arising from the supine to the standing position, with or without tachycardia, depending on the status of autonomic function. A patient's autonomic function can be assessed by evaluating blood pressure and heart rate responses to Valsalva maneuver and by tilt testing. These tests should be performed before any invasive studies unless a cardiac etiology is suspected.

Cardiogenic syncope can occur after an obstructive vascular event or arrhythmia. Vascular mechanical problems that can cause syncope include aortic stenosis, pulmonary stenosis, hypertrophic obstructive cardiomyopathy, and obstruction of the mitral valve, often exertional or postexertional. Disorders of cardiac automaticity (e.g., sick sinus syndrome), cardiac conduction disorders (e.g., atrioventricular blocks), and tachyarrhythmias (ventricular and supraventricular tachycardia) are also causes of cardiac syncope. Evaluation of these patients includes a thorough history and physical examination. In addition, the cardiac physical examination includes an orthostatic blood pressure evaluation and resting electrocardiogram (ECG). The ECG may reveal the cause, but some patients require longer periods of monitoring (e.g., Holter) or stress testing.[2,3]

PATHOPHYSIOLOGY

Vasodepressor syncope, or common fainting, is characterized by a transient loss of consciousness and postural tone. It is the most common type of syncope observed in the dental office. The syncope may recur and tends to take place during stressful situations, injuries or accidents, and

Table 12-1	Types of Syncope	
Cause	**Type**	**Features**
Peripheral vascular or circulatory	Vasodepressor	Prodrome, often precipitated by stress or pain
	Micturition	With urination
	Hypovolemia (orthostatic hypotension)	Occurs with vomiting, diarrhea, or hemorrhage
	Posttussive	Paroxysm of coughing
	Drugs	Orthostatic hypotension; occurs with antihypertensives, tricyclic antidepressants, and phenothiazines
	Carotid sinus syndrome	Bradyarrhythmia, vasodepressor or cardioinhibitory response
	Autonomic dysfunction	Occurs in diabetes, alcoholism, and Parkinson's disease
Central nervous system	Cerebrovascular	Transient ischemic attacks, stroke
	Seizures	Warning aura, postictal confusion
	Emotional	Disturbances, anxiety, hysteria
Metabolic	Hypoglycemia	Confusion, "jitteriness"
	Anemia	
	Hypoxia	
Cardiac	Obstructive	Often exertional; may result from mechanical problems (e.g., cardiac valve stenosis), embolism, and myocardial infarction
	Arrhythmias	Sudden dizziness, bradycardia or tachycardia, atrioventricular blocks

pain. Minor blood loss, poor physical condition, anemia, fever, organic heart disease, and fasting also increase the possibility of syncope in susceptible individuals. Events typically progress in three definitive phases: presyncope, syncope, and postsyncope.

Presyncope

Presyncope leads up to a syncopal event. The presyncopal phase can be triggered by stress, anxiety, or a specific painful event. In response the body releases increased amounts of epinephrine and norepinephrine. Catecholamine release results in a decrease in peripheral vascular resistance and an increase in blood flow to skeletal muscle. If skeletal muscle activity follows, the blood diverted to the skeletal muscle during catecholamine release is pumped back to the heart. No pooling of blood occurs, and vital signs (blood pressure, heart rate) remain at levels that do not allow syncope to develop. If the patient does not move and muscle activity does not occur, the blood pools in the skeletal muscle

and does not return to the heart. The resulting relative decrease in circulating blood volume, decrease in arterial blood pressure, and decrease in cerebral blood flow (CBF) are responsible for the signs and symptoms typically observed during presyncope. The presyncopal phase may include nausea, perspiration, epigastric distress, hyperpnea, tachypnea, weakness, confusion, pupillary dilation, and tachycardia (Box 12-1).

The pooling of blood in the peripheral vessels of skeletal muscle and the resultant decrease in arterial blood pressure activate compensatory mechanisms to maintain CBF. Baroreceptors act by constricting the peripheral blood vessels, activating the carotid and aortic arch reflexes, and increasing heart rate, blood return to the heart, and cardiac output. A near-normal blood pressure is present early in the presyncopal phase. Subsequently the compensatory baroreceptor mechanism decompensates, and bradycardia develops. Bradycardia leads to a significant drop in cardiac output, which causes a fall in blood pressure below the level required for conscious-

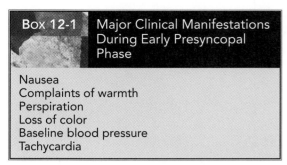

Box 12-1 Major Clinical Manifestations During Early Presyncopal Phase

Nausea
Complaints of warmth
Perspiration
Loss of color
Baseline blood pressure
Tachycardia

Modified from Fast TB, Martin MD, Ellis TM: Emergency preparedness: a survey of dental practitioners, *J Am Dent Assoc* 112:449-501, 1986.

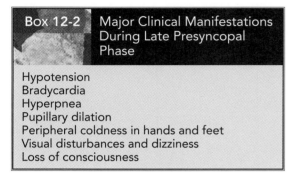

Box 12-2 Major Clinical Manifestations During Late Presyncopal Phase

Hypotension
Bradycardia
Hyperpnea
Pupillary dilation
Peripheral coldness in hands and feet
Visual disturbances and dizziness
Loss of consciousness

ness (Box 12-2). After loss of consciousness the patient enters the syncopal phase.

Syncopal Phase

True vasodepressor syncope occurs in the erect or sitting position, rarely in the supine position. During syncopal attacks, CBF, cerebral oxygen utilization, and cerebrovascular resistance are greatly reduced. An average human brain in a medium-size adult weighs approximately 1400 g. Normal CBF is 50 to 55 ml per 100 g of brain tissue per minute. The estimated critical level for CBF to maintain consciousness is 30 ml/100 g/min. The systolic blood pressure necessary to maintain CBF to prevent loss of consciousness may vary by patient. Normotensive patients are usually able to tolerate a drop in systolic blood pressure better than hypertensive patients. An electroencephalogram (EEG) reveals high-voltage slow waves, 2 to 5 seconds, coincident with the loss of consciousness. If the cerebral ischemia lasts only a few minutes, there are no lasting effects on the brain. If ischemia persists, however, necrosis of the border zone may occur between the major cerebral and

cerebellar arteries. Cerebral ischemia of 10 seconds with the onset of syncope can result in seizure activity. The degree of convulsive movement usually depends on the degree and duration of cerebral ischemia.

Postsyncope

The postsyncopal phase is the return of consciousness, which is usually rapid if management is adequate and expedited by proper positioning of the patient with feet slightly elevated (Trendelenburg position). To improve blood return to the heart and brain after return of consciousness, signs and symptoms (e.g., sweating, pallor, weakness) may persist for hours.[2,4]

DIFFERENTIAL DIAGNOSIS

The health care provider must differentiate between syncope and alternate conditions involving episodic weakness and fainting. *Anxiety attacks* and *hyperventilation syndrome* can be confused with syncope. The giddiness of anxiety is often interpreted as a feeling of faintness without actual loss of consciousness. No facial pallor is present, and the condition is not relieved by placing the patient in a Trendelenburg position. Hyperventilation is part of the event leading to hypocapnia, along with release of epinephrine. Alkalosis, increased cerebrovascular resistance, and decreased CBF follow.

Hypoglycemia may also lead to a vasodepressor syncopal event. Insulin-dependent diabetic patients most often lose consciousness from a hypoglycemic event. The patient's history is critical in making the diagnosis documenting a reduced blood sugar during an attack. The clinical picture is usually confusion progressing to loss of consciousness. Hypoglycemia resulting in a loss of consciousness is a potential life-threatening event and must be managed quickly. If hypoglycemia is suspected, glucose should be administered early during the attack.

Most typical varieties of syncope must also be distinguished from other disturbances of cerebral function, most often some form of *epilepsy*. Again, seizure activity is infrequently a part of vasodepressor syncope. In contrast, the epileptic attack may occur at any time of day or night, independent of the patient's posture. The patient's color does not usually change in epilepsy. Epilepsy is more sudden in onset, and if an aura is present, it rarely lasts longer than a few seconds before loss of consciousness. Injuries from

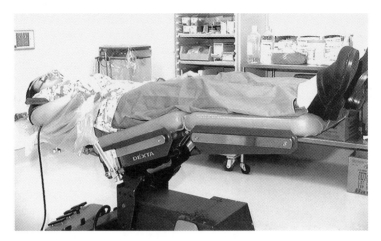

Figure 12-1. Syncopal patient in Trendelenburg position after syncopal attack. The feet are positioned slightly above the head. Oxygen is administered, and vital signs are monitored.

falling are more common in epilepsy because protective reflexes are instantaneously abolished. The period of unconsciousness is usually longer in epilepsy than in syncope. Placing the patient in a Trendelenburg position does not promote quicker recovery in the epileptic patient. Mental confusion and drowsiness are common postseizure sequelae but are rare with syncope. The patient's history, characteristics of the attack, and EEG documentation will distinguish the two conditions.[3,4]

PREVENTION

Vasodepressor syncope may be prevented because known predisposing factors can be controlled. Because syncope is recurrent in some patients, the dental care provider can identify potential problem patients and modify treatment. Some factors should be modified before the patient enters the treatment area, including thorough preprocedural instructions and making certain the patient has eaten recently. Having a comfortable environmental temperature and humidity in the office will also reduce the incidence of syncope in patients with significant anxiety. Stress reduction modalities can be employed. Sedation through a variety of drugs and routes of administration, including oral, intravenous, intramuscular, and inhalational, is available. The decision to use sedation is based on the patient's previous experiences, the planned procedure, the dentist's experience in administering sedation, patient monitoring equipment

in the procedure area, and the patient's health status.

Once the patient enters the treatment room, anxiety reduction is of utmost importance. In addition to sedation, simpler techniques include music headphones and proper positioning. True vasodepressor syncope cannot occur if the brain is adequately perfused with oxygenated blood. Ensuring proper positioning with the patient supine and receiving supplemental oxygen (with a nasal cannula) will reduce the incidence of syncope. Because the presyncopal phase is relatively long, the dental care provider can anticipate the impending event. Early recognition, quick positioning of the patient into the Trendelenburg position, and administration of oxygen should prevent the patient from progressing to a loss of consciousness.[2]

TREATMENT

Vasodepressor syncope is usually a benign process in the absence of underlying cardiac disease. Once the patient becomes syncopal and loses consciousness, quick and proper treatment will result in a prompt and full recovery.

The first step after identification of the syncopal event is to place the patient in the Trendelenburg position with the feet slightly elevated over the head (Figure 12-1). The correct position for the unconscious pregnant patient is the left lateral decubitus position, decreasing pressure from the fetus on the diaphragm, improving respiration, and on the inferior

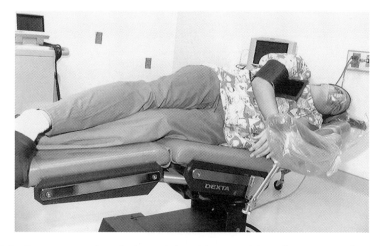

Figure 12-2. Pregnant patient in lateral decubitus position after syncopal attack. This position relieves pressure from the fetus on the diaphragm and the inferior vena cava.

vena cava, improving venous blood return (Figure 12-2).

The next step is to assess consciousness. If loss of consciousness is confirmed, the emergency protocol for the office should be activated. Every office should have an emergency protocol with defined responsibilities for the staff. Basic life support techniques (e.g., CPR) should be started. This includes assessing the airway, breathing, and circulation (ABCs). The head tilt should be utilized to establish a patent airway. After the adequacy of the airway is established, breathing is checked. Spontaneous respiration is usually present during vasodepressor syncope. Oxygen administration by face mask can hasten recovery. If spontaneous respiration is not present, artificial ventilation should be initiated.

Most patients regain consciousness quickly and progress to complete recovery. Monitoring of vitals signs (blood pressure, heart rate, respiratory rate) and comparison with baseline values should be continued until full recovery. Oxygen administration should also be maintained until full recovery. An ammonia vaporole can be used as an adjunct to aid in recovery. Once consciousness has returned, it is important to reassure and relax the patient. After loss of consciousness the patient should not undergo further dental treatment. Arrangements should be made to have the patient accompanied home. Weakness often follows a syncopal event, and patients should be assisted, especially when loss of consciousness

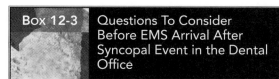

| Box 12-3 | Questions To Consider Before EMS Arrival After Syncopal Event in the Dental Office |

1. What are the patient's vital signs? Does the patient have a history of syncope?
2. Did the patient lose consciousness or just feel faint?
3. How long was the patient unconscious? Is the patient still unconscious?
4. What is the patient's medical history?
5. Did the patient have a seizure before the loss of consciousness? Does the patient have a history of epilepsy?
6. Did the patient fall and sustain other injuries?

has occurred. Full recovery should take less than 20 minutes. If the loss of consciousness is greater then 5 minutes or complete recovery takes longer than 20 minutes, the EMS system should be activated.

If the clinical course is not progressing as expected, the health care provider must continue to assess the situation to ascertain other possible causes (Box 12-3).

If the patient continues to have symptoms and bradycardia, atropine (0.5 to 1.0 mg intravenously) can be administered and repeated every 5 minutes to a maximum dose of 3 mg (0.3 to 0.4 mg/kg). Dental care providers should

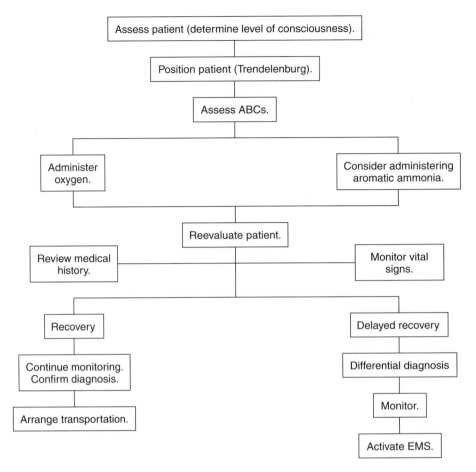

Figure 12-3. Patient assessment flowchart. *ABCs,* Airway, breathing, and circulation protocols; *EMS,* emergency medical services.

administer drugs only if they have completed specialized training (Figure 12-3).[1,2,4]

SUMMARY

Vasodepressor syncope is a common, benign process comprising muscle weakness and loss of consciousness. Prevention is the goal, with identification of patients at risk, elimination of predisposing factors, and modifications in treatment. In a syncopal attack, proper treatment usually results in prompt and complete recovery.

REFERENCES

1. Schroeder SA, Krupp MA, Tierney LM, McPhee SJ: *Current medical diagnosis and treatment,* Saddle River, NJ, 1990, Appleton & Lange.
2. Malamed SF: *Medical emergencies in the dental office,* ed 4, St Louis, 1993, Mosby.
3. Bennett JC, Plum F: *Cecil textbook of medicine,* ed 20, Philadelphia, 1996, Saunders.
4. Wright KE, McIntosh HD: Syncope: a review of pathophysiological mechanisms, *Prog Cardiovasc Dis* 13:58, 1971.

Altered Mental Status

A. Omar Abubaker
Robert J. Lesny

The occurrence of altered mental status (AMS) generally presents a formidable challenge because it does not suggest a discrete diagnosis but rather represents a symptom of a wide variety of possible medical conditions. In a dental setting, AMS poses a greater challenge because additional factors must be considered in the differential diagnosis, ranging from anxiety and fear about treatment to an interaction involving a drug used for pain control. The differential diagnosis in these patients may be more complicated if the event occurs before the patient is seen or before an adequate history is obtained.

Because homeostasis protects the brain at all costs, regardless of the etiology, acute AMS should be considered a severe physiologic problem, and timely diagnosis and treatment are critical. The challenge of both the initial approach and the definitive management of AMS is well recognized even in an emergency department (ED) setting. As a result, clinical policies based on vast experience and expert clinical opinions are often developed to evaluate and treat these conditions

AMS encompasses a spectrum of altered levels of homeostasis, with different management approaches for the various conditions causing the complaint. Different terms are used to distinguish these conditions. Although management of AMS focuses on documenting the specific physical findings rather than using descriptive terms, clinicians must be familiar with these common terms, as described by the American College of Emergency Physicians (Box 13-1).

PATHOPHYSIOLOGY

The state of consciousness depends on excitation of cortical neurons by impulses through the reticular activating system. Centers in the brainstem reticular formation receive impulses from components of the central nervous system (CNS), including the spinal cord, cerebral cortex, and lower region of the brain (thalamus, hypothalamus, midbrain, medulla). Any process that affects the components of consciousness can generally cause changes in mental status. Because physiologic insult to these components can change mental status, any process that affects one of these regions should be included in the differential diagnosis of AMS.

Conditions affecting these CNS regions and ultimately leading to a change in mental status generally fall into one of two broad categories: intracerebral processes and extracerebral processes. *Intracerebral processes* include conditions that affect the brain both locally and globally and influence neurologic functions through effects on the regions of consciousness, causing focal neurologic deficits and symptoms of AMS. These processes include brain tumor, infarcts, intracranial hemorrhages, and infection of the meninges. The regions of consciousness can also be affected indirectly through increased intracranial pressure (ICP), causing edema and a diffuse decrease in blood flow and leading to focal symptoms and AMS. Intracerebral processes usually manifest as variable degrees of AMS and as focal neurologic deficits (e.g., aphasia, unilateral motor or sensory deficit).

Extracerebral processes affect mental status indirectly through their effects on brain physiology and neurologic functions. These processes include respiratory and cardiovascular conditions associated with metabolic factors that affect metabolism of brain tissue, including hypoxia, hypoperfusion, fluid and electrolyte imbalances, and toxic conditions. These processes may indirectly inhibit CNS functions, initially with AMS and then proceeding to shock or even death if the condition is not treated promptly.

The classification of AMS into intracerebral or extracerebral is somewhat arbitrary, and events of AMS in the dental office can be caused by a variety of factors that fall in either of these two categories. The major types of conditions likely to cause AMS in the dental office can be metabolic, toxic, neurogenic, and cardiovascular (Box 13-2 and Table 13-1).

Text continued on p. 195

Box 13-1 | Terms Associated with Altered Mental Status (AMS)

altered mental status Collective, nonspecific term to denote any acute or chronic change in the subject's vigilance, mental content, or attentiveness.

cognition Mental faculty and process by which knowledge is gained, as through perception, reasoning, or intuition (i.e., cortical function).

coma State of unarousable unresponsiveness; subject cannot be aroused by external stimuli.

vigilance Graded state of wakefulness ranging from low degree in all stages of sleep to high degree in the awake state.

mental content Subject's present and past experiences bound by memory systems and integrated into the self with a constant flow of messages from the internal and external world.

attention Subject's capacity to select from the total stream of mental contents and focus on those stimuli appropriate to a given point and situation in time.

delirium Acute, transient, fluctuating, potentially reversible organic brain disorder characterized by globally impaired consciousness and attention. Also known as *acute confusional state*.

dementia Progressive organic brain disorder of insidious onset characterized by impaired memory, abstract thinking and judgment, personality changes, and disturbance of cortical function. Consciousness and attention remain intact in dementia, which is not associated with other central nervous system problems.

lethargy Depressed mental status in which the subject has the appearance of wakefulness but has global depression of awareness of self and environment.

stupor Unresponsiveness from which the subject can be aroused only by vigorous and repeated stimuli but does not return to a normal baseline of awareness.

Box 13-2 | Causes of Altered Mental Status

I. Metabolic
   A. Hypoxia/anoxia, hypoperfusion
   B. Hypoglycemia
   C. Hyperglycemia
   D. Fluid and electrolytes disorders
      1. Hypocalcemia
      2. Hypercalcemia
      3. Hyponatremia
      4. Hypernatremia
      5. Hyperkalemia
      6. Hypomagnesemia
      7. Acid-base disturbances
      8. Nutritional deficiencies
         a. Thiamine
         b. Vitamin B_{12}
II. Toxic
   A. Endogenous
      1. Sepsis
      2. Uremia, renal failure
      3. Hepatic encephalopathy
      4. Hypercarbia
      5. Reye's syndrome
      6. Porphyria
   B. Exogenous
      1. Opiates
      2. Barbiturates
      3. Benzodiazepines
      4. Neuroleptics
      5. Anticholinergics (e.g., tricyclics)
      6. Phenothiazines
      7. Aspirin overdose
      8. Alcohol
III. Neurogenic
   A. Seizure
   B. Intracranial infection, sepsis
   C. Trauma, concussion

IV. Cardiovascular
   A. Vascular
      1. Ischemic
         a. Reflex-mediated ischemia
            1. Vasovagal attack
            2. Carotid sinus syncope
            3. Micturition syncope
            4. Tussive syncope
            5. Blood loss, hypovolemia
         b. Vascular obstruction
            1. Thrombosis
            2. Embolism
            3. Vasospasm
            4. Subclavian steal syndrome
      2. Hemorrhagic
         a. Hypertensive event
         b. Aneurysm
         c. Bleeding diathesis
         d. Amyloid angiopathy
         e. Arteriovenous malformation
         f. Subdural/epidural hemorrhage
         g. Vascular tumors
   B. Cardiac
      1. Cardiac obstruction
      2. Aortic stenosis
      3. Mitral stenosis
      4. Arrhythmia
         a. Sick sinus syndrome
         b. Heart block
         c. Ventricular tachycardia
         d. Ventricular fibrillation
         e. Paroxysmal supraventricular tachycardia, atrial fibrillation, Wolff-Parkinson-White syndrome
         f. Long QT syndrome

Table 13-1	Causes of Altered Mental Status				
Cause	Precipitating Factor	Finding	Vital Signs	Physical Examination	Laboratory Testing
Hypoxia/anoxia, hypoperfusion	MI, arrhythmia Barbiturates, narcotics, benzodiazepines Asthma, bronchospasm, pulmonary embolus	History of MI, severe anemia, arrhythmias, asthma, history of COPD	Hypotension, tachycardia, bradyarrhythmia (ominous sign)	Cyanosis, pallor May have chest pain with acute MI, tachypnea, expiratory wheeze, and diaphoresis Use of accessory muscles of respiration	ABGs: ↑P_{CO_2}, ↓P_{O_2}, ↓pH
Hyperglycemia	New-onset DM or DM with insulin or oral medications	DM or history of polyphasia, polydipsia, polyuria	Dehydration, hypotension, tachycardia Kussmaul breathing Rapid, weak pulse Normal to low BP	N/V Abdominal pain/tenderness	↓Glucose levels in blood and urine, urine ketones, serum glucose >300 mg/dl, HCO_3 <15 mEq/L, pH <7.3
Hypoglycemia	Insulin therapy without oral intake	DM with insulin therapy		Sweating, shaking, anxiety, nausea, confusion, bizzare behavior, headache, lethargy, coma	Serum glucose <50 mEq/L, with symptoms
Fluid/electrolyte imbalances, hyponatremia	Trauma, sepsis, cardiac failure, cirrhosis, renal failure	CHF, hepatitis, alcoholic cirrhosis, renal insufficiency/failure		Abdominal pain, headache, agitation, hallucinations, focal neurotogic signs, confusion, seizures	Na+ <120 mEq/L
Hypernatremia	Diarrhea, vomiting, hyperpyrexia ↓Intake ↑Insensible losses	Diabetes insipidus, thyrotoxicosis	Hypotension, tachycardia	Irritability, brain hemorrhage	Na+ >145 mEq/L
Hypokalemia	Loop diuretics most common cause			Weakness, ileus, N/V	K+ <3.5 mEq/L

MI, Myocardial infarction; *COPD,* chronic obstructive pulmonary disease; *DM,* diabetes mellitus; *CHF,* congestive heart failure; *BP,* blood pressure; *ABGs,* arterial blood gases; *HCO_3,* bicarbonate; *N/V,* nausea/vomiting.

Continued

Table 13-1	Causes of Altered Mental Status—cont'd				
Cause	Precipitating Factor	Finding	Vital Signs	Physical Examination	Laboratory Testing
Hyperkalemia	Renal failure with oliguria most common	History of renal failure or worsening insufficiency, Addison's disease, sickle cell SLE, renal transplant	ECG: peaked T waves, prolonged PR and QT segments ECG: depressed ST segment, widened T waves	Weakness, ↑DTR, confusion	K^+ >5.0 mEq/L
Hypercalcemia		Addison's disease, multiple myeloma, Paget's disease, cancer, sarcoidosis, hyperthyroidism	Brady arrhythmias	"Stones, bones, moans, groans"	Ca^+ >10.5 mEq/L
Hypocalcemia		Parathyroid or thyroid surgery		Paresthesias, DTR spasms, cramps, weakness, confusion, seizures, Chvostek's sign, Trousseau's sign	Ca^+ <8.5 mEq/L
Hypomagnesemia		Alcoholism, cirrhosis, pancreatitis, excessive GI fluid loss	May have arrhythmias	CNS depression, vertigo, ataxia, seizures, DTR, tetany, arrhythmias	Mg <1.6 mg/dl
Thiamine	Can occur in 7 weeks in chronic alcoholism	Alcoholism		Wernicke's encephalopathy: gait ataxia, nystagmus Korsakoff's psychosis: short-term memory disturbance (permanent)	
Vitamin B_{12} deficiency		Pernicious anemia, gastrectomy, vegetarian diet, small-bowel bacterial overgrowth, sprue, alcoholism		Paresthesias, gait abnormalities, psychoses, DTR, smooth tongue, pallor, mild icterus, anorexia, bowel disturbances	Megaloblastic anemia, MCV >115 μm^3, large RBCs, poikilocytosis Varying degrees of anemia: thrombocytopenia, neuropenia, pancytopenia

TOXIC

Exogenous	Acute ETOH intoxication / Drug overdose / Withdrawal: ETOH, benzodiazepines, narcotics / Carbon monoxide exposure	Alcoholism, drug abuse: narcotics, barbiturates, benzodiazepines, phenothiazines, phencyclidine	ETOH withdrawal, fever, tachycardia, diaphoresis 72-96 hours after last drink / Narcotic overdose—hypotension, bradycardia	Miosis, narcotic overdose, needle marks, ETOH on breath, delirium, trismus, hallucinations, agitation, confusion, autonomic overactivity, seizures	Anion gap metabolic acidosis / Serum ETOH level >100 mg/dl (determine legal intoxication) / 200 ml/dl →drowsy, confused / >400 mg/dl →respiratory depression with death
Endogenous Hypercarbia	COPD→asthma, bronchospasm aspiration, laryngospasm, narcotic overdose, ETOH overdose, hypoglycemia	COPD, ETOH abuse, narcotic/drug abuse, DM, neuromuscular disorders	Pulse oximetry may be normal, cardiovascular collapse with Pco_2 >100 mm Hg	Headache, confusion, lethargy, seizures, coma	Pco_2 >45 mm Hg / ABGs: acute respiratory acidosis (low pH, high Pco_2, low Po_2, normal HCO_3)
Sepsis	Gram-positive/negative bacteria / Proliferation/invasion/release of exogenous toxins / Host response release of endogenous medications	DM, lymphoproliferative disease, cirrhosis, burns, invasive procedures, chemotherapy	Tachycardia, tachypnea / Hypotension: bradycardia, respiratory failure, poor prognosis / Hyperventilation / Temperatures: >38°C, <36°C	Lethargy, irritability, ↓ peripheral pulses, ↓ urine output, wide pulse pressure	Neutrophilic leukocytosis: neutropenia less frequent but associated with higher mortality / Thrombocytopenia (30%) / Liver enzymes: transaminases, alkaline phosphatase, bilirubin, hyperglycemia
Ketoacidosis	Relative insulin deficiency causing hypoglycemia + ketonemia from noncompliance with insulin therapy / Infection, stroke, MI, trauma, pregnancy, other physiologic stress / Alcoholic ketoacidosis from heavy ETOH use with minimum food intake	DM, alcohol abuse	Myocardial depression, vasodilation, Kussmaul breathing hypotension, tachycardia	N/V, abdominal pain, fruity breath, odor from acetone	↑Serum glucose >300 mg/dl urine ketones, ↓Na+/Cl/Ca/P/Mg from osmotic diuresis ↓K+ / Anionic gap metabolic acidosis HCO_3 <15 mEq/L pH <7.3

ECG, electrocardiogram; DTR, deep tendon reflexes; SLE, systemic lupus erythematosus; CNS, central nervous system; GI, gastrointestinal; ETOH, ethanol, alcohol; MCV, mean corpuscular volume; RBCs, red blood cells.

Continued

Table 13-1	Causes of Altered Mental Status—cont'd				
Cause	Precipitating Factor	Finding	Vital Signs	Physical Examination	Laboratory Testing
NEUROGENIC					
Seizure	Status epilepticus: toxicologic etiology Hypoglycemia, stroke, CNS infection, withdrawal syndromes, trauma, mass lesions, hypoxia	History of head trauma, seizure disorder, anticonvulsant meds, new onset headache, paranasal sinus infection, mastoiditis	↓Pulse oximetry measurements possible	Tonic-clonic seizures, aura that lasts seconds, urinary/fecal incontinence, postictal lethargy and confusion	↓HCO_3 ↑Creatine kinase possible
Bacterial meningitis	Blood-borne spread of infection, especially in children Direct spread of infection from paranasal sinuses, otitis media, mastoiditis, and skull fracture	History of head trauma, sinusitis, otitis media, mastoiditis, contact with infected patient	↑Temperature	↑Temperature, headache, stiff neck, photophobia, seizures (25%) Brudzinski's sign (flexion of hips and knees in response to passive neck flexion) Kernig's sign (contraction of hamstrings in response to knee extension while hip is flexed) Purpuric rash with meningococcemia Lumbar puncture mandatory	↑CSF protein ↓CSF glucose Positive Gram's stain
	Nausea/vomiting	Hyperglycemia, hypoglycemia, hypokalemia, toxicologic etiology, ketoacidosis, brain abscess/hemorrhage			ABGs, serum glucose, toxicologic screen, serum ketones, CT scan of head if brain abscess suspected
	Diaphoresis	Syncope, anoxia/hypoperfusion, hypoglycemia, cocaine intoxication	Airway maneuvers O_2 supplementation Trendelenburg position if syncopal BP, ECG		O_2 saturation, ABGs, toxicologic screen

	Syncope, near syncope, anoxia/hypoperfusion, orthostatic hypotension, hypoperfusion, anxiety, toxicologic etiology, hypoglycemia		Airway maneuvers, O$_2$ supplementation, Trendelenburg position if syncopal, BP, ECG	Lightheadedness	O$_2$ saturation, ABGs, serum glucose, toxicologic screen
Viral meningitis and encephalitis	Primary viral infection, HSV-1, enteroviruses, mumps, measles, rubella, varicella, HIV, CMV, EBV, influenza, vaccinia, yellow fever, rabies, pertussis	Vast majority associated with enteroviruses or mumps		Meningeal irritation: stiff neck, headache, photophobia. Findings related to specific virus, lethargy. Encephalitis has similar presentation, but with AMS ranging from inability to calculate to complete unresponsiveness. Seizures common with encephalitis. Hemiparesis possible	CSF protein. Normal CSF glucose. CSF WBC <1000 negative Gram's stain
Cerebral abscess	Direct extension of infection from chronic middle ear, mastoid, or paranasal sinus infections. Compound skull fracture, penetrating head wound	History of chronic infection, otitis media, mastoiditis, sinusitis, history of head trauma, endocarditis, lung infection, dental abscess, tonsillar abscess		Fever (50%), severe headache (70%), nausea and vomiting, papilledema, seizures (30%), focal neurologic signs (>50%)	Head CT. Routine blood tests of little value. Lumbar puncture contraindicated
CARDIOVASCULAR					
Arrhythmia	Hypoxia, pain, anxiety, fluid overload after surgery, electrolyte disturbances, acid-base imbalance, acute MI, increased ICP. New cardiac medications	History of MI, renal failure, CHF, cardiomegaly, thyroid dysfunction. Change in cardiac medication	Potential cardiac collapse. ABCs monitored at all times. Arrhythmia possible	12-lead ECG, monitor BP	

CNS, Central nervous system; HCO_3, bicarbonate; CSF, cerebrospinal fluid; ABGs, arterial blood gases; CT, computed tomography; BP, blood pressure; ECG, electrocardiogram; HSV-1, herpes simplex type 1; HIV, human immunodeficiency virus; CMV, cytomegalovirus; EBV, Epstein-Barr virus; WBC, white blood cells; ICP, intracranial pressure; AMS, altered mental status; MI, myocardial infarction.

Continued

Table 13-1 Causes of Altered Mental Status—cont'd

Cause	Precipitating Factor	Finding	Vital Signs	Physical Examination	Laboratory Testing
Aortic stenosis, mitral stenosis	Syncope, outflow obstruction, exertion, anemia, infection	Rheumatic valvular disease, calcification/fibrosis of congenitally bicuspid aortic valve, Kawasaki disease, unexplained change in exercise tolerance		Mid-to-late-peaking systolic murmur, dizziness, lightheadedness, dyspnea on exertion, angina	Antiarrhythmic drug levels, electrolytes (K^+, Ca^{++}, Mg), thyroid panel
Idiopathic hypertrophic subaortic stenosis (hypertrophic cardiomyopathy)	Anxiety, pain, physical exertion	Family history of death from cardiovascular disease		Dyspnea on exertion, palpitations, syncope, chest pain, sudden death, S_4 heart sound with systolic ejection murmur	
Stroke	Blood vessel occlusion (85%), blood vessel rupture (15%)	History of TIA-like symptoms, atherosclerosis, HTN, DM, bleeding diathesis, vascular malformations, cocaine use		Neurologic: level of consciousness, visual assessment, motor function, sensation/neglect, cerebellar function, cranial nerves	Head CT

TIA, Transient ischemic attack; *HTN,* hypertrophic tubular necrosis; *DM,* diabetes mellitus; *CT,* computed tomography.

ETIOLOGY AND DIFFERENTIAL DIAGNOSIS
Metabolic Causes

Metabolic causes of AMS include mechanisms that change essential elements of brain tissue metabolism, including oxygen (hypoxia), blood flow (hypoperfusion), and glucose (hypoglycemia, hyperglycemia). Other metabolic causes include abnormalities in acid-base balance and electrolyte levels and deficiencies in certain essential metabolic substrates (e.g., thiamine, vitamin B_{12}).

Hypoxia/Anoxia and Hypoperfusion

Decreased blood flow to the brain (hypoperfusion) secondary to thromboembolism, ruptured aneurysm, decreased cardiac output, or cardiac arrest may lead to hypoxic brain injury. Decreased oxygen supply to the brain (hypoxia) has many causes. Decreased oxygenation of the blood may result from acute respiratory distress secondary to laryngospasm, bronchospasm, anaphylaxis, aspiration of a foreign body, asthmatic attack, and acute exacerbations of chronic conditions (e.g., cystic fibrosis). These conditions may also lead to a significant decrease in cerebral oxygenation with resultant brain hypoxic injury, manifested initially as AMS, which may lead to coma or even death if untreated. In the dental office, hypoxia may be caused by an overdose of medications used to control anxiety and pain. If the dose is too high or the metabolism of the drug is altered, significant CNS depression and AMS may occur.

Hypoglycemia

Hypoglycemia may occur in diabetic patients taking insulin and may cause AMS or brain damage and death. Hypoglycemia is usually sudden in onset and can lead to AMS in a short time. Typical symptoms of hypoglycemia include diaphoresis (sweating), changes in vital signs, shakiness, anxiety, nausea, dizziness, confusion, slurred speech, lethargy, headache, and coma. Other, more unusual manifestations include cranial nerve palsies, hemiplegia, and seizures. These manifestations should be differentiated from those in patients with psychiatric disturbances, syncope, or stroke. Patients with low blood glucose may be unaware of their condition, and the diagnosis is therefore based on both clinical symptoms and blood glucose levels. The dangers of hypoglycemia warrant appropriate perioperative assessment, which may ne-

cessitate monitoring of blood glucose levels on the diabetic patient.

Both pretreatment and posttreatment situations may increase the potential for a hypoglycemic episode. The patient who has altered oral intake before a dental appointment and who has not appropriately adjusted or been instructed to adjust the morning insulin dosage is at risk. The patient may be anxious, with associated gastric distress altering the desire to eat, or may want to present an image of optimal hygiene. At times the dentist may request that the patient not eat or drink (NPO status) before a sedation procedure. Confusion associated with the physician's instructions may result in an inappropriate administration of the morning dose of insulin. Dental treatment, especially extensive surgical procedures, can alter the patient's ability to eat normally after dental treatment. Adherence to the normally prescribed insulin regimen may result in hypoglycemia. Appropriate care must be planned with the patient's physician to prevent hypoglycemia or hyperglycemia (see Chapter 24).

Hyperglycemia

Hyperglycemia is a state of elevated blood glucose, which is usually a manifestation of diabetes mellitus. Pancreatic or other endocrine abnormalities, trauma, and drugs are other causes. Precipitating factors include pregnancy, drug overdose, exercise, epinephrine, steroid therapy, and infection.

Symptoms of hyperglycemia usually manifest slowly, in contrast to the rapid onset of hypoglycemia. Prolonged hyperglycemia results in ketoacidosis and coma, the usual causes of an emergency situation. Symptoms include fatigue, headache, abdominal pain, nausea, vomiting, dyspnea (respiratory compensation for metabolic acidosis), acetone breath (sweet or fruity), weak thready pulse, loss of mental activity, coma, and death.

A history of signs and symptoms of diabetes mellitus, including polydipsia, polyphagia, polyuria, and weight loss, should alert the practitioner to AMS from hyperglycemia.

Fluid and Electrolyte Disorders

Common electrolyte disturbances that cause AMS are hypercalcemia, hypocalcemia, hypomagnesemia, and potassium and sodium abnormalities.
Hypercalcemia.   Hypercalcemia (serum calcium: 10.5 mg/dl) presents with multiple symptoms, best remembered by the mnemonic "stones,

bones, psychic moans" (lethargy, weakness, fatigue, confusion), "and abdominal groans." The physiologically active form of calcium is the ionized fraction, which is about 40% to 50% of the total calcium. The biologically inactive form is bound to albumin. In hypoalbuminemia the total calcium may be low but with normal levels of physiologically active ionized calcium. Parathyroid hormone increases calcium and decreases phosphate, and calcitonin decreases calcium levels. Hyperparathyroidism, Addison's disease, multiple myeloma, Paget's disease, sarcoidosis, cancer, milk-alkali syndrome, and vitamin D overdose are possible causes of hypercalcemia.

Hypocalcemia. Hypocalcemia (serum calcium <8.5 mg/dl) is manifested as weakness, perioral paresthesias, confusion, and seizures. These patients may also demonstrate *Chvostek's sign*, which is a twitching of the corner of the mouth when stimulating the seventh cranial nerve (CN VII, facial nerve) at the zygomatic arch. The patient may also show *Trousseau's sign*, which is carpal spasm of the arm when a blood pressure cuff is left inflated above the patient's systolic blood pressure for more than 3 minutes. Hypocalcemia is usually seen in patients after parathyroid or thyroid surgery, renal failure, sepsis, and pancreatitis.

Hyponatremia. Signs and symptoms of low serum sodium (hyponatremia) occur when serum sodium level is less than 120 mEq/L (normal range, 135 to 145 mEq/L). These symptoms include headache, abdominal pain, confusion, hallucination, and seizures. The most common cause of hyponatremia is a dilutional mechanism (i.e., increase in extracellular fluid). Other causes include trauma, cardiac failure, adrenal insufficiency, renal failure, hepatic failure, and sepsis. The sodium imbalance may be secondary to hyperglycemia, increased protein, or hyperlipidemia.

Hypernatremia. Hypernatremia may cause irritability, brain hemorrhage, and AMS. Neurologic symptoms begin when serum sodium (Na^+) concentration is greater than 158 mEq/L. Common causes of hypernatremia include decreased total body water from decreased intake or increased water loss from dehydration, usually caused by diarrhea, vomiting, fever, and increased sweating. To determine the significance and treatment of a serum Na^+ excess or deficit, the patient's volume status must be evaluated. Determination of serum osmolarity and urine Na^+ levels also assist in evaluation and treatment.

Hyperkalemia. Signs and symptoms of hyperkalemia include confusion, weakness, and increased deep tendon reflexes and are usually seen when serum potassium (K^+) is greater than 5.0 mEq/L (normal range, 3.3 to 4.9 mEq/L). On the electrocardiogram (ECG), peaked T waves are characteristic. If K^+ levels reach 8 mEq/L, heart rate becomes irregular, ECG patterns change to a sine wave pattern, and cardiac arrest soon follows. The patient taking a digitalis preparation is more sensitive to fluctuations in K^+ level and more susceptible to adverse cardiac arrhythmias.

Renal failure and hyperglycemia are the most common causes of hyperkalemia. The complexity in managing a medically compromised patient thus becomes evident. "Keeping the patient sweet," as in managing the diabetic patient during treatment, can have other adverse effects in the "brittle" patient. Other causes of hyperkalemia include hemolysis, thrombocytosis, leukocytosis, increased dosage of potassium-sparing diuretics, adrenal insufficiency, muscle damage secondary to trauma, and succinylcholine administration.

Hypomagnesemia. Hypomagnesemia is most often caused by alcoholism and poor nutrition. Signs of hypomagnesemia include neurologic abnormalities (e.g., vertigo, ataxia, increased deep tendon reflexes, tetany, seizures), cardiac dysrhythmias, and depression.

Acid-Base Disturbances

Acid-base disorders include metabolic and respiratory acidosis and metabolic and respiratory alkalosis. Acid-base disturbances are often seen in patients with renal problems, acute and chronic respiratory problems, diabetes mellitus, ketoacidosis, and possible drug ingestion (e.g., aspirin). These patients have a disordered bicarbonate–carbonic acid system, the most important buffering system in the body for acid base regulation, primarily through the lungs and kidneys. Acid-base homeostasis involves buffering mechanisms to prevent gross deviation from the normal pH of about 7.4. *Acidosis* is caused by an increase of acid or loss of alkali. *Alkalosis* is caused by loss of acid or addition of alkali. Both processes can occur through metabolic or respiratory mechanisms. Acute signs of acid-base changes include vomiting, diarrhea, tachypnea, cyanosis, respiratory failure, shock, and ultimately AMS.

Nutritional Deficiencies

Nutritional deficiencies that can cause AMS are often seen with chronic alcohol abuse and include thiamine (vitamin B_1) and vitamin B_{12}

deficits. *Thiamine deficiency* can occur within 7 weeks in chronic alcoholism, leading to an acutely evolving alcohol-related encephalopathy. *Wernicke's encephalopathy* initially manifests as a gait ataxia (stumbling) from cerebellar atrophy and involuntary eye movements (nystagmus) from brainstem lesions. Without treatment the disease will eventually progress to *Korsakoff's psychosis*, a disturbance in new memory formation caused by thalamic damage, at which point the disease is usually refractory to treatment. Tissue necrosis and atrophy with blood vessel changes occur within the hypothalamus and the thalamus. When intravenous (IV) thiamine (100 mg daily) is administered to the patient with Wernicke's encephalopathy, the eye movement abnormalities usually improve within 2 to 5 hours. However, gait ataxia takes longer to improve and often does not resolve completely. Treatment may reverse all mental changes, with persistent memory loss a sign of Korsakoff's psychosis. The patient's long-term memories are usually intact, whereas short-term memory is disturbed. It is imperative to treat chronic alcoholic patients against alcohol withdrawal while they are hospitalized.

Vitamin B$_{12}$ deficiency can result in pernicious anemia and megaloblastemia. Neurologic abnormalities manifest as paresthesias, gait and coordination abnormalities, psychosis, and AMS. Mural degeneration of the posterior and lateral columns of the spinal cord are manifested by decreased position sense, increased deep tendon reflexes, ataxic gait disturbance, and bowel and bladder dysfunction. Physical findings of vitamin B$_{12}$ deficiency include smooth tongue, pallor, mild icterus (jaundice), and splenomegaly. Causes of vitamin B$_{12}$ deficiency include lack of intrinsic factor, malabsorption, gastrectomy, strict vegetarian diet, small-bowel bacterial overgrowth secondary to diverticulosis, fistulas, and scleroderma. Drugs such as alcohol, neomycin, and colchicine can also impair absorption of vitamin B$_{12}$. All symptoms of pernicious anemia are reversible with vitamin B$_{12}$ therapy.

Toxic Causes

Toxic causes of AMS generally result from exogenous intake of agents (e.g., alcohol, opiates, barbiturates, anticholinergics, neuroleptics, carbon monoxide/cyanide poisoning) or endogenous production of toxins (e.g., sepsis, renal failure/uremia, hepatic encephalopathy, hypercarbia, Reye's syndrome, porphyria).

Exogenous toxic agents can have a profound metabolic effect on brain tissue, often leading to AMS. Toxicity may be induced through accidental or intentional administration or ingestion of medications, drugs, or poisonous substances. Common dental agents that may lead to overdose, toxicity, and AMS are local anesthetic agents and drugs used for sedation and pain control, including sedative-hypnotics and narcotics. Adverse or toxic effects of the drugs occur when excessive doses are administered or when metabolism of the agent is decreased, as in hepatic or kidney failure or from interactions with other drugs.

In the dental office, especially in the pediatric or geriatric patient, local anesthetic toxicity must be included in the differential diagnosis of an abrupt change in mental status. The first manifestation of an adverse anesthetic effect may be drowsiness. Other symptoms of mild toxicity from local anesthetic agents include slurred speech, confusion, nausea, vertigo, tinnitus, paresthesias, irritability, and muscular twitching. Serious symptoms then follow, including psychosis, seizures, respiratory depression, and sinoatrial and atrioventricular node blockade.

Narcotics may also cause CNS and respiratory depression and will present with decreased respiratory rate, hypotension, pinpoint pupils (miosis), stupor, and AMS. Naloxone will antagonize the effects of narcotics but can potentiate withdrawal symptoms (see Chapter 28). Acute narcotic withdrawal may cause combativeness initially (acutely with naloxone administration), restlessness, insomnia, yawning, hallucinations, diarrhea, mydriasis (ablation of pupils), piloerection ("goose flesh"), hypertension, tachycardia, and lacrimation.

Ethanol intoxication affects cognitive function and predisposes patients to trauma and accidental injury, as well as hepatic problems and AMS. It is also a leading cause of hypoglycemia. Signs and symptoms of ethanol intoxication are slurred speech, CNS and respiratory depression, and decreased motor control. The patient with respiratory depression may require airway management with oxygen supplementation and possibly intubation. Patients with a history of alcohol abuse can also present with agitation, tremors, anxiety, tachycardia, seizures, and hallucinations. Such patients should be hospitalized immediately and monitored under medical supervision and treated for possible withdrawal. Symptoms of alcohol withdrawal usually peak within 48 hours of the last ethanol ingestion. Treatment of these patients includes fluid and nutritional support and prophylaxis for delirium tremens with thiamine, benzodiazepines, phenobarbital, or alcohol.

Patients with a history of alcohol abuse and liver failure may also present with *hepatic encephalopathy* due to increased levels of ammonia in the blood. Severe cases may progress to coma and result in permanent brain damage. Hepatic encephalopathy is characterized by fluctuation in the levels of consciousness, increased deep tendon reflexes, spasticity, and seizures. Asterixis ("liver flap," flapping tremor of hands when arms are extended) is characteristic but not specific.

Neurogenic Causes

Neurologic causes of AMS range from a brief syncopal episode to seizure, cerebrovascular accident (CVA, stroke) or transient ischemic attack (TIA), and other intracranial processes (e.g., brain tumor, trauma, concussion, hypertensive encephalopathy). Neurogenic AMS may also include intracranial infection (bacterial, viral, fungal, parasitic). In an acute setting such as the dental office, however, the most likely cause of AMS is seizure disorder or CVA/TIA.

Seizures

A seizure is a period of altered neurologic function caused by abnormal neuronal electrical activity (see Chapter 15). Seizures can manifest in various types of seizure activity. Approximately 1% to 2% of the general population has some form of recurrent seizure activity. E*pilepsy* is a neurologic disorder that manifests as spontaneously occurring seizures. It may develop secondary to trauma, intracranial abscess, or brain tumor and may have a genetic link. Even patients without a history of epilepsy can experience seizures leading to AMS. The seizure may result from toxic doses of local anesthesia given during dental treatment or episodes of syncope, from intracranial hemorrhage, or from increased ICP.

Seizure activity falls into three broad categories: (1) generalized, (2) partial, and (3) complex. Patients experiencing *generalized seizures* have loss of consciousness. This category includes tonic-clonic (grand mal), absence (petit mal), myoclonic, and atonic seizures. A patient experiencing a grand mal seizure may experience a preictal *aura*. This visual, auditory, gustatory, or olfactory sensation directly precedes the loss of consciousness, and thus the patient may be able to anticipate an oncoming seizure. After loss of consciousness the patient experiences tonic-clonic phases of seizure activity. During the tonic phase the patient becomes rigid in extension.

The clonic phase is characterized by rhythmic contraction and extension of extremities, during which the patient may sustain injuries and requires protection. Then, during the postictal stage, the patient may become somnolent and may sleep for hours.

The patient with *partial* (focal) *seizures* has no loss of consciousness, but motor, sensory, or autonomic seizures may occur. *Complex* (psychomotor or temporal lobe) *seizures* are associated with impaired consciousness but rarely unconsciousness.

Infections

Bacterial meningitis is a CNS infection involving the leptomeninges that leads to AMS. Meningitis may develop through blood-borne spread of infection, especially in children, but may also result from direct spread of infection from the paranasal sinuses, as well as from spread of infection secondary to otitis media, mastoiditis, and skull fractures. The patient with bacterial meningitis classically presents with fever, headache, stiff neck, myalgia, photophobia, and AMS. Seizures occur in approximately 25% of cases. The elderly patient may present with only confusion and fever. Most symptoms develop over several days to a week, with a 25% mortality rate. About 10% of patients with symptoms advance to coma in less than 24 hours, with a 50% mortality rate.

Organisms important in the etiology of bacterial meningitis vary and depend on the patient's age. In neonates the most common infectious agents are *Escherichia coli*, *Streptococcus agalactiae*, and *Salmonella* species; in children ages 2 to 5 years, *Haemophilus influenzae*; ages 5 to 30, *Neisseria meningitidis*; and over age 30, *Streptococcus pneumoniae*. Close family contacts and sleeping partners are especially susceptible to contraction of the disease through the spread of H. *influenzae* or of meningococci, which are the most common cause of outbreaks. Exposure of health care personnel may require long-term antibiotic therapy.

Viral meningitis is an infection of the meninges and is a recognized complication of many common viral illnesses. Causes of viral encephalitis are usually mild and self-limited, although some conditions can result in extensive CNS damage and even death (e.g., herpes simplex type 1, rabies). Viral meningitis is acute in onset and usually has less severe clinical manifestations than bacterial meningitis. Most cases are caused by hematogenous spread to the CNS. Clinical symptoms are generally ambiguous, with fever, headache, and stiff neck most common.

Viral encephalitis can have a similar presentation to meningitis. AMS ranges from mild changes to complete unresponsiveness, frequently with seizures. Encephalitis associated with herpes simplex type 1 is characterized by bizarre behavior, olfactory hallucinations, and aphasia.

Cerebral abscess may also cause AMS through direct spread of infection from the paranasal sinuses and middle ear (otitis media), or blood spread secondary to infectious endocarditis emboli. The most common symptom of cerebral abscess is headache, and 50% of patients will present with fever, vomiting, confusion, and obtundation. Neck stiffness, hemiparesis, and seizures are present in less than half of patients.

Stroke

AMS, stroke, and brain damage invariably result from neuronal hypoxia. Two main mechanisms of stroke are blood vessel occlusion (ischemic causes, 86%) and aneurysm or blood vessel rupture leading to intracranial hemorrhage, mass effect, and direct neurologic damage (hemorrhagic causes, 14%). Common risk factors of cerebrovascular disease include atherosclerotic vessel disease, heart disease, high blood pressure, and diabetes mellitus.

Ischemic stroke is most often caused by large-vessel occlusion by thrombosis or embolism. Causes of thrombosis are atherosclerosis, vasculitis, polycythemia, syphilis, and trichinosis. Heart valve vegetations, mural thrombosis, and cardiac tremors can also cause emboli. Signs and symptoms of ischemic stroke are contralateral weakness or numbness, contralateral visual deficits, and aphasia.

Hemorrhagic conditions may cause local tissue damage that affects state of consciousness. Causes include hemorrhage from hypertensive events, aneurysm, bleeding diathesis, and amyloid angiopathy. Signs of *hemorrhagic stroke* are similar to those of ischemic stroke but may also include vomiting, nausea, dizziness, and headache. Hemorrhagic stroke occurs in a younger patient population and is divided into intracerebral and subarachnoid hemorrhages. Clinical presentation of CVA will depend on the location of and nature of the neural damage.

Subarachnoid hemorrhage usually occurs after berry aneurysm rupture, trauma, hypertensive crisis, vasculitis, and coagulation disorders. It presents as a severe headache, vomiting, and progressive loss of consciousness. Hemorrhage accumulates in the basal cisterns and around the brainstem and is instantly fatal in approximately 15% of patients. Risk factors for *intracerebral hemorrhage* are hypertension, older age, prior CVA, and cocaine use. Intracerebral hemorrhage occurs primarily in hypertensive patients over age 50. Dizziness, vomiting, ataxia, inability to walk, rapid progression to coma, and herniation may occur; mortality is greater than 80%. *Intracerebellar hemorrhage* is most often caused by hypertensive vascular disease, with bleeding usually in the basal ganglia (80%).

Patients suspected of stroke should be administered supplemental oxygen and placed on a cardiac monitor, with the chair back slightly elevated. IV access should be established if personnel are experienced. The patient's hydration status must be assessed; dehydration can cause decreased perfusion, and overhydration can cause cerebral edema with increased neurologic damage. Glucose-containing solutions should be avoided because of increased neural damage from hyperglycemia. Access to the emergency medical services (EMS) system is critical to optimize patient outcome.

Cardiovascular Causes

Cardiovascular causes of AMS generally result from vascular, hemorrhagic, or cardiac events. Vascular causes may result from infarction of brain tissue in the cerebral cortex, thalamus, hypothalamus, brainstem, or pons. This infarct may be caused by thrombotic, embolic, vasculitic, vasospastic, or venous thrombotic events.

Cardiac causes of AMS can lead to intracranial processes, which directly affect the brain tissue, or extracranial processes, which lead to decreased blood flow and hypoxia of the brain tissue. These processes vary from benign conditions (e.g., reflex-mediated episodes) to life-threatening disorders (e.g., hypertension-related stroke, intracranial hemorrhage). Reflex-mediated mechanisms include vasovagal epi-sode, carotid sinus reflex, micturition syncope, and tussive syncope. More serious causes of decreased blood flow include hypovolemia from blood loss or dehydration. Decreased blood flow to the brain can also be caused by vascular obstruction from pulmonary embolus or thrombus or by subclavian steal syndrome.

Cardiac obstruction from mitral or aortic stenosis and, more often, cardiac arrhythmias also can cause AMS. These arrhythmias include sick sinus syndrome, second- and third-degree heart blocks, ventricular tachycardia, ventricular fibrillation, paroxysmal supraventricular tachycardia, premature atrial contraction, Wolff-Parkinson-White (WPW) syndrome and long QT syndrome.

Eclampsia, a pregnancy-induced hypertension that usually occurs in the third trimester, may lead to AMS. This condition should be suspected if a pregnant patient with hypertension manifests epigastric pain, increased deep tendon reflexes, confusion, and headache. Eclampsia is a true hypertensive emergency and requires immediate admission and management by an obstetric-gynecologic specialist. CNS signs related to eclampsia can lead to seizures, progressive AMS, and coma if not aggressively treated.

MANAGEMENT APPROACH

AMS may be the initial manifestation of a life-threatening disease process. Therefore the initial treatment often precedes the diagnostic process; evaluation and management occur simultaneously, with immediate initiation of life-sustaining measures if needed. This phase of management of AMS should proceed in a similar manner to those during CPR measures: establish unresponsiveness, check and manage airway, and support circulation and breathing. Once the patient is stabilized, additional therapies may be indicated, followed by a complete history, physical examination, and additional studies, if needed. If a specific diagnosis is established, definitive treatment is administered, with appropriate disposition of the patient.

Establish Unresponsiveness

As in other life-threatening emergencies with loss of consciousness, unresponsiveness is checked by asking the patient, "What is your name?" "Open your eyes," or "Are you okay?" If there is no response, a painful or noxious stimulus is attempted. If a response is obtained, the level of consciousness is established in accordance with Glasgow Coma scale scores.

Manage Airway and Cervical Spine

Assessment and immediate management of the airway are important in all patients with AMS. Examine for airway obstruction by tongue, vomitus, or other objects. Determine whether the patient's decreased level of consciousness is profound enough to require active airway control, such as assisted ventilation and Combitube/endotracheal intubation. When trauma is the cause of AMS, or vice versa, precautions should be taken to protect the cervical spine.

Support Breathing and Circulation

Once airway patency is ensured or secured using airway maneuvers, breathing is assessed. If the patient is breathing spontaneously, effectiveness of respiration is assessed. If ventilation is ineffective or absent, breathing is controlled using a face mask, bag-valve-mask device, or airway device. Assessment of the circulation can be accomplished by evaluating the pulses, capillary refill, and blood pressure.

PATIENT ASSESSMENT AND DIFFERENTIAL DIAGNOSIS

The development of a differential diagnosis is best based on an orderly and systematic review of the history and physical examination of the patient. The information from the history and physical examination is then correlated with findings from preliminary laboratory tests and radiographic studies to formulate a working differential diagnosis. This preliminary diagnosis can be used to obtain any additional studies and specific laboratory tests to confirm or establish a final diagnosis. This diagnostic approach uses information from all components of the diagnostic work-up and provides a basis for effective treatment (Table 13-2).

History

Once the patent with AMS is stabilized, obtaining the history is essential in providing further therapy. Since obtaining an adequate history from patients with AMS may be difficult or impossible, however, information often must be obtained from other sources, including relatives and friends. If available, previous records can be reviewed to check the patient's medical history for past or current illnesses or medications that may provide clues to the causes of the AMS.

Accounts of the event from different sources, including others in the immediate area and office personnel, should be used to aid in the establishment of a differential diagnosis. Information in wallets or purses, on medical identification tags, in medical records, or from other medical personnel should be used. Salient points that can aid in the differential diagnosis include the onset and speed of symptoms, fluctuation of symptoms, and premonitory symptoms. The duration of the AMS and time until recovery should also be used.

The patient's age is also important to develop possible etiologies. AMS in a young patient is often the result of a toxin (alcohol or drug),

Text continued on p. 205

Table 13-2	Clinical Findings and Recommended Actions in Patients with AMS		
History	**Finding**	**Significance**	**Action**
Past medical history	HIV positive	CNS infection, space-occupying lesion	Assess and maintain airway, O_2 administration, MRI or head CT, LP (including syphilis test, fungal, mycobacterial)
	Seizure disorder	Nonconvulsive status epilepticus, antiepileptic drug intoxication	Antiepileptic drug levels, EEG, neurologic consultation
Current medications	Anticoagulants	Intracranial hemorrhage	PT/INR/PTT, head CT
	Opioids	Opioid intoxification	Naloxone
	Antiepileptic drugs	Antiepileptic drug intoxication, seizure	Antiepileptic drug levels
Social history	Chronic alcohol use	Withdrawal syndromes, subdural hematoma, Wernicke's encephalopathy, hepatic encephalopathy, infection, sepsis	Septic work-up, ammonia level, CBC, head CT, thiamine administration, pharmacologic management of withdrawal
	Chronic drug use	Withdrawal syndromes	Pharmacologic management of withdrawal syndomes
Associated symptoms	Headache	Toxicologic etiology (salicylates, carbon monoxide), intracranial hemorrhage, CNS infection, mass lesion	Carboxyhemoglobin level, salicylate level, head CT, LP if CT negative or not available
	Seizure	Nonconvulsive status epilepticus, toxicologic etiology, hypoglycemia, stroke, CNS infection, withdrawal syndromes	Assess and maintain airway, place in supine position and protect from self-injury, antiepileptic drug levels, toxicology screen, electrolytes, serum glucose, head CT, pharmacologic management if withdrawal
Blood pressure	Hypotension	Hypovolemia, MI, ETOH/barbiturate intoxication, Wernicke's encephalopathy, sepsis	Supplemental O_2, IV fluids, monitor VS, ACLS algorithm if MI, cardiac monitors, thiamine administration, septic work-up (blood cultures, LP, UA, chest film, other cultures if appropriate)

See Table 13-1 for additional abbreviations. *LP,* Lumbar puncture; *EEG,* electroencephalogram; *CBC,* complete blood count; *VS,* vital signs; *ACLS,* advanced cardiac life support; *UA,* urinalysis; *DIC,* disseminated intravascular coagulation; *ITP,* idiopathic thrombocytopenic purpura.

Continued

Table 13-2	Clinical Findings and Recommended Actions in Patients with AMS—cont'd		
History	**Finding**	**Significance**	**Action**
Blood pressure—cont'd	Hypertension	HTN encephalopathy, ↑ ICP, toxicologic (sympathomimetics), thyrotoxicosis, intracranial hemorrhage, pregnancy-induced HTN	Monitor BP, funduscopy, assess for end-organ damage, assess for pregnancy-induced HTN, thyroid screen, toxicology screen, head CT, LP if CT negative or unavailable, manage HTN
Heart rate	Bradycardia	Toxicologic (β-blockers, calcium channel blockers), ↑ICP, hypothyroidism	Cardiac monitors, assess for ↑ICP, toxicology screen, thyroid screen, ECG, manage bradycardia
	Tachycardia	Toxicologic (tricyclic, sympathomimetics, anticholinergics), sepsis, thyrotoxicosis, ↓cardiac output, withdrawal syndromes, hypoxia, hypoglycemia	O_2 saturation/O_2 supplementation, cardiac monitor, electrolytes, thyroid screen, toxicology screen, septic workup, CBC, ECG, manage withdrawal pharmacologically
Respiration	Hypoventilation	Toxicologic (opioids, barbiturates), stroke, ↑ICP	Assess airway, administer O_2, assess ↑ICP, toxicology screen, ABGs, head CT, naloxone
	Hyperventilation	Toxins or drugs causing metabolic acidosis, hypoxia, hypercapnia, acidosis, fever, liver disease, sepsis, pulmonary emboli, central neurogenic hyperventilation, salicylism	Assess airway, administer O_2, toxicology screen, ABGs, septic work-up, liver enzymes, liver function tests, serum ammonia, pulmonary embolism work-up
Temperature	Hyperthermia	CNS infection, sepsis, neuroleptic malignant syndrome, serotonin syndrome, toxicologic (anticholinergics, salicylates, sympathomimetics), stroke, heat stroke, thyrotoxicosis, withdrawal syndromes	Investigate source: septic work-up, toxicology screen, environmental exposures, thyroid screen, CBC, temperature reduction, antibiotics
	Hypothermia	Sepsis, toxicologic (ETOH, barbiturates), hypothyroidism, environmental exposure, hypoglycemia	Rewarming, investigate source: septic work-up, toxicology, screen, environmental exposure, thyroid screening, CBC, antibiotics

See Table 13-1 for additional abbreviations. *LP,* Lumbar puncture; *EEG,* electroencephalogram; *CBC,* complete blood count; *VS,* vital signs; *ACLS,* advanced cardiac life support; *UA,* urinalysis; *DIC,* disseminated intravascular coagulation; *ITP,* idiopathic thrombocytopenic purpura.

Table 13-2	Clinical Findings and Recommended Actions in Patients with AMS—cont'd		
History	**Finding**	**Significance**	**Action**
Mental status	Unarousable or difficult to arouse	Intracranial hemorrhage, stroke, space-occupying lesion, CNS infection, sepsis, seizure: nonconvulsive status epilepticus, prolonged postictal period; metabolic: hypoxia, hypercapnia, hypoglycemia, electrolyte abnormality, hypercalcemia, Wernicke's encephalopathy, uremia, hepatic encephalopathy; toxic ingestion drug ETOH, withdrawal, drug interaction; ↓cerebral perfusion, hypovolemia, anemia, ↓cardiac output	IV access, cardiac monitor, assess airway, O_2 administration, rapid glucose determination, dextrose administration, assess for ↓ICP, electrolytes, serum calcium, thyroid serum, septic work-up, CBC, head CT, EEG/ECG, thiamine, naloxone, cervical spine immobilization
	Depressed level of consciousness	Same as above	Mini–mental status exam, assess airway, O_2, electrolytes, serum Ca^+ levels, BUN/creatinine, thyroid screen, septic work-up, CBC, head CT, EEG/ECG, thiamine
	Hyperalterness/agitation	Toxicologic etiology (drug or toxic ingestion, exposure, withdrawal), psychiatric etiology, hyperthyroidism, hypoxia, hypoglycemia	Rapid glucose determination, dextrose administration, O_2 saturation and administration, thyroid screen, toxicology screen, thiamine administration. Consider potential for patient violence; chemical or physical restraint as needed
	Acute cognitive abnormalities: disorientation, language difficulties, impaired learning and memory	Toxicologic etiology, psychiatric etiology, CNS infection, sepsis, stroke, mass lesion	Rapid glucose determination, dextrose administration, mini–mental status exam, electrolytes, BUN/creatinine, toxicology screen, septic work-up, CBC, head CT, EEG/ECG, thiamine administration
Breath odor	Acetone smell	Ketoacidosis, toxic ingestion	Assess for isopropranolol, ABGs, electrolytes, serum glucose/ketones

Continued

History	Finding	Significance	Action
Table 13-2	**Clinical Findings and Recommended Actions in Patients with AMS—cont'd**		
Breath odor—cont'd	Fetor Hepaticus	Hepatic encephalopathy	Liver function tests, serum ammonia, PT/INR
	Ethanol smell	Ethanol or other volatile, chemical ingestion	Ethanol tests, assess for other alcohols
	Cheyne-Stokes breathing	Cerebral disease, impending transtentorial herniation, upper brainstem lesions, metabolic encephalopathy, CHF, ↑ICP, posterior fossa lesion, pontine lesion, transtentorial herniation, metabolic coma, medullary lesion	Assess airway, serial reassessment, consultation, admit as appropriate
	Cluster breathing	↑ICP, posterior fossa lesion	
	Apneustic breathing	Pontine lesion, transtentorial herniation, metabolic coma	
	Atoxic breathing	Medullary lesion	
Skin	Needle tracks	Drug overdose (opioids)	Naloxone
	Cyanosis	Hypoxia	Assess airway, administer O_2
	Cherry red	Carbon monoxide poisoning	100% O_2 administration, carboxyhemoglobin level
	Jaundice	Hepatic encephalopathy	Liver function, ammonia level, PT/INR
	Pallor	Anemia	CBC with differential
		Hemorrhage	Crystalloid challenge, blood transfusion when appropriate
	Petechiae	DIC	PT/PTT/INR
		ITP	Fibrin levels
		Drugs	CBC, toxicology screen
	Maculopapular rash	Toxic shock syndrome	Investigate source
		Subacute bacterial endocarditis	Septic work-up
		SLE	Blood cultures, antibiotics, antinuclear antigen test
	Bullous lesions	Drugs, especially barbituates	Assess airway, supplemental O_2, toxicology screen
Head	Head trauma	Intracranial hemorrhage	Heat CT, cervical spine immobilization
	New asymmetry or fixed pupil	Stroke, space-occupying lesion	Head CT, LP

See Table 13-1 for additional abbreviations. *LP*, Lumbar puncture; *EEG*, electroencephalogram; *CBC*, complete blood count; *VS*, vital signs; *ACLS*, advanced cardiac life support; *UA*, urinalysis; *DIC*, disseminated intravascular coagulation; *ITP*, idiopathic thrombocytopenic purpura.

Table 13-2	Clinical Findings and Recommended Actions in Patients with AMS—cont'd		
History	**Finding**	**Significance**	**Action**
Head—cont'd	Bilateral pinpoint pupils, bilaterally dilated pupils	Toxicologic (opioids, clonidine, organophosphates), pontine stroke, toxicologic (sympathomimetics, anticholinergics, hallucinogenics), brain death	Head CT, naloxone, directed toxicology screening
Neck	Nuchal rigidity or other meningeal signs, no fever	Subarachnoid hemorrhage, CNS infection	CT, LP if CT negative or not available, antibiotics if bacterial etiology suspected
	Nuchal rigidity or other meningeal signs, fever	CNS infection, subarachnoid hemorrhage	LP, antibiotics, blood cultures, CT, antipyretics
Eyes	Icterus (jaundice)	Hepatic encephalopathy	Liver function tests, serum ammonia, PT/INR
Funduscopic examination	Papilledema	Space-occupying lesion	Head CT
	Retinal (subhyaloid) hemorrhage	HTN encephalopathy, subarachnoid hemorrhage	Head CT, LP if CT is negative or unavailable
Heart	Arrhythmia	Cardiac arrest	ACLS algorithm
Gastrointestinal	Fecal incontinence	Seizure, postictal coma	Assess and manage airway, place patient supine and protect from self-injury, head CT if new-onset seizures, antiepileptic drug levels
Genitourinary	Urinary incontinence	Seizure, postictal coma	Assess and manage airway, place in supine position and protect from self-injury, head CT if new-onset seizures, antiepileptic drug levels

postictal state, or traumatic injury, whereas AMS in elderly persons is more likely to be of cardiovascular etiology or secondary to stroke or dehydration.

During the initial assessment of a patient with AMS, the clinician should inquire about symptoms associated with the event, including headache, fever, seizure, hallucination, change in speech, and motor activity changes (e.g., gait, equilibrium). Other areas for evaluation include alertness, visual changes, memory loss, and changes in bowel and bladder functions. Accessibility of the patient to drugs or poisons before the occurrence of symptoms is relevant. The history of present illness (HPI) includes the patient's present health status, similar events underlying chronic disease (e.g., neurologic, cardiovascular, endocrine, metabolic, and psychiatric deficits), and substance abuse.

Findings from the circumstances surrounding the event should be checked. For example, if the event occurred during an emotionally charged situation, a psychological or neurocardiogenic cause should be suspected. In rare instances, the event occurring after isolated arm use may suggest subclavian steal syndrome. Knowing the patient's position immediately before the onset of AMS may be helpful to the differential diagnosis. For example, prolonged standing, especially in a warm crowded environment, may suggest orthostatic syncope from venous pooling.

Orthostatic syncope should also be suspected if the event occurred after changing to the upright position. Presence of incontinence or focal neurologic signs, such as myoclonic jerking or lateralizing, are indicative of seizure. In the patient with a history of trauma, intracranial hemorrhage should be suspected, and head computed tomography (CT) may be urgently needed. If AMS occurred after head turning or any situation that put pressure on the neck, a carotid sinus cause should be suspected.

Premonitory symptoms are also helpful in the differential diagnosis of AMS. For example, nausea, diaphoresis, and lightheadedness are common in neurocardiogenic episodes. Presence of antecedent chest pain, rapid heartbeat, or skipped beats suggests a cardiac origin. On the other hand, presence of an aura or focal sensory or motor disturbances is more indicative of a neurogenic cause.

The past medical history should be checked for conditions associated with a potential change in mental status, such as a history of "fainting," diabetes, seizure disorders, Addison's disease, cardiovascular and cerebrovascular disease, substance abuse, recent infection, or trauma. The history should be checked for any recent changes in the patient's health before the event. Use of specific medications, recent changes in these medications, dosage, and compliance are important factors. Specific medications include hypoglycemics, antihypertensives, nitrates and other cardiovascular agents, antileptics, antidepressants, opioids, anticholinergics, neuroleptics, steroids, sedative-hypnotics, miotics, mydriatics, and over-the-counter medications. A history of anticoagulant use suggests intracranial hemorrhage.

Questioning during the period of assessment must be both direct and inclusive of all potential etiologies. The responses to the initial questions will dictate the specificity and direction of subsequent questions. No detail is insignificant. For example, a recent history of fever with vomiting and diarrhea may indicate dehydration, whereas a history of melena may suggest anemia. The latter may be secondary to the use of analgesics for odontogenic pain. A history of a headache with associated AMS may also be secondary to salicylate overdose. Do not be hesitant to inquire about alcohol use. The intoxicated patient may be easy to identify secondary to the smell of alcohol. However, AMS in the patient with a social history of alcohol may indicate possible withdrawal syndromes, subdural hematoma, or hepatic encephalopathy.

Physical Examination

Priority should be given to performing resuscitative measures if needed. Once the patient is stable, the physical examination of patients with AMS should be performed systematically. The physical examination should consist of (1) checking the vital signs, (2) performing a quick general survey, (3) assessing the level of response and mental status, and (4) conducting a focal neurologic examination.

Vital Signs

Temperature, respiratory rate, heart rate, and blood pressure measurements should be taken, documented, and repeated as necessary. Findings of significance should be analyzed and used in developing the differential diagnosis. Automatic blood pressure equipment is becoming more readily available. If pulse oximetry and ECG are available, oxygen saturation should be monitored and any major arrhythmia identified.

Temperature. *Fever* suggests infection, heat stroke, thyroid storm, malignant hypothermia, hypothalamic lesion, anticholinergic drug ingestion, salicylate or sympathomimetic toxicity, and withdrawal syndromes. *Hypothermia* may be indicative of alcoholic or barbiturate intoxication, hemorrhage, shock, cold exposure, myxedema, coma, hypoglycemia, hypopituitarism, and peripheral circulatory collapse.

Heart rate. *Bradycardia* suggests heart block, myocardial infarction, intoxication, and hypothyroidism. Bradycardia can also be caused by drug overdose, such as from β-blockers and calcium channel blockers. If bradycardia is associated with periodic breathing and hypertension, increased ICP should be considered.

Tachycardia may be indicative of hypovolemia, hypoglycemia, hypoxia, thyrotoxicosis, cocaine overdose, and sepsis. Tachycardia may also be secondary to overdose or drug interactions associated with tricyclic antidepressants, sympathomimetics, and anticholinergics. If tachycardia is severe (>140 beats/min) ectopic paroxysmal tachyarrhythmia should be suspected.

Blood pressure. *Hypotension* is often found in barbiturate or alcoholic intoxication, hemorrhage, shock, myocardial infarction, sepsis, and Wernicke's encephalopathy. *Hypertension* usually occurs early in shock, with intracranial hemorrhage, increased ICP, and hypertensive encephalopathy. It can also be caused by sympathomimetics, thyrotoxicosis, and pregnancy-induced hemorrhage.

Respiration. Significant information can be gained from evaluating the respiratory rate, pattern, and rhythm in patients with AMS.

Hypoventilation is an indicator of alcohol intoxication, drug overdose (opioids, barbiturates), and myxedema. The sedative overdose may be an inadvertent adverse effect secondary to a planned sedation. CVA or increased ICP may also be associated with hypoventilation. *Hyperventilation* in AMS patients may be indicative of a metabolic acidosis, as in hyperglycemia with a resultant diabetes ketoacidosis or aspirin overdose that results in hyperventilation from a metabolic acidosis.

Cheyne-Stokes respiration is indicative of an intracranial lesion, metabolic disorder, or congestive heart disease. Central neurogenic breathing (deep and rapid), pneustic breathing (prolonged inspiration followed by expiratory pause), and ataxic breathing (irregular) are indicative of some form of intracranial lesions at different levels of the CNS.

General Survey

Once vital signs are obtained and recorded, an immediate quick survey should be performed to evaluate for evidence of trauma or head injury, acute or chronic illness, and needle tracks or other signs of drug ingestion.

Breath odor. Certain odors suggest certain disorders, as follows:

- Odor of alcohol: ethanol intoxication
- Fruity odor: diabetic ketoacidosis
- Musty odor: hepatic coma
- Uriniferous odor: uremia
- Garlic odor: arsenic poisoning

Skin. Certain skin manifestations are indicative of specific disorders, as follows:

- Skin tracks: drug overdose
- Cyanosis: hypoxia
- Cherry-red skin: carbon monoxide (CO) poisoning
- Jaundice: hepatic encephalopathy
- Pallor: anemia or hemorrhage
- Petechiae: disseminated intravascular coagulation or drug ingestion
- Bullous ulcers: drug overdose, especially barbiturates

In addition, examination of the skin should evaluate skin turgor, whether the skin is dry or moist, and for bruises as evidence of trauma.

Level of Consciousness and Mental Status Examination

Level of consciousness is best assessed using the Glasgow Coma scale for responsiveness (Box 13-3). In assessing the level of consciousness, reduced awareness but with appropriate re-

---

Box 13-3 Glasgow Coma Scale Scores

EYE OPENING
4: Spontaneous
3: To verbal command
2: To pain
1: No response

MOTOR RESPONSE
6: To verbal command
5: Localizes pain (e.g., moves hand to push examiner's hand away)
4: Withdraws
3: Flexor response
2: Extensor response
1: No response

VERBAL RESPONSE
5: Oriented
4: Confused conversation
3: Inappropriate
2: Incomprehensible sounds
1: No response

---

sponse to verbal or physical stimulation indicates *lethargy*, whereas limited responsiveness to noxious stimulation is found in *stupor*. On the other hand, complete absence of responsiveness to stimulation is diagnostic of *coma*. If the patient is not responsive to verbal commands, response to pain can be tested by rubbing the knuckles on the sternum or by vigorous pressure on the supraorbital notch with a fingertip.

In assessing mental status, the examination should be performed to determine whether a psychiatric cause of the AMS is likely. Physical examination may also include evaluation for gross motor and sensory functions of extremities and for Babinski's sign.

Focal Neurologic Examination

The head should be examined for any subtle or obvious signs of head or craniofacial injury. This is followed by examination of the eyes and cranial nerves, then gross motor and sensory examination of the extremities. Evidence of head trauma includes scalp lacerations, edema, Battle's signs, "raccoon eyes," hemotympanum, retinal hemorrhage, papilledema, and cerebrospinal fluid otorrhea or rhinorrhea. The neck should be examined for stiffness, which may signify meningitis, CNS infection, cerebellar tonsillar herniation, or subarachoid hemorrhage.

The examination of the eyes is especially important because findings may reflect the status of the brain. Examination includes evaluation of pupils, eye movements, and fundi. Reactive pupils are usually indicative of an intact midbrain. Reactive pupils with absent oculocephalic and corneal reflexes generally indicate metabolic encephalopathy or drug overdose. Pinpoint pupils may indicate opiate overdose, use of certain drugs (e.g., pilocarpine), or a pontine dysfunction. Bilateral dilated and fixed pupils may indicate a toxic etiology (sympathomimetic, anticholinergic, hallucinogenic), impending complete brain herniation, severe brain lesion, or death. A unilateral fixed or dilated pupil and oculomotor nerve paralysis are seen in patients with uncal herniation or aneurysm.

Eye movements can only be tested in the cooperative awake patient. In the comatose patient, eye movements can be tested using the oculocephalogyric ("doll's eye") maneuver if the cervical spine is not injured. In the comatose patient without neural pathway dysfunction affecting eye movements, the eyes are often directed straight ahead or display slow, roving movements. Sustained involuntary conjugate deviation of the eye usually suggests a hemispheric lesion in the brain. Testing for corneal response is also indicative of the status of cranial nerves V and VII. Absence of the doll's eye movement and corneal reflexes indicates positive dysfunction.

Funduscopic examination can reveal signs of increased ICP through the presence of specific types of retinopathy.

Additional aspects of a focal neurologic examination should include examination of cranial nerves V, VI, VII, IX, and X by testing for certain sensory and motor functions and for different associated movements, such as yawning, swallowing, lip licking, multifocal myoclonic jerking, multifacial myoclonic seizures, jacksonian seizures, tremors, and asterixis. These movements can be signs of metabolic or anoxic encephalopathy, such as uremia, coma, and metabolic disease.

Laboratory Tests and Imaging Studies

Unless the cause of the AMS is determined from the history and physical examination, a battery of tests may be necessary to establish or confirm the diagnosis (Box 13-4). Also, if a history of trauma is detected, chest/skull films and head/abdominal CT scans should be obtained.

TREATMENT
Immediate Therapies and Tests

In some patients the preliminary clinical signs and initial tests provide a basis for administration of immediate therapies as a part of the management of AMS. Accordingly, any patient with an acute mental status abnormality should have oxygenation checked with a pulse oximeter and serum glucose checked with a finger-stick glucose test. If these tests are unavailable, oxygen and 50 ml of 50% dextrose solution should be administered empirically. Children's dextrose dose is 1 ml/kg of a 50% solution. If oxygen saturation and serum glucose tests are available, oxygen should be given to any patient with oxygen saturation of 92% or lower, and dextrose is given if measured glucose level is less than 60 mg/dl. Although there is no contraindication to administering oxygen for all patients with AMS, in patients who show classic signs of acute stroke, it is prudent to avoid dextrose infusion unless hypoglycemia is documented.

In patients suspected of drug overdose, administration of naloxone should be considered; criteria include one or more of the following: pinpoint pupils, respirations of 12 or less, and suspicion of drug overdose. If a benzodiazepine is believed to be the ingested drug, flumazenil should be given. The administration of a reversal agent must be balanced with the adverse side effects associated with its administration.

Finally, in patients with a history of heavy alcohol use and in those who appear malnourished, 100 mg of IV thiamine should be immediately given. In patients with Wernicke's encephalopathy, IV thiamine may reverse the acute symptoms. In patients who are to receive dextrose, thiamine should be given first to prevent precipitation of Wernicke's encephalopathy by administration of glucose.

Box 13-4	Laboratory Testing for Disorders in Patients With AMS	
TEST	**DISORDER**
BC, platelet count	Dehydration
Electrolytes	Renal function
BUN, creatine kinase	Diabetes
Serum glucose	Hyperparathy-
Calcium	roidism
PT/INR/PTT	Coagulopathy
Toxicology	Drug ingestion
ABG	Acid-base status
Lumbar puncture	Neurologic
Anemia, infection	infection

Initial interventions can be given in the early phases of management of patients with AMS. These interventions can be remembered with the mnemonic DON'T, as in "Don't forget these": *dex*trose, *o*xygen, *n*aloxone, and *t*hiamine.

Definitive Treatment and Disposition

Once immediate therapeutic measures are administered or considered and the life-threatening status is stabilized, the patient can be referred or transferred for definitive management of the cause of AMS in a more controlled setting, such as the hospital or physician's office. During the transfer period, frequent observation and examination of the patient and continuous administration of supportive therapy are important until the cause of the AMS is determined and definitive therapy administered. If the cause is immediately determined and the appropriate therapy administered with resolution of the emergency, a decision must be made as to whether the patient should be discharged home, transferred to the ED, or referred to the primary physician for additional work-up or therapy.

For example, if the cause of AMS is thought to be benign, such as mild alcohol overdose, the patient should not be treated and may be discharged with an appropriate escort. If the AMS is thought to be associated with illicit drugs, a similar course of action may be taken. Before discharging the patient, the clinician must ensure that the AMS is a drug side effect rather than an underlying cause associated with use of the drug (e.g., respiratory depression, circulatory abnormality). If the abused drug is not known and the full extent of the effect may not have

been defined, the patient may warrant transportation to a tertiary care facility.

The final decision as to the disposition of the patient with AMS must take into account severity of symptoms, length of episode, patient's age, previous episodes, medical history, and degree of residual findings.

SUGGESTED READINGS

1. American College of Emergency Physicians: Clinical policy for the initial approach to patients presenting with altered mental status, *Ann Emerg Med* 33:251-281, 1999.
2. Brown MM, Hachinski VC: Acute confusional states, amnesia, and dementia. In Wilson JD, editor: *Harrison's principles of internal medicine*, New York, 1991, McGraw-Hill.
3. Duman S, Ginsburg S: Coma. In Friedman HH, editor: *Problem-oriented medical diagnosis*, ed 2, Boston, 1975, Little, Brown.
4. Handlwer JA, Hunt DM: Altered mental status and syncope. In Rund DA, Barkin RM: *Essentials of emergency medicine*, ed 2, St Louis, 1997, Mosby.
5. Harner RN: Alterations in consciousness. In *Internal medicine for dentistry*, ed 2, St Louis, 1990, Mosby.
6. Henry GL: Altered mental status and coma. In Harwood AL, editor: *The clinical practice of emergency medicine*, ed 2, Philadelphia, 1996, Lippincott-Raven.
7. Henry GL: Coma and altered states of consciousness. In Tintinalli J, editor: *Emergency medicine: a comprehensive study guide*, ed 3, New York, 1992, McGraw-Hill.
8. Husk GT: The confused patient. In Kravis TK, Warner CG, editors: *Emergency medicine: a comprehensive review*, ed 2, Rockville, Md, 1987, Aspen.
9. Mickel HS: Approach to altered mental status and coma. In Howell AL, editor: *Emergency medicine*, vol 1, Philadelphia, 1988, WB Saunders.
10. Pruitt AA: Approach to the patient with altered consciousness. In Wilkins EW Jr, editor: *Emergency medicine: scientific foundations and current practice*, ed 3, Baltimore, 1989, Williams & Wilkins.
11. Schraeder PL: Central nervous system intoxications. In *Internal medicine for dentistry*, ed 2, St Louis, 1990, Mosby.

Cerebrovascular Accident (Stroke)

Anthony R. Petito
Albert E. Carlotti, Jr.

A stroke or cerebrovascular accident (CVA) describes a group of brain disorders involving loss of brain function. This loss of function occurs when blood supply to the brain has been interrupted. The end result of this event can range from a minor neurologic deficit to serious debilitation and death.

ANATOMY

The paired vertebral arteries and internal carotids give rise to the cerebral circulation (Figure 14-1). The vertebral arteries give rise to the posterior circulation and the carotid arteries the anterior circulation.

The vertebral arteries enter the skull and give off the posterior cerebellar arteries. The vertebral arteries continue cephalad and connect in the midline to form the basilar artery. The basilar artery gives off the paired anterior inferior and superior cerebellar arteries. The basilar artery then divides at its apex to become the left and right posterior cerebral arteries. The posterior intracranial circulation provides blood supply to the brainstem, thalmus, and posteromedial aspects of the cerebral hemispheres.

Each internal carotid enters the skull and gives off the posterior communicating artery, then divides into the anterior and middle cerebral arteries. The anterior cerebral arteries supply the medial surface of the hemispheres, and the middle cerebral arteries supply the lateral surfaces as well as the basal ganglia.

The circle of Willis is an intracranial anastomotic pathway that can compensate for localized reductions in blood flow. Distal to the circle, intracranial arterial beds anastomose over the surface of the brain through tiny arterioles. These arterioles are not large enough to compensate for major arterial occlusions.[1]

PATHOPHYSIOLOGY

The brain requires 20% of the total body circulation. Even a brief interruption of blood flow and oxygenation to the brain can result in neurologic deficit. If blood flow is decreased for longer than a few seconds, brain cell death and brain infarction begin, resulting in permanent brain damage.

A *focal* ischemic stroke is caused by occlusion of a major artery in the neck or head. A *global* ischemic stroke is caused by a total failure of blood supply, as in cases of cardiac arrest.

EPIDEMIOLOGY

In developing countries, CVA is the third most common cause of death. It is the second most common cause of neurologic deficit, after Alzheimer's disease. Over the last three decades the incidence of stroke has been decreasing. In the last few years, however, this decrease appears to have leveled off. Stroke remains the most common reason for institutionalization and long-term care.[2]

A stroke strikes 4 of every 1000 people. The incidence rises significantly with age; for each decade over age 35, the risk of stroke doubles. Approximately 5% of persons over age 65 have had at least one stroke. The incidence of disease has traditionally been more common in men, although the risk in women is increasing secondary to increased risk factors. An estimated 500,000 Americans have a stroke each year, with 25% of these cases resulting in death.[3]

CLASSIFICATION

CVAs are classified into two major categories. *Ischemic strokes* are secondary to occlusion of a blood vessel. *Hemorrhagic strokes* are caused by cerebral artery rupture. Both forms can be life

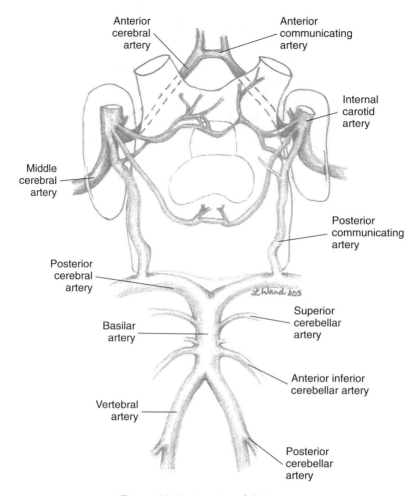

Figure 14-1. Arteries of the brain.

threatening, although ischemic strokes are rarely fatal within the first hour. Modern therapy aimed at reversing the vessel occlusion can be extremely effective if instituted early. If vessel occlusion is not reversed, permanent cell death and anoxic brain injury can ensue. A hemorrhagic stroke can be fatal at onset, and treatment has little effect on its natural course. Prevention is the most important goal in reducing the morbidity and mortality associated with a hemorrhagic stroke.[3]

Ischemic Syndromes

Ischemic syndromes include *transient ischemic attacks* (TIAs) and ischemic strokes. In the nonpathologic state, adequate cerebral blood supply is ensured by an efficient collateral system. This system includes the carotid and vertebral arteries via their anastomoses at the circle of Willis, as well as collaterals at the level of the cerebral hemispheres. If a vessel becomes occluded and collaterals are impaired, cerebral ischemia will result. The occlusion may be transient, as in TIAs.

A TIA is a reversible episode of focal dysfunction of the brain or eye caused by a temporary occlusion of an artery. The signs and symptoms of a TIA resemble those of a nonreversible ischemic stroke, although the patient recovers within minutes to hours. A TIA is the most important predictor of eventual brain infarction. As many as 5% of patients who have had a TIA will experience an irreversible event within 1 month. The risk at 1 year is 12%, and the risk increases by 5% each year thereafter.[4] Cerebral infarct can be prevented by prompt evaluation and treatment in patients with TIA.

Hemorrhagic Syndromes

Hemorrhagic strokes are usually more serious and more rapidly life threatening than ischemic syndromes. Subarachnoid hemorrhage is most often caused by head trauma. Spontaneous hemorrhage can result from rupture of a congenital intracranial aneurysm. The most common symptom is intense headache. An intracerebral hemorrhage often presents with focal neurologic deficits, similar to an ischemic stroke.

ETIOLOGY AND RISK FACTORS

Age is the most important risk factor for CVA. In patients over age 55, the risk of stroke increases for both men and women. Men overall are at a greater risk for stroke. The group most at risk is African-American males, who have more than twice the chance of a stroke compared with Caucasian males. The risk of stroke is higher for people with a family history of disease. It is difficult to assess this risk because many other risk factors also run in families. A history of a prior stroke increases the risk of a recurrent stroke up to 10% a year. The risk is highest within 30 days of the first stroke.[5]

Atherosclerosis

Atherosclerosis accounts for two thirds of all ischemic strokes. Atherosclerosis causes stroke by two possible mechanisms. The plaque buildup can cause it situ occlusion or stenosis of a vessel. The plaque can also embolize and cause occlusion at a distal site. The degree of symptoms will depend on collateral circulation and the rapidity of the process. If occlusion develops slowly so that collaterals have time to develop, little or no symptoms may be seen initially.

The risk factors for atherosclerosis are similar to those for stroke and can be divided into modifiable and nonmodifiable forms. The nonreversible factors include increasing age, male gender, and family history. Other factors, such as personality type, have also been proposed. The reversible risk factors for atherosclerosis include high cholesterol, hypertension, diabetes mellitus, obesity, hyperhomocysteinemia, and cigarette smoking.[1,2,6]

Hypertension

In addition to a risk for atherosclerosis, hypertension is an independent risk factor for both ischemic and hemorrhagic stroke. The risk of hemorrhagic stroke increases significantly with increases in systolic blood pressure. Blood pressure control has been shown to decrease the risk of CVA.[7]

Cigarette Smoking

Cigarette smoking causes several pathologic changes that significantly increase the risk of CVA. Smoking accelerates the development of atherosclerosis, and transient changes in blood pressure may cause endothelial damage. Enzyme release associated with smoking may increase the risk of aneurysms. Platelet alterations and decreased life span may increase coagulability. All these factors have been linked to an increased risk of stroke.[1,8] Smoking cessation has been shown to reduce the risk of stroke in women.[9]

Emboli

Emboli that originate from the heart and cause CVA may account for up to one third of ischemic strokes. Thromboemboli from the heart are likely to develop in the presence of arrhythmias, valvular lesions, and cardiac wall abnormalities.

Mural thrombi most often form under areas of dyskinetic myocardium. A dyskinetic myocardium usually results from myocardial infarction (MI) or cardiomyopathy. A third of patients with an anterior wall MI will harbor mural thrombi. If not anticoagulated, 40% will embolize within 4 months. *Cardiomyopathy* is characterized by cardiac enlargement, embolization, and arrhythmias. In one study, 15% of patients with cardiomyopathy harbored emboli. If atrial fibrillation is also present, the risk of embolization and stroke is even higher.

Valvular heart disease can predispose to systemic emboli. Valve disease is usually associated with lesions of the left side of the heart because the microcirculation in the lungs prevents right ventricular emboli from entering the circulation. Although less common today, rheumatic heart disease with resultant mitral stenosis was the most common valvular lesion giving rise to systemic emboli. Other possible valvular lesions that can increase the risk of stroke include bacterial endocarditis, Libman-Sacks endocarditis (seen in systemic lupus erythematosus), mitral valve prolapse, and prosthetic valve infection.[1,7]

Atrial fibrillation is a significant risk factor for stroke, especially in patients over age 60. This risk is highest immediately after the initial onset of atrial fibrillation. Therapeutic cardioversion also increases the risk. Approximately one third of patients with atrial fibrillation will develop an ischemic stroke.[1,2,6]

Vasculitides

Vasculitic disorders cause focal or multifocal cerebral ischemia through autoimmune-mediated inflammation and necrosis of extracranial and intracranial vessels. The inflammation causes platelet aggregation acutely and fibrinoid necrosis chronically. Both processes result in narrowing of vessel lumen. The many forms of vasculitis include temporal arteritis, Wegener's granulomatosis, infectious vasculitis, and the vasculitides associated with collagen vascular diseases (e.g., rheumatoid arthritis, scleroderma, Sjögren's syndrome).[1,6]

Hematologic Abnormalities

Hemoglobinopathy is a common cause of ischemic stroke. Sickle cell disease is by far the most common form of hemoglobinopathy; the hemoglobin S molecule deforms and polymerizes under deoxygenated conditions. This alteration increases blood viscosity and results in microvascular infarction.[10]

Hyperviscosity syndrome results from many disease states and can lead to "sludging" and ischemic stroke. Cellular hyperviscosity may be caused by polycythemia, thrombocytosis, and leukocytosis. Plasma hyperviscosity usually results from elevated plasma proteins, often seen in multiple myeloma and macroglobulinemia.[11]

Acquired hypercoagulable states include cancer, especially adenocarcinoma, and pregnancy. Congenital abnormalities can also result in a hypercoagulable state. Proteins C and S are naturally occurring anticoagulants made in the liver that inactivate factors V and VIII. Deficiency of these proteins is rare but can result in hypercoagulability and risk of ischemic stroke. Antiphospholipid antibodies associated with systemic lupus erythematosus (lupus anticoagulant) and other disease states may also cause cerebral ischemia.[1,2]

Drug-Related Causes

Many illicit drugs have been associated with stroke. The first problem is the use of nonsterile injectables, which increases the risk of endocarditis and systemic emboli. Drugs such as cocaine are potent vasoconstrictors that can lead to cerebral vasospasm. When crushing and injecting oral preparations, particles in the pills can result in microemboli.

Prescribed medications and over-the-counter preparations can increase the risk for stroke. Cold preparations often contain sympathomimetics such as phenylpropanolamine and ephedrine. High-dose estrogen contraceptives can significantly increase the risk of stroke, especially in woman over age 35 who smoke, are hypertensive, and have a history of migraine and long-term use of oral contraceptives.[1,2]

RECOGNITION AND ASSESSMENT

Significant morbidity and mortality can often be prevented if the early signs and symptoms of CVA are recognized. This can be accomplished at three basic levels: (1) recognition, evaluation, and treatment of modifiable risk factors for stroke; (2) recognition of the warning signs of stroke, with their reversal before a major event occurs; and (3) immediate recognition and treatment of a patient who has had a major stroke. In this way the devastating effects of brain infarction can be minimized or even avoided.

Transient Ischemic Attacks

A TIA begins suddenly and lasts 2 to 30 minutes or rarely up to 2 hours. The symptoms then resolve completely without sequelae. The patient is conscious throughout this event but may have slurred speech (dysarthria). The symptoms are identical to CVA but are transient. When the carotid artery is involved, ipsilateral blindness or contralateral hemiparesis, usually with paresthesias, is classic. The presence of aphasia indicates that the dominant hemisphere is involved. If the vertebrobasilar system is involved, symptoms will reflect brainstem dysfunction. Confusion, vertigo, binocular blindness, diplopia, and weakness of the extremities may be present. With bilateral weakness of the lower extremities, the patient's legs may buckle. The appearance of a drop attack (a conscious patient suddenly falling due to leg weakness) reflects vertebrobasilar involvement.[2,3]

Carotid Bruit

A carotid bruit indicates atherosclerosis of the carotid artery and a high risk for CVA. In patients with significant stenosis (greater than 70% blockage) a carotid endarterectomy can reduce the risk of stroke. Routine evaluation and examination for carotid bruit are critical in high-risk patients.[1,2]

Arterial Occlusion

An ischemic stroke occurs when an area of the brain is deprived of blood supply. An *evolving stroke* is when neurologic symptoms continue to worsen and spread over 24 to 48 hours. This progression is usually stepwise with intervening periods of stability. The worsening of symptoms correlates with an enlarging brain infarct. A *completed stroke* is seen when the neurologic deficits signify a stable injury. This is much more common than an evolving stroke. Symptoms develop quickly and usually hit a maximum within a few minutes. Consciousness is usually maintained unless a large infarct causes cerebral edema.[1,2]

Internal Carotid Artery

Occlusion of the internal carotid artery (ICA) leads to infarction in the central lateral portion of the cerebral hemisphere. Symptoms are often identical to middle cerebral artery (MCA) occlusion, except for ipsilateral ocular symptoms and occasionally a bitemporal headache. Focal motor or generalized seizures can occur during the acute stage in about 5% of large ICA-MCA infarcts.

Middle Cerebral Artery

The MCA or one of its deep penetrating branches is the most commonly occluded vessel, usually from systemic embolism. The onset of symptoms is rapid and typically silent. A contralateral paralysis is the most obvious initial finding. The degree of paresis depends on the occlusion's location along the MCA. Hemiplegia is most common with major strokes. If the dominant-side MCA is affected, aphasia is seen. Confusion, spatial disorientation, and sensory and emotional neglect will result if the nondominant MCA is affected.

Anterior Cerebral Artery

The anterior cerebral has two major portions. The proximal basal portion extends from the ICA to join the anterior communication artery. Proximal occlusion in the basal portion may not cause any symptoms as long as a patient anterior communicating artery carries blood flow for the contralateral ICA. If this collateral is not present and the ischemia is in the dominant hemisphere, Broca's aphasia can result. The interhemispheric portion supplies the ipsilateral medial frontal lobe posteriorly to the sensorimotor foot area. Occlusion of the interhemispheric portion produces a sensorimotor defect in the contralateral foot and distal leg. Occlusion of the anterior cerebral artery is an uncommon event, and TIAs in this area are even more uncommon.

Vertebrobasilar Disorders

The vertebrobasilar or posterior circulation is made up of the basilar artery and two intracranial vertebral arteries. Emboli are less common in the posterior circulation compared with the anterior circulation. Atherosclerotic occlusion, however, is seen more frequently in the posterior system than in the carotid systems. TIAs in the posterior circulation tend to be varied based on the variable anatomic distribution of the ischemia. This is in contrast to carotid TIAs, which tend to show the same signs and symptoms when recurrent.[2]

Occlusion of vertebrobasilar vessels and their main tributaries can cause a myriad of symptoms. The manifestations will depend on the level of the occlusion and whether the involvement includes the paramedian vessels and circumferential arteries.

Unilateral vertebral artery occlusion is asymptomatic in about 50% of patients. When they occur, symptoms resemble stroke of the vertebral artery and its posterior inferior cerebellar artery branch, resulting in a characteristic syndrome; there is pain and temperature loss to the ipsilateral face and contralateral body. Paralysis of cranial nerves IX, X, and XII affects the tongue and throat. Patients may also present with ipsilateral Horner's syndrome, ataxia, and vomiting.

Acute cerebellar infarct can occur when any of the cerebellar arteries becomes occluded. Blockage of the posterior, anteroinferior, or superior cerebellar artery can result in an acute cerebellar infarct. The infarct causes brain edema, which can distort the brainstem and block cerebrospinal fluid (CSF) outflow. Initial symptoms include ipsilateral headache and ataxia. Increased headache, vomiting, and ipsilateral cranial nerve defects soon follow. The patient may progress to drowsiness and stupor within 12 to 36 hours.

Symptoms caused by basilar artery involvement depend on the occlusion's location. Blockage in the *lower* portion will affect the vertebrobasilar junction. Manifestations include paraplegia of the legs or complete tetraplegia. Bizarre eye movements and pupillary miosis are also seen. The patient may have breathing irregularities and may progress to coma. Blockage at the basilar *apex* affects the junction of the posterior cerebral artery distribution. Symptoms depend on the extent of occlusion and the contralateral communication. Symptoms may include hemiplegia, paralysis of cranial nerve III, visual defects, and amnesia. Signs and symptoms can rapidly progress to stupor or coma. *Complete* basilar occlusion affects both paramedian and circumferential vessels and results in incomplete ischemic transection of the brainstem. Patients are usually comatose, with pinpoint pupils and conjugate gaze paralysis. Most patients succumb within a few days.

Manifestations caused by blockage in the posterior cerebral artery distribution depend on where along the artery the occlusion occurs. Interruption of blood flow in the distal branches will result in quadratic or hemianopic visual field loss. Proximal occlusion will result in thalamic ischemia, causing memory loss and sensorimotor hemiplegia.[1,2]

Hemorrhagic Stroke

Many manifestations of ischemic stroke overlap signs and symptoms of hemorrhagic stroke. Some findings, however, may point to the diagnosis of hemorrhagic stroke. Patients with hemorrhagic stroke usually are sicker and deteriorate more rapidly. Spontaneous cerebral hemorrhage generally occurs in two major areas. Bleeding can occur into the brain itself, causing an intracerebral or parenchymal injury. Bleeding can also occur over the surface of the brain, giving rise to a subarachnoid hemorrhage.[1-3,6]

Subarachnoid Hemorrhage

The most common symptom seen with subarachnoid hemorrhage is a severe headache. This headache is often described as "the worst headache ever felt" and prompts the patient to seek medical attention. The headache occurs suddenly, usually during maximal exertion, and reaches maximum severity quickly. The pain is generalized about the head and usually radiates to the neck and back; this may be the only symptom initially. Other symptoms may include vomiting, altered mental status, and intolerance to noise and light. A brief loss of consciousness is an ominous sign.[1,2]

Intracerebral Hemorrhage

Patients with intracerebral hemorrhage often present with the sudden onset of focal neurologic deficits much like those seen with an ischemic stroke. Unlike ischemic stroke, however, these patients are more likely to have a decreased level of consciousness, headache, and vomiting.

THE STROKE "CHAIN OF SURVIVAL"

The "chain of survival" is used to describe the sequence of events necessary to prevent sudden cardiac death in a patient with CVA. The stroke chain of survival and recovery strives to prevent or at least reduce brain death when a stroke occurs.[3] The recognition phase requires rapid assessment of stroke signs and symptoms, rapid activation of the emergency medical services (EMS) system, and rapid transport. The treatment phase includes prehospital interventions as well as rapid diagnosis and definitive care in a hospital setting. Time is crucial in recognizing and treating stroke. For example, thrombolytic therapy can reverse a clot and prevent brain infarct but must be initiated within 3 hours of the onset of symptoms to be effective. All health care professionals must be able to assess the signs and symptoms of stroke rapidly so "brain-saving" treatment can be quickly delivered (Box 14-1).

Initial Intervention

When a stroke occurs, prevention of permanent brain injury depends on rapid detection and assessment. The signs and symptoms of stroke can be subtle, especially early on. For this reason the American Heart Association (AHA) and other

---

Box 14-1	Seven-Step Stroke "Chain of Survival"*

1. Detection of the onset of stroke signs and symptoms
2. Dispatch of EMS system and rapid response
3. Delivery of patient to receiving hospital, providing prehospital care and prearrival notification
4. Door (emergency department triage)
5. Data (emergency department evaluation)
6. Decision about potential therapies
7. Drug therapy

Modified from Hazinski MF: *Curr Emerg Cardiac Care* 7:8, Winter 1996.
*Based on cardiac care chain and national program on heart attack awareness.

groups have increased the public's awareness of stroke. In this way, untrained people can recognize stroke and initiate emergency interventions early.

Once a stroke has been identified, the goal is to admit the patient to the hospital, where innovative therapies can be instituted (Figures 14-2 and 14-3). The speed of transport and the therapies instituted before transport are crucial to a stroke patient. Because CVA can occur anywhere and at any time, dental practitioners must be able to recognize and treat stroke in the prehospital setting.

When a patient is suspected of having a stroke in the office setting, a prompt diagnosis and treatment regimen should be available. As with all emergencies, the initial intervention is to establish responsiveness, then airway, breath-

ing, and circulation (ABCs) in a rapid and efficient manner. As the physician performs the primary assessment, staff members place anesthetic monitors, bring emergency equipment to the room, and activate the EMS system.

Paralysis of the muscles of the throat and tongue can cause airway obstruction. Saliva will not be swallowed and can be aspirated. Vomiting is another risk for aspiration, and the patient requires aggressive suctioning. In an awake patient, turning the patient to the lateral decubitus position may be helpful. Maintenance of an airway may require head repositioning or use of an oropharyngeal or nasopharyngeal airway. Oxygen should be administered. If basic airway management is ineffective, positive-pressure ventilation or tracheal intubation may become necessary (Figure 14-4).

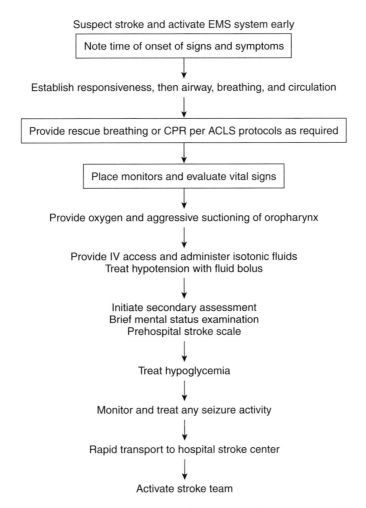

Figure 14-2. Recognition and management of patients with suspected stroke in the dental office. *CPR,* Cardiopulmonary resuscitation; *ACLS,* advanced cardiac life support.

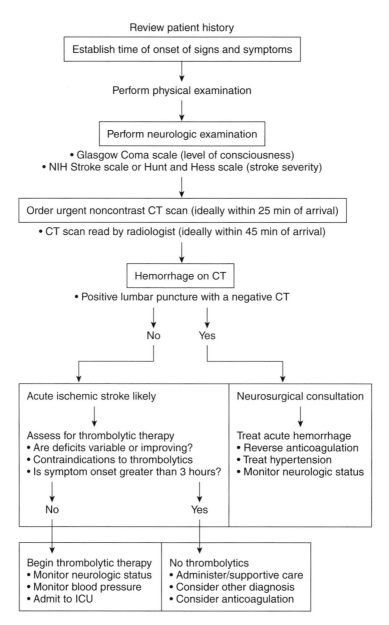

Figure 14-3. Management of stroke patients in the hospital. *CT,* Computed tomography; *ICU,* intensive care unit.

Breathing abnormalities are uncommon, except in severe stroke with brain edema. In these patients and others who are nonresponsive or comatose, rescue breathing may become necessary. Irregular breathing may include prolonged pauses, Cheyne-Stokes breathing, neurogenic hyperventilation, or ineffectual breathing secondary to paralyzed muscles. The onset of coma and breathing irregularity is always an ominous sign.

Circulatory monitoring should include assessment of pulse, blood pressure, and cardiac rhythm. Cardiac arrest is rare with stroke; it most often results from hypoxia and respiratory arrest. Hypertension is a common circulatory problem with stroke. It should not be treated in the prehospital setting; hypertension typically subsides and requires no treatment. Cardiac arrhythmia may point to an underlying cause for stroke, such as atrial fibrillation. Bradycardia may indi-

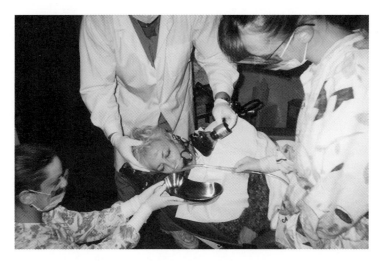

Figure 14-4. Patient with suspected stroke in lateral decubitus position. Airway support, supplemental oxygen, and aggressive suctioning are required to control secretions and maintain a patent airway.

cate hypoxia or elevated intracranial pressure (ICP).

Secondary Intervention

The secondary assessment should include a brief mental status examination and use of a prehospital stroke scale. The Cincinnati stroke scale is a useful tool in identifying patients with CVA. The major physical findings evaluated include facial droop, arm drift, and speech abnormalities.[13]

While the secondary assessment is being conducted, other interventions should be started. Intravenous (IV) access should be obtained and isotonic fluids given. Bolus therapy is only started if hypotension is documented. Glucose-containing fluids should be used only if hypoglycemia is found. Another concern is the development of seizures, which may require treatment.

Neurologic Stroke

When a patient with suspected CVA arrives in the emergency department (ED), primary and secondary assessments and therapies are revisited. As part of the secondary survey, an emergency stroke assessment focuses on the patient's level of consciousness (LOC) and the type, location, and severity of the stroke.

Decreased LOC implies a severe brain injury with increased ICP, more often associated with hemorrhagic stroke than an ischemic disorder. A comatose state is caused by bilateral hemi-spheric damage or brainstem dysfunction. Coma at the onset of a stroke usually indicates massive bleeding or basilar artery occlusion. Patients with depressed LOC are evaluated using the Glasgow Coma scale and other signs of brainstem function. Testing size, equality, and reactivity of pupils assesses function at the level of the oculomotor nerves. Unilateral pupillary dilation may be the first sign of uncal herniation. A fixed dilated pupil in a patient complaining of a headache suggests a ruptured aneurysm. The corneal reflexes reveal function at the levels of the trigeminal and facial nerves. The gag reflex demonstrates function at the level of the glossopharyngeal and vagus nerves. An absent "doll's eye" reflex suggests severe brainstem dysfunction.[3]

The type of CVA may be apparent based on signs and symptoms. The only definitive test to determine a hemorrhagic versus ischemic stroke is a non-contrast-enhanced computed tomography (CT) scan of the head. The location of the stroke can be assessed by neurologic signs in an alert patient. Unilateral paralysis, numbness, aphasia, and monocular blindness indicate an anterior circulation infarct. Vertigo, diplopia, dysarthria, ataxia, and sensory motor disturbance suggest a posterior circulation infarct. Contralateral or bilateral neurologic signs, especially effecting cranial nerves, suggest a brainstem infarct.

The severity of a stroke is best measured by the National Institutes of Health Stroke Scale (NIHSS), which correlates stroke severity with outcome for ischemic stroke patients (Box 14-2).

Box 14-2	National Institutes of Health Stroke Scale (NIHSS)

Administer stroke scale items in the order listed. Scores should reflect what the patient does, not what the clinician thinks the patient can do. Except where indicated, the patient should not be coached (i.e., repeated requests to patient to make a special effort).

INSTRUCTION

1a. Level of Consciousness (LOC)
The investigator must choose a response, even if a full evaluation is prevented by such obstacles as an endotracheal tube, language barrier, orotracheal trauma/bandages. A **3** is scored only if the patient makes no movement (other than reflexive posturing) in response to noxious stimulation.

1b. LOC Questions
The patient is asked the month and his or her age. The answer must be correct—there is no partial credit for being close. Aphasic and stuporous patients who do not comprehend the questions will score **2**. Patients unable to speak because of endotracheal intubation, orotracheal trauma, severe dysarthria from any cause, language barrier, or any other problem not secondary to aphasia are given a **1**. It is important that only the initial answer be graded and that the examiner not "help" the patient with verbal or nonverbal cues.

1c. LOC Commands
The patient is asked to open and close the eyes and then to grip and release the nonparetic hand. Substitute another one-step command if the hands cannot be used. Credit is given if an unequivocal attempt is made but not completed due to weakness. If the patient does not respond to command, the task should be demonstrated to them (pantomime) and score the result (i.e., follows none, one, or two commands). Patients with trauma, amputation, or other physical impediments should be given suitable one-step commands. Only the first attempt is scored.

2. Best Gaze
Only horizontal eye movements will be tested. Voluntary or reflexive (oculocephalic) eye movements will be scored but caloric testing is not done. If the patient has a conjugate deviation of the eyes that can be overcome by voluntary or reflexive activity, the score will be **1**. If a patient has an isolated peripheral nerve paresis (CN III, IV, or VI), score a **1**. Gaze is testable in all aphasic patients. Patients with ocular trauma, bandages, preexisting blindness, or other disorders of visual acuity or fields should be tested with reflexive movements and a choice made by the investigator. Establishing eye contact and then moving about the patient from side to side will occasionally clarify the presence of a gaze palsy.

SCALE DEFINITION

0 = Alert; keenly responsive
1 = Not alert, but arousable by minor stimulation to obey, answer, or respond
2 = Not alert, requires repeated stimulation or painful stimulation to make movements (not stereotyped)
3 = Responds only with reflex motor or autonomic effects, or totally unresponsive, flaccid, areflexic

0 = Answers both questions correctly
1 = Answers one question correctly
2 = Answers neither question correctly

0 = Performs both tasks correctly
1 = Performs one task correctly
2 = Performs neither task correctly

0 = Normal
1 = Partial gaze palsy. This score is given when gaze is abnormal in one or both eyes, but where forced deviation or total gaze paresis is not present.
2 = Forced deviation or total gaze paresis not overcome by the oculocephalic maneuver.

From American Heart Association: *ACLS*, Dallas, 1997-1999, The Association.

| **Box 14-2** | National Institutes of Health Stroke Scale (NIHSS)—cont'd |

3. Visual

Visual fields (upper and lower quadrants) are tested by confrontation, using finger counting or visual threat as appropriate. Patient must be encouraged, but if he or she looks at the side of the moving fingers appropriately, this can be scored as normal. If there is unilateral blindness or enucleation, visual fields in the remaining eye are scored. Score **1** only if a clear-cut asymmetry, including quadrantanopia, is found. If patient is blind from any cause, score **3**. Double simultaneous stimulation is performed at this point. If there is extinction, patient receives a **1** and the results are used to answer question 11.

0 = No visual loss
1 = Partial hemianopia
2 = Complete hemianopia
3 = Bilateral hemianopia (blind including cortical blindness)

4. Facial Palsy

Ask or use pantomime to encourage the patient to show teeth or smile and close eyes. Score symmetry of grimace in response to noxious stimuli in the poorly responsive or noncomprehending patient. If facial trauma/bandages, orotracheal tube, tape, or other physical barrier obscures the face, these should be removed to the extent possible.

0 = Normal symmetrical movement
1 = Minor paralysis (flattened nasolabial fold, asymmetry on smiling)
2 = Partial paralysis (total or near total paralysis of lower face)
3 = Complete paralysis (absence of facial movement in the upper and lower face)

5 and 6. Motor Arm and Leg

The limb is placed in the appropriate position: extend the arms 90° (if sitting) or 45° (if supine) and the leg 30° (always tested supine). Drift is scored if the arm falls before 10 seconds or the leg before 5 seconds. The aphasic patient is encouraged using urgency in the voice and pantomime but not noxious stimulation. Each limb is tested in turn, beginning with the nonparetic arm. Only in the case of amputation or joint fusion at the shoulder or hip may the score be **9**, and the examiner must clearly write the explanation for scoring as a **9**.

0 = No drift; limb holds 90° (or 45°) for full 10 seconds.
1 = Drift; limb holds 90° (or 45°) but drifts down before full 10 seconds; does not hit bed or other support.
2 = Some effort against gravity; limb cannot get to or maintain (if cued) 90° (or 45°), drifts down to bed but has some effort against gravity.
3 = No effort against gravity; limb falls.
4 = No movement
9 = Amputation, joint fusion; explain:
5a = Left arm
5b = Right arm
0 = No drift, leg hold 30° position for full 5 seconds.
1 = Drift; leg falls by the end of the 5-second period but does not hit bed.
2 = Some effort against gravity; leg falls to bed by 5 seconds but has some effort against gravity.
3 = No effort against gravity; leg falls to bed immediately.
4 = No movement
9 = Amputation, joint fusion; explain.
6a = Left leg
6b = Right leg

Continued

Box 14-2	National Institutes of Health Stroke Scale (NIHSS)—cont'd

7. Limb Ataxia

This item is aimed at finding evidence of a unilateral cerebellar lesion. Test with eyes open. In case of visual defect, ensure testing is done in intact visual field. The finger-nose-finger and heel-shin tests are performed on both sides, and ataxia is scored only in present out of proportion to weakness. Ataxia is absent in the patient who cannot understand or is hemiplegic. Only in this case of amputation or joint fusion may the item be scored **9,** and the examiner must clearly write the explanation for not scoring. In case of blindness, test by touching nose from extended arm position.

0 = Absent
1 = Present in one limb
2 = Present in two limbs
If present, is ataxia in
Right arm: 1 = Yes 2 = No
9 = Amputation or joint fusion;
explain:
Left arm: 1 = Yes 2 = No
9 = Amputation or joint fusion;
explain:
Right leg: 1 = Yes 2 = No
9 = Amputation or joint fusion;
explain:
Left leg: 1 = Yes 2 = No
9 = Amputation or joint fusion;
explain

8. Sensory

Sensation or grimace to pin prick when tested or withdrawal from noxious stimulus in the obtunded or aphasic patient. Only sensory loss attributed to stroke is scored as abnormal, and the examiner should test as many body areas (arms [not hands], legs, trunk, face) as needed to accurately check for hemisensory loss. A score of **2,** "severe or total,"' should only be given when a severe or total loss of sensation can be clearly demonstrated. Stuporous and aphasic patients will therefore probably score **1** or **0.** The patient with brain stem stroke who has bilateral loss of sensation is scored **2.** If the patient does not respond and is quadriplegic, score **2.** Patients in coma (question 1a = 3) are arbitrarily given a **2** on this item.

0 = Normal; no sensory loss
1 = Mild to moderate sensory loss; patient feels pin prick is less sharp or is dull on the affected side, or there is a loss of superficial pain with pin prick but patient is aware of being touched.
2 = Severe to total sensory loss; patient is not aware of being touched.

9. Best Language

A great deal of information about comprehension will be obtained during the preceding sections of the examination. The patient is asked to describe what is happening in the attached picture, to name the items on the attached naming sheet, and to read from the attached list of sentences. Comprehension is judged from responses here as well as to all of the commands in the preceding general neurologic exam. If visual loss interferes with the tests, ask the patient to identify objects placed in the hand, repeat, and produce speech. The intubated patient should be asked to write a sentence. The patient in coma (question la = 3) will arbitrarily score **3** on this item. The examiner must choose a score in the patient with stupor or limited cooperation, but a score of **3** should be used only if the patient is mute and follows no one-step commands.

0 = No aphasia, normal
1 = Mild to moderate aphasia; some obvious loss of fluency or facility of comprehension, without significant limitation on ideas expressed or form of expression. Reduction of speech and/or comprehension, however, makes conversation about provided material difficult or impossible. For example, in conversation about provided materials examiner can identify picture or naming card from patient's response.
2 = Severe aphasia; all communication is through fragmentary expression; great need for inference, questioning, and guessing by the listener. Range of information that can be exchanged is limited; listener carries burden of communication. Examiner cannot identify materials provided from patient response.
3 = Mute, global aphasia; no usable speech or auditory comprehension

From American Heart Association: *ACLS,* Dallas, 1997-1999, The Association.

Box 14-2	National Institutes of Health Stroke Scale (NIHSS)—cont'd

10. Dysarthria
If the patient is thought to be normal, an adequate sample of speech must be obtained by asking the patient to read or repeat words from the attached list if the patient has severe aphasia, the clarity of articulation of spontaneous speech can be rated. Only if the patient is intubated or has other physical barriers to producing speech may the item be scored **9,** and the examiner must clearly write an explanation for not scoring. Do not tell the patient why he or she is being tested.

0 = Normal
1 = Mild to moderate; patient slurs at least some words and, at worst, can be understood with some difficulty.
2 = Severe; patient's speech is so slurred as to be unintelligible in the absence of or out of proportion to any dysphasia, or is mute/anarthric
9 = Intubated or other physical barrier; explain:

11. Extinction and Inattention (formerly Neglect)
Sufficient information to identify neglect may be obtained during the prior testing. If the patient has severe visual loss preventing visual double simultaneous stimulation, and the cutaneous stimuli are normal, the score is normal. If the patient has aphasia but does appear to attend to both sides, the score is normal. The presence of visual spatial neglect or anosagnosia may also be taken as evidence of neglect. Since neglect is scored only if present, the item is never untestable.
Additional item, not part of the NIH Stroke Scale score.

0 = No abnormality
1 = Visual, tactile, auditory, spatial, or personal inattention or extinction to bilateral simultaneous stimulation in one of the sensory modalities
2 = Profound hemi-inattention or hemi-inattention to more than one modality; does not recognize own hand or orients to only one side of space

12. Distal Motor Function
The patient's hand is held up at the forearm by the examiner, and patient is asked to extend his or her fingers as much as possible. If the patient can't or doesn't extend the fingers, the examiner places the fingers in full extension and observes for any flexion movement for 5 seconds. The patient's first attempts only are scored. Repetition of the instructions or of the testing is prohibited.

0 = Normal (no flexion after 5 seconds)
1 = At least some extension after 5 seconds but not fully extended; any movement of fingers that is not commanded is not scored.
2 = No voluntary extension after 5 seconds; movement of the fingers at another time is not scored.
a. Left arm
b. Right arm

The NIHSS has also been used to guide decisions about the need for thrombolytic therapy. It is easily used by physicians and nurses and allows for standardized evaluation of patients over time. The scale is broken down into five major categories: (1) LOC, (2) visual assessment, (3) motor function, (4) sensation and neglect, and (5) cerebellar function. However, the NIHSS is not comprehensive. Further neurologic evaluation may be required in some patients.[14]

Hemorrhagic stroke is graded by the Hunt and Hess scale, which correlates survival with severity of subarachnoid hemorrhage. The five grades are (1) asymptomatic, (2) severe headache with nuchal rigidity but no neurologic deficit, (3) drowsy with minimal neurologic deficit, (4) stu-

porous with hemiparesis, and (5) deep coma with decerebrate posturing.[15]

DIAGNOSTIC STUDIES

Further diagnostic studies are required to (1) establish stroke as the cause of the patient's symptoms, (2) determine the type of stroke, and (3) determine the most likely etiology. CT, the most important diagnostic test, is performed without contrast so that the contrast and blood cannot be confused. Drug therapy must be held until the CT scan is evaluated and hemorrhagic stroke ruled out. Hemorrhagic stroke appears hyperdense on CT, whereas an ischemic stroke is hypodense. Brain infarction secondary to an ischemic stroke may not be noted on initial CT. Definite evidence of brain infarction is rarely seen within 3 hours of a stroke.[16]

Hemorrhagic strokes are usually noted on the initial CT scan. Approximately 5% of patients with subarachnoid hemorrhage have a normal scan, however, and lumbar puncture is indicated when no neurologic deficits are present but subarachnoid bleeding is strongly suspected. Lumbar puncture is contraindicated in patients with a positive CT scan, those with neurologic signs, and patients who may benefit from thrombolytic therapy.

Other diagnostic tests are conducted to establish the cause of a stroke and prepare for medical or surgical intervention. At a minimum, complete history and physical examination, electrocardiogram, chest radiograph, and blood work are done. Blood tests must include coagulation studies if thrombolytic therapy is anticipated. Serum electrolyte and glucose levels and toxicology screen are used to rule out other causes of symptoms and detect complications.

DIFFERENTIAL DIAGNOSIS

A stroke patient can present with a variety of signs and symptoms. Manifestations may be subtle and overlooked, or focal brain dysfunction may point directly to the diagnosis of stroke. The patient may have a decreased LOC or may be comatose. In these patients the diagnosis may be difficult, with a more extensive differential diagnosis.

The differential diagnosis of sudden-onset, focal neurologic deficit is limited. Hemorrhagic or ischemic stroke tops the list. Other vascular conditions may result in strokelike symptoms. Severe migraine can cause persistent neurologic symptoms. Severe and sustained hypertension may result in an encephalopathic picture that mimics a stroke.

Hypoglycemia or hyperglycemia, especially in diabetic patients, can cause focal signs with or without a change in LOC. Seizure activity, especially when the patient is postictal, can mimic a stroke if neurologic signs and symptoms persist.

Drug overdose can cause signs and symptoms that may appear as a stroke. A toxicology screen is a mandatory test when any neurologic signs are present. Trauma, infection, and neoplasia can also cause signs and symptoms that may be confused with a CVA. A diagnosis of head trauma is based on mechanism of injury and CT scan. Meningitis or encephalitis can be ruled in by blood studies and CSF examination. A tumor that causes neurologic symptoms can be diagnosed by CT or magnetic resonance imaging (MRI).

MANAGEMENT

The goals of management are to prevent or minimize brain death and to prevent complications. ABCs must be monitored and evaluated. The patient should be constantly assessed for oxygenation, ventilation, pulse, blood pressure, and cardiac rhythm. IV access is necessary for fluid and medication requirements. Hypotonic fluids will cause an intracellular shift of fluid and the potential for brain cell edema. Normal saline or lactated Ringer's solution should be used. Bolus therapy is only required if the patient is hypotensive. Fluid management should be monitored using at least careful recording and Foley catheterization. Severe hypoglycemia or hyperglycemia should be treated. In addition to dextrose, thiamine should be provided to hypoglycemic patients.

Grand mal seizures are a common complication of stroke. Severe seizures can be potentially life threatening. *Status epilepticus* is defined as seizures occurring for longer than 30 minutes or seizures occurring too frequently for the patient to regain consciousness. Permanent central nervous system injury can occur within 60 minutes of seizure activity, which is independent of brain injury secondary to a stroke. Initial treatment includes ABCs and protecting the patient from injury. Diazepam (Valium) is the first-line drug, given intravenously at 2 mg/min to a total of 10 mg. This dose can be repeated two more times at 20-minute intervals. Diazepam is followed by a longer-acting anticonvulsant given concurrently. A loading dose of phenytoin can be followed by a maintenance drip. Phenobarbital and diazepam can also be used in maintenance drip form. If seizures are still not controlled, a pentobarbital coma with mechanical ventilation in an intensive care setting may be required.[17]

Stroke, especially the hemorrhagic type, can cause an increase in ICP. As ICP rises, cerebral blood flow becomes impaired. If this process is allowed to progress untreated, irreversible brain damage or death can occur. Treatment includes intubation and mechanical hyperventilation. As carbon dioxide is blown off, the cerebral vasculature constricts. The diuretics mannitol and furosemide are used to decrease intravascular volume rapidly. Care should be taken not to dehydrate the patient to a serum osmolarity greater than 310 osmol/L. Severe hypertension must be controlled. Agitation should be managed with narcotics, barbiturates, or propofol. In young patients with a good initial examination, a pentobarbital coma may be of benefit. If a dangerous rise in ICP is noted, CSF drainage and neurosurgical decompression may be lifesaving.

Blood Pressure

Blood pressure management in patients with CVA is controversial. An elevated pressure may be required to maintain collateral flow to ischemic areas after stroke. Treatment of the agitation, vomiting, and increased ICP associated with stroke may adequately treat transient blood pressure elevation.

Specific indications exist for drug treatment of hypertension in the patient with ischemic stroke. If thrombolytic therapy is planned, aggressive control of blood pressure is required to minimize the risk of bleeding. Thombolytic therapy is contraindicated in patients who do not respond to transdermal nitroglycerin or IV labetalol. Other indications for strict blood pressure control include cardiac disease when afterload reduction is required. Acute MI and severe left ventricular failure can worsen in the patient with severe hypertension. Other conditions, such as aortic dissection and hypertensive encephalopathy, may also require acute blood pressure control.

The goals of blood pressure control in patients with a hemorrhagic stroke are to prevent rebleeding and minimize the extent of bleeding. Sodium nitroprusside is used for severe hypertension because of its immediate onset and short duration of action. A drawback to nitroprusside is vasodilation, which can increase ICP. For mild to moderate hypertension, labetalol is the drug of choice.[3]

Thrombolytic Therapy

Acute therapy for the management of ischemic stroke underwent a significant change in 1995. The National Institute of Neurological Disorders and Stroke (NINDS) trial showed benefits for ischemic stroke patients treated with *tissue plasminogen (t-plasminogen) activator* (TPA). Patients treated within 3 hours of the onset of an ischemic stroke were 30% more likely to have little or no disability than those treated with placebo. The treated patients, however, did have a significant incidence of hemorrhage, but without an increase in overall mortality. Therefore the U.S. Food and Drug Administration (FDA) approved IV TPA for acute ischemic stroke. Any patient who arrives in the ED within 3 hours of an ischemic stroke should be considered for TPA administration.[18]

Because of the strict time limit associated with CVA, hospitals have implemented systems for rapid diagnosis and treatment both in the field and the hospital. TPA is not recommended until an experienced physician has made the diagnosis clinically and an experienced radiologist has made the diagnosis using head CT. Also, the AHA recommends that TPA be given as a bolus, followed by a 60-minute infusion. TPA is not indicated after 3 hours or when the time of stroke cannot be determined. There is no information regarding the use of TPA in children.[19]

The exclusion criteria for TPA are absolute. Any patient with minor or rapidly improving symptoms does not require TPA. Most other concerns relate to the potential for bleeding. Patients with intracranial hemorrhage or suspected subarachnoid bleeding are excluded. Patients who are actively bleeding or who have a bleeding diathesis (platelets less than 100,000, recent anticoagulation, or inherited bleeding disorder) are not candidates for TPA. Patients with major surgery in the last 2 weeks or head trauma in the last 3 months are also excluded. Other exclusion criteria include recent lumbar puncture, recent acute MI, uncontrollable hypertension, or a witnessed seizure at the onset of stroke symptoms.

Thrombolytic therapy should only be considered in centers prepared for bleeding complications. After initiation of thrombolysis, every attempt must be made to prevent bleeding. Arterial lines, central venous pressure monitors, Foley catheters, and nasogastric tubes should be avoided in the first 24 hours, if possible. Any drug with the potential to cause bleeding should be avoided during this time. Neurologic worsening after thrombolytic therapy is most likely caused by intracranial bleeding.[18,19]

Subarachnoid Hemorrhage

Emergency arteriography is indicated to detect an aneurysm. Finding a saccular aneurysm necessitates emergency neurosurgery to clip the aneurysm.[20] Fluid management with close attention to plasma sodium and osmolarity is critical. The calcium channel blocker nimodipine has been shown to improve outcome in patients with subarachnoid hemorrhage.[21]

SUMMARY

Stroke is the third leading cause of death in the United States. Many patients who survive an initial stroke have severe neurologic dysfunction. The ultimate goal of therapy is to recognize and treat symptoms early so that permanent brain injury can be minimized or prevented. This system of recognition might begin in the hospital, in the dental office, or in the field. Rapid assessment, stabilization, and immediate transfer to an ED for thrombolytic therapy can be lifesaving.

REFERENCES

1. Andreoli TE, Carpenter CC, Bennett JC, Plum F, editors: *Cecil essentials of medicine*, ed 4, Philadelphia, 1997, WB Saunders.
2. Beers MH, Berkow R: *The Merck manual*, Whitehouse Station, NJ, 1999, Merck Research Laboratories.
3. Cummins RO: *Advanced cardiac life support*, Chicago, 1997, American Heart Association.
4. Viitanen M, Eriksson S, Asplund K: Risk of recurrent stroke, myocardial infarction and epilepsy during long-term follow-up after stroke, *Eur Neurol* 28:227-231, 1988.
5. Sacco RL, Hauser WA, Mohr JP, Foulkes MA: One-year outcome after cerebral infarction in whites, blacks, and Hispanics, *Stroke* 22:305-311, 1991.
6. Myers AR: *Medicine*, ed 2, National Medical Series for Independent Study, Baltimore, 1996, Harwal.
7. Whisnant JP: Effectiveness versus efficacy of treatment of hypertension for stroke prevention, *Neurology* 46:301-307, 1996.
8. Siess W, Lorenz R, Roth P, Weber PC: Plasma catecholamines, platelet aggregation and associated thromboxane formation after physical exercise, smoking or norepinephrine infusion, *Circulation* 66:44-48, 1982.
9. Kawachi I, Colditz GA, Stamfer MJ, et al: Smoking cessation and decreased risk of stroke in women, *JAMA* 265:232-236, 1993.
10. Ogle OE, Hernandez AR: Management of patients with hemophilia, anticoagulation, and sickle cell disease, *Oral Maxillofac Surg Clin North Am* 10:414-416, 1988.
11. Murphy GP, Lawrence W, Lenhard RE, editors: *American Cancer Society textbook of clinical oncology*, Atlanta, 1995, American Cancer Society.
12. Hazinski MF: Demystifying recognition and management of stroke, *Curr Emerg Cardiac Care* 7:8, Winter 1996.
13. Kolthari R, Hall K, Broderick J, Brott T: Early stroke recognition: developing an out of hospital stroke scale, *Acad Emerg Med* 4:986-990, 1997.
14. Brott T, Adams HP Jr., Olinger CP, et al: Measurements of acute cerebral infarction: a clinical examination scale, *Stroke* 20:864-870, 1989.
15. Hunt WE, Hess RM: Surgical risk as related to the time of intervention in the repair of intracranial aneurysms, *J Neurosurg* 28:14-20, 1968.
16. Davis KR, Ackerman RH, Kistler JP, Mohr JP: Computerized tomography of cerebral infarction: hemorrhagic, contrast enhancement, and time of appearance, *Comput Tomogr* 1:71-86, 1977.
17. Berry S: *The Mont Reid surgical handbook*, ed 4, St Louis, 1997, Mosby.
18. National Institute of Neurologic Disorders and Stroke, rt-PA Stroke Study Group: Tissue plasminogen activators for acute ischemic stroke, *N Engl J Med* 333:1581-1587, 1995.
19. Adams HP, Brott TG, Furlan AJ, et al: Guidelines for thrombolytic therapy for an acute stroke: a supplement to the guidelines for the management of patients with acute ischemic stroke, *Stroke* 27:1711-1718, 1996.
20. Kassell NF, Torner JC, Haley EC Jr., et al: The International Cooperative Study on the Timing of Aneurysm Surgery. I. Overall management results, *J Neurosurg* 73:18-36, 1990.
21. Petruk KC, West M, Mohr G, et al: Nimodipine treatment in poor-grade aneurysm patients: results of a multicenter, double blind placebo-controlled trial, *J Neurosurg* 68:505-517. 1988.

Seizures and Epilepsy

Roger S. Badwal

A *seizure* is a temporary stoppage of brain function caused by the excessive hypersynchronous discharge of cortical neurons and the recruitment of neighboring neurons into an abnormal firing mode. A seizure is a manifestation of brain dysfunction, which may be associated with an underlying pathologic condition. E*pilepsy* refers to a pathologic condition associated with recurrent unprovoked seizures, usually two or more.[1]

Seizures may also be a manifestation of brain derangement secondary to various toxins, drug overdose or withdrawal, cerebral hypoxia, or metabolic disturbances (Box 15-1).

EPIDEMIOLOGY AND ETIOLOGY

Up to 1 in 20 persons experience a seizure at some point in their lifetime.[2] The age distribution of seizure is bimodal, with increased frequency in children under 11 years of age and in adults over age 60. The incidence is higher in older adults, with risk of a seizure approaching 10% if the adult lives to be 80 years old.[3]

Not all individuals who have a seizure will develop epilepsy. The incidence of epilepsy in the general population is less than 1%. However, the occurrence of a second seizure is a reliable indication of epilepsy.[4]

Seizures can arise from a variety of conditions. The etiology may be associated with an underlying pathologic condition or metabolic disturbance or may be unidentifiable. The differential diagnosis for the patient presenting with a first-time seizure is the same for any age group, but the frequency of etiologies is altered.

Pediatric Patients

Sixty percent of childhood seizures are classified as primary, or *idiopathic*. Heritable factors play a significant role. Other common causes in the pediatric population include idiopathic epilepsy, congenital anomalies, chronic encephalopathies, infection, or hypoxic or metabolic disturbances.[5]

Adult Patients

In the adult patient, idiopathic seizures, or those with genetic etiology, generally arise during childhood. Most new-onset seizures in adults are reactive and are secondary to identified conditions (see Box 15-1). For adults under age 60, cessation or withdrawal of *anticonvulsants* or subtherapeutic anticonvulsant levels is the most common cause of seizures. In patients between ages 30 and 60, alcohol- and drug-related seizures predominate; *drug effects* are the second most common reason for seizures. Alcohol-related seizures may result from acute inebriation but are more frequently associated with cessation of alcohol consumption. Alcohol withdrawal seizures may occur 6 to 48 hours after cessation of alcohol consumption. The most common illicit drugs associated with ictal activity are cocaine, amphetamines, and phencyclidine.

Elderly Patients

Elderly patients over age 60 are at risk for seizures from several common conditions (Box 15-2). About 15% of patients who survive a cerebrovascular accident (stroke) will have unprovoked seizures within 5 years of the initial stroke. Those patients experiencing seizures within 1 month of the initial event are at an increased risk. I*nfarction* or *hemorrhagic stroke* accounts for approximately 50% of new-onset seizures in the elderly patient and is the leading cause of seizures in the elderly population. T*umors* are the second most common etiology for seizures in those older than 60. Neurodegenerative diseases also account for an increased risk factor for the development of seizures.

Focal or generalized seizures occur in 5% of patients with multiple sclerosis. Alzheimer's dementia is associated with a sixfold to tenfold

Box 15-1 Causes of Seizure in the Dental Patient

Vasovagal/vasodepressor syncope
Psychogenic (e.g., hyperventilation, breath holding)
Narcolepsy
Cerebrovascular accident
Neurodegenerative disease (e.g., Alzheimer's disease)
Brain neoplasm
Metabolic derangement (e.g., hypoglycemia)
Movement disorders (e.g., tic disorders)
Drug/alcohol withdrawal
Drug overdose (e.g., local anesthetic)
Extrapyramidal reactions
Trauma

Box 15-2 Increased Risk of Epilepsy in Elderly Patients with Predisposing Conditions

Cerebrovascular disease: 20×
Neurodegenerative: 5-10×
Trauma: 3×
Advanced age: 0.3×
Alcohol: 3×
Infection: 3×
Neoplasm: 30% present with seizure as initial symptom

increase in unprovoked seizures. The pathology is presumably related to the alterations of neurons and glia in the hippocampus and neocortical areas. Elderly patients often are taking many medications, including anxiolytics and sedatives (barbiturates, benzodiazepines), and abrupt cessation from various causes (e.g., forgetfulness, lack of money) can lead to withdrawal seizures.

Metabolic Disorders

Metabolic disturbances can initiate a seizure in all age groups. The most common is *hypoglycemia*. Plasma glucose levels below 45 mg/dl are usually associated with ictal activity, which should be suspected in the diabetic patient. Therapy is directed to increasing the plasma glucose levels (see Chapter 24). Loss of consciousness and ictal activity secondary to hypoglycemia are also common in the alcoholic patient. Thiamine should be administered to the alcoholic patient before the administration of dextrose to avoid the development of Wernicke's encephalopathy.

Several electrolyte abnormalities can also cause ictal activity. *Hyponatremia* is the most common electrolyte disorder in the hospitalized patient. Plasma sodium levels below 120 mEq/L (normal, 136 to 145 mEq/L) frequently incite ictal activity. The rate of change, in addition to the absolute value, is a contributing factor to the onset of ictal activity. Hyponatremia may result from intravenous administration of hypotonic solutions or excess consumption of water. Children are especially sensitive to the effects of hyponatremia in the perioperative period. The former should not be overlooked when managing a young child in the office for an ambulatory anesthetic. Alternatively, dehydration resulting in *hypernatremia* (sodium ≥160 mEq/L) may also cause ictal activity.

Drugs

Seizures may also occur secondary to the overdose of medications. Elevated plasma levels secondary to an overdose or the inadvertent intravascular administration of local anesthetic agent has been reported (see Chapter 29). Several antibiotics, including metronidazole and the newer quinolones, can lead to seizures. Penicillin and other β-lactam antibiotics are renally excreted and in high doses can provoke seizures, compounded by renal failure. Meperidine (Demerol), a synthetic opioid, has a metabolic byproduct (normeperidine) with a half-life of 15 to 30 hours and is known to induce seizures when it accumulates due to repetitive dosing. The kidneys eliminate meperidine, and patients with renal disease are at particular risk.

Elevated plasma levels of prescribed medications (e.g., cyclosporine, lithium, tricyclic antidepressants, carbamazepine, theophylline) and over-the-counter medications (e.g., aspirin) can provoke seizures. Increased levels may be secondary to an intentional overdose, impaired metabolism, or elimination due to underlying systemic disease or associated with a drug-drug interaction.

Trauma

Patients with head trauma have a twelvefold increase in the incidence of seizures compared with the general population.[2]

CLASSIFICATION
Seizures

The most common method used to classify seizures is based on the type of clinical manifestation. This system classifies a seizure as either generalized or partial (Box 15-3).

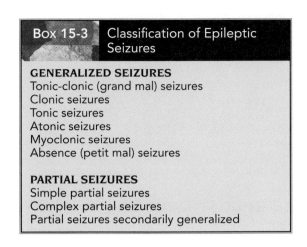

Box 15-3 Classification of Epileptic Seizures

GENERALIZED SEIZURES
Tonic-clonic (grand mal) seizures
Clonic seizures
Tonic seizures
Atonic seizures
Myoclonic seizures
Absence (petit mal) seizures

PARTIAL SEIZURES
Simple partial seizures
Complex partial seizures
Partial seizures secondarily generalized

Generalized Seizures

Generalized seizures are diffuse, and the ictal discharge involves both cerebral hemispheres simultaneously. This results in an altered consciousness. The seizures are frequently accompanied by abnormal motor activity but may be convulsive or nonconvulsive. Categories of generalized seizures are usually distinguished based on the extent of conscious activity and ictal motor activity (see Box 15-3).

Generalized tonic-clonic seizures result from paroxysmal neuronal discharge that is spread diffusely through the brain. The seizure may or may not be preceded by an *aura*. The prodromal warning associated with a generalized seizure is nonspecific and lacks the focal characteristics (e.g., olfactory hallucinations) associated with partial seizures that may become secondarily generalized. These warnings, if present, may manifest as mood changes or minor twitching, which abruptly progresses to loss of consciousness with muscular hypertonicity. The initial muscular hypertonicity results in a rapid expulsion of air from the lungs. This causes a loud vocalization, the "epileptic cry," followed by the actual tonic-clonic sequence, consisting of rhythmic extension and flexion of the trunk and limbs. These contractions may be quite vigorous and result in orthopedic injuries, such as shoulder dislocation or vertebral fractures. Tongue biting with resultant intraoral hemorrhage and increased salivations may occur and impair airway patency.

Systemic symptoms may include hypertension, tachycardia, diaphoresis, hypoxia, apnea, and less often, vomiting and pulmonary aspiration. Urinary and rarely fecal incontinence may occur with muscular relaxation on seizure cessation. Prolonged ictal activity can result in rhabdomyolysis and lactic acidosis, resulting in cardiac arrhythmias and death. The ictus is usually self-limiting, lasting no more than 5 minutes and in most cases less than 2 minutes. As they recover, patients are usually lethargic, confused, and disoriented for the first 15 to 30 minutes, although this may last hours. Confusion, headache, and muscle tenderness may last for hours to days. Patients are amnestic to the event.

Nonconvulsive seizures include both absence (petit mal) and myoclonic seizures. *Absence seizures* occur most often in children but can occur in adults. They are characterized by a brief period of dissociation or unconsciousness and usually last less than 10 seconds. The patient maintains gross body tone but may demonstrate muscle relaxation, dropping a held object or allowing the body to slouch. *Automatisms* (repetitive purposeless movements), such as eyelid fluttering, lip smacking, and facial twitching, may also be evident. Absence seizures may recur numerous times each minute or may occur as a prolonged episode. With cessation of the seizure, no postictal period occurs, and patients resume their normal activity as if nothing happened.

Myoclonic seizures also are most often seen in children. They are characterized by sudden brief muscle jerks, which may be repetitive. They may be unilateral or bilateral. Myoclonic seizures may be subtle, involving minor twitching in the face or extremities, or may be vigorous. Consciousness is not lost.

Partial Seizures

Partial seizures may be defined as either simple or complex. *Simple partial seizures* are limited and confined to a circumscribed area of the brain. The clinical manifestations of the seizure reflect the area in which the ictal event originated. Clinical features may be sensory (e.g., auditory or visual hallucinations), psychoillusory (e.g., déjà vu, unexplained fear or sensation of doom), autonomic (e.g., nausea, salivation), or motor (rhythmic jerking of discrete muscle groups). A rhythmic jerking of a discrete body part may spread progressively to involve the entire ipsilateral body (*jacksonian march*). Consciousness is not impaired in a simple partial seizure.

Complex partial seizures produce impairment of consciousness but not loss of consciousness. Complex seizures produce auras similar to those seen with simple complex seizures. The most common behavior is a motionless, absent stare. Automatisms are common and include such repetitive movements as lip smacking, swallowing, or picking at clothes. Individuals may also demonstrate strange behavior, such as pelvic thrusting and loud vocalizations. Individuals may retain some ability to react to their surroundings and perform tasks requiring higher cortical function. However, the individual's interactions are often clumsy and inappropriate. The seizure generally lasts less than 2 minutes. Postictally the patient is confused and disoriented, which may last from minutes to hours. Individuals may also demonstrate a focal weakness of the trigger area, which may last up to 48 hours. Clinically this may appear as a strokelike paralysis, called *Todd's paralysis*. Individuals are amnestic to the ictal event.

A partial seizure can spread to involve the entire brain, referred to as a *secondarily generalized seizure*. The clinical features are similar to those of a generalized tonic-clonic seizure. It may be difficult to distinguish between a primary generalized seizure and a secondarily generalized seizure. Features that may distinguish between the two classifications include auras and Todd's paralysis, both of which are more typical of secondarily generalized seizures.

Epilepsy

In 1989 an International Classification of Epilepsies and Epileptic Syndromes was proposed to categorize epilepsies according to seizure seismology, anatomic localization, electroencephalogram (EEG) and physical findings, and epidemiologic data. This approach allowed a better understanding of the prognosis and treatment of the condition. The syndromic approach classifies epilepsies into generalized, localization-related, and indeterminate focus subtypes (Box 15-4).

EPILEPTIC SYNDROMES
Febrile Seizures

Febrile seizures occur in 3% to 5% of children between 6 months to 6 years of age, representing the most common form of seizures in infancy and accounting for 30% of all childhood seizures.[3,6] They occur between 1 and 2 years of age, peaking from 18 to 24 months. Febrile seizures tend to recur in one third of patients, 50% of whom will have a third seizure. The risk

---

Box 15-4	Classification of Epilepsy

GENERALIZED EPILEPSY
Idiopathic. Patients with idiopathic epilepsies have normal neurologic status, with seizures beginning in childhood or adolescence and a hereditary component. They are more responsive to medical therapy and can remit spontaneously. Epileptic syndromes in this category include childhood absence epilepsy, juvenile absence epilepsy, juvenile myoclonic epilepsy, benign neonatal convulsions, and benign neonatal familial convulsions.
Symptomatic. The symptomatic classification implies the presence of a central nervous system lesion causing the seizures. These disorders include infantile spasms (West's syndrome), Lennox-Gastaut syndrome, and epilepsy with myoclonic-astatic seizures. In another category, seizures are a component of a previously defined nonepileptic syndrome (e.g., Tay-Sachs disease, phenylketonuria).
Cryptogenic. The cryptogenic classification suggests that the condition has a symptomatic cause, but the etiology remains unidentified.

LOCALIZATION-RELATED EPILEPSY
Idiopathic. The epileptic focus usually involves areas in both hemispheres. Examples include benign (rolandic) childhood epilepsy with centrotemporal spikes, childhood epilepsy with occipital paroxysms, and primary reading epilepsy.
Symptomatic. The epileptic focus is usually confined to a single hemisphere from lesions such as tumors, infarctions, and cerebral malformations. It is becoming clearer, with improved imaging techniques (MRI, PET), that focal cortical dysplasias (neuronal migration defects) are responsible for many of these lesions and have a genetic component. The localized nature of the lesions allows an anatomic classification. The types best characterized are the *temporal lobe seizures*.

EPILEPSY OF INDETERMINATE FOCUS
Epilepsies with indeterminate foci include neonatal seizures, severe myoclonic epilepsy in infancy, and acquired epileptic aphasia (Landau-Kleffner syndrome). The most common cause of neonatal seizures is hypoxic-ischemic encephalopathy. Other causes include intracranial hemorrhage, infection, hypoglycemia, hypocalcemia, drug withdrawal, and developmental defects.

Modified from Zupanc ML: *Mayo Clin Proc* 71(9):899, 1996.

of recurrence is related to the patient's age at the initial seizure, positive family history, and lower temperature at the initial seizure.[7] The child less than 1 year old at the time of the initial seizure event has a 50% chance of additional seizures, whereas the child older than 3 years has a 20% risk of recurrent seizures.

Most febrile seizures occur in association with common illnesses (e.g., tonsillitis, upper respiratory infections, otitis media). Coupled with the low seizure threshold and high fevers, preschool children are at increased risk for seizures. There is a possible link to human herpesvirus 6 (HHV-6), which is postulated to infect the brain during an acute illness and is reactivated during subsequent fevers. HHV-6 is the etiologic agent for roseola.

Most seizures last less than 6 minutes. Children usually present for medical evaluation after the febrile seizure has ceased. A careful history and physical examination involve looking for altered level of consciousness, signs of meningismus, bulging fontanelles, Kernig's or Brudzinski's sign, and muscle tone. A low threshold for performing lumbar puncture is indicated, particularly in those of toddler age or younger, unless elevated intracranial pressure is suspected. The EEG is not of use for the evaluation of febrile seizures.

Other causes of seizures include *Shigella* gastroenteritis, roseola, electrolyte abnormalities secondary to dehydration, and such drugs as tricyclic antidepressants, amphetamines, cocaine, diphenhydramine, phenylpropanolamine.

In up to 10% of children with a history of febrile seizures, seizures may occur when afebrile, particularly in those experiencing complex febrile seizures. A child has a 6% chance of developing permanent epilepsy, in which two or more signs of complex febrile seizures occur, versus less than 1% with no features. Anticonvulsant therapy is rarely instituted after a single febrile seizure. Prolonged febrile convulsions can be aborted very effectively with rectal diazepam (Diastat), which can be easily administered by parents.

Generalized Epilepsies

Generalized epilepsies consist of episodes of staring and behavior interruption followed by rapid return to normal awareness. Focal motor signs are minimal, usually consisting of a mild twitching of extremities or facial muscles. These signs do have a characteristic pattern during EEG investigations. Motor signs are typically treated with ethosuximide (Zarontin) or valproic acid/divalproex (Depakote).

Childhood absence epilepsy has its onset between 4 and 8 years of age. They are clinically categorized as absence seizures. Children have normal neurologic status. The prognosis is debatable, but seizures remit by midadolescence. These seizures may be induced by hyperventilation. Treatment with ethosuximide or valproate sodium (Depacon) is effective in suppressing 80% of these seizures.

Juvenile absence epilepsy has its onset between 10 and 17 years of age. Generalized tonic-clonic seizures occur in 60% to 80% of patients. Treatment with valproate sodium is usually successful in controlling the seizures.

Juvenile myoclonic epilepsy has its onset between 12 and 18 years of age. The epilepsy is characterized by seizures involving brief jerky motion of shoulders and arms occurring in the morning. The majority of individuals also have generalized tonic-clonic seizures.

Approximately one third of patients have absence seizures. Sleep deprivation or alcohol use can provoke seizures. Valproic acid is usually the drug of choice. Genetic linkage in some families has been related to the short arm of chromosome 6.

Lennox-Gastaut syndrome is a severe condition that has its onset in infancy. The syndrome is associated with severe mental retardation. The ictal activity is variable and manifested as atonic, atypical absence and tonic seizures. Polyanticonvulsant therapy is usually instituted with poor response to therapy.

Localization-Related Epilepsies

Benign rolandic epilepsy is the most common childhood epilepsy and has a strong hereditary component. Patients are neurologically normal. The seizure activity consists of focal activity coupled with sensorimotor symptoms, typically affecting the face and oropharynx, including hypersalivation and speech arrest. Occasionally the patient has generalized tonic-clonic activity. Seizures stop by midadolescence. Treatment is with carbamazepine.

Benign occipital epilepsy demonstrates a strong genetic and family relationship. The seizure focus occurs most frequently in the occipital lobe with visual symptoms and can generalize to tonic-clonic seizures. Severe pulsatile headaches mimicking childhood migraines are common postictally. The seizures are controlled with carbamazepine.

Temporal lobe epilepsy has presenting symptoms that depend on the patient's age, as reflecting the development of the brain and synapse formations. In very young children, features include simple automatisms (e.g., blinking) followed by dystonic posturing. In older children the most common symptom is an epigastic fullness sensation that begins as a simple partial seizure with associated olfactory or auditory sensations. This can progress to altered consciousness and automatisms (e.g., lip smacking, repetitive swallowing).

Epilepsies of Indeterminate Focus

There are two known but relatively rare epilepsies of indeterminate focus that are quite treatable. The first disorder involves a mutation in the molecule that binds *pyridoxine* (vitamin B_6). The apoprotein of glutamic acid decarboxylase needs pyridoxine to produce gamma-aminobutyric acid (GABA). With an insufficient production of the inhibitory neurotransmitter GABA, seizures occur. This diagnosis is usually made in the neonatal period, and lifelong pyridoxine supplementation of 100 mg or more is required daily.

The second epilepsy is characterized by medically refractory seizures. The *ketogenic diet* was developed in the 1920s to treat these children with difficult-to-control seizures. The diet effectively reduced the seizure occurrences by 90%, in approximately 30% of the population. The ketogenic diet is a high-fat, low-carbohydrate, low-protein diet with an imprecisely understood mechanism of action. This diet mimics the body's response by starving the brain of *glucose*, the preferred energy source. This forces the neurons to substitute *ketones* as an energy source. Currently, one known molecular defect in glucose transport in the central nervous system prevents adequate levels of glucose in the cerebrospinal fluid (CSF). The affected glucose co-transporter molecule disrupts the maintenance of CSF glucose levels across the blood-brain barrier. The ketogenic diet forces the brain not to rely on glucose. This presumably maintains neuronal homeostasis without disruption in energy supply.[8,9]

RECOGNITION AND MANAGEMENT

The first step in emergency intervention for seizure in the dental patient is recognition of the situation. Although seizure is often envisioned as a violent convulsive episode, numerous clinical presentations are possible, which may require the astute clinician to recognize subtle changes. In the elderly patient, for example,

seizures (or status epilepticus) may not present as the classic, physically convulsing patient with tonic-clonic manifestations. Instead, it often presents as a confusional state without overt generalized tonic-clonic activity. Failure to recognize these signs and symptoms for acute seizures or status epilepticus in the older population leads to misdiagnosis and delays in treatment. The delay in treatment contributes to a high mortality rate.[10]

Nonconvulsive epilepsy or status epilepticus should always be considered in the differential diagnosis in the patient who demonstrates altered level consciousness. Alternatively, other altered states of consciousness and abnormal movements may be confused for a seizure. Disorders in the differential diagnosis include vasodepressor syncope, vasovagal syncope (see Chapter 12), hyperventilation (see Chapter 6), breath-holding episodes, drug overdose (e.g., local anesthetic), hypoglycemia (see Chapter 24), transient ischemic attack, cardiovascular arrhythmias, psychogenic conditions, narcolepsy, movement disorders, and extrapyramidal reactions. Astute observation of the event and the sequences leading up to the event will assist in determining the diagnosis. The patient's response to therapy and recovery will support the diagnosis or suggest a different diagnosis.

Emergency Management of Seizures (In the Patient without a History of Seizures)

Management of any emergency in the dental office requires initial recognition of the abnormal condition, initial stabilization, diagnosis, diagnosis-directed therapy, and transfer (especially whether to transfer the patient to the emergency department [ED]). Of the medical emergencies just listed, the common "faint" (vasodepressor syncope or vasovagal syncope) and hyperventilation are the most common seizure-associated conditions that occur in the dental office. The patient who has "fainted" occasionally may manifest minor tremulous activity, as well as incontinence. The hyperventilating patient loses consciousness and manifests activity that could be construed as a seizure less often than the syncopal patient. Considering the increased likelihood of a vasodepressor or vasovagal syncopal episode in the dental office compared with a "seizure," the clinician must consider syncope ("fainting") as a primary differential diagnosis. Recognizing the appropriate diagnosis will avoid unnecessarily activating the local emergency medical services (EMS) system.

Airway Assessment/Intervention

Initial stabilization requires removing all objects from the patient's mouth, positioning the patient into the supine ("syncopal") position, removing all objects away from the patient, and passively restraining the patient to prevent self-inflicted trauma. Care must be taken to minimize injury to the dental team as well. For a first-time seizure the EMS system should be activated. It is essential that both the dentist and the staff remain perceptive and note all the features of the event. This may facilitate the physician's ability to make a rapid diagnosis.

Objects such as padded tongue blades should not be placed in the mouth because they will not minimize the risk of the patient biting the tongue. Placement of an object into the mouth of a seizing patient may traumatize the dentition and oropharyngeal tissues and puts the caregiver at risk for injury. Patients do not swallow their tongue. However, relaxation of the airway musculature with the displacement of the tongue against the posterior pharyngeal wall can result in airway obstruction. Airway repositioning using the chin-forehead tilt may be beneficial. The seizing patient may also have a brief period of apnea. Increased oxygen consumption secondary to the increased muscular activity in addition to respiratory impairment may result in hypoxia. Supplemental oxygen and rarely positive-pressure ventilation may be indicated.

The majority of seizures last less than 2 minutes. Early pharmacologic intervention is not indicated. If the seizure lasts more than 5 minutes or recurs, drug treatment is indicated (see Status Epilepticus).

The postictal state that follows a tonic-clonic seizure is characterized by lethargy, disorientation, confusion, and amnesia to the event. Supportive therapy should adhere to airway, breathing, circulation, and defibrillation protocols (ABCDs) of advanced cardiac life support. While assessing airway patency and breathing, the dentist confirms that all objects that were within the mouth are accounted for, if not already done. Airway opening may be required secondary to the patient's obtunded state. The administration of a benzodiazepine to control seizures may increase central nervous system and respiratory depression. The oral cavity is inspected for trauma to the tongue with resultant hemorrhage, displacement of dental prostheses, and tooth fracture. If all objects cannot be accounted for or a tooth is fractured and cannot be found, a chest radiograph may be indicated.

Patients actively seizing have copious secretions, but regurgitation is rare. Adequate tonsillar suction should be immediately available to remove these from the oral pharynx. McGill forceps can be used to remove a foreign object. Suctioning during the actual tonic-clonic seizure may cause injury to the oral cavity and pharynx. If the patient did not fall, the likelihood of cervical injury is low. During the postictal period when the patient is lethargic, they can then be placed into the lateral decubitus position to promote passive drainage of secretions.

If available, a pulse oximeter is used to assess for *hypoxemia*. Hypoxemia may be secondary to neurogenic pulmonary edema and will be assessed further in the ED. Initial management of hypoxemia in the breathing patient within the office is the administration of supplemental oxygen. If the patient is not breathing, positive-pressure ventilation using an Ambu bag should be initiated. Intubating the airway with an endotracheal tube or an esophageotracheal tube (Combitube) is rarely indicated and increases the risk of gastric regurgitation and pulmonary aspiration.

Cardiovascular Assessment/Intervention

After managing the airway, the dentist should proceed to the cardiovascular examination, taking the blood pressure and pulse. If no pharmacologic agents were administered, the patient should have an elevated pulse and pressure. Rhythm of the heart is assessed as well. Hypotension and arrhythmias suggest a diagnosis other than a "seizure."

Neurologic Assessment

With respiratory and cardiovascular systems managed, the patient's neurologic status is assessed. This is actually done from the initial point of involvement by continuously attempting to solicit responses from the patient. The clinician mentally notes the patient's progression from (1) unresponsive, (2) responds to pain, (3) responds to voice, and (4) awake. At this time, however, the clinician may consider assessing the symmetry and reactivity of the pupils.

Incontinence and tongue biting are suggestive of a seizure. Incontinence may also be seen with vasovagal syncope and breath holding in the child. The dentist and staff should complete their physical examination by assessing for other injuries (e.g., orthopedic injuries).

When the patient arrives in the ED of the hospital, the diagnostic work-up includes an EEG, brain imaging (preferably MRI), electrolytes and blood glucose, and toxicology screen. The emergency physician also looks for focal findings or deficits, which may indicate the etiology of the seizure. Careful questioning of the patient and family may reveal prior episodes that were not appreciated as seizures at the time (Box 15-5).

Disposition

If the patient is healthy without systemic illnesses as potential contributing factors and has recovered from the postictal state, hospitalization is not necessary and the patient can be discharged home from the emergency department. The patient can be discharged to the care of a reliable caregiver, who will observe the patient for recurrent episodes or deterioration and ensure medical transport to the hospital if necessary.

Management of a Patient with a History of Seizure Disorder

The basic tenets of seizure management apply to both the patient with a first-time seizure and the patient with a known seizure disorder, although some differences exist in the management approach. First, the dentist must distinguish the patient with a known seizure disorder who has the disorder controlled from the patient who is refractory to medical intervention.

Disorder Controlled

The patient whose disorder is effectively controlled and who has a seizure should be managed in the dental office as if having a first-time seizure. This entails activating the EMS system immediately on diagnosing the condition. In the ED the physicians will investigate why the patient developed a recurrent or breakthrough seizure. The most likely explanation is a low therapeutic blood level of anticonvulsant. This may be secondary to noncompliance, unintentional missed dosing, or a change in the pharmacologic preparation (brand name, which generic) of the prescribed agent. The physician will also complete a history and physical examination, looking for findings that may suggest an alteration in the patient's disorder, as well as assessing for other medical illnesses. A patient with a seizure disorder may sustain a seizure that is incited from a condition other than their seizure disorder.

| Box 15-5 | Health History Questions for the Dental Patient with Seizure Disorder* |

- What type of seizure disorder do you have?
- Are you prescribed any medication?
- Are you compliant with the medication, or do you occasionally miss a dose?
- Have you had serum levels of your anti-epileptic medication determined? If so, when was the blood work done, and what were the levels?
- When was the last time that you had a seizure?
- Are there any specific stimuli that may evoke a seizure?
- Were seizures related to missed doses of medication?
- Do you have an aura? If so, what does it consist of?
- Can you describe the clinical manifestation of the ictal (tonic-clonic, seizure) event?
- How long does the postictal (recovery, postseizure) period last?

*A family member or friend may be better able to answer some of these questions for the patient whose seizures are not well controlled by medication.

Disorder Not Controlled

The patient whose disorder is not effectively controlled has restrictions (e.g., inability to drive), and a friend or relative probably accompanied them to the office. If this patient suffers a seizure while in the dental office, the dentist may request the caregiver's assistance. This person most likely will be able to provide details as to the pattern and features of the patient's seizure (see Box 15-5). Transportation to the ED is generally not indicated.

Pharmacologic Intervention

The patient who has experienced only one seizure may not be medicated after this first and sole event. One reason for not treating the patient after the first seizure is that antiepileptic drugs may have adverse side effects (Table 15-1). Also see Chapter 29.

Regardless of whether patients are taking an antiepileptic drug, they must adhere to certain lifestyle restrictions. If patients are taking a prescribed antiepileptic and have remained seizure free, a decision must be made to continue or discontinue their medication. If patients remain seizure free and continue the medication, they will be able to resume most normal activities. If

Table 15-1	Antiepileptic Drugs for Seizure Patients and Common Side Effects	
Drug	**Indication**	**Side Effects**
Carbamazepine	SPS,CPS,GTC	Diplopia, dizziness, idiosyncratic aplastic anemia, rash, hyponatremia
Diazepam	Acute seizures	Hypotension, respiratory depression, sedation tolerance
Clonazepam	Myoclonic, atonic	Hypotension, respiratory depression, sedation
Ethosuximide	Absence	Sedation, GI distress
Felbamate	SPS,CPS,GTC, absence	Dizziness, headache, insomnia, weight loss
Gabapentin	SPS,CPS,GTC	Fatigue, transient GI distress, dizziness
Lamotrigine	SPS,CPS,GTC	Dizziness, rash, headache, weight gain
Phenobarbital	SPS,CPS,GTC	Cognitive effects, respiratory depression, sedation Connective tissue effects, sexual dysfunction
Phenytoin	SPS,CPS,GTC	Ataxia, gingival hyperplasia, hirsutism, nystagmus, osteoporosis, lymphadenopathy
Primidone	SPS,CPS,GTC	Sedation, depression, dizziness, connective tissue effects, behavioral effects
Tiagabine	SPS,CPS,GTC	GI distress, cognitive effects, dizziness
Topiramate	SPS,CPS,GTC	Cognitive effects, weight loss, ataxia, paresthesias
Vigabatrin	SPS,CPS,GTC	Cognitive effects, depression, rash, visual field constriction

From Sirven G: *J Am Geriatric Soc* 46:1291, 1998.
SPS, Simple partial seizures; *CPS,* complex partial seizures; *GTC,* generalizes tonic-clonic seizures; *GI,* gastrointestinal.

they decide to discontinue the medication, however, they must again tolerate a period of restricted activities.[11]

The First Seizure Trial Group assessed the risk of not administering an antiepileptic drug to the patient with a first tonic-clonic seizure.[12] Of patients prescribed an antiepileptic, approximately 25% had a recurrent seizure, whereas 51% of those not prescribed an antiepileptic had another seizure. This finding would suggest that antiepileptics should be prescribed. However, the investigation revealed that approximately 50% of the patients did not require antiepileptic drugs and therefore did not need to expose themselves to the potential adverse effects. The patient who decides not to take medication is at increased risk of a seizure, which in itself may not be harmful. If a patient suffers a seizure during dental therapy, medical emergency intervention is initiated as described in the previous section.

Disposition

The patient will need follow-up medical consultation. Most likely the patient has a physician or neurologist who is familiar with the prior event. If possible the dentist should contact this person and discuss the patient's disposition.

Although the dentist may want to transport the patient to the ED, such transfer may not be necessary.

STATUS EPILEPTICUS

Status epilepticus is defined as either prolonged seizure or recurrent seizures without full recovery. Traditionally it has been defined as ictal activity that exceeds 30 minutes, although shorter periods are now being suggested. This is a critical time period in which increased morbidity and mortality are reported. Complications result from hypoxemia, aspiration pneumonia, neurogenic pulmonary edema, autonomic dysfunction with hypotension and bradycardia resulting in organ hypoperfusion, hypoglycemia, metabolic acidosis, and rhabdomyolysis with acute renal failure. Mental function may also decline secondary to direct neuronal injury at the cellular level. Both convulsive and nonconvulsive status epilepticus can lead to brain damage.

Management Protocol

Most seizures last less than 2 minutes. Therefore it is recommended that if the seizure lasts longer than 2 minutes, the EMS system should be activated. Furthermore, once the patient goes into status epilepticus, the disorder may be more refractory to pharmacologic management.[5]

Up to 5 Minutes
Standard Seizure Management

- Position patient and passively restrain to minimize self-inflicted injury.
- Ensure that the dental team takes appropriate actions to minimize injury to themselves.
- Institute airway management, with supplemental oxygen if necessary.
- Monitor vital signs, including pulse, blood pressure, and oxygen saturation.
- Monitor cardiac rhythm with electrocardiogram, if available.
- Obtain a detailed history and evaluate neurologic status.

Dental Management

- Remove all objects from oral cavity.
- Activate the local EMS system if the seizure lasts longer than 2 minutes, unless the history suggests otherwise.
- When the seizure stops, examine the oral cavity for injury (e.g., fractured tooth) and displacement of objects.
- If all objects or teeth cannot be accounted for, consider chest and abdominal radiographs.

5 to 10 Minutes

- If not previously done, activate EMS system.
- Establish intravenous access, if skilled; avoid overhydration becaue status epilepticus can cause cerebral edema.

Pharmacologic Management: Benzodiazepines

Diazepam
- Adult: 5 to 10 mg/dose intravenously (IV)
- Pediatric: 0.2 to 0.5 mg/kg IV
  Rectal gel formulation
- Adult: 0.2 mg/kg (maximum 20 mg)
- Pediatric: 0.3 to 0.5 mg/kg (maximum 20 mg)

Midazolam
- Intravenous: 0.05 to 0.1 mg/kg
- Intramuscular: 0.2 mg/kg (maximum 10 mg)
  Benzodiazepines may complicate the patient's respiratory status. The dental staff must be prepared to intervene and administer appropriate respiratory support.

Suspected Hypoglycemia

- Administer thiamine (vitamin B_1), 100 mg IV, to adult patients.
- Administer dextrose, 50-ml bolus of 50% glucose solution (adult) or 2 ml/kg of 25% solution (pediatric).

Emergency Department Management

- Draw blood for complete blood count, electrolytes (sodium, potassium, chloride, bicarbonate, calcium, phosphorus, magnesium), glucose, blood urea nitrogen, creatinine, and other tests.
- Obtain urine or blood sample for toxicology screen.

10 to 30 Minutes

At this point a longer-acting anticonvulsant is required, and either phenobarbital or phenytoin must be administered IV. These drugs have important side effects, and the patient must be closely monitored.
- *Phenobarbital* (barbiturate), 20 mg/kg in neonates
- *Phenytoin*, 20 mg/kg at maximum rate of 50 mg/min
- *Fosphenytoin* is a phenytoin prodrug without many of the serious side effects of phenytoin and can be administered intramuscularly. It is given at phenytoin equivalents of 1.5 mg of fosphenytoin = 1 mg of phenytoin, or 30 mg/kg. Fosphenytoin can also be administered IV up to 150 mg/min.

30 to 45 Minutes

- Consider intubation.
- Evaluate blood work for metabolic causes.
- Consider additional doses of medications, with addition of phenobarbital, 20 mg/kg.

45 Minutes or Longer

- Institute mandatory intubation.
- Administer general anesthesia, either inhalation or intravenous drip with phenobarbital.

SUMMARY

The dentist can safely treat patients with seizure disorders. A complete history is the most important factor in determining the course and location of treatment. The patient with well-controlled seizures can be treated in the dental office. In the patient whose disorder is not well controlled, the dentist may elect to perform dental treatment with a sedative technique, depending on the planned intervention. The severity of the patient's disorder in conjunction with the necessary treatment also is a factor in deciding whether the airway should be intubated. The dentist must also be cognizant of the adverse effects associated with antiepileptics.

REFERENCES

1. Stafstreom CE: The pathophysiology of epileptic seizures: a primer for pediatricians, *Pediatr Rev* 19:342, 1998.
2. Hauser WA, Hesdorffer DC: *Epilepsy: frequency, causes and consequences*, New York, 1990, Demos.
3. Bradford JC, Kyriakedes CG: Evaluation of the patient with seizures: an evidence based approach, *Emerg Med Clin North Am* 17:203, 1999.
4. Bennett JC, Plum F, editors: *Cecil textbook of medicine*, Philadelphia, 1996, WB Saunders.
5. Sabo-Graham T, Seay AR: Management of status epilepticus in children, *Pediatr Rev* 19:306, 1998.
6. Hulihan JF: Seizures in special populations: children, the elderly and patients with coexistent medical illness, *Postgrad Med* 102(1):165, 1997.
7. Hirtz DG: Febrile seizures, *Pediatr Rev* 18:5, 1997.
8. Zupanc ML: Update on epilepsy in pediatric patients, *Mayo Clin Proc* 71(9):899, 1996.
9. Freeman JM: The efficacy of the ketogenic diet, 1998: a prospective evaluation of intervention in 150 children, *Pediatrics* 102(6):1358, 1998.
10. Sirven JI: Epilepsy in older adults: causes, consequences and treatments, *J Am Geriatr Soc* 46:1291, 1998.
11. Blum DE: Seizures. In Wachter RM, Goldman L, Hollander H, editors: Hospital medicine, Philadelphia, 2000, Lippincott-Williams & Wilkins.
12. Musicco M, Beghi E, Solari A, et al: Treatment of first tonic-clonic seizure does not improve the prognosis of epilepsy, First Seizure Trial Group (FIRST Group), *Neurology* 49:991, 1997.

Headache and Facial Pain

Steven Ganzberg

Dentists are increasingly being called on to evaluate and manage head and face pains of various etiologies, not just related to dentoalveolar sources. In addition to temporomandibular disorders, specially trained dentists are managing various primary headache and neuropathic pain problems. With this added responsibility comes the need to recognize not only head and face pains that indicate life-threatening conditions (e.g., subarachnoid hemorrhage), but also those that can produce significant morbidity (e.g., temporal arteritis). Both types of conditions frequently present as headache or face pain, which the patient may misinterpret as having masticatory origin. Headache is an extremely common complaint, with more than 300 conditions that may produce head or face pain.[1] Headache accounts for 1% to 16% of all emergency department (ED) visits.[2-5]

The first health care provider to see the patient may be a dentist. The dentist must determine if the headache is a sign of a serious medical problem. The dentist may also evaluate patients for pain of supposedly masticatory origin caused by a medical problem that requires prompt attention. Although not a true "emergency," it is important for the dentist to include these conditions in the differential diagnosis of pains being evaluated.

ETIOLOGY

The dentist first must determine if headache is caused by an organic disease or a benign process. Primary headaches include the so-called neurovascular headaches—migraine and cluster headache—as well as tension-type headache. Although painful and often debilitating for brief periods, these headaches are benign and not life threatening. During primary headaches, alterations in brain neurochemistry cause pain and associated symptoms. During headache-free periods, however, the patient is "normal" and usually displays no sign of headache disorder. An underlying neurotransmitter imbalance likely underlies these processes, but there is no overt disease process.

Organic headaches are associated with a specific pathologic process. Common organic causes of headache include cerebrovascular accident (CVA, stroke), infection, inflammation, tumor, and hypertension (Box 16-1). Diagnostic signs and symptoms can aid in the differential diagnosis of headache (Table 16-1).

PRIMARY HEADACHE

Although a patient may have symptoms indicative of migraine, cluster headache, or tension-type headache, this does not rule out an organic cause of headache. Criteria used for diagnosis of headache specifically include eliminating any organic cause for headache (Boxes 16-2 to 16-4). A history of multiple similar headaches helps establish the diagnosis of primary headache rather than organic headache.

Migraine

Migraine headache is a common problem worldwide. Approximately 17.6% of women and 5.7% of men in the United States ages 12 to 80 years experience more than one migraine headache per year.[6] The peak prevalence is between ages 20 and 40 years. Approximately 11 million people in the United States are moderately to severely disabled by migraine.[7] Migraine is frequently undiagnosed.[8]

Migraine headache occurs with or without aura (i.e., headache preceded by neurologic symptoms). Typically the aura gradually develops over 5 to 20 minutes and may last as long as 60 minutes. Common visual disturbances include convex figures with scintillating edges, scotomas, areas of lost vision, and flashing lights or colors. Less common sensory or motor symptoms include paresthesias, unilateral weakness, and speech difficulty. Typical headache features

Box 16-1 Organic Causes of Headache

CEREBROVASCULAR ACCIDENT (CVA, STROKE)
Embolic stroke
Thrombotic stroke
Hemorrhagic stroke

INFECTION
Meningitis
Encephalitis
Sinusitis
Brain abscess

INFLAMMATORY DISORDERS
Vasculitis
Temporal arteritis
Temporomandibular arthritis
Cervical arthritis

CARCINOMA
Primary tumor
Metastatic tumor

HYPERTENSION
Essential
Secondary

then ensue. Other migraineurs have a prodrome, which may occur up to 24 hours before headache and is not associated with frank neurologic changes, and they know headache will occur in the near future. This prodrome has a variety of presentations, from cervical muscle tightness to a feeling of increased energy and productivity.

Regardless of whether migraine occurs with or without aura, the headache phase has a characteristic presentation: unilateral or bilateral head pain, frequently throbbing and accompanied by nausea and vomiting, photophobia (sensitivity to light), and phonophobia (sensitivity to noise). The International Headache Society (IHS) provides criteria for the classification of headache and facial pain criteria (Box 16-2). Migraine headache can last 4 to 72 hours if untreated. The migraineur will often lie down in a dark room. Sleep, if possible, will frequently abort migraine.

Pathophysiology

The pathophysioloy of migraine is not completely understood but likely involves a central nervous system (CNS) neurotransmitter imbalance, especially in regard to serotonin and nor-

epinephrine. Certain initiating factors (e.g., ingestion of ethanol, exposure to bright lights, alteration of natural circadian rhythms, stress) cause release of chemical mediators, resulting in neurogenic inflammation of intracranial blood vessels. This sterile inflammatory process triggers and then is perpetuated by nociceptor activation, primarily of the trigeminal system. Depending on the blood vessel(s) involved, the pain is referred to some head or face location, most often the orbits or temples.

Treatment

Treatment of migraine and other primary headaches is divided into symptomatic, abortive, and preventive therapies. Adjunctive treatments, such as biofeedback, cognitive-behavioral therapies, and avoidance of headache triggers, may be appropriate, but pharmacologic interventions remain the mainstay of therapy.

Symptomatic therapy. Pain is treated with either nonsteroidal antiinflammatory drugs (NSAIDs) or opioids, and if present, nausea and vomiting are managed with antiemetics. Frequent use of opioids, some NSAIDs, barbiturates, caffeine, ergotamines, benzodiazepines, and other agents may perpetuate and worsen migraine and tension-type headache, so care must be taken to ensure proper patient use of these drugs. As a general rule, limiting use to less than 6 to 8 days per month is ideal. Cluster headache poses a unique challenge in that oral medications may only begin to take effect when headache is already declining.

Abortive therapy. Abortive therapy refers to specific medications that interrupt the processes thought to be responsible for headache pain generation. The agents typically chosen today are the "triptans:" sumatriptan (Imitrex), zolmitriptan (Zomig), naratriptan (Amerge), and rizatriptan (Maxalt). When taken early in headache onset, or even once headache is established, these drugs frequently eliminate headache, as well as associated symptoms (e.g., nausea, vomiting) and parasympathetic effects, in many migraineurs and cluster headache sufferers. These medications are generally less effective for tension-type headache. All these drugs are related structurally to serotonin and affect specific subsets of serotonin receptors (e.g., 1B, 1D). Because these receptors also reside on the cardiac vasculature, there is some risk of coronary vasoconstriction. Although it is unlikely that a headache sufferer taking a triptan that day would keep a dental appointment, the dentist should

Table 16-1	Differential Diagnosis of Headache						
	SAH	**Meningitis**	**TA**	**HTN**	**Migraine**	**Cluster**	**TTH**
Onset	Acute	Acute or chronic	Acute or chronic	Acute or chronic	Acute	Acute	Chronic
Location	Global	Global	Localized	Occipital frontal	Unilateral	Unilateral	Global
Associated symptoms	N, V, decreased LOC, meningismus, focal neurologic signs	N, V, fever, photophobia, meningismus, focal signs, seizures	Weight loss, PMR, fever, decreased vision, jaw claudication	N, V, focal neurologic signs	N, V, fever, photophobia, phonophobia	Rhinorrhea, lacrimation of ipsilateral side	Multisomatic complaints
Pain character	Worse ever	Severe throbbing	Severe throbbing over affected area	Throbbing	Throbbing	Sharp stabbing	Ache
Duration	Brief	Brief	Prolonged	Brief	Prolonged	30 min to 2 hours	Daily
Prior history	(−)	(−)	(−)	(+)	(+)	(+)	(+)
Diagnostic test	CT, 80%-90%	LP (+) CBC	ESR (+)	CT scan to rule out bleeding	—	—	—
Physical examination	Focal signs, decreased LOC, meningismus	Focal signs, decreased LOC, irritability, rash	Tender temporal arteries, myalgias, fever	Papilledema, decreased venous pulsations, decreased LOC, cardiovascular changes	N, V, photophobia, phonophobia	Rhinorrhea, lacrimation, partial Horner's	(−)

From Diamond ML: *Headache* Q 3(suppl 1): 28-33, 1992.
SAH, Subarachnoid hemorrhage; *TA,* temporal arteritis; *HTN,* hypertension; *TTH,* tension-type headache; *N,* nausea; *V,* vomiting; *LOC,* level of consciousness; *CT,* computed tomography; *LP,* lumbar puncture; *CBC,* complete blood count; *ESR,* erythrocyte sedimentation rate; *PMR,* polymyalgia rheumatica.

<table>
<tr><td>

Box 16-2   **IHS Criteria for Migraine Headache and Common Features**

WITHOUT AURA
A. Two of the following:
 • Unilateral headache pain location
 • Headache pain has pulsating quality
 • Nausea
 • Photophobia or phonophobia
B. Both of the following:
 • Similar pain in the past
 • No evidence of organic disease

WITH AURA
Headache pain is preceded by at least one of the following neurologic symptoms:
A. Visual
 • Scintillating scotoma
 • Fortification spectra
 • Photopsia
B. Sensory
 • Paresthesia
 • Numbness
 • Unilateral weakness
 • Speech disturbance

COMMON CHARACTERISTICS
 • Duration: usually 12-72 hours
 • Gender: >2:1 female/male ratio
 • Neurologic aura: ~40%
 • Bilateral:unilateral: 60:40

</td><td>

Box 16-3   **IHS Criteria for Cluster Headache and Common Features**

CRITERIA
A. Severe unilateral headache with orbital, supraorbital, or temporal pain lasting 15 to 180 minutes*
B. At least one of the following on the headache side:
 • Conjunctival injection
 • Facial sweating
 • Lacrimation
 • Miosis
 • Nasal congestion
 • Ptosis
 • Rhinorrhea
 • Eyelid edema
C. No evidence of organic disease

COMMON CHARACTERISTICS
 • Gender: predominantly male
 • Frequency: up to eight per day
 • Quality: throbbing, stabbing
 • Intensity: severe

</td></tr>
</table>

*Frequently in posterior maxillary dentoalveolar region as well.

be aware that excessive use of vasoconstrictors, as with local anesthetic solutions, at least theoretically can augment undesirable coronary vasoconstriction. The same applies to traditional abortive medications, such as ergotamine tartrate, now available as a nasal spray (Migrainal), and DHE-45.

Preventive therapy. Daily preventive medications, generally for patients with more than four headaches per month, include these first-line agents: tricyclic antidepressants, (β-blockers, and the anticonvulsant divalproex (Depakote). Second-line agents include selective serotonin reuptake inhibitors, various anticonvulsants, calcium channel blockers, and cyproheptadine (Periactin).

Cluster Headache

Cluster headache may present as pain in the teeth and jaw, usually the posterior maxillary quadrants. Most often, pain is experienced in the orbit or temple (Box 16-3). This is an almost ex-

clusively unilateral headache, extremely severe in intensity, lasting 15 to 180 minutes, and associated with autonomic dysfunction, usually tearing or nasal congestion. Men are affected much more often than women. The pathophysiology of cluster headache is less well understood than for migraine, but their mechanisms overlap, with neurogenic inflammation of trigeminal afferents playing a major role in pain transmission.

Therapy for cluster headache is medical. Preventive treatment is with verapamil, lithium salts, methysergide, and prednisone. Abortive treatment includes high-flow oxygen early, then ergots and triptans. Surgical treatment can be effective on chronic cases.

Tension-Type Headache

Episodic tension-type headache (TTH), also referred to as stress headache or muscle contraction headache, is the most common form of headache. Stress and muscle contraction are not always present, however, and the current IHS classification reflects previous criteria for "tension" and "muscle contraction" headaches in earlier classifications (Box 16-4). Most TTH sufferers do not have elevated pericranial muscle tension levels.

Box 16-4 IHS Criteria for Episodic Tension-Type Headache

A. Headache pain accompanied by two of the following symptoms:
- Pressing/tightening (nonpulsating) quality
- Bilateral location
- Not aggravated by routine physical activity

B. Headache pain accompanied by both of the following symptoms:
- Photophobia and phonophobia not present or only one present

C. Fewer than 15 days per month with headache (if more than 15 days/month, termed chronic tension-type headache)

D. No evidence of organic disease

TTH is frequently a pressing or squeezing sensation in the region of the temples and forehead. Some patients describe it as a "hatband" headache. It is generally bilateral and, unlike migraine, is not intensified by physical exertion. Patients do not experience nausea or vomiting but may report photophobia. When headache is present less than 15 days per month, it is termed *episodic*, and more than 15 days per month, *chronic*. The pathophysiology of TTH is poorly understood but may be similar to migraine, with TTH on the milder end of the migraine spectrum in intensity.

Antidepressants, particularly the tricyclics, are the mainstay of treatment for TTH, although many other preventive migraine therapies can provide relief. Psychological therapies can be effective for many patients, especially if stress is implicated in the etiology of TTH.

Analgesics

The dentist must understand that analgesic medication may worsen or perpetuate both migraine and TTH. Agents that may be involved in *analgesic rebound headache* include opioids, aspirin, acetaminophen, NSAIDs, barbiturates (e.g., proprietary combinations containing butalbital), benzodiazepines, and excessive caffeine. When used more than 6 to 8 days per month for at least 2 to 3 months, these agents may produce a clinical picture of increasingly severe or frequent headache unresponsive to traditional treatments. TTH may easily be confused with masticatory myofascial pain, and migraine may be precipitated by temporomandibular disorders or

may aggravate these conditions, depending on presentation. The dentist may unknowingly contribute to worsening head pain, leading to increasing analgesic use and a patient more refractory to otherwise successful interventions.

ORGANIC HEADACHES

Organic headache processes should be recognized by the dentist, and in contrast to primary headaches, rapid medical evaluation and treatment can lead to decreased morbidity and mortality (see Table 16-1).

Hemorrhagic Stroke

Hypertension is a common etiologic factor in hemorrhagic stroke. Although rupture of an aneurysm or arteriovenous malformation may occur, most intracerebral hemorrhages are caused by hypertension. Hemorrhagic stroke is often associated with exertion and is more common in persons over 50 years of age. There is no warning, and the patient is typically awake. At the time of stroke, headache may be severe but is absent in at least half of cases. Vomiting is common. Hemorrhagic stroke can be subdivided based on localization of the bleeding.

Intraparenchymal Hemorrhage

Intraparenchymal bleeding generally produces headache and focal neurologic symptoms. Weakness, aphasia, dysarthria, ataxia, and diplopia are potential symptoms, depending on where the bleed occurs.[9] These hemorrhages may not be large, and healed sequelae may be seen on brain imaging.

Subarachnoid Hemorrhage

Subarachnoid bleeding produces the "thunderclap" headache, the most excruciating headache pain. The pressure of blood on the meningeal blood vessels is a profound irritant to the pain receptors in the area. Focal signs may or may not be present. Approximately 50% of patients with subarachnoid hemorrhage experience a warning headache days to months before the major event. These headaches tend to resolve after 1 or 2 days but may last as long as 2 weeks. One of three cases of subarachnoid hemorrhage is associated with exertional effort. Accompanying symptoms may include nausea, neck pain, visual disturbances, and sensory abnormalities.[10,11]

Subdural Hematoma

Subdural hematomas result directly from intracranial bleeding but are best viewed as mass lesions that produce direct pressure on pain-sensitive structures. They usually manifest after trauma and rarely produce focal neurologic deficits. Overt changes in mental status or varying levels of consciousness are more common signs of subdural hematomas.[6]

Ischemic Stroke

Headaches associated with ischemic stroke occur most often with occlusion of the larger cerebral vessels and less often with embolic phenomena. Atherosclerotic disease is frequently present. Normal cerebral blood flow delivers about 55 ml/100 g/min, with oxygen and glucose in concentrations exceeding the brain's requirement. If blood flow is decreased, homeostatic mechanisms induce cerebral vasodilation. Total or near-total deprivation of needed substrates results in ischemia, hypoglycemia, and infarction. Cerebral infarcts may increase over 4 or 5 days because of cerebral ischemia. As brain swelling subsides, neurologic function may improve. Approximately 50% of potential recovery is present at 1 month, with almost 100% of potential recovery at 1 year. Headache is usually of mild intensity and is usually not clinically relevant. Transient ischemic attacks (TIAs), which may herald the onset of ischemic stroke, frequently present as headache typically lasting less than 24 hours.[12-14] Other focal neurologic signs may occur and must be distinguished from migraine with aura, Meniere's disease, and peripheral vestibulopathy. Early intervention with thrombolytics is critical to limiting permanent neurologic compromise.

Intracranial Venous Thrombosis

Intracranial venous thrombosis is a relatively rare condition. When the superior sagittal sinus is involved, headache and focal leg symptoms may occur. Involvement of the cavernous sinus may result in headache, irregularities in eye movement, and diplopia. Intracranial venous thrombosis is more common in women prone to a hypercoagulable state, such as during pregnancy, while taking oral contraceptives, or with protein C deficiency.[15-19]

Meningitis

The classic presentation of meningitis is headache, fever, and meningismus (sore and stiff neck). Because of profound constitutional symptoms, a patient with acute meningitis is unlikely to be seen for a dental appointment. Milder or chronic forms of meningitis may be more difficult to identify. In children, *Haemophilus influenzae* is the most common precipitating organism. Pneumococci, meningococci, and *Listeria monocytogenes* are the most common causes of adult, community-acquired meningitis.[20]

Brain Abscess and Other Infections

Infectious agents may be transferred to the brain parenchyma by trauma, or infection may extend from contiguous structures, such as the oral cavity, paranasal sinuses, ears, or lungs. As in meningitis, concomitant constitutional symptoms probably would not allow a patient with brain abscess to keep a dental appointment. Similar to other mass lesions, brain abscesses cause headache by pressure on pain-sensitive meningeal structures. Most patients present with headache, vomiting, mental status changes, and focal neurologic deficits.[21] Slower-growing organisms, such as fungi or tuberculosis, usually affect immunocompromised patients, such as those with human immunodeficiency virus (HIV), transplantation, or cancer. Headache frequently accompanies HIV infection. In one series, 82% of HIV-infected patients had an identifiable cause for headache.[22,23]

Temporal (Giant Cell) Arteritis

Temporal arteritis (TA) should be suspected in any patient over age 50 years who presents to the dentist with nonodontogenic head or face pain. TA is caused by giant cell infiltration of the cranial artery system and is frequently associated with polymyalgia rheumatica. TA carries a significant risk of stroke and visual loss. Although an elevated erythrocyte sedimentation rate (ESR) and positive temporal artery biopsy are confirmatory, negative testing does not rule out TA. The temporal arteries are frequently tender and indurated. Symptoms include headache and *jaw claudication*, literally "jaw limping," which manifests as pain and cramping of the jaw muscles during use. Jaw claudication occurs shortly after mastication starts, as when blood flow is decreased to the masticatory muscles. Extension of the arterial inflammation to the ophthalmic artery leads to blindness in 7% to 60% of patients. If TA is suspected, the physician should initiate prompt treatment with high doses of prednisone.[24-27]

Neoplasm

Tumors usually present with focal symptoms or seizures but may start simply as headache that worsens over weeks to months. Focal neurologic deficits may also occur and worsen over time. When the tumor extends to include pain-sensitive intracranial structures, such as the larger cerebral blood vessels and the meninges, headache or face pain may result. The location of perceived pain depends on the location of the mass and the pain referral pattern of the structure involved. Pain is typically felt ipsilateral to the site of the tumor. The most frequent primary brain tumors are gliomas, meningiomas, and pituitary adenomas. The most common source of brain metastases is from the lung or breast, although the kidney, gastrointestinal tract, and skin (malignant melanoma) are other sources.[28-30]

Hypertensive Headache

Although highly variable in presentation, hypertensive headache does not generally occur at diastolic blood pressures less than 110 mm Hg. Hypertensive headaches are generally throbbing or "bursting" in quality, and the intensity is not reliably correlated with degree of diastolic blood pressure elevation above 110 mm Hg. The pain is generally bilaterally occipital in distribution and may be worse on awakening, with improvement during the day.

PATIENT EVALUATION

Two factors alerting the dentist that a pain in the head or the face (headache) is a potential emergency and not a benign common headache are (1) acuity of onset and (2) presence of other symptoms or findings. The abrupt onset of a severe headache in a person without a prior history of headache or in a patient with a history of headache who states that this headache is different or more severe than prior headaches ("worst headache of my life") deserves close attention and possible referral to a hospital ED. As a general rule, the "first or worst" headache requires prompt medical evaluation.

If a patient has symptoms of neurologic dysfunction, even if transient, the patient should be immediately evaluated. Symptoms of neurologic dysfunction include focal weakness (e.g., in extremities, facial droop), focal numbness, speech difficulty, incoordination, gait difficulty, changes in level of consciousness, and decreased alertness. Visual phenomena and mild dizziness, al-

though also important, must be distinguished from acute migraine with or without aura, which may also present with these signs. Photophobia may be present in primary headaches (e.g., migraine) or may herald an emergency situation. Acral paresthesias, involving the fingertips and bilateral perioral region, that are not clearly localized to defined neuroanatomic boundaries are less serious symptoms, usually associated with hyperventilation. Meningismus (severe headache, neck pain and stiffness) should prompt immediate attention (Box 16-5).

Although these symptoms indicate the need to consider serious medical problems associated with a complaint of headache, one third to one half of ED headache patients present with primary headaches, such as migraine and TTH.[1-3] Therefore the most important component of the evaluation of the emergency patient with headache is the history, since the general medical and neurologic examinations are usually normal.[31]

History

The dentist must decide whether the patient has a benign headache (migraine, TTH, cluster headache) or headache caused by organic disease. The history focuses on the following areas (see Table 16-1):

1. Onset of the headache (e.g., did the onset follow exertion?)
2. Character, severity, duration, and location of the pain
3. Associated gastrointestinal and neurologic symptoms (e.g., vomiting, blurred vision)
4. Prior history of headache, including family history of headache (e.g., Have imaging studies been used to evaluate patient with history of headache?)
5. Medications currently or previously taken for headache

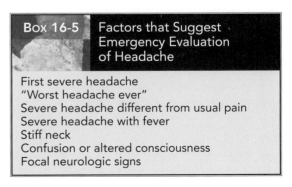

Box 16-5 Factors that Suggest Emergency Evaluation of Headache

First severe headache
"Worst headache ever"
Severe headache different from usual pain
Severe headache with fever
Stiff neck
Confusion or altered consciousness
Focal neurologic signs

Physical Examination

Ideally a complete neurologic and focused physical examination is done, with emphasis on vital signs and facial, neck, and funduscopic examination. Although the neurologic examination skills of most dentists are limited, it is easy to assess if the patient's pupils are equal and reactive to light or the patient is photophobic by use of the dental light. The dentist may simply elicit information from the patient regarding facial or extremity paresthesias and test this with pinprick relative to the contralateral side. Disturbed gait is disturbed or the patient's inability to grip both the dentist's hands with equal force may indicate motor deficit. Percussion over the sinuses may be performed if sinus pathology is suspected. Tightness of the cervical musculature and decreased cervical range of motion may indicate meningismus. Indurated superficial temporal arteries with poor pulsations in an elderly patient should suggest TA.

Although these may be incomplete evaluation measures (e.g., formal ophthalmoscopic examination is unlikely to be performed), this type of examination is the mainstay of the physical evaluation. The ability to obtain advanced imaging modalities and perform lumbar puncture, if indicated, significantly contributes to the complete patient evaluation.

TREATMENT

As a general rule, dental office treatment of the patient with severe headache is supportive, especially with suspected organic disease. The only exception may be the patient being treated by an orofacial pain dentist whose practice includes management of primary headache. Oxygen is always appropriate for any patient in distress. The patient is positioned comfortably in the dental chair. The lights may be dimmed if the patient is photophobic. The dentist should continually assess mental status through verbal communication. Periodic monitoring of vital signs is prudent. In the unconscious patient, basic life support is required. If serious organic pathology is suspected, rapid transport to the nearest ED via emergency medical services (EMS) is appropriate if readily available (Box 16-6).

DIFFERENTIAL DIAGNOSIS

Although not true "emergencies," many serious medical and dental conditions can present with headache and facial pain. Dental and periodontal *infection*, including major space infections of the face and neck, is the most common cause of

---

Box 16-6	Triage and Emergency Management of Patient with Headache (Head or Face Pain)

A. Assess for imminent emergency.
   1. Is the patient rapidly losing consciousness?
   2. Is the patient developing motor or cognitive dysfunction?
   3. Is the patient in profound distress?
B. Evaluate the patient.
   1. History (see Box 16-5)
      a. Activate EMS.
      b. Continue with physical evaluation.
   2. Physical examination
      a. Vital signs
      b. Neurologic survey
      c. Sensory and motor examination
C. Initiate treatment measures.
   1. Headache secondary to suspected organic pathology
      a. Provide supportive care as necessary; be prepared to perform basic life support measures if needed.
      b. Administer supplemental oxygen.
      c. Position patient for comfort.
      d. Periodically monitor vital signs.
      e. Await EMS transport for definitive diagnosis and treatment.
   2. Primary headache similar to past treated headaches
      a. Defer dental treatment if possible.
      b. Arrange for transport to ED or home as appropriate.
      c. Consider notification of family physician or neurologist.

---

facial pain and should be apparent to most dentists. Likewise, all dentists should include *jaw fractures* and local *jaw tumors* in the differential diagnosis of pain and limitation in jaw function.

This section highlights serious medical conditions presenting with pain in the masticatory region. All these conditions require prompt, although not necessarily emergency, work-up. *Any facial pain not responsive to therapy should prompt the dentist to reassess the working diagnosis and expand the work-up to include less common, but frequently more serious, conditions.*

Pain and Associated Mandibular Hypomobility

The most common nondental causes of jaw pain and mandibular hypomobility are associated with *temporomandibular disorders* (TMDs). Common

TMDs that may present in this way include temporomandibular joint (TMJ) synovitis with secondary muscle splinting, TMJ anterior disk displacement without reduction, coronoid hypertrophy (usually with minimal pain when an isolated entity), masticatory myositis or spasm, and masticatory myofascial pain syndromes. Forward pressure on the dislocated TMJ disk causes pain associated with stretching of diskal collateral and other ligaments. Muscular symptoms may be associated with primary benign headache syndromes (e.g., migraine, TTH). Masticatory muscle splinting may be associated with severe pharyngeal pain (e.g., tonsillitis, irritation from endotracheal intubation). Other, more serious conditions may have similar presentations.

Oropharyngeal carcinomas, including the tongue base, may present with pain and mandibular hypomobility, depending on the location of tumor infiltration. Decreased tongue movement is frequently evident on cranial nerve testing, and musculoskeletal findings may not follow basic principles of temporomandibular joint mechanics. Typically there is invasion of the floor of the mouth and the medial pterygoid muscle. *Nasopharyngeal carcinomas* may also present with limited mandibular opening, although facial pain is the more common primary symptom.

Trigeminal neuralgia and *glossopharyngeal neuralgia* are severely painful conditions that may be associated with limited mandibular movement. These sharp, lancinating, or "electric shock" pains may be associated with central nervous system (CNS) convergence phenomena manifesting as masticatory muscle hyperactivity or spasm.[32,33]

A rare cause of pain and mandibular hypomobility that should not be overlooked is related to *tetanus*. Infection caused by *Clostridium* may require prompt treatment with antitoxin. A history of recent penetrating wound or fever, abdominal pain, and nausea suggests *Clostridium* infection.[34]

Because of potentially life-threatening sequelae and blindness, TA requires prompt medical care (see earlier discussion).

Other Facial Pains

Trigeminal and other cranial neuralgias typically arise without clear etiology but may be associated with an identifiable cause (e.g., tumor, arteriovenous malformation, aneurysm) or as the initial presenting symptom of multiple sclerosis (MS). Cranial neuralgia presenting in a patient under age 40 should suggest MS. *All* facial pain of neuropathic origin requires brain imaging to rule out serious underlying disease. The severity of pain in typical trigeminal neuralgia (*tic douloureux*) requires immediate treatment, although this would not be considered an emergency in the classic sense.

Nasopharyngeal, dermatologic, cranial, primary, and metastatic carcinomas that invade the trigeminal nerve may produce pain in the face or mouth. The symptoms may mimic TMDs, or a TMD may coexist. When clinical testing is inconclusive or trial therapy is ineffective, especially when the patient presents with significant risk factors for oral cancer (e.g., smoking, ethanol abuse), neoplasm should be included in the differential diagnosis.[35-40]

Lung cancer and acute myocardial infarction (MI) can present as facial pain in some patients. In lung cancer, pain is typically ipsilateral to the tumor, on the right side, and perceived in the ear, jaw, or temporal regions. Digital clubbing, recent unintended weight loss, and elevated ESR may provide diagnostic clues. The presumed mechanism is compression of the vagus nerve by the tumor, with CNS convergence causing referred trigeminal distribution of pain symptoms. This same mechanism of vagus-trigeminal interaction likely accounts for reports of jaw pain associated with acute MI.[7,41-44]

Acoustic neuroma, or vestibular schwannoma, is a benign tumor of cranial nerve VIII. Although rare, case reports detail acoustic neuroma with facial pain as the primary presenting symptom. Acoustic neuroma should be suspected in a patient with a relatively recent history of hearing loss, ear fullness, or vestibular dysfunction.[45,46]

SUMMARY

Most head and face pains, or headaches, whether of primary masticatory or other etiology, are benign processes. However, certain conditions that present with headache or masticatory dysfunction may herald a serious medical condition. The dentist must promptly refer patients presenting with suggestive signs or symptoms to an ED for further physician evaluation.

REFERENCES

1. Silberstein SD: Evaluation and emergency treatment of headache, *Headache* 32:369-404, 1992.
2. Dhorest V, Anwar R, Herring G: A retrospective assessment of emergency department patients with complaint of headache, *Headache* 19:37-42, 1979.
3. Leight MJ: Non-traumatic headache in the emergency department, *Am J Emerg Med* 9:404-409, 1980.

4. Dickman RL, Masten T: The management of non-traumatic headache in a university hospital emergency room, *Headache* 19:391-396, 1979.

5. Diamond ML: Emergency department treatment of the headache patient, *Headache Q* 3(suppl 1):28-33, 1992.

6. Stewart WF, Lipton RB, Centano DD, Reed ML: Prevalence of migraine headache in the United States: relation to age, income, race, and other sociodemographic factors, *JAMA* 267:64-69, 1992.

7. DesPrez RD, Freemon FR: Facial pain associated with lung cancer: a case report, *Headache* 23:43-44, 1983.

8. Lipton RB, Stewart WF, Centano DD, Reed ML: Undiagnosed migraine headaches: a comparison of symptom based and reported physician diagnosis, *Arch Intern Med* 152:1273-1278, 1992.

9. Stieg PE, Kase CS: Intracranial hemorrhage: diagnosis and emergency management, *Neurol Clin North Am* 16:373-390, 1998.

10. Duffy GB: The warning leak in spontaneous subarachnoid hemorrhage, *Med J Aust* 28:514-516, 1983.

11. Leblanc R: The minor leak preceding subarachnoid hemorrhage, *J Neurosurg* 66:35-39, 1987.

12. Portenoy RK, Abissi CJ, Lipton RB, et al: Headache in cerebrovascular disease, *Stroke* 15:1009-1012, 1984.

13. Edmeads J: Headache in cerebrovascular disease. In Rose CF, editor: *Handbook of clinical neurology*, vol 4, Amsterdam, 1986, Elsevier.

14. Gorelick PB: Ischemic stroke and intracranial hematoma. In Olesen J, Tfelt-Hansen P, Welch KMA, editors: *The headaches*, New York, 1993, Raven.

15. Monton F, Rebollo M, Quintana F, Berciano J: Cerebral arterial occlusion and intracranial venous thrombosis in a woman taking oral contraceptives, *Postgrad Med J* 60:426-428, 1984.

16. Parsons M: Intracranial venous thrombosis, *Postgrad Med J* 43:409-414, 1967.

17. Biller J, Adams HP Jr: Cerebrovascular disorders associated with pregnancy, *Am Fam Physician* 33:125-132, 1986.

18. Wintzen AR, Broekmans AW, Bertina RM, et al: Cerebral haemorrhagic infarction in young patients with hereditary protein C deficiency: evidence for "spontaneous" cerebral venous thrombosis, *Br Med J* 290:350-352, 1985.

19. Estanol B, Rodriguez A, Conte G, et al: Intracranial venous thrombosis in young women, *Stroke* 10:680-684, 1979.

20. Francke E: The many causes of meningitis, *Postgrad Med* 82:175-188, 1987.

21. De Marinis M, Kurdi AA, Welcj KMA: Headache associated with intracranial infection. In Olesen J, Tfelt-Hansen P, Welch KMA, editors: *The headaches*, New York, 1993, Raven.

22. Ramadan NW: Unusual causes of headache, *Neurology* 48:1494-1499, 1997.

23. Lipton RB, Ferarru ER, Wiess G, et al: Headache and HIV-1 related disorders, *Headache* 31:518-521, 1991.

24. Allen NB, Studenski SA: Polymyalgia rheumatica and temporal arteritis, *Med Clin North Am* 70:369-384, 1986.

25. Boghen DR, Glaser JS: Ischaemic optic neuropathy: the clinical profile and natural history, *Brain* 98:689-708, 1975.

26. Ellis ME, Ralston S: The ESR in the diagnosis and management of the polymyalgia rheumatica/giant cell arteritis syndrome, *Ann Rheum Dis* 42:168-170, 1983.

27. Solomon S, Cappa KG: The headache of temporal arteritis, *J Am Geriatr Soc* 35:163-165, 1987.

28. Forsyth PA, Posner JB: Intracranial neoplasms. In Olesen J, Tfelt-Hansen P, Welch KMA, editors: *The headaches*, New York, 1993, Raven.

29. Posner JB, Chernick NL: Intracranial metastasis from systemic cancer, *Adv Neurol* 19:579-592, 1978.

30. Rushton JG, Rooke ED: Brain tumor headache, *Headache* 2:147-152, 1962.

31. Newman LC, Lipton RB, Solomon S: Headache history and neurologic examination. In Tollison CD, Kunkel RS, editors: *Headache: diagnosis and treatment*, Baltimore, 1993, Williams & Wilkins.

32. Jannetta PJ: Outcome after microvascular decompression for typical trigeminal neuralgia, hemifacial spasm, tinnitus, disabling positional vertigo, and glossopharyngeal neuralgia, *Clin Neurosurg* 44:331-383, 1997.

33. Thompson TP, Jannetta PJ, Lovely TJ, Ochs M: Unilateral trismus in a patient with trigeminal neuralgia due to microvascular compression of the trigeminal motor root, *J Oral Maxillofac Surg* 57:90-92, 1999.

34. George L, Finegold SM: Clostridial infections. In Kelley WN, editor: *Textbook of internal medicine*, Philadelphia, 1992, Lippincott.

35. Wong JK, Wood RE, McLean M: Pain preceding recurrent head and neck cancer, *J Orofac Pain* 12:52-59, 1998.

36. Marshall JA, Mahanna GK: Cancer in the differential diagnosis of orofacial pain, *Dent Clin North Am* 41:355-365, 1997.

37. Su CY, Lui CC: Perineural invasion of the trigeminal nerve in patients with nasopharyngeal carcinoma: imaging and clinical correlations, *Cancer* 78:2063-2069, 1996.

38. Epstein JB, Jones CK: Presenting signs and symptoms of nasopharyngeal carcinoma, *Cancer* 75:32-36, 1993.

39. Boyczyk EM, Solomon MP, Gold BD: Unremitting pain to the mandible secondary to metastatic breast cancer: a case report, *Compendium* 12:104-110, 1997.

40. Ruff T, Lenis A, Diaz JA: Atypical facial pain and orbital cancer, *Arch Otolaryngol* 111:338-339, 1985.

41. Schroeder TL, MacFarlane DF, Goldberg LH: Pain as an atypical presentation of squamous cell carcinoma, *Dermatol Surg* 24:263-266, 1998.

42. Shakespeare TP, Stevens MJ: Unilateral facial pain and lung cancer, *Australas Radiol* 40:45-46, 1996.

43. Capobianco DJ: Facial pain as a symptom of non-metastatic lung cancer, *Headache* 35:581-585, 1995.

44. Schoenen J, Broux R, Moonen G: Unilateral facial pain as the first symptom of lung cancer: are there diagnostic clues? *Cephalagia* 12:178-179, 1992.

45. German DS: A case report: acoustic neuroma confused with TMD, *J Am Dent Assoc* 122:59-60, 1991.

46. Payten RJ: Facial pain as the first symptom in acoustic neuroma, *J Laryngol Otol* 86:523-534, 1972.

Psychiatric Emergencies

Mark D. Litt
William H. Wood

Mental health problems are increasingly appearing in the general medical practice setting.[1,2] Less is known about the prevalence of psychiatric disturbances in the general dental practice. If trends in dentistry follow those in medicine, however, dentists also are seeing patients who have significant psychiatric disturbances that can affect the success of dental treatment and even the health and life of the patient. Therefore dentists must develop an awareness of the detection and management of psychiatric problems to prevent difficulties of emotion, thought, and behavior from becoming full-scale emergencies in the dental office. This is not an easy or familiar role for the dentist; most dentists receive little psychiatric training in dental school, and they may be uncomfortable with problematic patients. To be a true health care provider, however, the dentist must be prepared to manage even difficult patients.

This chapter describes a screening process for psychiatric problems, discusses the major classes of psychiatric problems that may appear in a dental practice, and offers guidelines for management. Although many dentists may find it difficult "managing" their patients, the advantage is that virtually all patients are treatable once their particular needs are met.

As the sample case illustrates, overlooking a psychiatric problem can have serious consequences (Box 17-1). Ample information was available to prompt a more thorough assessment of the patient's emotional and psychiatric status. Such an assessment might have resulted in actions that would have prevented the patient's panic attack. The first actions would have been (1) to keep the patient informed about procedures and consultations and (2) to ensure that the patient understood and consented. If necessary, the patient could have been allowed to go home. In future visits the patient might have been given a sedative agent or nitrous oxide sedation to help manage anxiety. A program of desensitization to specific dental procedures should have been incorporated in the treatment plan.

The fact that these steps were not taken highlights not only a discomfort in dealing with such issues, but also a basic lack of tools by which to do so. Therefore this chapter emphasizes screening and assessment as well as management. The dentist should always know what type of person comes into the office as a new patient. Dentists are trained to examine the patient's history routinely for evidence of medical problems that might compromise or complicate dental care. As the case illustrates, the same care must be taken to identify psychological or psychiatric problems that can also compromise care.

GENERAL SCREENING PROCESS

A short, general screening process should consist of three phases: (1) a dental fears index, (2) a review of the patient's medications and medical history, and (3) a targeted interview.

Dental Fears Index

Although a dental fears index is best suited to screen for dental anxiety, it will also highlight unusual behavior in the dental environment that may be attributable to other psychiatric conditions. For example, a patient may avoid the dentist, which would be picked up on most dental fear indexes. However, the reason for the avoidance may have less to do with a dental phobia than with a *body dysmorphic disorder* in which patients are ashamed of their teeth. Any index that asks patients about their thoughts, feelings, and behaviors in the dental environment is useful to help screen for psychiatric disturbances that can impact dental care when appropriate follow-up questions are asked.

An example of a fears index is the Dental Experience Survey (DES, Figure 17-1).[3] The instrument is straightforward and includes questions that are likely to be given high scores by patients

---

Box 17-1 Psychiatric Case Study

Ms. Green, a 38-year-old single white female whose medical history includes a left pulmonectomy and multiple medical problems, including asthma, presented to the dental emergency department of a university hospital on a Wednesday complaining of pain in a right maxillary premolar. The dentist took her history and discovered that she was extremely anxious about dentistry. Indeed, she was anxious about all invasive medical procedures and admitted to a particular fear of needles. The resident on call noted these facts in the chart and returned to an examination of her mouth, which was in need of much dental work. He gave the patient a prescription for pain medication and scheduled a follow-up appointment in the dental clinic for comprehensive treatment planning. At the appointed time the patient was seen in the dental clinic. Numerous consultations were sought, and the patient was ultimately referred to the endodontic clinic for management of the situation.

As the consultations progressed, the patient was becoming increasingly agitated over the prospect of procedures being performed without her input or comprehension. Additionally, no one since the first resident had noted that the woman was fidgety, short of breath, and close to tears. No one had read the chart or knew that she was anxious about dentistry. When the endodontist tried to give her an injection of local anesthetic in preparation for a pulpectomy, the woman screamed and went into a full-scale panic attack, prompting bronchospasm and acute asthma attack and causing her to fall unconscious. She regained consciousness after a few minutes with oxygen. Fortunately, a crash cart was not needed. It required another 2 hours to settle the patient sufficiently to obtain a more thorough history and make plans for her to complete her dental care. Additional history revealed a long-standing panic disorder in addition to the phobic anxiety reactions to medical and dental procedures.

---

with notable dental anxiety. Any item that is scored at 5 or 6 should elicit a follow-up question by the dentist. If five or more items are given a score of 4 or greater, clinically significant dental anxiety should be suspected. The dentist should always ask questions similar to those shown in items 9 and 10 of the DES. Asking the patient directly about what makes the dental visit more difficult and what makes it easier takes advantage of the experiences of the patient's previous dentists.[4]

It is recommended that the dentist use an actual index or questionnaire and not rely on the interview process to elicit this information. Patients are more likely to be truthful on questionnaires than they would be with a new dentist, and dentists frequently forget to ask all the pertinent questions.

Review of Medications and History

After a review of a dental fears checklist, the dentist should review the patient's listed medications. Several classes of drugs will alert the dentist to the presence of current or past psychiatric illness (see following sections).

A review of the medical history may show anomalies indicative of psychiatric problems. For example, a hospital stay may be listed but no medical condition recorded. A long gap in the patient's dental treatment history should always be explored. A long history of any chronic illness should be noted, with follow-up later.[4]

Targeted Interview

The dentist should follow-up a review of the patient's chart with an interview targeted at items of concern in the previous assessment. This part of the patient interview should be straightforward and direct. The dentist should address any high score on a fears checklist and any medication the patient is taking that is typically prescribed for a psychiatric condition. The patient may acknowledge a psychiatric problem but state that it does not interfere with dentistry. The patient may even acknowledge fear but assert that that fear does not represent a significant problem for care. In these situations the patient may require very little intervention. Often, patients appreciate the dentist's effort to evaluate the patient's problem, and the screening process can often help build rapport. In patients with psychiatric problems that may interfere with care, the dentist should find out how it was handled by past dentists and must be prepared

DENTAL EXPERIENCE SURVEY
(to be completed by patient)

Date _____   Patient Name/ Chart # _____

The following questions ask about your past dental experiences and your feelings about dental treatment. Your answer may help us find ways to make your dental treatment a more pleasant experience. Answer questions 1 through 9 by circling the best number that describes your feelings. Be sure to answer questions 10 and 11 if they apply to you.

1. How often have you avoided calling for a dentist appointment?	1 Never	2	3	4	5 Often	6	
2. How often have you canceled dentist appointments?	1 Never	2	3	4	5 Often	6	
3. In general, how would you describe your experiences with dentists?	1 Very Pleasant	2	3	4	5 Very Unpleasant	6	
4. In general, how do you feel when you first arrive at the dentist's office?	1 Very Relaxed	2	3	4	5 Very Nervous	6	
5. In general, how do you feel when you are in the dental chair?	1 Very Relaxed	2	3	4	5 Very Nervous	6	
6. In general, how satisfied have you been with your past dental care?	1 Very Satisfied	2	3	4	5 Very Dissatisfied	6	
7. Do you ever take anything to calm your nerves before dental treatment?	1 Never	2	3	4	5 Often	6	
8. Do you ever have trouble with gagging while getting dental work done?	1 No Trouble	2	3	4	5 Lots of Trouble	6	

9. Have you ever been given anything to make you go to sleep or feel more relaxed for dental treatment?

   1. **Yes**   2. **No**

10. What are things that dentists do that make the dental visit harder for you? _____
_____
_____

11. What could the dentist do to make your dental visit better? _____
_____
_____

Figure 17-1. Dental Experience Survey (DES) screening instrument for dental anxiety. *From Litt MD: The Dental Experience Survey: a screening instrument for dental anxiety for use in the dental clinic, 1994, University of Connecticut School of Dental Medicine.*

for possible complications in the provision of dentistry.

ANXIETY DISORDERS

Anxiety disorders are the most common cause of disruptions in dental practice. Recent surveys of the prevalence of extreme dental anxiety in general population samples have produced estimates ranging from 4.2% to 23%, depending on the scale and cutoff value used.[5-7] Some estimates place the rate of significant nonphobic dental anxiety in adults at 50%.[8]

Anxious dental patients tend to be management problems for the dentist, requiring more time and preparation to treat effectively.[9,10] They also complain of greater discomfort during and after dental procedures.[8] It is important to identify and manage anxious patients before their psychological status interferes with dental care. Some severe anxiety disorders can leave patients vulnerable to panic attacks or posttraumatic stress syndrome (PTSD) flashbacks. Anxiolytic medications taken for these disorders can interact with sedation or may make the patient appear under the influence of alcohol or illicit drugs. Patients with the most common anxiety disorders have distinguishing characteristics (Box 17-2).

Apprehension

Identification.   In one study, 44% of adults acknowledged canceling dental appointments because of fear.[4] Apprehensive dental patients, or those who are fearful of the dentist but whose fear does not interfere with dental care, express some fear on a screening instrument (e.g., DES) but otherwise show no behavioral or physiologic signs of distress.

Management.   Management of apprehensive patients is based on the assessment, history, and interview. For most patients, simply avoiding behaviors and practices that are anxiety provoking is sufficient for effective management. Adopting practices that have proven useful to the patient (e.g., offering the patient a means to stop dental work, such as by raising a hand) and attending to the patient's dental concerns will increase the patient's overall satisfaction with the visit and keep procedure-related pain in check.[11] This will entail specifically inquiring about the ways the dentist can help the patient feel more comfortable, then following through on the patient's comments.

Dental Fears and Phobias

Identification.   Patients with phobic anxiety are those whose fear of dentistry in particular has interfered with dental care, usually by prompting the patient to avoid the dentist. Such patients may only appear in a dentist's office in emergency situations. These patients admit on screening instruments and in interviews that they are extremely nervous about seeing the dentist. Their fears take specific forms, including fear of needles, fear of pain, fear of medical catastrophes in the dental office, and fear of being humiliated for poor dental health.[12] In extremely anxious patients, sleep is disturbed the night before the dental visit. Dental history is either nonexistent or sparse, with many missed appointments and long intervals between appointments (see Box 17-2).

Management.   Management should start with environmental modifications. The dental office should be nonthreatening; there should be no loud noises, and unpleasant odors should be eliminated before the patient arrives. The operatory should be cleared of instruments until they are used.

Pharmacologic management may also be considered, with premedication using short-acting sedative-hypnotics (e.g., triazolam). Nitrous oxide sedation or other conscious sedation should also be considered. If the patient is to be premedicated, the dentist should consider prescribing a dose of sedative to be taken the night before the next dental visit, as well as a dose to be taken an hour or so before the visit.

Behavioral management should start with scheduling. Anxious patients should be scheduled as the first appointment in the morning to minimize the time the patient can spend ruminating about the visit to come. Morning is also when patients are freshest and best able to concentrate on coping with dentistry. Visits should be scheduled to be as predictable as possible. The dentist should have specific and limited goals for each visit.

Basic management consists of the shorthand behavioral prescription learned in dental school: "tell, show, do." The patient should be seated comfortably and given information about the procedures to follow. Information should be complete, but needless detail should be avoided. Both *procedural* information (what will take place) and *sensory* information (what the patient will feel) should be provided. Euphemisms may be used in place of terms that might arouse anxiety (e.g., "You'll feel a pinch when I administer the local anesthetic" vs. "You'll feel a little

| Box 17-2 | Characteristics of Dental Patients with Anxiety Disorders |

ANXIETY/DENTAL PHOBIA
Dental fears index: High overall score; avoidance items endorsed; nervousness endorsed
Typical medications: Diazepam (Valium), lorazepam (Ativan), triazolam (Halcion); often as premedication
Presentation/history: Presents with emergent problem; delayed seeking care; spotty or absent dental records; long time between visits; missed appointments; lack of follow-up care; temporary procedures never completed; dental care delivered in emergency department
Interview: Admits high degree of nervousness; describes specific fears (e.g., needles, catastrophes, drill, rubber dam); may have issues about control of situation or fears of being "out of control"; may use alcohol or other drug to reduce anxiety before appointment

GENERALIZED ANXIETY DISORDER
Dental fears index: Moderate overall score; some avoidance; high nervousness
Typical medications: Alprazolam (Xanax), buspirone (Buspar), venlafaxine (Effexor)
Presentation/history: Nervous on presentation; irregular visits to dentist
Interview: No specific fear of dentist; reports feeling "wound up," chronically worried; all medical/dental visits difficult; restlessness; fatigue; difficulty concentrating; sleep disturbance; irritability; anxiety is disruptive

POSTTRAUMATIC STRESS DISORDER (PTSD)
Dental fears index: Moderate overall score; some avoidance; high nervousness; may endorse 1 or 2 items at maximum on scale
Typical medications: Phenelzine (Nardil), fluoxetine (Prozac), buspirone, venlafaxine, sertraline (Zoloft), amitryptiline (Elavil), clonidine

Presentation/history: Nervous on presentation; normal dental history; avoidance behavior
Interview: May reveal recent trauma (e.g., abuse, serious accident, loss of a loved one); associated flashbacks, memories of trauma; periods of high anxiety; restlessness; fatigue; difficulty concentrating; sleep disturbance; irritability; hypervigilance; exaggerated startle response

PANIC DISORDER
Dental fears index: Normal range of scores except for high nervousness in dental office
Typical medications: Alprazolam, imipramine, paroxetine (Paxil)
Presentation/history: Normal dental history until development of panic disorder
Interview: Recurrent attacks of anxiety with palpitations, sweating, hyperventilation, chest pain, dizziness, shortness of breath, fear of dying; dentistry usually not a problem, but certain situations may provoke anxiety or panic attack (e.g., "hovering" by dentist, discussion of extensive unexpected work, unexplained delays)

OBSESSIVE-COMPULSIVE DISORDER
Dental fears index: Normal range of scores
Typical medications: Clomipramine (Anafranil), fluvoxamine (Luvox), sertraline, paroxetine
Presentation/history: May present with damaged gums or teeth from compulsive brushing, flossing; obsessions about mercury amalgams
Interview: Obsessions (recurrent distressing thoughts, ideas, or impulses) and/or compulsions; repetitive intentional behaviors in response to obsessions; obsessions or compulsions about dentistry, especially dental hygiene

pain when I inject the local anesthetic"). The patient should be encouraged to ask questions.

The dentist should be prepared to "show" the patient any visual aids, including radiographs, models, drawings, and illustrations, that will help convey what is to be done. Patients should be given as much information as they want. The dentist should be aware, however, that some patients may prefer less information, and that too much information makes some persons more anxious.[13] The patient should determine the level of information exchange.

For the "do" portion of patient management, the dentist should work quickly and confidently.

Conversation with assistants should be restricted to the procedures being done. The dentist should periodically check the patient's condition, and frequent breaks should be scheduled. The patient should never have to "endure" the dental procedure. The dentist should give occasional updates regarding time left for completing a procedure.

A relaxation procedure can be used to keep anxious patients calm during preparation and dental work. An additional benefit of relaxation is that it requires the patient's attention and thus provides a distraction from the dental work. An effective deep-breathing relaxation procedure can be taught to a patient in less than 3 minutes

Box 17-3	Relaxation Instructions for the Dental Patient

1. Focus on a point in space.
2. Take a deep breath through the nose and hold it.
3. Slowly release the breath with a sigh; let all air out of the lungs, and let the muscles go limp, "like a rag doll."
4. Take another deep breath and hold it, then again release slowly.
5. Take another breath through the nose and slowly release it; let eyes close, let limbs go limp, and mentally suggest tension release.
6. Suggest feelings of heaviness and warmth.

(Box 17-3). Having the patient breathe through the nose is recommended to avoid aspiration of water or materials during dental work. During dental work the dentist should monitor the patient's level of relaxation; for example, clenched hands and a stiff jaw are good indicators of patient tension. The dentist should provide occasional reminders to relax, as well as reassurance and updates on time left. Reassurance should continue throughout the dental visit.

Generalized Anxiety Disorder

Identification.   Generalized anxiety disorder (GAD) is characterized by chronic and uncontrollable worry about multiple life circumstances. This constant worry may be manifested in symptoms of restlessness, fatigue, difficulty concentrating, irritability, muscle tension, and sleep disturbance. The lifetime prevalence of GAD in the adult population is 4% to 7%. Dental patients with GAD may not score as being highly anxious on a dental fears index and may report being fairly satisfied with past dental work. However, they may show significant nervousness in the dentist's office. These patients may appear histrionic at times and may report unlikely dental symptoms. The drug most widely prescribed at present for GAD is alprazolam (Xanax), a long-acting benzodiazepine-like anxiolytic (see Box 17-2). Patients with GAD may have a varied history with dentists, often reporting many providers. The interview may indicate that the patient is not fearful of any particular procedure but is generally fearful of any "doctor" and has had a variety of complaints.

Management.   Management should begin with an assessment of the areas of dentistry the patient finds most difficult to tolerate and of the procedures that have been used successfully in the past to calm the patient. In extremely anxious patients, pharmacologic management may be advisable, particularly if the patient is not taking medication. As with phobic patients, premedication is best done with a short-acting, benzodiazepine sedative-hypnotic with a short half-life. Nitrous oxide may also be used, but the dentist must be careful that it does not disinhibit the patient and prompt a panic attack. Deep-breathing relaxation or progressive muscle relaxation may help calm and distract the patient. As with phobic patients, visits should be made as predictable as possible, with defined and limited goals so as not to exhaust the person. Emphasis should be placed on normalizing the dental experience for the patient (i.e., presenting the dental visit as nonthreatening). Some dentists alert the staff to ensure that they greet the patient properly.

Posttraumatic Stress Disorder and Abuse

Identification.   PTSD is an anxiety disorder defined by a reexperiencing of a psychologically traumatic event. The reexperiencing can take one of the following forms: (1) recurrent and intrusive distressing recollections of the event, (2) recurrent distressing dreams of the event, (3) suddenly feeling as if the event were recurring, or (4) intense psychological distress in situations that symbolize or resemble an aspect of the traumatic event.[14] Other symptoms include flashbacks, use of alcohol or other drugs as self-medication, avoidance of activities or situations that recall the trauma, amnesia related to the event, obvious decreased interest in daily activities, and sleep disturbance. In many patients with PTSD the traumatic event consists of sexual abuse or sexual assault. Close dental work with the patient increases the chances of prompting a PTSD-related panic. On a dental fears index the patient may score moderately overall, with avoidance of dentistry indicated and one or two items scored at the maximum. Medications prescribed for PTSD include phenelzine (Nardil), a monoamine oxidase inhibitor (MAOI) antidepressant, sertraline (Zoloft), and others (see Box 17-2). When interviewed the patient may disclose the nature of the flashbacks and may indicate a preference for a male or female dentist. Issues of control and feeling trapped may be raised, as in panic disorder.

Management.   The dentist should accommodate patient preferences to the extent possible, particularly regarding the choice of male or female dentist. Care must be taken to avoid circumstances that would prompt a panic attack or lead to a dissociative state. Typically the patient will know what situations to avoid. Many patients report a feeling of claustrophobia if the dentist hovers, and a change of patient position (e.g., more upright) might be helpful. Dissociative states can result from use of sedative-hypnotics. Nitrous oxide should be used with care. Suggestions of relaxation and reassurance (e.g., "Just let yourself relax a bit") and specific suggestions to let hands and mouth be loose and relaxed ("As we work, just keep paying attention to your hands; make sure they stay nice and relaxed") may be safer than actual relaxation induction.

Panic Disorders

Identification.   Panic disorder is characterized by recurrent attacks of anxiety that can occur at any time but more often occur in certain situations, especially in crowded and enclosed places. The dental office or operatory may also be a situation in which panic attacks occur. Patients may complain of bouts of intense fear and apprehension, a feeling of not being in their own body, or an intense fear of death. This may be accompanied by shortness of breath, diaphoresis, and complaints of dizziness. Patients usually acknowledge that their fears are unfounded but claim an inability to control them. On a structured index of dental fears, patients usually score in the normal range on most items but may display extreme nervousness in the dental environment, with a history that includes receiving premedication for dental work. Common medications for panic include alprazolam, imipramine, and increasingly, paroxetine (Paxil). An interview may reveal what circumstances are likely to prompt panic attack. Common problematic situations in the dental environment include instances of hovering or of the patient feeling trapped or out of control.

Management.   Panic attacks may be avoided if the dentist ensures that the patient does not feel out of control or trapped. The dentist should brief the patient as to procedures and provide information while working. The dentist should check the patient's understanding before any work is started (e.g., "Do you understand everything that I have just told you? Do you have any questions? Does all this sound OK to you?"). The dentist should make sure that the patient is ready before beginning a new procedure or a new phase of work. Frequent breaks should be given. A signal should be arranged (e.g., raise a hand) to allow the patient to stop dental work if necessary. The interview may indicate what procedures have worked well for the patient in the past. Distractions such as conversation may help, but care must be taken with such interventions as use of headphones or premedication. Some panic disorder patients react with panic attacks in response to dissociating interventions such as nitrous oxide sedation or even relaxation instruction. If sedative premedication is to be attempted, the lowest dose available should be tried first.

Obsessive-Compulsive Disorders

Identification.   Obsessions are recurrent thoughts or impulses, often of a distressing nature, that are perceived as *both* distressing and irresistible. Compulsions are repetitive intentional behaviors that occur in response to obsessions. Obsessive-compulsive disorder (OCD) may consist of either obsessions or compulsions, or both together. Although the compulsions may be recognized as senseless (e.g., repetitive handwashing), they are perceived as virtually uncontrollable. Some compulsions may take the form of repetitive oral hygiene behaviors, such as repetitive flossing or brushing.[15]

The obsessions and compulsions in OCD are accompanied by extreme levels of anxiety. The anxiety escalates into a state of panic if the obsessions or compulsions are interrupted. On a dental fears index, a person with mild OCD will score in the low-to-moderate range on most items, with possible elevations on selected items that may relate to obsessive or compulsive behaviors. For example, an individual may report feeling very nervous in the dental chair because a certain compulsive behavior (e.g., fingernail chewing) is restricted. Although the score on that item may be elevated, scores on other items would be in the normal range. A person with severe OCD will have a history of few dental visits; the anxiety involved in possible interruptions of compulsive routines often results in restriction of activities. Common medications taken for OCD include the tricyclic antidepressant (TCA) clomipramine (Anafranil) and the selective serotonin reuptake inhibitors (SSRIs) fluvoxamine (Luvox), sertraline (Zoloft), and paroxetine. The interview should indicate under what circumstances obsessions or compulsions appear. Compulsions seen in the dental environment may include repetitive handwashing, picking at clothing, or other cleaning or grooming behavior.

Management. Mild OCD usually does not present a management problem. Serious problems can develop, however, if compulsive routines are disrupted during the course of dental work. For example, a patient with a time-checking compulsion may develop a panic attack if not allowed to check his watch while having a restorative procedure done. If OCD is detected, the dentist must be sure to determine the seriousness of the symptoms and the circumstances under which compulsions occur. Usually the dentist can work around the compulsion, allowing breaks during which the patient may engage in the anxiety-reducing behavior. For lengthy procedures, conscious sedation may be required to keep the patient comfortable throughout the work.

MOOD DISORDERS AND THE SUICIDAL PATIENT

Mood disorders constitute a group of disorders whose primary feature is a disturbance in affect. The best known and most prevalent mood disorder is major unipolar depression, but the group also encompasses bipolar disorders, also called manic-depressive illness. Estimated lifetime prevalence of depressive disorders is up to 24% for women and 15% for men.[16]

Major Depression

Identification. Depression is characterized by a profoundly dysphoric or sad mood, often accompanied by a loss of interest in many activities and presence of at least five of the neurovegetative signs of depression, including depressed mood (Box 17-4). Major depression is considered to be a time-limited disorder, resolving in 9 to 36 months. Some cases may last longer, however, and become reclassified as dysthymia, an enduring depressive disorder. Given the high degree of overlap between depression and anxiety, a person with depression may score in the moderate range on several items of a dental fears index. In severe depression, dental hygiene may suffer, and the person's history may show long gaps between dental visits. Mild to moderate depression typically does not affect dental care seeking.

The current medications of choice for depression are the SSRIs, including fluoxetine (Prozac), sertraline, and paroxetine.[17] TCAs such as amitriptyline (Elavil), imipramine (Tofranil), doxepin (Sinequan), and desipramine (Norpramin) are still in widespread use. MAOIs such as

| Box 17-4 | Neurovegetative Signs of Depression* |

- Depressed mood
- Inability to experience pleasure or marked loss of interest in activities
- Appetite changes (increase or decrease)
- Weight change within past month (increase or decrease)
- Sleep disturbance (late onset, early awakening, or multiple awakenings)
- Psychomotor agitation or retardation
- Fatigue, loss of energy
- Feelings of worthlessness, excessive guilt
- Difficulty concentrating, indecisiveness
- Recurrent thoughts of death or of suicide

Modified from American Psychiatric Association: *Diagnostic and statistical manual of mental disorders*, ed 4, Washington, DC, 1994, The Association.
*At least five are present, including depressed mood, in clinically diagnosable depression.

tranylcypromine (Parnate) and phenelzine are still used, but much more rarely, and usually in the treatment of recalcitrant depression (Table 17-1).

The patient interview should uncover the extent to which depression has complicated dental care in the past, including periods in which the patient has not taken care of his or her teeth or has missed appointments. Special attention should be paid to the assessment of adverse reactions to medications.

Management. Patients with depression rarely pose an immediate safety threat in the dental operatory. The exception is an adverse drug interaction that can precipitate a cardiovascular crisis. These severe adverse reactions are unusual, however, particularly with the SSRIs. If the patient is being treated with an MAOI (e.g., phenelzine), however, neither epinephrine nor morphine should be used because of the possibility of triggering a hypertensive or hypotensive crisis.

The Suicidal Patient

The most significant threat presented by patients with depression is suicidal ideation. If a patient confides to the dentist that he or she is contemplating suicide, the dentist should assess the risk and be prepared to refer the patient to his or her therapist or to an appropriate care provider. Assessment of suicide risk includes determining whether the patient actually has *intent*

Table 17-1	Medications Used in Treatment of Depression	
Drug	Daily Adult Dose (mg)	Common Side Effects
SELECTIVE SEROTONIN REUPTAKE INHIBITORS		
Fluoxetine	20-80	Insomnia, tremor, anxiety, gastrointestinal complaints, reacts with ketorolac (Toradol)
Sertraline	50-200	Gastrointestinal complaints, insomnia, male sexual dysfunction
Paroxetine	10-50	Headache, sedation, dry mouth, insomnia, dizziness
Nefazodone	300-600	Dry mouth, nausea, somnolence, dizziness, blurred vision
Citalopram	20-40	Dry mouth, nausea, somnolence
TRICYCLICS/TETRACYCLICS		
Amitriptyline	150-300	Dry mouth/eyes, drowsiness, hypotension
Desipramine	75-200	Dry mouth/eyes, sedation, nausea/vomiting
Imipramine	150-300	Dry mouth/eyes, confusion, cardiovascular effects
Doxepin	25-75	Dry mouth/eyes, drowsiness, seizures
Trazodone	150-600	Dry mouth, drowsiness, hypotension
MONOAMINE OXIDASE INHIBITORS		
Phenelzine	45-90	Hypotension, drowsiness, dizziness, reactive with vasoactive agents (including epinephrine and morphine)
Tranylcypromine	30-60	Agitation, hypertension, headaches, reactive with vasoactive agents
NOVEL AGENTS		
Venlafaxine	37.5-225	Nausea, headache, insomnia

Modified from Janicak PG: *Handbook of psychopharmacotherapy,* Philadelphia, 1999, Lippincott–Williams & Wilkins.

to commit suicide and a *plan* by which to do it (Box 17-5). If the patient expresses no intent or plan, the risk is considered small, and the patient should be referred and seen by an appropriate mental health care provider at the earliest possible time. If the patient has both intent and a plan (e.g., a gun in the car, a bottle of medication, a length of rope), the dentist must try to contain the patient and contact someone to take charge of the person (e.g., significant other, therapist, hospital ED).

Bipolar Disorder

Identification. Bipolar disorder is characterized by the presence of mania or hypomania and usually a history of depression or a depressive episode. Mania is a mood disturbance featuring a distinct period of abnormally elevated, expansive, or irritable mood.[18] Hypomania also refers to elevated mood, but not so extreme as that seen in mania. Some patients with bipolar disorder have psychotic features. A patient in a manic episode may be agitated and constantly moving and thus difficult to treat.

No clear picture of a bipolar patient is likely to be revealed in a dental fears index. Likewise, a review of the dental history is unlikely to show evidence of bipolar disorder per se. The medical history, however, may show that the patient has had episodes of involuntary commitment or hospitalizations. Medications prescribed for bipolar disorder include lithium (usually lithium carbonate, 900 to 1800 mg/day), carbamazepine (600 to 1600 mg/day in divided doses), and occasionally antipsychotic medications, such as risperidone. If any of these medications is listed by the patient, the interview should focus on the degree of mania and the frequency of manic episodes. The dentist may also want to consult briefly with the patient's therapist or psychiatrist regarding control of mania and likelihood for disruption of care.

Management. If the patient is manic or hypomanic in the dental operatory, no attempt should be made to carry out dental treatment;

Box 17-5   Management of the Suicidal Patient in the Dental Office

STEP	SPECIFIC QUESTION/ACTION
I. Assess suicide risk.	
A. Is there intent?	"Do you think you could really go through with hurting yourself?"
B. Is there a plan?	"Have you thought about ways you would hurt yourself?"
II. Implement course of action.	
A. There is neither intent nor a plan.	Refer patient to mental health care provider, to be seen at earliest possible time.
B. There is intent, but no plan.	Arrange for patient to be seen by a mental health care provider the same day.
C. There is a plan, but no intent.	Urge patient to dispense with plan (e.g., get rid of pills, take rope out of car, give gun to police) and to see a mental health care provider as soon as possible.
D. There is both intent and a plan.	Keep the patient in the office if possible; phone patient's mental health care provider or family member to take charge of patient. If necessary, have patient taken to an emergency department by friends or family.

---

the restriction of patient movement necessitated by dental treatment may cause the manic episode to escalate. The dentist should be prepared to contact the patient's mental health care provider. If a manic episode does become violent, the dentist should not try to restrain the patient but should withdraw and call the police (see following section). Extreme manic episodes are very rare, however, and even those are seldom violent, and most bipolar patients are "normal" or average looking. The most significant consideration is a drug interaction with the medication being used to manage the disorder. Lithium alone may cause nausea and vomiting and may interact with nonsteroidal antiinflammatory drugs (NSAIDs), as may carbamazepine. The dentist should specifically question the patient on reactions to medications and, if applicable, should consult the patient's psychiatrist before prescribing medications.

VIOLENCE AND PSYCHOSIS
The Violent Patient

Several conditions can prompt violence or violent outbursts in patients. This violence may occur as part of a disease process (e.g., dementias), as a reaction to medication or to illicit drug use, or as a result of a combination of drugs and a vulnerability to violence caused by illness.

Identification.   Except when prompted by medications, most violent episodes are preceded by a period of increasing restlessness or pacing. Patients who clench their fists or jaws or who are verbally profane, belligerent, abusive, or threatening to others in the office are at high risk for being violent.[19] Little in a patient's history may indicate potential for violence; even a history of psychiatric hospitalization is not predictive of violence. The level of cooperation seen in completing paperwork, obtaining radiographs, or completing other administrative chores of the dental office, however, is predictive. If the patient angrily refuses to complete such tasks, violence is possible.

Management.   If a patient becomes violent in the dental office, the most important action for the dentist is to keep away from the patient. The dentist must try to be reassuring and to acknowledge the patient's state of mind; for example, "I can see that you're really upset. I'm truly sorry about that. But I think we can fix this." At times it may be helpful to offer the patient a drink of water and suggest that the patient sit down and talk over the problem. The most serious threat comes from the patient with weapons. If a patient admits to having a weapon, the dentist should not immediately ask for it but may ask the patient to keep it concealed or to put it down. The dentist might suggest that the patient give the weapon to the dentist later. Patients who have violent potential may be engaged in discussion (e.g., "Let's talk about what's upsetting you"), but patients who have become vio-

Box 17-6	"Dos and Don'ts" of Managing Violent Patients

"DO"

Anticipate possible violence from hostile, threatening, agitated, restless, or abusive patients or from those who appear to lack control for any reason.

Heed your "gut feeling." If you feel frightened or uneasy, discontinue treatment and get help.

Summon as much help (e.g., police, security guards) as you can find at the first sign of violence. Patients who see that you take them seriously often will not act out further. If they do, you will be prepared.

Ask if the patient is carrying a weapon. These must be surrendered to security personnel. Never treat an armed patient.

Offer help, food, and medication. Bolster patients by commenting on their strength and self-control.

If restraint becomes necessary, summon police as quickly a possible; always have assistance or wait for help to restrain a patient.

Keep constant watch on restrained patients.

Summon help if a patient states an intent to harm others, refuses to answer questions about intent to harm, or refuses to cooperate with treatment.

Notify the police of threatened violence, and remind them to warn potential victims.

Document everything.

"DON'T"

Don't see angry, threatening, or restless persons right away; have them wait so that their behavior may be observed outside the operatory.

Don't ignore your gut feeling that a patient may be dangerous.

Don't compromise your ability to escape a dangerous situation. Don't place yourself so that the dental chair or another person is between you and the door.

Don't antagonize the patient by responding angrily or being patronizing.

Don't touch or startle the patient or approach quickly without warning.

Don't try to restrain a patient single-handedly.

Don't bargain with a violent person about the need for others to help control the person.

Don't wait to see if a violent person will "just calm down."

Don't neglect any details of what a violent person may have said regarding threats to others.

Don't forget to secure witnesses for notes in chart.

Modified from Weissberg MP: *Dangerous secrets: maladaptive responses to stress,* New York, 1983, WW Norton.

lent must be handled by professionals (i.e., police, security guards).[20] "Dos and Don'ts" are important in managing violent patients (Box 17-6).

Psychotic Disorders

Identification. The term *psychotic* refers to a loss of contact with reality. Psychosis is most often seen in thought disorders such as schizophrenia. Psychotic symptoms, however, may occur in multiple medical, neurologic, and substance abuse disorders. Psychotic symptoms present as distorted cognitions, or delusions. Delusions may be paranoid or grandiose. With paranoid delusions, events are interpreted to have special personal meaning for the individual (e.g., messages heard on the car radio are directed specifically at the patient). Grandiose delusions have a theme of inflated worth or power. Psychotic symptoms frequently include a decline in social functioning, employment, and

self-care. The affect of a person with psychosis is often flat and unusually nonresponsive. Finally, hallucinations may accompany the other psychotic symptoms. Hallucinations refer to the sensing of things that are not really there. In schizophrenia, auditory hallucinations are common, and visual hallucinations are rare. Hallucinations in the other senses (olfactory, tactile, gustatory) most often have nonpsychotic, neurologic causes.

Responses on a dental fears index may be fairly sensible and ordinary if the person's symptoms are well controlled. If the person is floridly psychotic, however, the responses on the index are likely to appear very odd, with notes written in the margins, multiple responses, nonsense scribbling on the page, or no response at all. A review of medications may show a variety of drugs being used to control symptoms. Common medications for psychotic symptoms are the neuroleptic drugs, such as haloperidol or chlorpromazine. Increasingly, nonneuroleptic drugs are being used to manage psychotic symptoms, including clozapine, risperidone, olanzapine, and quetiapine, all of which have greater effects on the serotonergic system than do the neuroleptics. Other psychoactive drugs may be added to deal with specific additional symptoms, including benzodiazepines, antidepressants, or mood stabilizers (e.g., lithium, carbamazepine).

A review of the patient's history will show average dental care seeking until the time of onset of the psychotic disorder. Dental care seeking and dental hygiene are often the first aspects of self-care affected. There may be long periods between dental appointments. Severely disturbed patients will usually be in the care of a guardian or escort, who may have knowledge of the patient's condition. Those with psychotic disorders are typically poor historians, and thought disorder will impair a patient's ability to communicate. The dentist should confirm information about medications with the guardian and should ask about the nature of the patient's symptoms and how well they are controlled. The dentist should also contact the patient's psychiatrist.

Management. Most patients with psychotic disorders pose no threat in the operatory. The most serious consideration is dental drugs interacting with the patient's medications. The neuroleptics are sedating and may interact with both sedatives and amphetamines. Care should be taken if sedation is required, and the patient's psychiatrist should be consulted. Severely affected patients are best managed with the help of the patient's caregiver. It is likely that a psychotic patient would be ruled unable to give consent for treatment, so consent must be obtained from the patient's legal guardian. Patients who present on their own for dental work are presumed sound and able to give consent.

Even well-controlled psychotic patients may have difficulty coping with the dental environment. Delusional patients may be distrustful and may accuse the dentist of trying to attack or control them. These patients are manageable if the dentist proceeds slowly, explains procedures carefully as they come up, and asks the patient's permission to proceed. These patients cannot be "bullied" into treatment; a firm approach works poorly. Rather, they must be engaged in treatment. Although some may be distrustful, an approach of openness is likely to be most successful.

DELIRIUM AND DEMENTIAS

Several psychiatric conditions are associated with cognitive impairments that may significantly complicate dentistry. Dementia and delirium occur predominantly in elderly persons and are among the most common psychiatric disorders encountered in medical practice. Their incidence will continue to increase as the population ages.

Delirium

Identification. Delirium is generally an acute disorder characterized by an altered state of consciousness (e.g., hyperalert or obtunded, unfocused periods fluctuating with lucid periods). Onset of delirium is usually abrupt, and the cause is usually traced to medication side effects, intoxication or withdrawal, or metabolic abnormalities[21] (Box 17-7). A delirious patient in the operatory will frequently appear to be intoxicated. If administered, patient checklists will be incomplete or incorrectly completed. Words may be slurred and gait unsteady. The patient may suddenly become agitated and disruptive or even abusive. The administration of benzodiazepines in particular can result in behavioral disinhibition. It is important to distinguish delirium from intoxication by alcohol. An episode of

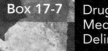

Box 17-7 Drug Classes and Specific Medications that May Cause Delirium

Antiarrhythmics/antidysrhythmics: lidocaine, mexilitene, quinidine
Anticholinergics: diphenhydramine
Anticonvulsants: beclamide, carbamazepine
Antihistamines: triprolidine
Antimigraine drugs: methysergide
Antineoplastic agents: asparaginase, methotrexate, vincristine, fluorouracil
Antivirals: acyclovir, interferon
Benzodiazepines: diazepam, lorazepam
β-Blockers: propranolol, atenolol
Corticosteroids: prednisone, dexamethasone
Dopamine agonists: L-dopa, bromocriptine, amantadine
Histamine receptor antagonists: cimetidine, ranitidine
Muscle relaxants: baclofen, cyclobenzaprine
Opiates: meperidine, pentazocine
Tricyclic antidepressants: amitriptyline, desipramine

MISCELLANEOUS
Aldehyde dehydrogenase inhibitor (alcohol deterrent): disulfiram
Antimalarials: quinidine

delirium often resolves completely with proper, timely treatment.

Management. The management of the patient with delirium primarily involves treating the underlying cause. The dentist often is not in a position to manage the delirious patient definitively. If a patient should become delirious in the operatory, the dentist should use personal judgment as to the best way to subdue the person; restraints may be necessary in some cases. The dentist should call the patient's primary physician, then an ambulance. If the cause of the delirium is unknown, antipsychotic agents, particularly haloperidol, may be administered orally or intramuscularly to help control the patient's behavior.

Dementia

Identification. An estimated 6% of the U.S. population over age 65 have a dementia syndrome; about half of these have Alzheimer's disease.[22] Dementia is a deterioration of multiple cognitive functions, although consciousness and alertness are unimpaired. The cardinal feature of dementia is impaired memory, both long term and short term. Judgment and ability to plan may also be affected. Noncognitive disorders may also occur, including disorders of mood, perception, belief, and behavior. A sustained depressive syndrome accompanies dementia in 10% to 60% of patients, depending on the type.[23] Pathologic laughing or crying may occur. Irritability and explosiveness may also be part of a given patient's profile, particularly after task failure. Those in the early stages of dementia will be noticeable only because of memory lapses and occasional bouts of frustrated anger. Nothing in a normal screening protocol can reveal early dementia. Patients in later stages of dementia almost always are accompanied to the dentist's office by a caregiver.

Management. Unlike the psychotic person, who seldom poses a risk to the dentist, the delirious patient and the patient suffering from dementia can present significant physical risks in terms of disruptive behavior and even physical attacks on the dentist and staff. In patients with dementia, excessive emotional outbursts after task failure or memory lapse can be avoided by not challenging the patient and by providing support. Memory lapses should not be exposed or confronted. For example, a patient may state that he does not have his dentures with him because they have been "stolen." The dentist should sympathize with the patient's plight and express hope that the stolen dentures may later

be recovered with the caregiver's help. Given the memory lapses of patients with dementia, all instructions for dental care should be written out for both the patient and the caregiver.

DEVELOPMENTAL DISABILITIES

Identification. A variety of developmental disabilities may be seen in the dental office. They range in severity of impairment from severe autism to the mild retardation sometimes seen in Down syndrome. Autism occurs in about 1 of every 10,000 live births. Down syndrome occurs about 10 times as often, or about 10.2 cases per 10,000 live births.[24] In autism, all aspects of functioning may be affected, including social behavior, self-care, language, and intellectual functioning. In other developmental delays the primary area of impairment is intellectual functioning, although social behavior may also be erratic or inappropriate in fetal alcohol syndrome and in attention deficit disorder.

Although developmental delays are often thought of as affecting children, the life span of these children is normal or close to normal for the population. Therefore significant numbers of developmentally disabled adults also are seeking dental care. Highly functioning individuals often have no difficulty with dentistry. Seriously affected adults and children, however, may be quite afraid of dentistry. Although an anxiety checklist may not be completed, the patient will often readily admit to feeling uncomfortable at the dentist's office. Developmentally disabled individuals present few serious problems for the dentist but may be uncooperative. In adults this lack of cooperation may become problematic, even violent.

Management. In profoundly impaired individuals it may be necessary to use sedation to immobilize the patient. This is preferable to the use of restraints and papoose boards, which, although often effective, may simply retraumatize the patient at each dental visit. If present, the caretaker should be included in discussions of treatment to explain the dental plan to the patient later. The dentist therefore becomes a trusted partner with the patient and the caregiver. Dentists should avoid "tricks" and deceptions intended to accomplish limited goals (e.g., promising a patient that an injection will not hurt at all). The dentist must ascertain beforehand if an impaired adult has a history of acting out aggressively with the physician or dentist. If so, the dentist should ask the caregiver the best means to manage the person, such as conscious sedation. Nitrous oxide may be used, but many intellectually or developmentally impaired adults have a fear of the nasal hood used with nitrous oxide. Some individuals may be taking medication, including methylphenidate for attention deficits or phenobarbital, phenytoin (Dilantin), or divalproex (Depakote) for seizures. The medication should be taken before the dentistry begins to aid in concentration and cooperativeness and reduce the risk of complications. If the patient becomes agitated, all work must be stopped and the patient reassured. If the patient becomes violent, the dentist must withdraw (see The Violent Patient).

ALCOHOL AND DRUG INTOXICATION AND WITHDRAWAL
Intoxication

The history or a checklist may offer little to indicate that a particular patient is abusing drugs or is presenting to the dentist in a state of intoxication or withdrawal. A patient under the influence of drugs or alcohol may have difficulty concentrating, slurred speech, glassy eyes or unfocused gaze, and lack of coordination. Alcohol is the most dangerous and unpredictable of the drugs of abuse seen in dentistry. Those intoxicated with alcohol may display affective lability, ranging from bouts of crying to overt belligerence and even violence. Extreme agitation, hallucinations, and delusions are also seen in intoxication from cocaine, amphetamines, or phencyclidine (PCP). In cocaine intoxication, hallucinations, paranoid delusions, and aggressive behavior may develop, and the person may become dangerous. The patient's pupils become dilated, and the drug's sympathomimetic effect increases heart rate, respirations, and blood pressure (Table 17-2).

Withdrawal

Alcohol withdrawal usually begins 12 to 48 hours after cessation of drinking. The typical withdrawal syndrome includes tremor, weakness, sweating, irritability, and gastrointestinal disturbances. Some patients have generalized seizures, and all patients in alcohol withdrawal have lowered seizure threshold.[25] The withdrawal syndrome from an opioid generally includes symptoms and signs of central nervous system hyperactivity, including sweating, tremor, and nausea. Severity of the syndrome increases with the size of the opioid dose and the duration of dependence. Symptoms appear as early as 4 to 6 hours after withdrawal and, for heroin, peak within 36 to 72 hours. Also present are marked anxiety and a craving for the drug.

Differential Diagnosis

Intoxication and withdrawal from drugs or alcohol are serious medical concerns, but the signs and symptoms are not unique. A variety of medical conditions can appear similar to those from drugs. Hypoxia induced for any reason (e.g., pulmonary embolus, coronary insufficiency, stroke) will appear exactly like alcohol intoxication. Likewise, apparent withdrawal symptoms may actually be symptoms of a medical problem (e.g., diabetic crisis, seizure disorder) or a result of overdosage of prescribed medication.

Management

If drug or alcohol intoxication or withdrawal is suspected, the dentist should try to rule out other causes, such as symptoms stemming from a medical condition or from a prescribed medication. The patient must be asked again about their medications, and vital signs should be taken. If a patient admits to using a drug or to drinking alcohol, the times of ingestion and the amounts taken should be noted. The dentist must be careful to avoid appearing judgmental or critical; this can trigger belligerence or violence in some patients. *Under no circumstances should the dentist attempt any procedure, nor should the patient be allowed to leave the office.* In cases of mild alcohol intoxication, the patient may be seated in the waiting room (under supervision) until blood alcohol declines to safe levels (at least 2 hours). If a patient refuses to wait, efforts should be made to call a family member or friend who can take the patient home or to a hospital emergency department if signs of withdrawal appear. If a patient shows any sign of violence, the dentist and staff should withdraw; no attempt should be made to restrain a patient unless an overt attack is made (see The Violent Patient). Any patient who appears in the dentist's office intoxicated should be given a referral for substance abuse treatment.

EATING DISORDERS
Anorexia Nervosa

Anorexia nervosa is characterized by a disturbed sense of body image, a morbid fear of obesity, a refusal to maintain a minimally normal body weight, and in advanced cases in women, amenorrhea. Anorexia may be mild and transient or severe and long-standing. About 95% of persons

Table 17-2	Signs of Intoxication and Withdrawal with Selected Drugs of Abuse	
Drug	**Intoxication**	**Withdrawal**
Alcohol	Difficulty concentrating Slurred, indistinct speech Ataxia, lack of coordination Glassy eyes Difficulty focusing or holding gaze Affective lability Potential for violence	Tremor Weakness Sweating Irritability Gastrointestinal disturbance
Cocaine	Dilated pupils Dry mouth Increased heart rate and blood pressure Agitation Hallucinations Delusions Aggressive behavior Potential for violence	Somnolence Agitation Hallucinations Delusions
Opiates	Pinpoint pupils Euphoria Flushing Itching (particularly with morphine) Drowsiness Hypotension	Sweating Tremor Nausea Anxiety Drug craving Yawning Muscle twitching Hot and cold flashes Complaints of aching muscles
Amphetamines	Dilated pupils Dry mouth Agitation Aggressive behavior Potential for violence	Somnolence Agitation Hallucinations Delusions
Phencyclidine	Euphoria with low doses Anxiety or mood lability Catatonia or ataxia in high doses Excessive salivation Unusual nystagmus Risk of coma, convulsions	Somnolence Agitation Hallucinations Delusions Prolonged psychotic states

with this disorder are female. Onset usually occurs during adolescence, occasionally earlier, and less often in adulthood. Mortality rates of 7% to 20% have been reported.[26] Patients have no characteristic attitude toward dentistry and are average in dental care seeking. However, because of the tendency to deny the disorder and to avoid confrontations over their weight, they likely have avoided seeing a physician. Therefore the dentist is often in the best position to detect severe eating disorders. Scores on screening instruments (e.g., DES) are likely to be in the normal range. Similarly, review of the dental history and medication use is unlikely to yield abnormal findings, in part because patients will not reveal use of emetics or laxatives that may be used to restrict weight gain. The most obvious sign is emaciation, which may be noticed by a dentist who sees a patient on a regular basis over many years. Other indicators include bradycardia, low blood pressure, hypothermia, and edema. Emaciation can reach the point of cachexia, but even then the patient's overall health may be remarkably good. Depressive symptoms and clinical depression are common. In advanced cases, heart rhythm abnormalities may be noted, and dehydration will be evident.

Bulimia

Bulimia is characterized by recurrent episodes of binge eating followed by purging. Bulimics may also use laxatives or diuretics, vigorous exercise, or fasting in an effort to compensate for eating binges. Bulimic patients are aware of their abnormal eating pattern, feel a lack of control over eating behavior, are overly concerned with body weight, and have depressed mood accompanied by self-deprecating statements. Bulimics may never become as emaciated as anorectics, and the mortality rates from bulimia are much lower. Dentists are often the first to detect bulimia because of the erosion of the enamel of the front teeth or evidence of acid etching on the lingual surfaces of the teeth, which results from repeated vomiting. Painless salivary gland enlargement may also occur.

Management

If an eating disorder is suspected, the dentist should be diligent about taking vital signs and should contact the patient's physician at the earliest opportunity. If the patient is a minor, the dentist should inform the parents. On occasion an adolescent patient with bulimia may be persuaded to discuss the problem with parents or counselors. Typically, however, a patient with an eating disorder, especially anorexia, will deny that anything is wrong and will express resentment. The dentist's only course is to suggest that the patient may want to seek advice or counseling from an eating disorders program. The dentist should be prepared to refer to a specific program or individual. Although patients with eating disorders present no threat of disruption in the dental office, the patient's physical condition may be precarious, depending on the degree of the condition. Any sedation or surgical procedure should be carefully considered and monitored.

SUMMARY

Various psychiatric problems can arise in the dental office. If quickly identified and handled properly, these situations and conditions will never become psychiatric emergencies. As the diversity of the dental patient population increases, the dentist should consider instituting systematic procedures for assessing and planning for the behavioral and psychological aspects of their patients as well as the medical and dental aspects.

REFERENCES

1. Goldberg D, Blackwell B: Psychiatric illness in general practice: a detailed study using a new method of case identification, Br Med J 2:439-443, 1970.
2. Kerwick S, Jones R, Mann A, Goldberg D: Mental health care training priorities in general practice, Br J Gen Pract 47:225-227, 1997.
3. Litt MD: The Dental Experience Survey: a screening instrument for dental anxiety for use in the dental clinic, Farmington, Conn, 1994, University of Connecticut School of Dental Medicine.
4. Milgrom P, Weinstein P, Kleinknecht R, Getz T: Treating fearful dental patients. In A patient management handbook, Reston, Va, 1985, Prentice-Hall.
5. Hakeberg M, Berggren U, Carlson SG: Prevalence of dental anxiety in an adult population in a major urban area in Sweden, Community Dent Oral Epidemiol 20:97-101, 1992.
6. Locker D, Shapiro D, Liddell A: Who is dentally anxious? Concordance between measures of dental anxiety, Community Dent Oral Epidemiol 24:346-350, 1996.
7. Vassend O: Anxiety, pain and discomfort associated with dental treatment, Behav Res Ther 31:659-666, 1993.
8. Klepac RK, Dowling J, Hauge G: Characteristics of clients seeking therapy for the reduction of dental avoidance: reactions to pain, J Behav Ther Exp Psychiatry 13:293-300, 1982.
9. Kleinknecht R, Bernstein D: The assessment of dental fear, Behav Ther 9:626-634, 1978.
10. Milgrom P, Fiset L, Melnick S, Weinstein P: The prevalence and practice management consequences of dental fear in a major U.S. city, J Am Dent Assoc 116:641-647, 1988.
11. Mackenzie R: Psychodynamics of pain, J Oral Med 23:75-83, 1968.
12. Kleinknecht RA, Klepac RK, Alexander LD: Origins and characteristics of fear of dentistry, J Am Dent Assoc 86:842-848, 1973.
13. Litt MD, Nye C, Shafer D: Preparing for oral surgery: evaluating elements of coping, J Behav Med 18:435-459, 1995.
14. Stoudemire A: Clinical psychiatry for medical students, ed 3, Philadelphia, 1998, Lippincott-Raven.
15. Echeverria JJ, Lasa I, Ramon BJ: Compulsive brushing in an adolescent patient: case report, Pediatr Dent 16:443-445, 1994.
16. Kessler RC, McGonagle KA, Zhao S, et al: Lifetime and 12-month prevalence of DSM-III-R psychiatric disorders in the United States, Arch Gen Psychiatry 51:8-18, 1994.
17. Janicak PG: Handbook of psychopharmacotherapy, Philadelphia, 1999, Lippincott–Williams & Wilkins.
18. American Psychiatric Association: Diagnostic and statistical manual of mental disorders, ed 4, Washington, DC, 1994, The Association.
19. Lion JR: Evaluation and management of the violent patient, Springfield, Ill, 1972, Thomas.
20. Dwyer B, Weissberg M: Treating violent patients, Psychiatr Times, December 1998, p 11.
21. Trzepacz P: Delirium: advances in diagnosis, pathophysiology, and treatment, Psychiatr Clin North Am 19:429-448, 1996.
22. Rocca WA, Amaducci LA, Schoenberg BS: Epidemiology of clinically diagnosed AD, Ann Neurol 19:415-424, 1986.
23. Rovner BW, Kafonek S, Filipp L, et al: Prevalence of mental illness in a community nursing home, Am J Psychiatry 143:1446-1449, 1986.
24. Olsen CL, Cross PK, Gensburg LJ, Hughes JP: The effects of prenatal diagnosis, population aging, and changing fertility rates on the live birth prevalence of Down syndrome in New York State, 1983-1992, Prenat Diagn 16:991-1002, 1996.
25. Greenblatt DJ, Shader RI: Treatment of the alcohol withdrawal syndrome. In Shader RI, editor: A manual of psychiatric therapeutics, Boston, 1977, Little, Brown.
26. Crow S, Praus B, Thuras P: Mortality from eating disorders: a 5- to 10-year record linkage study, Int J Eat Disord 26:97-101, 1999.

Nausea, Vomiting, and Abdominal Pain

Alan L. Felsenfeld
Earl G. Freymiller

Manifestations of gastrointestinal (GI) disorders are frequently seen as part of dental disease or in concert with dental treatment. In addition, patients may present with a history of GI distress or develop acute problems during dental therapy. GI diseases have a definite impact on dental patients and treatment. The two most likely problems that will be encountered in the dental office are nausea and vomiting and acute abdominal pain.

NAUSEA AND VOMITING

Nausea and vomiting are not diseases but rather signs and symptoms of underlying maladies or disorders that manifest through GI malfunction. The implications for dental treatment mandate consideration of nausea and vomiting in the dental office. The problems associated with nausea and vomiting are best understood if nausea and vomiting is divided into two forms, acute and chronic.

In the *acute* form, nausea and vomiting is a manifestation of a reactive process to a noxious stimulus. This is a protective mechanism for ingested toxins, as in bacterial food poisoning. Nausea and vomiting can also occur with vestibular stimulation (e.g., motion sickness) and in inflammatory processes that affect the bowel (e.g., obstruction, peritonitis). In dental offices, nausea and vomiting (1) may be a manifestation of psychogenic stimuli, (2) may occur as an adverse effect associated with medications (e.g., opioids, nitrous oxide), or (3) may be associated with a gastric irritant (e.g., swallowed blood).

The *chronic* form of nausea and vomiting is more likely to relate to an underlying GI disorder that affects gastric motility. Patients with diabetes or idiopathic gastroparesis tend to have increased nausea and vomiting.

Epidemiology

The incidence of nausea and vomiting is diverse for different patient populations and difficult to predict. Nausea and vomiting associated with dental procedures depends on the general status of the patient, including stress level (manifest or occult); the dental procedures performed; and the anesthetic techniques used.

Although a specific incidence rate for nausea and vomiting cannot be determined, certain groups of patients are more susceptible (Box 18-1). Women, young children, obese patients, and those with a full stomach are more likely to develop nausea and vomiting in the dental office. Similarly, patients with gastroparesis, gastrointestinal reflux disease (GERD), pregnancy, history of motion sickness, and high stress levels are at risk for this problem.[1] Dental procedures that tend to produce bleeding with the potential for swallowing blood are more likely to cause nausea and vomiting. If large amounts of irrigation are not suctioned carefully, the potential for problems increases.

Finally, although their use is designed to minimize the stresses and potential for nausea and vomiting, anesthetic and sedative medications may cause intraoperative and postoperative nausea and vomiting.

Etiology

The precise etiology for nausea and vomiting is not always known, although it can be caused by a number of events in many cases. Nausea and vomiting can be mediated by central, peripheral, and local factors. This reactive process that rids the body of locally ingested toxins (e.g., microorganisms in food poisoning) does not explain the reason for nausea and vomiting in patients who receive chemotherapeutic medications, radiation therapy or L-

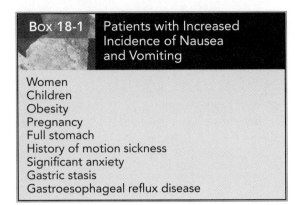

Box 18-1 Patients with Increased Incidence of Nausea and Vomiting

Women
Children
Obesity
Pregnancy
Full stomach
History of motion sickness
Significant anxiety
Gastric stasis
Gastroesophageal reflux disease

dopa. Additional *local* factors include gastric outlet obstruction, gastric stasis, and gastric irritation from noxious chemicals.[2]

Peripheral causes of nausea and vomiting are seen in pregnant patients and in those with significant liver disease, metabolic derangements, or motion sickness. *Central* etiology of nausea and vomiting includes such disorders as increased intracranial pressure. Vagal stimulation produces vomiting as well as bradycardia, hypersalivation, reverse peristalsis of the small intestine, and the urge to defecate.[2] Stimulation of the auricular branch of the vagus nerve (Arnold's nerve) and stimulation of ventricular cardiac afferents also lead to dental office nausea and vomiting.[3]

Other diverse sources of nausea and vomiting include bad tastes or smells associated with the dental office. Stimulation of pharyngeal afferent nerves is a critical cause in dental offices. Pharyngeal stimulation or suctioning and injection of local anesthetic medications, which may alter the sensation of the pharyngeal area, may contribute to emesis in the office. Anxiety, with or without aerophagia (swallowing air), may exacerbate nausea. Anesthetic and sedative medications intended to minimize the anxiety may contribute to nausea. If general anesthetic or sedation agents are used during the dental procedure, the depth of anesthesia, class of agents, and duration of the anesthetic all influence the possibility of postoperative nausea and vomiting. Nitrous oxide has the therapeutic effect of calming patients by its sedative properties and thereby reducing psychogenic incidents of nausea and vomiting. In doses greater than 40%, however, nitrous oxide can create paradoxical nausea and vomiting in many patients. Presence of food in the stomach may contribute to nausea, especially with anesthetic, sedative, and opioid medications, but the lack of food associated with a prolonged wakeful fast may lead to nausea as well.

In the immediate postoperative period, other factors can create nausea and vomiting in the dental patient. Inadequate pain control, the use of narcotic medications and swallowing of blood are most likely precipitants of the problem. Premature movement with attendant dizziness or ingestion of significant quantities of fluids in the immediate postoperative period may also contribute to nausea and vomiting.

Pathophysiology and Anatomic Considerations

Anatomic and physiologic factors contribute to the process of nausea and vomiting. Wang and Borison[4] described the original pathways in 1952. They noted that the site where humoral substances act in the brain is separate from the motor mechanism, making nausea and vomiting a complex interaction of neural pathways. Both humoral and peripheral afferents feed the central areas.

Multiple anatomic areas of the body centrally and peripherally are involved in the process of nausea and vomiting. Central receptors include the chemoreceptor trigger zone and the vomiting center. Peripherally, receptors within the gastric mucosa, when stimulated, send impulses via vagal afferents to the brain to initiate the nausea and vomiting process.[5] The physiologic relationship between the afferent and efferent areas is complex, but simplified for this discussion.

Chemoreceptor Trigger Zone

The chemoreceptor trigger zone (CTZ) is located in the *area postrema* adjacent to the vomiting center, serving as the receptor for afferent stimuli in the nausea and vomiting process.[6] The CTZ is unique in that it lies outside the blood-brain barrier, thus sensing potential toxins. It is rich in dopamine, serotonin, acetylcholine, and opioid receptors, which activate the vomiting center when stimulated. Some drugs that precipitate nausea and vomiting act centrally in the CTZ as well as peripherally in the GI tract.

Different types of stimuli can precipitate nausea and vomiting. Abdominal organ nerve endings respond to intraabdominal stimuli such as distention, infection, toxins, irritation, and inflammation. They send impulses to the vomiting center by parasympathetic and sympathetic fibers. Local nociceptors, chemoreceptors, and mechanoreceptors in the gut use afferent pathways via the vagus nerve and spinal dorsal root ganglia. Vagal afferent input summates in the dorsal motor nucleus of the vagus.[6]

In addition, the central nervous system has receptors that respond to input from the vestibular apparatus. Cerebellar areas and cerebral cortical areas respond to sensory input (e.g., taste, smell) as well as higher brainstem input. One of the most recently identified mediators of nausea and vomiting is *5-hydroxytryptamine* (serotonin, 5-HT, 5-HT$_3$), which is known to act peripheral to the brain, especially in the stomach, as well as centrally at the CTZ.[6]

Vomiting Center

The vomiting center is located in the lateral reticular formation of the medulla oblongata. It receives input primarily from the vestibular apparatus, higher brainstem, and cortical structures, with peripheral input from the GI tract, heart, and in men, testes. Most attention focuses on CTZ activation from stimuli delivered through blood or cerebrospinal fluid, but multiple sources of stimulation exist for the vomiting center.[7]

Three Phases

Nausea and vomiting can be subdivided into three phases.[2] The *preexcitation phase* is the prodromal feeling of nausea without active GI discharge. The patient has gastric relaxation, retroperistalsis, and hypersalivation, with vasomotor and behavioral changes that produce the short-term or long-term feeling of nausea.

As the problem progresses to the second phase, the patient experiences *retching*, which is the spasmodic contraction of the upper GI tract diaphragm, intercostal muscles, and abdomen against the resistance of the closed glottis. At this time, gastric contents can ascend into the esophagus from the stomach. This is frequently associated with excessive salivation, frequent swallowing, dizziness, pallor, and sweating. Gastric cramping and burping (eructation) may be seen as well.

The final stage is the *vomiting* or *ejection phase*, with the rapid projection of gastric contents up through the esophagus and out the mouth and nose. Abdominal and respiratory muscles are the most active propulsive agents; the stomach has a lesser role in the process. Increased intraabdominal pressures are mediated by the abdominal musculature and diaphragm. The fundus and lower esophageal (cardiac) sphincter lose tone, and the abdominal muscles spastically contract to propel gastric contents upward. Vomiting may be of short or long duration or may occur in waves. After ejection the patient

may have generalized muscle weakness, shivering, and lethargy.[2]

Treatment

It is axiomatic to suggest that the treatment of nausea and vomiting should be dictated by defining the etiology. The use of "shotgun cures" without a specific diagnosis reflects an ease of treatment rather than a lack of desire to identify the cause. From a practical standpoint, the practitioner needs to become familiar with a few medications useful in the management of this annoying problem for both patient and physician.

As with the treatment of malignancies, GERD or other GI disorders with reflux, and adverse reactions to long-term medications with gastric side effects, *chronic* nausea and vomiting generally does not fall within the purview of the dentist and is best left to the skill of the treating physician. Because of the classic signs of enamel erosion and gingival hyperemia, however, the dentist is ideally suited to identify the bulimic patient. The metabolic abnormalities associated with bulimia can have significant adverse effects. Additionally, for patients with hiatal hernias or GERD, positioning in the dental chair may be problematic. These patients may tolerate other positions better than the supine position and may need to be treated with the head elevated.

However, the dentist must address *acute* nausea and vomiting that results from dental procedures or related therapies. The problem may be best assessed as a pretreatment, intraoperative, or posttreatment event.

Prevention

Patients who exhibit significant signs of stress in the dental office are more likely to have acute nausea and vomiting as a sign of their fears. If these people can be identified early, the practitioner can take precautions to prevent undue problems for the patient. For example, for some form of sedation may be inherently a good approach to manage the very anxious patient.

Nitrous oxide should be considered to relieve stress. Alternatively, an oral benzodiazepine might be more beneficial. Benzodiazepines are excellent at allaying preoperative fears and have inherent antiemetic properties as well. Similarly, steroids are frequently administered to minimize postoperative swelling and also have antiemetic effects. Pain can precipitate postoperative nausea and vomiting. In procedures associated with significant levels of postoperative pain, long-acting local anesthetics decrease not only the sympathetic stimulation that may contribute to nausea and vomiting, but also the amount of pain medication needed, thus minimizing opioid-induced nausea and vomiting.

For the occasional patient who is resistant, or when these regimens fail, the practitioner should consider parenteral sedation or even general anesthesia.

Management Considerations

Nausea and vomiting during a procedure in the office is uncomfortable for the patient, staff and dentist. In the conscious dental patient, however, it is unusual for untoward sequelae to result from a patient vomiting. Sitting these patients up with a receptacle and allowing for the spontaneous termination of the event are sufficient in the vast majority of incidents. Once a patient vomits, a secondary episode will likely occur soon.

Intraoperative vomiting in obtunded or sedated patients is of greater concern. This subset of dental patients may not have full control of their protective pharyngeal and laryngeal reflexes, resulting in aspiration of the regurgitated gastric contents and making emesis a potentially life-threatening event. The increase in thoracic pressure that occurs during ejection of gastric contents is somewhat protective and prevents immediate aspiration of the contents into the lungs. Thus the clinician can minimize a significant complication but must be aggressive in the management of acute vomiting. The patient needs to be turned to the right side and placed in the Trendelenburg position. This allows the effluent to come out the mouth and, if impossible to prevent aspiration, preferentially allows the aspirate to enter the right lung, thus sparing the left lung. High-volume suction of the oropharynx with large-bore suction tubes (Yankauer tips) is important. Positive-pressure ventilation is contraindicated until the pharynx is cleared of the vomitus. Airway irritability, as manifested by cough, suggests aspiration. If the patient may have aspirated gastric contents, paramedic-assisted transfer to the hospital should be considered.

Fortunately for the patient, most acute post-treatment nausea and vomiting is brief and resolves spontaneously without significant medical intervention. For the patient with acute nausea and vomiting the practitioner must consider the effects of prescribed medications as the cause, such as narcotics for postoperative pain.

Codeine preparations frequently cause nausea and vomiting in susceptible patients. Although the use of nonsteroidal antiinflammatory drugs (NSAIDs) such as ibuprofen can cause some gastric upset, their role in nausea and vomiting is significantly less than the classic opioid medications and should be considered for analgesia in patients at risk. In addition, antibiotics can cause stomach upset and lead to nausea and vomiting. Aspirin compounds have similar effects. Patients who have had intraoral surgery may swallow blood, which irritates the gastric mucosa and causes nausea and vomiting. In patients who receive general anesthesia or intravenous (IV) sedation, the long-term effects of the anesthetic agents may result in gastric upset with nausea and vomiting.

In the simplest case, time may be the best medicine for most dentally related nausea and vomiting. The dentist may discontinue the potential etiologic agent (e.g., postoperative opioid) and allow sufficient time for the spontaneous diminution of the symptoms, recommending a bland, liquid diet. Pharmacies have numerous over-the-counter (OTC) medications for these purposes, and dentists should become familiar with one or two to recommend for patients (Table 18-1). These drugs, however, are administered orally. Since the patient is significantly nauseous or vomiting, it may be counterproductive to use a medication that depends on gastric absorption for uptake.

If the nausea and vomiting level is significant or the OTC medications are ineffective, the practitioner or patient may consider a prescription medication. The dentist must also consider an alternative route of delivery, such as rectal or intramuscular (IM) administration.

Antiemetic Medications

Pharmacologic management of nausea and vomiting has been developing in many areas over the last 50 years. Various stimuli for nausea and vomiting act in diverse ways and in different parts of the body. Therefore the pharmacologic management of these symptoms has variable effectiveness, depending on the etiology of nausea and vomiting. For example, medications that are efficacious in controlling drug-induced (cytotoxic) nausea and vomiting may not affect motion-induced nausea and vomiting.[4] The astute clinician will pinpoint the etiology of the problem and use antiemetic therapies designed to work at the sites of action. Regrettably, this is not the usual case because

Table 18-1 Over-the-Counter Antiemetic Medications

Drug	Manufacturer	Active Ingredient	Form
Cola	Unico	Phosphoric acid, corn syrup, sucrose	Syrup
Emecheck	Savage Labs	Phosphoric acid, dextrose, levulose	Liquid
Emetrol	Pharmacia, Upjohn	Phosphoric acid, dextrose, fructuose	Liquid
Nauzene	Alva-Amco Pharmacal	Diphenhydramine	Tablet
Rekematol Anti-Nausea	Reese Chemical	Phosphoric acid, dextrose, levulose	Liquid

From *Nonprescription products: formulations and features*, '97-98, Washington, DC, 1997, American Pharmaceutical Association.

Table 18-2 Classes of Antiemetic Drugs

Drug Class	Specific Agents	Site of Action
Phenothiazines	Prochlorperazine Thiethylperazine Promethazine Chlorpromazine	CTZ
Benzodiazepines	Lorazepam	Cerebral cortex, CTZ
Butyrophenones	Droperidol Haloperidol	CTZ
Antihistamines	Diphenhydramine Meclizine Dimenhydrinate	Gastrointestinal vestibular center, CTZ
Cannabinoids	Dronabinol Tetrahydrocannabinol	Cerebral cortex, CTZ
Prokinetics	Metoclopramide	Gastrointestinal, CTZ
5-Hydroxytryptamine (serotonin) receptor antagonists	Ondansetron Granisetron Dolasetron	Gastrointestinal, cerebral cortex, CTZ

CTZ, Chemoreceptor trigger zone.

clinicians tend to use the same drugs to treat nausea and vomiting regardless of the cause. Consequently the effectiveness of these drugs will vary with the patient. Table 18-2 and Boxes 18-2 and 18-3 summarize antiemetic medications by class, site of action, and indication.

Phenothiazines. The phenothiazines are prototypical drugs used to assist in the management of nausea and vomiting. Classically they are antipsychotic medications but also exhibit antiemetic properties by their antidopaminergic effect.[8] They act by blocking the postsynaptic mesolimbic dopaminergic receptors in the brain. Their use in chemotherapy-induced nausea and vomiting is not as widely accepted as in postoperative nausea and vomiting.[6,9] Additional antiemetic action is related to depression of the reticular activating system. Phenothiazines have a strong α-adrenergic blocking effect, which can lead to significant hypotension.

Prochlorperazine (Compazine) is the most popular of the phenothiazines. Other medications in this family include promethazine, perphenazine and loxapine. Various forms of these medications exist for oral, rectal, and IM administration.

A significant problem associated with phenothiazines is extrapyramidal effects. The patient with *tardive dyskinesia* undergoes muscle spasms with seizurelike contortions. Treatment with antihistamines (e.g., diphenhydramine) is successful,

Box 18-2	Sites of Action for Antiemetic Drugs

SITE OF ACTION	DRUG CLASS
Cerebral cortex	Benzodiazepines
	Phenothiazines
	Butyrophenones
	Cannabinoids
	5-Hydroxytryptamine (serotonin) antagonists
	Prokinetics
Gastrointestinal	Prokinetics
	Serotonin antagonists
	Steroids
	Anticholinergics
Vestibular apparatus	Anticholinergics
	Antihistamines
Chemoreceptor trigger zone (CTZ)	Benzodiazepines
	Phenothiazines
	Anticholinergics
	Antihistamines
	Prokinetics
	Serotonin antagonists
	Cannabinoids
	Steroids
Vomiting center	Phenothiazines
	Antihistamines
	Anticholinergics

Box 18-3	Indications for Antiemetic Drugs

INDICATION	DRUG CLASS
Motion sickness	Anticholinergics
	Antihistamines
Anticipatory nausea	Benzodiazepines
	Antihistamines
Chemotherapy-induced emesis	Phenothiazines
	Prokinetics
	Butyrophenones
	Cannabinoids
	5-Hydroxytryptamine (serotonin) antagonists
Postoperative sequelae	Butyrophenones
	Phenothiazines
	Prokinetics
	Antihistamines
	5-Hydroxytryptamine (serotonin) antagonists

but patients with tardive dyskinesia are reluctant to use this class of drugs.

Antihistamines. The use of antihistamines in the prevention and treatment of nausea and vomiting is well established. Primarily noted for their use in acute or chronic allergies, many of these drugs have an antiemetic side effect. Antihistamines work at the H_1 receptors and inhibit stimulation of the vomiting center by the vestibular center.[10]

Diphenhydramine (Benadryl), promethazine (Phenergan, a phenothiazine derivative with antihistamine properties), and hydroxyzine (Atarax, Vistaril) are classic examples of this class of drugs. These medications also possess a sedative effect that may aid in the prevention of psychologically induced nausea and vomiting. Antihistamines may be bundled with narcotics for IM injections in pain management to alleviate the nausea and vomiting that often occurs with opioid medications.

Other antihistamines are used for *motion sickness*, such as cyclizine, a piperazine derivative that acts on the labyrinthine apparatus and the CTZ. Other medications useful for motion sickness and vertigo but do not help with postoperative nausea and vomiting are meclizine, buclizine, thiethylperazine, and dimenhydrinate.

Prokinetics. The primary action of the prokinetic class of antiemetics is blocking dopamine receptors in the CTZ. Secondary actions of prokinetics are tightening the cardiac sphincter and emptying the stomach more rapidly than normal by enhancing the response to acetylcholine in the GI tract. Although the secondary function is not a truly antiemetic effect, the evacuation of gastric contents will minimize the amount of vomitus in some patients. Prokinetic drugs can be used prophylactically to prevent aspiration of gastric contents (in select patients) under sedation and anesthesia but have a short duration of action and do not provide long-term relief of nausea. A classic prokinetic is metoclopramide (Reglan).[6]

5-Hydroxytryptamine (serotonin) blockers. The 5-HT₃ blockers are a newer drug class aimed at the treatment of nausea and vomiting. They were developed for chemotherapy but there is widespread use of these drugs in the management of postoperative nausea and vomiting in patients that are refractory to routine antiemetic treatment.[10] The sites of action are the serotonin receptors located in the CTZ and cerebral cortex, limbic system and autonomic neurons of the vagus nerves. Recent literature supports the concept of combination of a serotonin receptor antagonist with other antiemetics such as steroids to enhance the efficacy of effect.[11]

The 5-HT₃ blockers are extremely expensive; health care facilities save them for use when more conventional and less expensive therapies are ineffective. Granisetron (Kytril) and ondansetron (Zofran) are the original drugs of this group and have equivalent efficacy. Similarly effective but less expensive, dolasetron (Anzemat) is one of the newest members of this drug class.
Butyrophenones. Butyrophenones are another group of agents effective in the management of nausea and vomiting. Classified as antipsychotic or neuroleptic medications, these drugs are antidopaminergics.[12] They are chemically related to the phenothiazines.

Butyrophenones are used frequently in the management of acute nausea and vomiting related to anesthesia. Droperidol (Inapsine) in small doses is one of the most common medications used by anesthesiologists and is very effective against postoperative nausea and vomiting when used intravenously.[6] Larger doses tend to increase the level and duration of sedation and would be used only in recalcitrant patients.
Benzodiazepines. Benzodiazepines are best known for their anxiolytic properties. This class of drugs is not only anxiolytic but antiemetic, which makes them quite effective in the anticipatory form of nausea and vomiting.[8] Butyrophenones have antiemetic and calming effects that are particularly helpful in the management of psychologically induced nausea and vomiting.[6] These medications are universally used for IV sedation but may also be given orally. Although not applicable to the dental office, the use of low-dose IV benzodiazepines is effective in controlling chronic nausea and vomiting in postoperative patients.[13] Lorazepam (Ativan) is a classic benzodiazepine with good antiemetic effects.

Drugs for Chronic Nausea and Vomiting

In addition to the more common drugs, other drugs used in the patient with chronic nausea and vomiting include steroids, cannabinoids (e.g., marijuana), anticholinergics, amphetamines, miscellaneous dopamine antagonists, benzamides, and even ibuprofen and progestogens.[6,14]

Complications

Although persistent nausea and vomiting are rare, lack of dietary intake may result in hypoglycemia (e.g., diabetic patient), dehydration, electrolyte imbalance, and inability to absorb drugs in the routine manner. Alternative agents (e.g., antibiotics) might be indicated if nausea and vomiting cannot be controlled with the usual medications. Other complications in the patient with severe postoperative nausea and vomiting include esophageal rupture (Boerhaave's syndrome), rib fracture, gastric herniation, muscle strain and fatigue, cutaneous vessel rupture, wound dehiscence, intraocular bleeding, and skin flap bleeding.

Prolonged recovery from dental procedures and anesthetics has other implications. The loss of work coupled with patient distress does not allow for a satisfactory experience for a patient who might have been anxious about the dental procedure at the outset, which compounds the problems for future encounters. Significant nausea and vomiting in the postsurgical patient may lead to a patient who is reluctant to undergo additional surgery regardless of the need.[3]

When nausea and vomiting is prolonged to the point that secondary side effects may be likely, it may be advisable to consult with the patient's physician and if necessary hospitalize the patient for IV fluids and more aggressive antiemetic therapy.

ABDOMINAL PAIN
Etiology

Myriad causes of abdominal pain exist. Some are relatively benign, whereas others are life threatening and require immediate medical or surgical intervention. Some instances of abdominal pain that occur in the dental office are directly related to the dental therapy. Other instances are unrelated, coincidental occurrences. Furthermore, abdominal pain may result from GI pathology or may be a symptom of cardiovascular, pulmonary, genitourinary, or gynecologic pathology. Making a definitive diagnosis often presents a difficult challenge to the emergency department (ED) physician. Five percent of ED presentations are for evaluation of nontraumatic abdominal pain.[15] Dentists occasionally encounter patients who either present with abdominal pain or develop abdominal pain in the office. Therefore the dentist must be prepared to evaluate these patients and make decisions regarding their disposition.

This section first discusses cases in which abdominal pain and dentistry are related (dentistry causes abdominal pain, abdominal pain disorders affect dentistry), then addresses abdominal pain unrelated to dentistry.

Pathophysiology and Anatomic Considerations

The peritoneal lining of the abdomen has two components: visceral peritoneum and parietal peritoneum. The visceral peritoneum surrounds the intraabdominal organs and receives autonomic innervation. The parietal peritoneum lines the overlying abdominal wall and receives somatic innervation. *Visceral pain* is perceived as dull, diffuse, and variable in intensity. Diaphoresis, nausea, vomiting, alteration in heart rate and blood pressure, and spasticity of the abdominal wall musculature may concurrently occur. These reflexes and hemodynamic changes are thought to result from the autonomic innervation of the visceral peritoneum.

Somatic pain is sharper and more well localized than visceral pain. Where mild stimulation of the visceral peritoneum does not frequently significantly aggravate the patient's symptoms, stimulation of the involved parietal peritoneum results in a significant increase in pain. The patient may actually attempt to minimize the discomfort by minimizing movement and flexing the thighs to relax the peritoneum. The difference between visceral and parietal pain symptoms has clinical importance, since it explains the changing patterns of pain associated with the progression of many intraabdominal conditions.

Many abdominal disorders begin with localized distention, inflammation, or ischemia of the involved organ and overlying visceral peritoneum. The initial presenting symptoms are characteristically a dull and poorly localized pain. Visceral pain refers to the *epigastric region* (middle of upper abdomen) for organs derived from the embryologic foregut (stomach, liver, bile ducts, gallbladder, pancreas, spleen, proximal duodenum) and to the *periumbilical region* for midgut-derived organs (distal duodenum, jejunum, ileum, cecum, appendix, ascending colon, proximal transverse colon). Visceral pain in the *hypogastric region* (suprapubic area) is referred from hindgut-derived organs (distal transverse colon, descending colon, sigmoid colon, rectum, anus).

As the disease process evolves over time, the adjacent parietal peritoneum becomes stimulated, causing sharp somatic pain to be felt at a well-localized area of the abdominal wall. Thus the pain may be noted to change in location and quality. *Acute appendicitis* is the classic example that demonstrates this progression of abdominal pain. As expected, the symptoms of appendicitis frequently begin as dull, diffuse, and poorly localized periumbilical pain while only the visceral peritoneum is stimulated. This later shifts to a severe, sharp, right lower quadrant pain as the overlying parietal peritoneum becomes involved.

Anatomically the abdomen consists of the peritoneal cavity, retroperitoneal space, and pelvis. The *peritoneal cavity*, or true abdominal cavity, contains hollow organs, including the stomach, small intestine, transverse colon, gallbladder, and bile ducts, as well as solid organs, including the liver and spleen. The *retroperitoneal space* contains the pancreas, kidneys, ureters, adrenal glands, ascending and descending colon, abdominal aorta, inferior vena cava, and part of the duodenum. The *pelvis* contains the rectum, prostate, female reproductive organs, and urinary bladder. Abnormalities developing in any of these cavities or spaces can result in abdominal pain.

Clinically the abdomen is divided into seven regions: the four abdominal quadrants and the epigastric, periumbilical, and suprapubic areas (Figure 18-1 and Box 18-4). Although pain from a specific organ may refer pain to a different region of the abdomen or even beyond the abdominal boundaries, these clinical demarcations are helpful and functional when making an examination.

Pain can be referred to or from the abdominal area. Not all organs of the GI tract are located within the abdomen; the esophagus, for example, is mainly a thoracic organ. Although conditions such as esophagitis and esophageal spasm can give rise to abdominal pain, they more frequently result in chest pain, which can easily be mistaken for pain of cardiac origin. Subdiaphragmatic irritation may refer pain to the ipsilateral shoulder, whereas pain from renal calculi in men may be referred to the ipsilateral testicle. Intrathoracic conditions (e.g., myocardial infarction, pneumonia) may refer pain to the abdomen.

Dental Therapy Causing Abdominal Pain and Abdominal Emergencies

The most likely reason for a dental patient to develop abdominal pain directly related to dental therapy is from a side effect of a prescribed medication. Many of the medications prescribed by dentists have either direct or indirect effects on the GI tract and can result in GI symptoms such as abdominal pain, nausea and vomiting, and diarrhea.

Nonsteroidal Antiinflammatory Drugs and Other Analgesics

Aspirin and other NSAIDs inhibit prostaglandin synthesis and disrupt the normal cytoprotective mechanisms and secretions of the stomach, re-

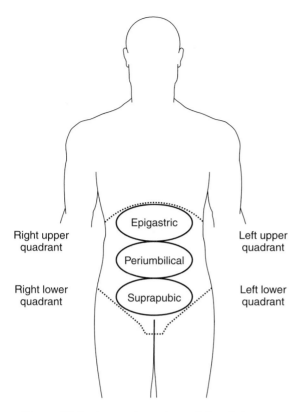

Figure 18-1. Anatomic regions of the abdomen.

Box 18-4	Abdominal Regions and Contents

REGION	CONTENTS
Right upper quadrant	Liver, gallbladder, parts of colon and small intestine
Left upper quadrant	Stomach, spleen, parts of colon (splenic flexure) and small intestine
Right lower quadrant	Appendix, parts of colon (ileocecal junction) and small intestine
Left lower quadrant	Parts of colon and small intestine
Epigastric area	Stomach, pancreas, duodenum, liver
Periumbilical area	Small intestine
Suprapubic area	Parts of colon and small intestine, pelvic organs

cance. However, these drugs can exacerbate bleeding or cause perforation of gastric or duodenal ulcers, which may be acute in onset and life threatening. The newer, more specific COX-2 inhibitors cause significantly less GI distress.

Management primarily involves prevention and recognition of an impending problem. While aspirin is contraindicated, the dentist should prescribe other NSAIDs cautiously for patients with a known history of peptic ulcer disease. Hemorrhage secondary to the development and progression of GI pathology associated with NSAIDs is not always preceded by gastric distress. If NSAIDs are to be administered to a patient at risk or over a prolonged period, the dentist should inquire about potential adverse effects. The dentist should ask the patient about a history of hematemesis, hematochezia, or melena. Postoperative assessment may be difficult because swallowed blood may contribute to nausea and vomiting as well as hematemesis. Changes in vital signs, such as hypotension or tachycardia, are of great concern because they may indicate a serious problem. GI hemorrhage is a cause of significant morbidity and mortality. If there is any question regarding the patient's signs and symptoms, immediate medical assessment is warranted.

Analgesics other than NSAIDs may also cause abdominal distress. Narcotic medications such as codeine may result in mild to moderate abdominal pain, frequently associated with nausea and vomiting, in susceptible patients. Fortunately, the treatment for abdominal pain caused by a side effect of a drug is relatively simple. Discontinuing the medication should result in resolution of the symptoms within 6 to 12 hours. For patients with a known history of an adverse reaction to these drugs, the problem can usually be avoided by prescribing alternative medications.

Antibiotics

Antibiotics can adversely affect the GI tract through direct irritation of the GI mucosa, stimulation of the endogenous receptor systems, or disturbance of the normal microbial flora. Erythromycin is an endogenous receptor stimulator that may cause abdominal cramping, nausea, and vomiting. The newer macrolide preparations are better tolerated and have a lower incidence of this complication. An alteration of the normal GI microbial flora may result in diarrhea. Changes in bowel movement and stool consistency occur in up to one third of patients prescribed antibiotics.

sulting in both minor and major adverse effects. These medications may cause GI distress, as manifested by abdominal pain and cramping. Occult bleeding may also occur. The quantity of blood loss is usually minimal and not of clinical signifi-

A serious form of antibiotic-induced superinfection is *pseudomembranous colitis*, which results from a toxin produced by the proliferation of a normally suppressed microorganism, *Clostridium difficile*. All antibiotics can cause pseudomembranous colitis, but several common antibiotics in dentistry are among the most frequent causes: broad-spectrum cephalosporins, ampicillin, and clindamycin.[16] Although more likely seen in dental patients requiring long-term antibiotic therapy for persistent infections (e.g., actinomycosis, osteomyelitis), cases of pseudomembranous colitis have been reported after only a single antibiotic dose and as late as 4 weeks after cessation of therapy.[17] The signs and symptoms are diarrhea, abdominal pain, fever, and blood and mucus in the stool.

For patients who develop mild diarrhea, often associated with abdominal pain, during or soon after completion of antibiotic therapy, the antibiotic should be stopped if possible or the patient switched to a different class of antibiotic. Depending on the severity of the presenting signs and symptoms or their persistence, patients should be referred to their physician.

Drug Toxicity

Medications can also cause abdominal pain through drug toxicity. In the pediatric patient a drug more frequently prescribed by dentists than physicians is *fluoride*. A common symptom of fluoride poisoning is abdominal pain.[18] Fluoride toxicity should be considered in any patient who develops abdominal pain after taking an excessive dose of fluoride tablets or drops. In this situation, immediate referral to an ED is indicated.

Aspiration of Foreign Objects

The accidental ingestion of a foreign object during dentistry puts patients at risk for developing complications that have abdominal pain as a symptom. The supine position for patients undergoing dental treatment places them at increased risk for aspiration or accidental ingestion of foreign objects. This is especially true if the patient's protective reflexes have been obtunded with sedation. Prevention is always the best policy. Rubber dams, throat screens, and floss ligatures on small instruments can be used to protect patients from accidentally swallowing a dental foreign object. Nevertheless, many different dental instruments and devices have been swallowed, including crowns,[19] inlays,[20] endodontic files,[21] barbed broaches,[22] rubber dam clamps,[23] air-water syringe tips,[24] drill bits,[25] and implant screwdrivers.[26]

If any foreign body is lost down the throat during a dental procedure and not retrieved, the object must be localized radiographically with chest and abdominal films. This is required even if the patient has no respiratory compromise. Although most dental objects that are accidentally swallowed pass uneventfully through the GI tract, the patient should be instructed to strain the stool until passage of the object can be confirmed. However, if the swallowed object is sharp, such as an endodontic file, immediate medical intervention is required. The patient should be instructed to take nothing by mouth and should be immediately transported to the nearest ED. Time is crucial. If the patient is seen immediately, a sharp object can be endoscopically removed from the stomach or proximal duodenum, before it has had time to pass beyond reach. If not removed, sharp objects can perforate the bowel anywhere along the GI tract.

For a patient who has recently swallowed any foreign object that has not yet passed, the onset of abdominal pain must be regarded as an emergency. The patient must be referred for immediate medical evaluation because bowel perforation can be life threatening.

Gastrointestinal and Other Abdominal Disorders Affecting Dental Care

In certain chronic GI disorders, dental therapy does not necessarily induce abdominal pain. However, delivery of care still needs to be modified to optimize patient care.

Gastroesophageal Reflux Disease

GERD is characterized by heartburn, dyspepsia, and regurgitation. It affects approximately 10% to 20% of Americans. When untreated, GERD may result in or contribute to esophagitis, GI hemorrhage, esophageal ulceration, esophageal stricture, and bronchospasm. Bronchospasm occurs as a result of regurgitation and aspiration of gastric contents. Placing patients into a supine position increases the risk of regurgitation and possible aspiration in patients with GERD. These patients may prefer to be treated in a more upright position.

In general, dental treatment does not cause significant complications in patients with GERD. At the onset of symptoms, however, the dentist must differentiate these symptoms from those of cardiac etiology, especially in individuals at risk for coronary artery disease. Also, the risk of regurgitation and aspiration is greatly increased during sedation or general anesthesia, and modifications in the patient's management may be required.

Aortic Abdominal Aneurysm

Abdominal aortic aneurysm (AAA) is another chronic disorder unrelated to the GI tract that can affect the delivery of dental care. Although an extremely rare occurrence in the dental office, a ruptured AAA is usually fatal. AAAs typically enlarge over time, and larger-diameter aneurysms are at much greater risk of rupture. The 2-year risk of rupture for AAAs less than 4 cm is less than 2%, which increases more than tenfold to 22% for those greater than 5 cm.[27] In good surgical candidates, AAAs greater than 5 cm are recommended for repair, and those greater than 4 cm are monitored every 6 months with ultrasound or CT scan.[27]

An abrupt increase in systolic blood pressure can lead to dissection or rupture of a large aneurysm, which is often associated with the sudden onset of abdominal pain. To maintain a lower blood pressure, measures should be taken to alleviate stress in these patients. Consideration should be given to blood pressure monitoring during dental treatment of patients with known large AAAs. Any patient with a known AAA who develops acute abdominal pain during therapy, especially if accompanied by hypotension, requires immediate medical assistance.

Diseases with Oral Manifestations

Patients with certain GI problems may seek dental consultation for evaluation of an oral manifestation of this medical condition. These situations may be known or unknown to the patient. The dentist has the ability as a primary care provider to make a significant contribution in the diagnosis and care of the patient. Patients with *Crohn's disease*, for example, may have associated oral lesions. If the severity of the GI symptoms is mild, the patient may not have sought medical consultation, or the physician still may not have made the diagnosis. GI disorders characterized by chronic vomiting may cause chemical erosion on the lingual aspects of the teeth. *Anorexia and bulimia* may be life threatening. The dentist's role in recognizing a problem is significant.

Abdominal Pain Unrelated to Dental Therapy

Often the dental patient complaining of abdominal pain has an underlying problem unrelated to dentistry. Acute abdominal conditions can occur at any time and at any place, including the dental office. A vast number of conditions cause abdominal pain, many of which are unrelated to the GI system. In addition to GI disorders, genitourinary, vascular, obstetric, and gynecologic problems frequently give rise to abdominal pain.

It is beyond the scope of this text to offer the dentist an exhaustive approach to evaluate and diagnose all conditions that present with abdominal pain. In fact, the dentist should not attempt to make a definitive diagnosis in most situations. Nevertheless, dentists should have sufficient familiarity with these conditions to know when immediate medical referral is indicated. Some causes of acute abdominal pain are life threatening and require immediate surgical intervention; for others, surgery is not indicated (Box 18-5).

Diagnosis and Treatment in the Dental Office

When a dental patient complains of abdominal pain during treatment, the dentist should not attempt to make a final diagnosis as to the etiology of the pain. Rather, the dentist must determine whether or not the problem is of sufficient severity to warrant medical evaluation, and if so, whether immediate medical evaluation or nonemergency medical consultation is indicated. This is not always a clear and easy decision.

History

The first step in establishing a diagnosis is to review the patient's medical history, looking for preexisting or chronic conditions that can give rise to abdominal pain. Nonabdominal sources of pain (e.g., cardiac) must also be considered. For the dental patient complaining of abdominal pain, nausea, and diaphoresis, even without frank complaints of concomitant chest pain, acute myocardial infarction should always be included in the dentist's differential diagnosis. A potential complication of pregnancy should be considered for any female of childbearing age.

The history should reveal the onset of the pain, activity associated with the onset, location of the pain (presently and at its onset), radiation or referral of pain to other locations, intensity and character of the pain, associated symptoms

| Box 18-5 | Medical Causes of Acute Abdominal Pain |

GASTROINTESTINAL
Appendicitis
Peptic ulcer (gastric, duodenal, with or
    without perforation)
Reflux esophagitis
Cholecystitis
Biliary colic
Pancreatitis
Diverticulitis
Hepatitis
Cholangitis
Gastroenteritis
Small bowel obstruction
Volvulus of cecum or sigmoid colon
Inflammatory bowel disease (ulcerative colitis,
    Crohn's)
Irritable bowel syndrome
Strangulated bowel (e.g., incarcerated hernia)
Bowel ischemia

GENITOURINARY
Pyelonephritis
Nephrolithiasis
Urinary tract infection

OBSTETRIC/GYNECOLOGIC
Pelvic inflammatory disease
Ruptured ovarian cyst
Ectopic pregnancy
Endometriosis
Threatened spontaneous abortion

VASCULAR
Abdominal aortic aneurysm (dissection,
    rupture)
Mesenteric thrombosis

REFERRED PAIN
Myocardial infarction
Pneumonia
Pleurisy
Endocarditis
Pericarditis

MISCELLANEOUS
Sickle cell crisis
Diabetic ketoacidosis
Porphyria
Acute adrenal insufficiency
Pernicious anemia
Heavy metal toxicity

(e.g., nausea and vomiting, diarrhea or constipation), and past episodes of similar distress. The relatively abrupt onset of moderate to severe abdominal pain that persists or even worsens, rather than diminishes in intensity, should be considered for immediate medical evaluation. For many acute conditions, nausea and vomiting often follows the onset of abdominal pain. Nausea and vomiting preceding the abdominal pain decreases the likelihood of an acute problem requiring surgical intervention.

The ability for the dentist to collect and relay this information is important. Signs and symptoms may change, and the initial presenting signs and symptoms may better define the involved organ.

Physical Examination

Physical examination begins with monitoring the patient's vital signs. Hypotension and tachycardia are ominous signs of potential intraabdominal hemorrhage or septic shock. Gentle palpation of the abdomen may elicit areas of tenderness. Tensing of the abdominal wall musculature (guarding) may be voluntary or involuntary and may indicate peritonitis. Rebound tenderness, another indication of peritonitis, occurs when sudden release of manual pressure on the abdomen results in exacerbation of the pain.

Patients presumed to have an acute abdominal process should be transported to the local ED for immediate medical evaluation. If the patient is thought to be unstable (e.g., writhing in excruciating pain, hypotensive, decreased mental status), transportation should be direct by ambulance. No specific treatment by the dentist is indicated, other than possibly supportive care, depending on the dentist's level of training and ability (e.g., IV fluids for the hypotensive patient). Narcotic pain medication should not be administered, since this can mask the signs and symptoms that will be crucial for making an accurate differential diagnosis during subsequent medical evaluation in the ED. Patients with an acute abdominal condition usually have loss of appetite. Nevertheless, they should be specifically informed to take nothing by mouth because emergency surgery may be required.

Evaluation in the Emergency Department

When a patient complaining of abdominal pain presents to the ED, an initial evaluation is made to determine if immediate surgical intervention is needed. Delay in surgery can result in a substantial increase in morbidity and mortality. Appendicitis is the most common surgical cause of abdominal pain in persons under 50 presenting to the ED, with cholecystitis the most common in persons older than 50.[27]

History

As in all medical evaluations, a thorough history is first obtained. Questions outlining the onset, progression, and character of the pain can aid in establishing the differential diagnosis (Box 18-6 and Figure 18-2). Prior episodes, if any, are reviewed. Associated symptoms include fever, chills, nausea and vomiting, loss of appetite, and change in frequency, consistency, and color of bowel movements. Questions focusing on the genitourinary system include any pain with urination, urgency, increased urinary frequency, and presence of visible blood in the urine. For women a complete menstrual history is obtained, along with questions concerning vaginal burning or discharge. A history of previous abdominal surgery increases the risk of small bowel obstruction, and heavy alcohol consumption is common in patients with acute pancreatitis.

Physical Examination

A complete physical examination is performed, with emphasis on the abdomen. Vital signs are taken first. The normal sequence of inspection, palpation, percussion, and auscultation is modified for the abdominal examination, since palpation can alter bowel sounds heard on auscultation.

The abdomen is first inspected for distention, gross hernias, and surgical scars. *Inspection* of the abdominal skin may reveal evidence of jaundice, which is evaluated better in other locations (e.g., sclera). *Auscultation* is performed next, listening for increased bowel sounds (e.g., early small bowel obstruction), absent bowel sounds (e.g., peritonitis, paralytic ileus), or abdominal vascular bruits. When the abdomen is percussed, tympanitic sounds may represent air in distended loops of obstructed small bowel. *Percussion* is also useful for evaluating organ size (e.g., liver) and for determining the presence of ascites. More forceful percussion on the back, at the costovertebral angle, may elicit renal tenderness. *Palpation* is performed last and often gives the most information. The abdomen is palpated lightly, searching for localized areas of tenderness. As discussed, guarding and rebound tenderness are signs of possible peritonitis. Deeper palpation is used to evaluate organ size and possible organ tenderness. Palpation can reveal the presence of an abnormal intraabdominal mass and is used to approximate the size of AAAs.

All patients receive a rectal examination, checking for masses and tenderness. In males,

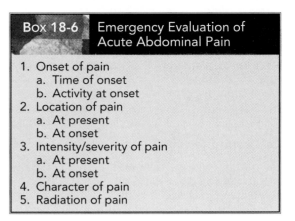

Box 18-6   Emergency Evaluation of Acute Abdominal Pain

1. Onset of pain
   a. Time of onset
   b. Activity at onset
2. Location of pain
   a. At present
   b. At onset
3. Intensity/severity of pain
   a. At present
   b. At onset
4. Character of pain
5. Radiation of pain

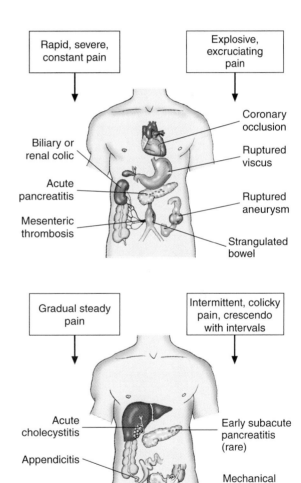

Figure 18-2. Differential diagnosis of acute abdominal pain by character. *Redrawn from Schwartz GR, Rothrock SG, Shea DJ, et al: Abdominal pain: evaluation. In Schwartz GR, editor:* Principles and practice of emergency medicine, *ed 4, Baltimore, 1999, Williams & Wilkins.*

tenderness or enlargement of the prostate is also examined. A stool guaiac test checks for occult blood. Special maneuvers are performed to identify hernias. Women undergo a pelvic examination to evaluate for vaginal discharge, cervical motion tenderness, ovarian tenderness, and masses.

Laboratory Testing

Laboratory tests are routinely ordered in the ED. A complete blood count is obtained to check for signs of hemorrhage or dehydration and an elevated white blood cell count. Electrolyte abnormalities may be identified, especially in persons with dehydration or chronic, prolonged vomiting. Blood urea nitrogen (BUN) and creatinine levels are checked to evaluate fluid status and renal function. Elevated serum amylase is common in pancreatitis. Liver function tests may be elevated in hepatitis, cholecystitis, and bile duct obstruction. Urinalysis is performed to check for white blood cells, bacteria, and occult blood. For women of childbearing age, a pregnancy test is performed.

Imaging of the abdomen is frequently performed. Upright plain films of the abdomen can reveal air-fluid levels in dilated loops of bowel or subdiaphragmatic free air if a ruptured viscus is present. Ultrasound can be used to evaluate for cholelithiasis, to determine the size of an AAA, and to evaluate the pelvic organs in women. An intravenous pyelogram (IVP) may be performed to evaluate the renal outflow system and to identify radiolucent stones. Upper and lower GI contrast studies may be useful to better visualize the bowels. Computed tomography (CT) scanning of the abdomen not only can provide images of the abdominal, pelvic, and retroperitoneal organs, but also can detect free fluid in the peritoneum.

Disposition

Once all available data are collected, a differential diagnosis is made and appropriate treatment instituted. However, the diagnosis may still not be readily apparent. Patients with acute abdominal pain may be held for observation because serial abdominal examinations often reveal important new information as the underlying disease process progresses.

Excellent references on the evaluation of the "acute abdomen" are available.[28]

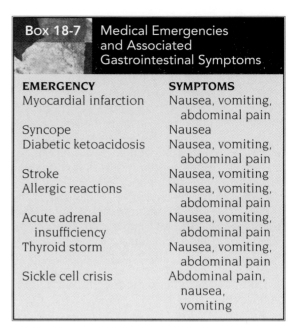

Box 18-7	Medical Emergencies and Associated Gastrointestinal Symptoms
EMERGENCY	**SYMPTOMS**
Myocardial infarction	Nausea, vomiting, abdominal pain
Syncope	Nausea
Diabetic ketoacidosis	Nausea, vomiting, abdominal pain
Stroke	Nausea, vomiting
Allergic reactions	Nausea, vomiting, abdominal pain
Acute adrenal insufficiency	Nausea, vomiting, abdominal pain
Thyroid storm	Nausea, vomiting, abdominal pain
Sickle cell crisis	Abdominal pain, nausea, vomiting

GASTROINTESTINAL SYMPTOMS ASSOCIATED WITH OTHER MEDICAL EMERGENCIES

Nausea, vomiting, and abdominal pain also occur in non-GI medical emergencies, as described elsewhere in this text (Box 18-7). The dentist should not overlook these conditions when evaluating the patient with these symptoms.

SUMMARY

Although relatively uncommon, emergencies associated with the gastrointestinal tract or with other abdominal, retroperitoneal, or pelvic organs can occur during dental treatment. Nausea, vomiting, and abdominal pain are frequently seen with these conditions. These symptoms may be directly related or may be unrelated to the dental therapy. Dentists should be familiar with possible underlying causes and must be prepared to offer appropriate treatment or medical referral if indicated.

REFERENCES

1. Yagiela JA: Review of antiemetic therapies, *Oral Maxillofac Surg Clin North Am* 11(4):647-658, 1999.
2. Andrews PLR, Hawthorn J: The neurophysiology of vomiting, *Baillieres Clin Gastroenterol* 2:141-168, 1988.
3. Andrews PLR: Physiology of nausea and vomiting, *Br J Anaesth* 69(suppl 1): 2S-19S, 1992.

4. Wang SC, Borison BC: A new concept of organization of the central emetic mechanism: recent studies on the sites of action of apomorphine, copper sulfate, and cardiac glycosides, *Gastroenterology* 22:1-12, 1952.

5. Becker DE: Management of nausea and vomiting: physiological, pharmacological, and therapeutic considerations, *J Am Dent Assoc* 115:292-294, 1987.

6. Allan SG: Antiemetics, *Gastroenterol Clin North Am* 21(3):597-611, 1992.

7. Carpenter DO: Neural mechanisms of emesis, *Can J Physiol Pharmacol* 68:230-236, 1990.

8. Axelrod RA: Antiemetic therapy, *Comp Ther* 23(8):539-545, 1997.

9. Marin J et al: Therapeutic management of nausea and vomiting, *Gen Pharmacol* 21(1):1-10, 1990.

10. Sanger GJ: New antiemetic drugs, *Can J Physiol Pharmacol* 68(2):314-324, 1990.

11. Wadibia EC: Antiemetics, *South Med J* 92(2):162-165, 1999.

12. Rowbotham DJ: Current management of postoperative nausea and vomiting, *Br J Anaesth* 69(suppl 1):46S-59S, 1992.

13. Di Florio T, Goucke CR: The effect of midazolam on persistent postoperative nausea and vomiting, *Anaesth Intensive Care* 27(1):38-40, 1999.

14. Leslie RA et al: The neuropharmacology of emesis: the role of receptors in neuromodulation of nausea and vomiting, *Can J Physiol Pharmacol* 68(2):279-288, 1990.

15. Powers RD, Guertler AT: Abdominal pain in the ED: stability and change over 20 years, *Am J Emerg Med* 13(3):301-303, 1995.

16. Goldman L, Bennett JC, editors: *Cecil textbook of medicine*, ed 21, Philadelphia, 2000, Saunders.

17. Kasper DL, Zaleznik DF: Gas gangrene and other clostridial infections. In Isselbacher HA et al, editors: *Harrison's principles of internal medicine*, ed 13, vol I, New York, 1994, McGraw-Hill.

18. Augenstein WL, Spoerke DG, Kulig KW, et al: Fluoride ingestion in children: a review of 87 cases, *Pediatrics* 88(5):907-912, 1991.

19. Kharbanda OP, Varshney P, Dutta U: Accidental swallowing of a gold cast crown during orthodontic tooth separation, *J Clin Pediatr Dent* 19(4):289-292, 1995.

20. Palmer GM, Shortsleeve MJ: Transient golden appendicolith, *South Med J* 1998.

21. Kaufman AY: Accidental ingestion of an endodontic instrument, *Quintessence Int* 9(5):83-84, 1978.

22. Faegenburg D, Chiat H, Ludman H: Accidental ingestion of endodontic instruments: barbed broach, *NY State J Med* 69(5):690-693, 1969.

23. Alexander RE, Delhom JJ Jr: Rubber dam clamp ingestion, an operative risk: report of a case, *J Am Dent Assoc* 82(6):1387-1389, 1971.

24. Pinkney HS, Greenbaum JB, Pelc M: Case report: ingestion of an air-water syringe tip, *J Mich Dent Assoc* 77(8):38-39, 1995.

25. Klingler PJ, Smith SL, Abendstein BJ, et al: Management of ingested foreign bodies within the appendix: a case report with review of the literature, *Am J Gastroenterol* 92(12):2295-2298, 1997.

26. Worthington P: Ingested foreign body associated with oral implant treatment: report of a case, *Int J Oral Maxillofac Implants* 11(5):679-681, 1996.

27. Schwartz GR, Rothrock SG, Shea DJ, et al: Abdominal pain: evaluation. In Schwartz GR, editor: *Principles and practice of emergency medicine*, ed 4, Baltimore, 1999, Williams & Wilkins.

28. Silen W: *Cope's early diagnosis of the acute abdomen*, ed 19, New York, 1996, Oxford University Press.

Hemorrhage and Bleeding Disorders

Robert Bona

U ncontrolled hemorrhage is rarely a complication associated with dental treatment. However, hemorrhage may occur and be related to a surgical wound, a prescribed or over-the-counter medication, or an underlying systemic problem. Bleeding may be mild or severe and in the worst case may cause airway obstruction and a true acute emergency. Managing hemorrhage requires an understanding of both normal and abnormal physiology as well as basic surgical principles.

This chapter discusses surgical principles of hemorrhage control, including use of hemostatic materials, and management of bleeding disorders, with attention to the physiology of hemostasis.

HEMORRHAGE

When a patient presents with bleeding, regardless of whether the patient has a known systemic disease or contributing factor, basic principles should be followed for hemorrhage control.

Patient Assessment

Simultaneous with initiating maneuvers to control the hemorrhage, the dentist must obtain an adequate history detailing both the event contributing to the patient's condition and the patient's past medical and family history (Box 19-1). A basic physical examination consists of obtaining both blood pressure (BP) and heart rate (HR) and performing a cursory assessment of the skin and mucosa. BP and HR measurements may either suggest an etiology or indicate the severity of the situation. BP should be taken in both supine and upright positions. Low BP, elevated HR, or abnormal change between supine and upright values suggests significant blood loss. Conversely, an elevated HR consistent with hypertension may be contributing to the hemorrhage. During examination of the skin and mucosal surfaces, identification of ecchymosis or petechia may suggest an underling systemic etiology.

Initial Intervention

The first step in managing hemorrhage is to apply firm and continuous pressure. Pressure is generally applied directly to the site (e.g., extraction socket). Alternatively, pressure to a vessel proximal to the site of hemorrhage may control or at least minimize the severity of the hemorrhage (Figure 19-1). This initially may be achieved by simply compressing the vessel, not necessarily with direct visualization of the vessel. This may afford more time to explore the wound and directly identify the vessel. When the vessel is fully visualized, a hemostat may be secured to both ends of the severed vessel, which then may be ligated or cauterized. A hemostat should never be blindly placed into a surgical wound.

Most cases of hemorrhage managed by a dentist are not secondary to large vessels. More frequently the hemorrhage is associated with an extraction site or traumatized gingiva. After the initial application of pressure to control the hemorrhage, a local anesthetic containing epinephrine should be injected. The α-agonist effect of the epinephrine provides local hemostasis. The potential for rebound hemorrhage secondary to the β_2-agonist effect of the epinephrine is more theoretic than clinical. Most importantly, the local anesthetic provides pain control, which allows surgical exploration and debridement of the wound.

It is important to determine if the hemorrhage is from the soft tissue or the bone. Hemorrhage from the *soft tissue* can frequently be controlled by debriding the tissue margins and any granulation tissue. Vessels often do not contract on themselves in granulation tissue, which is a common site for persistent bleeding. If soft tissue hemorrhage persists, the sites of bleeding can be cauterized. Electrocautery, although readily available in operating rooms, often is not available in typical dental offices. Chemical cauterization of the soft tissue can be achieved with silver nitrate sticks.

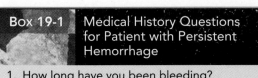

Box 19-1 Medical History Questions for Patient with Persistent Hemorrhage

1. How long have you been bleeding?
2. What have you done to stop the bleeding?
3. Have you or any member of your family had a problem with the following?
   a. Prolonged or excessive bleeding
   b. Excessive bruising
   c. History of liver disease
   d. History of cancer or treatment of cancer
   e. History of blood disorders
   f. History of alcohol abuse
4. Are you taking any of the following medications?
   a. Blood thinners (e.g., coumadin)
   b. Aspirin
   c. NSAIDs
   d. Antibiotics

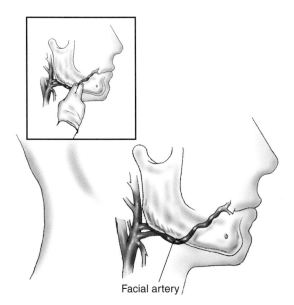

Facial artery

Figure 19-1. Control of hemorrhage may be obtained by compressing the facial artery and vein between the dentist's fingers and the patient's bony mandible.

If the hemorrhage is from the *bone* (e.g., extraction socket), attention should first be directed to finding the specific site of hemorrhage within the bone. This may be from a small vessel within the bone that did not retract on itself and thus resulted in the persistent bleeding. Burnishing the bone with a blunt instrument will frequently occlude the vessel and promote he-

mostasis. If the hemorrhage is diffuse such that hemostasis is not readily achieved, the application of topical hemostatic materials may assist in providing hemostasis.

Hemostatic Materials

Hemostatic materials that should be readily available in a dental office include gelatin sponges (Gelfoam), oxidized regenerated cellulose (Surgicel), fibrillar collagen (Avitene, Helistat), bone wax (beeswax and salicylic acid), and topical thrombin. When placed into the surgical site, both the Gelfoam and the Surgicel provide a scaffold to stabilize the blood clot. The Surgicel, because of its acidity, provides chemical cauterization as well. The collagen products (Avitene, Helistat) provide both an active stimulus for platelet activation and a scaffold on which the clot may form. These agents are advantageous in that they promote platelet activation; however, they are much more expensive and are not recommended unless necessary.

Bone wax is a very effective agent. It is burnished into the bony surfaces that are hemorrhaging and provides a mechanical block. The material is associated with a foreign body reaction and delays healing. Therefore it is not usually used as the initial hemostatic agent.

Thrombin is the coagulation factor that activates fibrinogen. Topical administration to the site of hemorrhage promotes the formation of fibrin (see following section). A gelatin sponge or sheet of collagen is frequently saturated with the thrombin, which is loosely applied to the wound. Topical thrombin is not applied in conjunction with Surgicel and should never be injected into the hemorrhaging site.

The dentist should consider obtaining primary soft tissue closure.

Secondary Intervention

If the hemorrhage persists after appropriate measures are taken, further medical assessment is immediately required. Laboratory studies should minimally include prothrombin time (PT)/international normalized ratio (INR), partial thromboplastin time (PTT), and complete blood count (CBC). The CBC provides both the platelet count as well as the hemoglobin and hematocrit values, which may indicate the severity of blood loss. The physician may also want to consider obtaining a bleeding time. If the PT, PTT, platelet count, and bleeding time are within normal limits, it is less likely that the patient has an underlying bleeding disorder.

Abnormal values suggest that the patient has either a congenital or an acquired bleeding disorder. Consultation and management in conjunction with a hematologist is strongly recommended. Despite the recommendation to seek consultation, however, it is important for the dentist to have a rudimentary understanding of hemostasis and the more common bleeding disorders and approaches to therapy.

BLEEDING DISORDERS
Normal Hemostasis

The formation of a normal blood clot requires the presence of adequate and functionally normal platelets, adhesive glycoproteins, and an intact coagulation system (Figure 19-2). Blood clot formation has been traditionally described as proceeding through an ordered process of (1) primary hemostasis, (2) coagulation activation, (3) clot formation and stabilization, and (4) clot dissolution by the process of fibrinolysis and tissue repair (Figure 19-3).

Primary hemostasis is the process by which platelets adhere to a damage vascular surface, followed by platelet aggregation. The initial adhesion of platelets to subendothelial collagen exposed by injury is mediated by von Willebrand's factor and a specific platelet integrin receptor for collagen ($\alpha_{2B}\beta_1$).[1] *Von Willebrand's factor* (vWF) is a large, adhesive glycoprotein synthesized by megakaryocytes and endothelial cells.[2] It is either secreted constitutively or stored in specialized granules in the endothelium and platelets, where release can occur in response to a number of chemical signals. The protein undergoes posttranslational modifications, including multimerization, and the mature protein has a molecular weight ranging from 1 to 20 million daltons. The protein has specific binding sites for coagulation factor VIII, collagen, the platelet–glycoprotein Ib/IX complex, and heparin. After initial tissue injury, vWF binding to collagen occurs, followed by binding to platelets via their glycoprotein Ib-IX receptor. In this way, vWF serves as the primary ligand allowing for platelet adhesion to subendothelial collagen.

Platelets can also adhere directly to collagen via the *platelet integrin receptor* $\alpha_2B\beta_1$. Platelets subsequently become activated in a complex biochemical process, resulting in platelet shape change, granule secretion, thromboxane synthesis, cell surface phospholipid exposure, and finally, exposure of $\alpha_{2B}\beta_{3A}$ (GP IIb-IIIa) in a conformation whereby it can bind to its ligand, fibrinogen or vWF. This process results in *platelet*

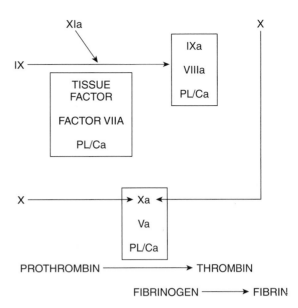

Figure 19-2. Coagulation cascade.

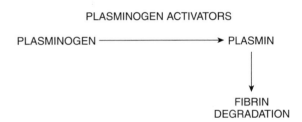

Figure 19-3. Elements of fibrinolytic system.

aggregation, a process by which platelets adhere to one another.

The vWF also binds to circulating factor VIII and significantly enhances its half-life in the blood, presumably by protecting the molecule from degradation by proteases. Thus the half-life of factor VIII in the absence of vWF is approximately 1 hour, which is prolonged up to 8 to 12 hours in the presence of vWF. By binding to factor VIII, vWF also serves to co-localize the factor VIII molecule to sites of tissue injury, thereby increasing its local concentration in areas where fibrin deposition is required.

The generation of a fibrin blood clot depends on the activation of a number of precursor proteins (zymogens) to serine esterases, each with specificity for a precursor substrate.[3] The ultimate substrate is *fibrinogen*, which is converted to a fibrin monomer by the enzyme thrombin. Current understanding of this process is that these reactions take place on a phospholipid cell surface, in vivo, supplied by the endothelium, the platelet, or other cells. These membrane enzyme complexes require the presence of a cofactor, a divalent cation (calcium), a substrate, and an enzyme for optimal kinetics. The process is initiated after tissue injury, thereby exposing the blood to small amounts of *tissue factor* (factor III), a lipoprotein and integral membrane protein found in many cells but not normally expressed by the endothelium. After tissue injury, tissue factor expressed on subendothelial adventitial cells is exposed to the flowing blood and causes a rapid activation of the coagulation system, with the generation of thrombin and the formation of fibrin monomer. The fibrin monomer dimerizes and multimerizes, then becomes cross-linked in a reaction involving *transglutaminase*, the active form of factor XIII.

Integral to tissue factor activity is its ability to bind factor VII or factor VIIa. This complex is able to convert factor X to factor Xa or factor IX to factor IXa. This latter reaction may be more important physiologically because there is a potent inhibitor of the TF-VIIa-Xa complex. Factor IXa is also able to convert factor X to factor Xa. Factor VIIIa serves as a cofactor in this latter reaction. Thus factor Xa can be produced by two different reactions: (1) the TF-VIIa complex cleaves factor X, and (2) factor X is cleaved by the complex of factor IXa and factor VIIIa, with factor IXa produced by either tissue factor–VIIa or activated factor XI (XIa).

Natural inhibitors of both platelet activation and fibrin formation provide balance to this system, where a low level of thrombin is generated under basal conditions. These inhibitory substances include endothelial-derived relaxing factor (EDRF), prostacyclins, antithrombin (formerly antithrombin III), protein C, protein S, and tissue factor pathway inhibitor (TFPI).

Another important regulator of fibrin deposition is the *fibrinolytic system*[4] (see Figure 19-3). This enzymatic system is capable of degrading the fibrin blood clot and ultimately allows for vessel recanalization and tissue repair. Plasminogen must be converted to the active enzyme, plasmin, by tissue plasminogen activators. When this occurs, fibrin degradation continues.

These procoagulant forces (e.g., platelets, vWF, coagulation proteins) and the anticoagulant forces (e.g., fibrinolytic system, protein C, protein S) serve to maintain homeostasis and blood fluidity. Because there is a low level of thrombin generation at basal conditions, the system can accelerate quickly in response to tissue injury.

Pathophysiology
Von Willebrand's Disease

Perhaps the most common congenital bleeding disorder is von Willebrand's disease (vWD), occurring in up to 1 in every 200 persons and usually inherited as an autosomal dominant disorder.[5] In its mildest and most common form, vWD presents as a mild bleeding disorder with predominantly mucosal and cutaneous bleeding.

There are four general categories of vWD. The most common variety, *type 1*, occurs in approximately 85% of individuals with vWD. It is an autosomal dominant disorder characterized by a minimal reduction in vWF and an equal reduction in all sizes of vWF multimers. Factor VIII levels often are mildly reduced, and bleeding time is frequently prolonged (Table 19-1).

Patients often present with signs and symptoms of a mild bleeding disorder, including epistaxis, menorrhagia, easy bruisability, gingival bleeding, and bleeding after mucocutaneous operative procedures. The signs, symptoms, and laboratory findings of type I vWD vary considerably, and some patients may have few or no symptoms, whereas others appear to be more severely affected. Plasma vWF levels vary greatly over time in any given individual and are affected by the hormonal milieu of the patient, epinephrine levels, medications, ABO blood type, and other unknown factors. This may make diagnosis difficult and also may cause variability in clinical bleeding symptoms. The genetic abnormal-

Table 19-1	Laboratory Results in Bleeding Disorders			
Diagnosis	Factor VIII	Factor IX	vWF	Bleeding Time
Hemophilia A	Low	Normal	Normal	Normal
Hemophilia B	Normal	Low	Normal	Normal
vWD	Low	Normal	Low	Prolonged
Platelet disorder	Normal	Normal	Normal	Prolonged

vWF, Von Willebrand's factor; *vWD*, von Willebrand's disease.

ity(ies) causing this bleeding disorder is not yet known.

The many variants of vWD are generally associated with more severe bleeding and may be more difficult to treat. Type 2 variants are associated with *qualitative* abnormalities of von Willebrand's protein, leading to either excessive proteolysis (*type 2a*), abnormal binding to platelet glycoprotein Ib (*type 2b*), abnormal binding to factor VIII (*type 2N*), or other functional abnormalities (*type 2M*). *Type 3* variant of vWD is associated with almost complete absence of the protein, very low levels of factor VIII, and a severe bleeding disorder. This is a very rare form of VWD.

Hemophilia

Hemophilia A and B are X-linked disorders caused by deficiencies in coagulation factors VIII and IX, respectively[6] (see Table 19-1). Hemophilia is seen in approximately 1 in 50,000 males. Hemophilia A is five times more common than hemophilia B, although these are clinically indistinguishable disorders characterized by soft tissue or muscle bleeding. The clinical severity parallels the residual factor remaining in the blood.

Patients are categorized as having *severe, moderate,* or *mild* disease, with factor levels of less than 1%, 1% to <5%, and 5% to 40%, respectively. Approximately half of patients have severe deficiencies. Patients with any degree of clinical severity are at risk for surgical bleeding, with the greatest risk seen in those with severe disorder. Before the availability of effective therapy, life-threatening bleeding was common in patients with severe hemophilia who underwent oral surgery, including simple extractions. With proper therapy, however, dental surgery can be performed safely in patients with hemophilia.

Carriers of hemophilia A or B. Mothers of individuals with hemophilia are obligate carriers of the disease, except in the unusual instance of a new mutation in the proband. On average, maternal carriers will have factor VIII or IX levels of approximately 50% of the normal range. Because of unequal inactivation of the X chromosome (Lyon hypothesis), however, the range of factor levels can be significant (22% to 116%).[7] Occasionally, levels can be low enough to cause significant bleeding after surgical procedures, including dental surgery.

Platelet Disorders

A number of platelet disorders that can cause excessive bleeding have been described. Rare dis-

orders, such as *Bernard-Soulier disease* (glycoprotein IB-IX abnormality) and *Glanzmann's thrombasthenia* (glycoprotein IIb-IIIa abnormality), cause severe bleeding and may be difficult to manage.[8] More common disorders include storage pool disorders, other platelet receptor abnormalities (adenosine diphosphate, collagen), or disorders of thromboxane secretion; these are much milder bleeding disorders that are seen frequently, although their exact incidence in the population is unknown. Many of these disorders are congenital, but *qualitative* platelet abnormalities may be seen with systemic disorders (e.g., uremia, hepatic failure), drug use (e.g., aspirin, nonsteroidal antiinflammatory drugs [NSAIDs], clopidogrel), or bone marrow disorders (e.g., myelodysplasia, myeloproliferative disorders).

The common disorders that lead to *quantitative* platelet disorders (e.g., thrombocytopenia) include autoimmune thrombocytopenia, hypersplenism secondary to liver disease, bone marrow failure secondary to hematologic malignancy, or treatment with chemotherapy or radiation therapy. Bleeding after oral surgical or dental procedures may range from inconsequential to clinically significant. The patient's bleeding history may help in predicting the outcome of a dental procedure.

Coagulation Deficiencies

Other coagulation deficiencies that lead to bleeding disorders occur less often. *Factor XI deficiency* is most common, inherited as an autosomal recessive condition. Patients have variable bleeding tendency, associated with the residual factor XI in the plasma.[9]

Blood Component Therapy
Factor Replacement

Replacement of factor VIII or factor IX is possible with direct intravenous (IV) infusion of purified, plasma-derived, or recombinant factor concentrates.[10,11] The practice of using plasma or cryoprecipitate has been abandoned in favor of the safer recombinant or virally inactivated plasma-derived products (Box 19-2). These concentrates can be given by IV bolus infusion or continuous infusion and are effective at preventing or treating bleeding episodes in the patient with hemophilia.

The factor required to raise the recipient's plasma level can be calculated based on the body weight of the patient, realizing that the body distribution of factor VIII is primarily intravascular

Box 19-2	Common Therapies for Patients with Bleeding Disorders

DRUGS	DOSE
Platelets	1 unit (U) of platelets raises platelet count by approximately 10,000/mm^3
Factor VIII	2 U/kg raises plasma level by 1%
Factor IX	1 U/kg raises plasma level by 1%
Desmopressin (DDAVP)	0.3 μg/kg intravenously
Intranasal DDAVP (Stimate)	1 spray (<50 kg) 2 sprays (>50 kg)
Tranexamic acid (Cyclokapreon)	25 mg/kg 3 or 4 times daily *or* 4.8% aqueous solution mouth rinse
Aminocaproic acid (Amicar)	Children: 100 mg/kg 4 times daily Adults: 4-6 g 4 times daily

and that of factor IX is both intravascular and extravascular. Thus 1 unit of factor VIII per kilogram of body weight raises the circulating factor VIII level by 2%, and the same dose of factor IX raises the circulating factor IX by 1%. The plasma half-life of factor VIII is approximately 12 hours, whereas that of factor IX is 24 hours.

The virally inactivated and recombinant products are virtually free of side effects, except for an occasional allergic reaction, which is generally easily treated. About 10% to 15% of patients, especially those with severe deficiencies, will develop antibodies to the factor. Most often these are transient and do not cause a clinical problem, but occasionally they can be of high titer and can render the infused factor VIII or IX ineffective. It is therefore essential to measure these inhibitor titers on all patients before surgical procedures to ensure treatment will be effective.

Desmopressin

Desmopressin (DDAVP) is an analog of vasopressin, a posterior pituitary hormone.[12] Desmopressin's therapeutic value in bleeding disorders is its ability to cause a transient increase in plasma vWf and factor VIII in patients with type 1 vWD and mild hemophilia.[13] DDAVP therefore is used to treat or prevent bleeding in patients with mild factor VIII deficiency or type 1 vWD, often

instead of or with factor or plasma concentrates. DDAVP has also been beneficial in patients with qualitative bleeding disorders.[14] Of particular dental relevance, DDAVP also causes release of plasminogen activators into the saliva, thereby stimulating fibrinolysis.[15]

The precise mechanism of action of DDAVP is unknown. The IV administration of DDAVP at a dose of 0.3 μg/kg of body weight reliably raises the vWF and factor VIII in most patients with type 1 vWD and mild hemophilia A and in some patients with moderate hemophilia A. The duration and magnitude of the response are variable but reproducible, and therefore the response must be measured in all patients undergoing a surgical procedure when DDAVP use is anticipated.

DDAVP is now also available as a nasal spray, and the results from IV and nasal administration are similar. The intranasal DDAVP available for the use in treatment of bleeding disorders is 100-fold more concentrated than the DDAVP formulated for use in the treatment of diabetes insipidus.[13] The dentist must ensure that the correct formulation is used: Stimate (DDAVP, 1.5 mg/ml). The correct dose for adults (>50 kg) is one spray (100 μl, 150 μg) in each nostril. The dose for children (<50 kg) is one squirt. The dose may be repeated every 8 to 12 hours, but excessive dosing (>3 or 4 doses in 48-hour period) may produce significant hyponatremia because of the drug's water-retaining properties. Additionally, tachyphylaxis may occur after repeated doses. Other common side effects include mild flushing and mild increase in BP. Unusual side effects include nausea, vomiting, significant hypotension, and ischemic pain.

Antifibrinolytics

Fibrinolysis occurs when plasminogen activators are released and convert plasminogen to the enzyme plasmin. Plasminogen and plasmin bind to the fibrin blood clot by way of lysine binding sites that interact with lysine residues on fibrin. This binding is essential for optimal activity and enzyme generation.

The synthetic compound *aminocaproic acid* (Amicar) is similar to lysine but lacks the alpha amino group. Another compound and synthetic amino acid was subsequently discovered, *tranexamic acid* (Cyclokapreon).[16,17] Both these compounds displace or block plasminogen and plasmin binding to the fibrin blood clot and are very effective inhibitors of fibrinolysis. This is particularly relevant to their use in dental surgery because saliva is enriched with plasminogen activators. Although circulating levels of the drugs can be measured after administration, tissue concentrations may be more important in predicting their efficacy.

Aminocaproic acid and tranexamic acid can be administered intravenously or orally. Cyclokapreon can also be given as a mouthwash.[18-20] Cyclokapreon is given at a dose of 25 mg/kg three or four times daily or as a mouth rinse formulated as a 4.8% aqueous solution given three to four times daily. Amicar is given at a dose of 100 mg/kg four times daily in children and 4 to 6 g four times daily for adults. Amicar is available as an elixir (250 mg/ml) or in pill form (500 mg/pill).

Amican and Cyclokapreon are well tolerated, with loose stools, diarrhea, and nausea reported as the most frequent side effects. Hypotension occasionally occurs. Neither drug should be given if disseminated intravascular coagulation (DIC) is suspected or if there is urinary bleeding from a site proximal to the bladder. In both instances, accelerated thrombosis may occur, producing tissue ischemia or ureteral obstruction, respectively.

Fibrin Sealants

In their most rudimentary form, fibrin sealants consist of partially purified, plasma-derived fibrinogen and thrombin.[21,22] When applied locally to a site of injury, the thrombin rapidly converts the fibrinogen to a fibrin clot. Some fibrin sealants also contain factor XIII as well as protease inhibitors (most often aprotinin) to inhibit fibrinolysis. There is no evidence that the addition of these latter two components confers greater efficacy compared with the simpler formulations.

The commercial fibrin sealants vary greatly in their composition and in the methods used to virally attenuate the plasma derived proteins. They may be beneficial in patients with coagulation disorders who are undergoing dental surgery or other invasive procedures.[23-26] Tiseel VH has been approved for use in the United States and is composed of partially purified fibrinogen from human plasma, bovine aprotinin, human thrombin, and calcium chloride. Virucidal treatment consists of a two-step vapor heat treatment process to kill envelope-coated viruses.[27]

MANAGEMENT
General Measures

Dental treatment of a patient with a bleeding disorder requires close communication between the dentist and a hematologist familiar with the diagnosis and management of these disorders. Patients with severe hemophilia are at greatest risk for hemorrhage after a dental procedure, whereas those with vWD, mild hemophilia, platelet abnormalities, or factor XI deficiency are at lower risk. A comprehensive dental plan that includes good oral hygiene and semiannual examination and prophylaxis are essential in the patient with a bleeding disorder, as in other individuals. Generally, prophylaxis does not require special attention to prevent excessive bleeding. Procedures that require regional anesthesia with inferior alveolar nerve block theoretically expose the patient to the greatest risk of hemorrhage compared with infiltrative anesthesia. Loose connective tissue and highly vascularized tissue at the site of the mandibular block make this procedure more likely to cause hematoma formation in the patient with a bleeding disorder.

The level of coagulation factor necessary to ensure a safe procedure has not been established. No specific treatment protocols have been shown to be superior in rigorously conducted clinical trials. It is clear, however, that the patient with a severe bleeding disorder will have excessive hemorrhage, which may be life threatening after a dental procedure in some patients. Many patients with less severe bleeding disorders will suffer needless hemorrhage after a dental procedure. Therefore the dentist should consider some form of hemostatic treatment in most patients with a documented bleeding disorder. Appropriate local measures to improve hemostasis, including the use of fibrin sealants, should be considered in all patients.[28] Drugs that inhibit the function platelets, such as aspirin and NSAIDs, should be avoided if possible.

Severe Hemophilia A or B

Patients with severe hemophilia should be treated with factor replacement therapy before (1 to 2 hours) the planned procedure and with an inhibitor of fibrinolysis. The antifibrinolytic decreases the amount of factor replacement therapy required.[29-36] Therapy should be started before the procedure and continued for 7 to 10 days. The appropriate level of factor replacement is controversial; some suggest that 10% plasma factor levels are sufficient, whereas others support a level of about 50% to 60%.[37] A common practice is to raise the factor level to approximately 50% if mandibular regional anesthesia will be used and to some lower level if infiltrative analgesia is being considered. The duration of fibrinolytic therapy and the need for further factor replacement are then based on the amount of trauma and blood loss at surgery.

Mild or Moderate Hemophilia A and Von Willebrand's Disease

DDAVP is often very useful treatment in these individuals and can often obviate the need for factor replacement therapy. The coagulation factor response to DDAVP should be well documented before the planned procedure, particularly in the patient with moderate hemophilia A who may or may not show a response to DDAVP. If an adequate response to DDAVP is not demonstrated in patients with mild or moderate hemophilia A, their care should follow that for patients with severe hemophilia. Maximum response and duration of response to DDAVP are important considerations. Because DDAVP often causes an increase in salivary plasminogen activator levels, inhibitors of fibrinolysis are often used with DDAVP in these patients. Again, duration of treatment with these agents depends on the type of procedure and the amount of tissue injury sustained during the surgery.

Mild or Moderate Hemophilia B

Patients with mild hemophilia B do not respond to DDAVP and should receive antifibrinolytic agents. They may also require factor replacement therapy, depending on the procedure and their residual plasma factor level.

Platelet Disorders

Patients with platelet abnormalities often have excessive oozing after dental procedures and occasionally have more severe hemorrhage. DDAVP and antifibrinolytics are effective treatments. Occasionally, platelet transfusions are required.

Factor XI Deficiency

Antifibrinolytics are often sufficient to prevent bleeding in patients with factor XI deficiency. Factor replacement, if necessary, should be done with fresh frozen plasma.

SUMMARY

Dental procedures can result in hemorrhagic complications. A basic understanding of surgical principles and physiology will optimize patient care.

REFERENCES

1. Ruggeri ZM: Old concepts and new developments in the study of platelet aggregation, J Clin Invest 105:699-701, 2000.
2. Ruggeri ZM: Structure and function of von Willebrand factor, Thromb Haemost 82:576-584, 1999.
3. Rapaport SI, Rao VM: Initiation and regulation of tissue factor–dependent blood coagulation, Arterioscler Thromb 12:1111-1121, 1992.
4. Collen D: The plasminogen (fibrinolytic) system, Thromb Haemost 82:259-270, 1999.
5. Ginsburg D: Molecular genetics of von Willebrand disease, Thromb Haemost 82:585-591, 1999.
6. Hoyer LW: Medical progress: hemophilia A, N Engl J Med 330:38-47, 1994.
7. Rizza CR, Rhymes JL, Austen DEG, et al: Detection of carriers of hemophilia: a "blind" study, Br J Haematol 30:447-456, 1975.
8. Liesner RJ, Machin SJ: ABC of clinical haematology: platelet disorders, BMJ 314:809-812, 1997.
9. Hancock JF, Wieland K, Pugh RE, et al: A molecular genetic study of factor XI deficiency, Blood 77:1942-1948, 1991.
10. Brettler DB, Levine PH: Factor concentrates for treatment of hemophilia: which one to chose? Blood 73:2067, 1989.
11. Furie B, Limentani SA, Rosenfield CG: A practical guide to the evaluation and treatment of hemophilia, Blood 84:3, 1994.
12. Mannucci PM: Hemostatic drugs, N Engl J Med 339:245-254, 1998.
13. Rose EH, Aledort LM: Nasal spray desmopressin (DDAVP) for mild hemophilia A and von Willebrand disease, Ann Intern Med 114:563-568, 1991.
14. Lethagen S, Tennvall GR: Self-treatment with desmopressin intranasal spray in patients with bleeding disorders: effect on bleeding symptoms and socioeconomic factors, Ann Hematol 66:257-260, 1993.
15. MacGregor IR, Roberts EM, Prowse CV, et al: Fibrinolytic and haemostatic responses to desamino-D-arginine vasopressin (DDAVP) administered by intravenous and subcutaneous routes in healthy subjects, Thromb Haemost 59:34-39, 1988.
16. Andersson L, Nilsson SM, Colleen S, et al: Role of urokinase + tissue activator in sustaining bleeding and management thereof with EACA + AMCA, Ann NY Acad Sci 146:642, 1968.
17. Andersson L, Nilsson IM, Nilehn J-E, et al: Experimental and clinical studies on AMCA, the antifibrinolytically active isomer of p-aminomethyl cyclohexane carboxylic acid, Scand J Haematol 2:230, 1965.
18. Sindet-Pedersen S, Ramstrom G, Bernvil S, et al: Hemostatic effect of tranexamic acid mouthwash in anticoagulant-treated patients undergoing oral surgery, N Engl J Med 320:844, 1989.
19. Sindet-Pederson S, Stenbjerg S: Effect of local antifibrinolytic treatment with tranexamic acid in hemophiliacs undergoing oral surgery, J Oral Maxillofac Surg 44:703, 1986.
20. Sindet-Pederson S: Distribution of tranexamic acid to plasma and saliva after oral administration and mouth rinsing: a pharmacokinetic study, J Clin Pharmacol 27:1005, 1987.
21. Spotnitz WD: Fibrin sealant in the United States: clinical use at the University of Virginia, Thromb Haemost 74:482-485, 1995.
22. Martinowitz U, Spotnitz WD: Fibrin tissue adhesives, Thromb Haemost 78:661, 1997.

23. Martinowitz U, Varon D, Heim M: The role of fibrin tissue adhesives in surgery of haemophilia patients, *Haemophilia* 4:443, 1998.

24. Tock B, Drohan W, Hess J, et al: Haemophilia and advanced fibrin sealant technologies, *Haemophilia* 4:449, 1998.

25. Martinowitz U, Schulman S, Horoszowski H, Heim M: Role of fibrin sealants in surgical procedures on patients with hemostatic disorders, *Clin Orthop Rel Res* 328:65-75, 1996.

26. Martinowitz U, Schulman S: Fibrin sealant in surgery of patients with a hemorrhagic diathesis, *Thromb Haemost* 74:486-492, 1995.

27. Fibrin sealant Tiseel VH product information, 1999, Deerfield, Ill, Baxter Healthcare.

28. Rakocz M, Mazar A, Varon D, et al: Dental extractions in patients with bleeding disorders, *Oral Surg Oral Med Oral Pathol* 75:280, 1993.

29. Walsh PN, Rizza CR, Matthews JM, et al: Epsilon-aminocaproic acid therapy for dental extractions in haemophilia and Christmas disease: a double blind controlled trial, *Br J Haematol* 20:463, 1971.

30. Forbes CD, Barr RD, Reid G, et al: Tranexamic acid in control of haemorrhage after dental extraction in haemophilia and Christmas disease, *Br Med J* 2:311, 1972.

31. Djulbegovic B, Marasa M, Pesto A, et al: Safety and efficacy of purified factor IX concentrate and antifibrinolytic agents for dental extractions in hemophilia B, *Am J Hematol* 51:168, 1996.

32. Tavenner RW: Epsilon-aminocaproic acid in the treatment of haemophilia and Christmas disease with special reference to the extraction of teeth, *Br Dent J* 124(1):19-22, 1968.

33. Sindet-Pederson S, Stenbjerg S, Ingerslev J: Control of gingival hemorrhage in hemophilic patients by inhibition of fibrinolysis with tranexamic acid, *J Periodont Res* 23:72, 1988.

34. Cooksey MW, Perry CB, Raper AB: Preliminary communications: epsilon-aminocaproic acid therapy for dental extractions in haemophiliacs, *Br Med J* 2:1633, 1966.

35. Reid WO, Lucas ON, Francisco J, et al: The use of epsilon-aminocaproic acid in the management of dental extractions in the hemophiliac, *Am J Med Sci* 24:81-84, 1964.

36. Tavenner RW: Use of tranexamic acid in control of haemorrhage after extraction of teeth in haemophilia and Christmas disease, *Br Med J* 2(809):314-315, 1972.

37. Steinberg SE, Levin J, Bell WR: Evidence that less replacement therapy is required for dental extractions in hemophiliacs, *Am J Hematol* 16:1, 1984.

Epistaxis

Bertrand Sorel

Epistaxis, or nose bleeding, is the most common bleeding disorder of the head and neck. Most people have a nosebleed at least once in their life, and although most episodes are treated at home and resolve spontaneously, some will present to health care professionals, usually emergency physicians and otolaryngologists. Epistaxis can occur in a variety of settings and for multiple reasons.

The incidence of epistaxis varies with age. It is rarely observed in infants, then becomes increasingly common in children as they age (with a peak between 3 and 8 years). It decreases in frequency after puberty, then increases again in older age. Most patients who require intervention can be managed in an outpatient setting, with only the most severe refractory bleeding necessitating hospitalization.

Severe nasal hemorrhages may lead to hypotension, hypoxia, and life-threatening aspiration. It is therefore important to be able to evaluate the problem properly, establish an appropriate diagnosis, treat appropriately, and eventually refer the patient to a hospital setting if necessary.

PATHOPHYSIOLOGY

Many reasons exist to explain nasal bleeding. Just as the mouth is the portal of entry of the digestive tract, the nose is the gateway to the respiratory tree. It is similarly the area most exposed to the environment and its multiple agents. The nose is an extremely vascular structure and usually the most prominent part of the face, exposing it frequently to trauma. The presence of multiple superficial vessels in the nasal mucosa makes it a prime area where hematologic (e.g., blood dyscrasias), coagulation, or vascular disorders may be initially revealed.

The nose also acts as a humidifier, bringing inspired air to 100% relative humidity and at the temperature of 37° C in the short course between nares and posterior nasopharynx. This water and warmth exchange exposes the nose to dryness when very dry air is inspired. The filtration role of the nose subjects it to multiple allergens, some of which will cause inflammation and engorgement of the blood vessels of the nasal mucosa, with frequent subsequent trauma and bleeding. The nasal mucosa has an intrinsic capacity for venous engorgement, with a submucosal plexus of veins (*cavernous nasal plexus*) that acts similar to erectile tissue under parasympathetic action. This autonomic response arises from chemical, mechanical, thermal, and psychogenic stimuli.

BLOOD SUPPLY TO THE NOSE

The rich arterial blood supply to the nose is derived from both the internal and external carotid artery systems. To simplify the model, the dual irrigation can be described as follows. Viewing the nose in sagittal cuts reveals a corresponding pattern between the lateral nasal wall and the septum (Figure 20-1). These areas supplied by the internal and external carotid systems can be approximated by triangles, with the external system having greater influence in the nasal septum.

Internal Carotid System

After branching from the common carotid, the internal carotid artery goes directly to the brain without further branching. It therefore has to reemerge from the cranium to irrigate facial structures, through the ophthalmic artery. The ophthalmic artery exits the cranium through the superior orbital fissure and divides into several branches, two of which will irrigate the superior portion of the nasal mucosa. These two branches are called anterior and posterior ethmoidal arteries because they pass through the ethmoidal sinus complex. After going through the sinuses, they reenter the anterior cranial fossa, then exit it again by descending through the cribriform plate to enter the nose. Each then divides into medial and lateral branches, to irrigate corresponding parts of the septum and lateral walls

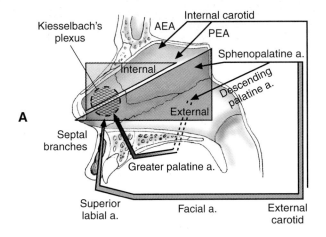

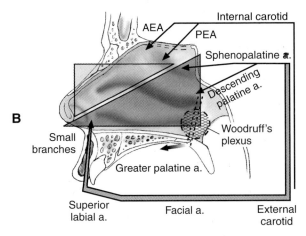

Figure 20-1. **A,** Blood supply to the nasal septum. **B,** Blood supply to the lateral nasal wall.

of the nose. The *anterior ethmoidal artery* (usually the larger of the two vessels) supplies the mucosa of the anterior one third of the lateral wall and a corresponding part of the septum. The *posterior ethmoidal artery* irrigates the superior turbinate and a small portion of the septum.

External Carotid System

Two of the main branches of the external carotid artery have minor and major roles in the irrigation of the nose. A major branch of the external carotid is the facial, or external maxillary, artery. In the minor role the *external maxillary artery* divides into the superior labial artery, which supplies the upper lip and then gives off a septal branch that courses cephalad to irrigate the anterior portion of the nasal floor and septum.

The external carotid has two terminal branches, the superficial temporal and internal maxillary arteries. After giving off multiple branches as it proceeds anteriorly to the pterygopalatine fossa, the *internal maxillary artery* divides into the infraorbital, posterior alveolar, pterygopalatine, and in its major vascular role for the nasal cavity, into the sphenopalatine, descending palatine, and pharyngeal arteries.

The *sphenopalatine artery* is the main blood supply of the nose. It enters the nasal cavity through the foramen bearing its name, located at the posterior edge of the middle turbinate. It divides there into several branches, grouped as medial and lateral divisions. Predictably, the medial division supplies the septum, and the lateral division vascularizes the lateral walls, which comprise the turbinate. The medial division (nasoseptal or nasopalatine) gives rise to the posterior septal artery, which courses all the way anteriorly along the septum. The lateral division is called the posterior, posterosuperior, or lateral nasal artery and supplies the middle and inferior turbinates.

The *descending palatine artery* is the other terminal branch of the internal maxillary artery. It has a minor role in nasal perfusion. It goes through the pterygopalatine canal, may divide in two or three branches, the largest one entering the buccal cavity through the greater palatine foramen, becoming the greater palatine artery. It supplies the palate going anteriorly, then reenters the nasal cavity by turning superiorly through the incisive foramen, to irrigate the septum and the floor of the nose.

The *pharyngeal artery* has a lesser role, primarily involved in irrigating the soft palate, although it contributes to Woodruff's plexus on its way there.

Plexuses and Anastomotic Areas

Regardless of the pattern associated with vascularization of the nose, a major feature is the vast amount of anastomotic areas that exist at every level. The internal and external carotid systems converge in multiple areas. In the area of the cavernous sinus, the internal carotid has communicating branches with the internal maxillary artery (via the artery of the pterygoid canal, and the ascending pharyngeal artery).

Kiesselbach's plexus (Little's area) is the space in the anterior septum where four sources of blood irrigation converge, forming multiple anastomoses. The superior labial (septal branch), sphenopalatine, and greater palatine arteries represent the external carotid system contribution, and the internal carotid supplies this area through the anterior ethmoidal artery from

---

BOX 20-1 Causes of Epistaxis

LOCAL

A. Inflammatory
1. Allergic rhinitis
2. Childhood exanthems
3. Foreign body reactions
4. Eosinophilic nonallergic rhinitis
5. Vasomotor rhinitis
B. Infections
1. Viral (cold, flu, mononucleosis)
2. Bacterial (sinusitis, furunculosis)
3. Fungal (rhinosporidiosis)
C. Trauma
1. Rhinitis sicca (low humidity, dry heat)
2. Self-induced (nose picking or rubbing)
3. Foreign body
4. Facial fracture, blunt trauma
5. Surgery (nasal/sinus procedures)
6. Nasotracheal or nasogastric tube placement
7. Nasal prong oxygen, continuous positive airway pressure
8. Barotrauma (scuba diving, flying)
9. Air pollution (indoor/outdoor)
10. Inhalants (chemical, caustic agents [e.g., tobacco, cannabis, ammonia, chlorine, wood dust])
D. Anatomic
1. Severe septal deviation
2. Unilateral choanal atresia
3. Septal perforation (trauma, surgery, granulomatous diseases)
4. Postsurgical adhesions
5. Idiopathic atrophic rhinitis
6. Pseudoaneurysm of internal carotid artery from prior trauma to neck
E. Medications
Rhinitis medicamentosus (chronic use of cocaine or topical decongestants [e.g., phenylephrine, oxymetazolone])
F. Benign lesions and neoplasms
1. Nasopharyngeal angiofibroma
2. Papillomas (inverted, squamous)
3. Pyogenic granuloma
4. Polyps
5. Meningocele, encephalocele, glioma (central nervous system lesions)
6. Necrotizing sialometaplasia
7. Hemangioma

G. Malignant neoplasms
1. Squamous cell carcinoma
2. Malignant melanoma
3. Rhabdomyosarcoma
H. Idiopathic (~10%)

SYSTEMIC

A. Bleeding disorders
1. Coagulopathies
a. Inherited (hemophilia A and B, von Willebrand's disease)
b. Acquired (vitamin K deficiency, liver disease)
2. Platelet disorders
a. Inherited (polycythemia vera, thrombocytopenic purpura, thrombasthenia, Bernard-Soulier syndrome, idiopathic aplastic anemia)
b. Acquired (heparin-induced thrombocytopenia, uremia, cirrhosis, aplastic anemia, vitamin B_{12} or folate deficiency)
3. Blood vessel disorders
a. Inherited (hereditary hemorrhagic telangiectasia)
b. Acquired (vitamin C deficiency)
B. Neoplasms
1. Leukemia
2. Lymphoma
C. Infections
1. Scarlet fever
2. Malaria
3. Typhoid fever
4. Sepsis
5. Granulomatous disease (sarcoidosis, syphilis, tuberculosis)
D. Drug induced
1. Aspirin
2. Anticoagulants (e.g., coumadin, heparin)
3. Antibiotics (e.g., chloramphenicol)
4. Antineoplastics (e.g., methotrexate)
E. Cardiovascular
1. Arteriosclerosis
2. Hypertension
F. Idiopathic inflammatory disorders
1. Wegener's granulomatosis
2. Lethal midline granuloma

---

above. Kiesselbach's area is by far the most common site for epistaxis.

Woodruff's plexus is in the area of the posterior tip of the inferior turbinate and nasal floor. The posterior nasal artery anastomoses with the pharyngeal branch of the maxillary artery.

ETIOLOGY

Epistaxis may be caused by a wide variety of events or factors, both local and systemic (Box 20-1). As with most other head and neck structures, the nose is extremely vascular and can bleed profusely if its integrity is breached.

Trauma, inflammation, and infection are by far the most common causes of bleeding. *Trauma* can be obvious (e.g., baseball or fist to nose, car accident, surgery) or more subtle (e.g., nose picking, putting objects in nasal cavity). *Inflammation* can arise from allergies, dryness of air, inhalants, drugs (recreational, prescribed), or a foreign body and is part of the infection process. *Infections* cause bleeding by several mechanisms, primarily inflammation and mechanical trauma (excessive blowing of nose in many cases). Infections also vary from some common sources (viruses) to rare ones (fungal).

Once the common causes likely have been eliminated, the practitioner must consider the rarer causes.

Anatomic characteristics of the nose have been studied to determine if certain elements (e.g., deviated septum) might help predict epistaxis and assist in its treatment by localizing the source faster. Results have been contradictory, although an associated anatomic landmark exists. Keisselbach's plexus is the site of approximately 90% of bleeding events and is easy to find and visualize in the anterior nose. This is practical for the physician who wants to control bleeding in that area. Keisselbach's plexus simply happens to be an anastomotic area of vessels located superficially in a site highly exposed to trauma, directly in the portal of entry of the airway.

Bleeding disorders are important to consider because of potential far-reaching implications. The problem might be found at any of several levels of the overall hemostatic mechanism: clotting factors, platelets, or blood vessels themselves. All these components may be disturbed genetically or altered secondary to some other process. Drugs must always be high on the list when looking for iatrogenic causes of epistaxis.

Neoplasm must also be considered. Although uncommon, the consequences of missing a malignant neoplasm may be significant. The epistaxis may be an initial sign of leukemia or lymphoma. Multiple systemic diseases may manifest as epistaxis, including uremia, liver disease (often secondary to alcoholism), and several disease processes that cause marrow failure. *Hypertension* as a cause of epistaxis is still debated in the literature but is supported by several authors. Rare causes include genetic disorders (e.g., Rendu-Osler-Weber disease), idiopathic or inflammatory diseases (e.g., Wegener's granulomatosis, lethal midline granuloma), or posttraumatic events (e.g., internal carotid pseudoaneurysm).

PATIENT EVALUATION
Initial Assessment

The evaluation of the care needed by the patient starts with a rapid assessment of the situation's seriousness. The person who presents with a severe hemorrhage (rare) must be treated like any patient with a life-threatening emergency. Advanced cardiac life support (ACLS) guidelines are applied, since the hemorrhage with direct airway involvement threatens both respiratory and cardiovascular systems. It is vital to assess properly the patient's airway, breathing, and circulation (ABCs).

Once the airway and breathing have been cleared, determination of the hemodynamic status is essential: how much blood has been lost, and is the patient unstable? If any doubt about patient stability exists, intravenous (IV) lines should be started, IV fluids given, and the patient's blood should be typed and cross-matched and sent to the laboratory for testing (complete blood count, prothrombin time, partial thromboplastin time).

The vast majority of cases will not represent ACLS emergencies. Patients typically present with mild to moderate bleeding, often stopped by the time the practitioner is reached.

History

An appropriate history is essential in all patients with epistaxis. Proper questioning will often help determine the probable etiology and guide the treatment. After inquiries about the person's overall medical condition, any prescribed or over-the-counter medications, and allergies, the bleeding itself can be investigated. How long has the patient been bleeding, and how much blood has been lost (estimate)? Which side is the blood coming from? Is it coming from the nose only, or also going in the throat? Spitting blood suggests posterior nosebleed. Is the patient feeling weak or dizzy (hypovolemia, orthostasis)? Is this the first nosebleed the patient has had? If not, how was bleeding treated previously, and with what success?

In the absence of an obvious cause, specific questions should be asked. Is there any recent history of trauma? Has the patient been blowing the nose frequently due to allergies or an upper respiratory infection? Is nose picking involved? Does the patient usually breathe well through the nose? Is any medication used in the nose? Admission of cocaine use might be difficult to elicit in patients, especially teenagers. Are there family members with the same problem or with any bleeding disorder? Does the patient bruise easily?

Physical Examination

The history questions usually help to identify the cause of bleeding. Physical examination comes next, unless the patient presented as an acute emergency (vital signs and overall assessment would then be the first priority). Vital signs should be taken. The skin should be examined for evidence of blood dyscrasia (petechia, ecchymosis, purpura). A complete head and neck examination should be made, including the neck nodes. Special attention would finally be given to the mouth, throat, and nose. In the mouth and pharynx, the presence of blood suggests posterior bleeding. The dentist should check for mucosal evidence of blood dyscrasia and determine the nasal side involved and amount of blood. The examination of the nose itself is described under Management.

Laboratory Testing

Unless a life-threatening situation is involved as described earlier, laboratory tests are usually not necessary. They can be useful to confirm a suspected bleeding disorder or in hematologic malignancies. Radiogaphs of the sinus and lateral neck and computed tomography (CT) scanning can be useful to localize tumors.

MANAGEMENT

The first important action is to calm and reassure the patient. Bleeding from the nose can be very frightening, especially for a young child. Localizing the bleeding site is important. In general the bleeding will be coming from one nostril only, indicating the side of the nasal cavity involved, and only one site will be responsible for the bleeding. Multiple simultaneous bleeding sites are improbable, except in trauma. The patient with profuse bleeding might have blood in both nostrils and mouth, by exchange through the nasopharynx and oropharynx.

Box 20-2 describes a list of useful items for examination and treatment of the bleeding nose. Availability will depend on where the intervention takes place.

A cooperative patient is needed for safe and proper intervention. Reassurance is important for the anxious patient, although sedation or even general anesthesia may be necessary, especially for children.

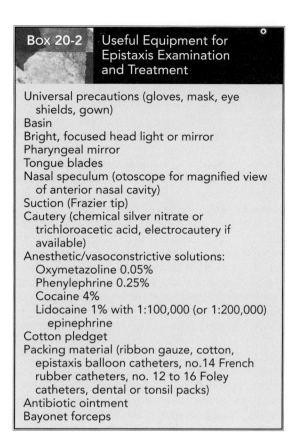

Box 20-2   Useful Equipment for Epistaxis Examination and Treatment

Universal precautions (gloves, mask, eye shields, gown)
Basin
Bright, focused head light or mirror
Pharyngeal mirror
Tongue blades
Nasal speculum (otoscope for magnified view of anterior nasal cavity)
Suction (Frazier tip)
Cautery (chemical silver nitrate or trichloroacetic acid, electrocautery if available)
Anesthetic/vasoconstrictive solutions:
   Oxymetazoline 0.05%
   Phenylephrine 0.25%
   Cocaine 4%
   Lidocaine 1% with 1:100,000 (or 1:200,000) epinephrine
Cotton pledget
Packing material (ribbon gauze, cotton, epistaxis balloon catheters, no.14 French rubber catheters, no. 12 to 16 Foley catheters, dental or tonsil packs)
Antibiotic ointment
Bayonet forceps

The examiner should follow universal precautions, using gloves, mask, eye shields, and gown. The patient's clothes should also be protected against his or her own bleeding with appropriate covering. A basin is used to collect the blood. Sitting reclined in the typical dental treatment position is not recommended. Blood dripping in the throat will increase the patient's discomfort, the incidence of gagging, and the risk of vomiting and aspiration. With the exception of the syncopal or orthostatic patient, the preferred position is sitting in a straight chair, with the head inclined forward. This will favor examination of the nasal vestibule; otherwise, only the roof of the nose will be seen. Extending the neck should be avoided because it also encourages bleeding in the pharynx.

With visualization so paramount, a good light source is important, whether external from a head mirror or light or internal from an otoscope or endoscope. A good way to start clearing the nasal cavity is to have the patient blow the nose, although this can occasionally increase the bleeding. A strong suction, using a Frazier tip, is useful for removing remaining blood and clots. Several solutions may be used for local anesthesia and vasoconstriction (see Box 20-2). These can be applied as spray (atomizer) or as a more prolonged contact through cotton tips, soaked cotton pledget, or neurosurgical cotton; these take effect in 5 to 10 minutes. Anesthesia improves patient comfort and may allow minor interventions. Vasoconstriction may help control or diminish the bleeding problems itself, improving visibility and creating the dry field needed for cauterization. Local infiltration using lidocaine with 1:200,000 epinephrine provides sphenopalatine or anterior ethmoidal blocks; the solution also can be infiltrated directly around the bleeding site.

After obtaining adequate visualization, the dentist can search for the bleeding site. The nasal speculum should be held in the horizontal position to allow an optimal view of the nasal septum, where most bleeding occurs. At this point an important distinction must be made. Although varying slightly depending on the authors, epistaxis is usually described as *anterior* when the bleeding site *can be visualized*; this usually means that it is anterior to the turbinate. *Posterior* epistaxis is then defined as a bleeding point that *cannot be visualized* on routine (nonendoscopic) intranasal examination. Again, about 90% of nasal bleeding is anterior in origin, most often in Kiesselbach's plexus, the roof of the septum, or the anterior end of the inferior or middle turbinate. These hemorrhages are usually venous in origin. Posterior nosebleeds represent approximately 10% of cases and most often originate from the posterior septum or Woodruff's plexus. They are more often arterial in origin and also present more complex treatment issues.

Anterior Epistaxis

Once the bleeding point is identified anteriorly, controlling it depends on the degree of hemorrhaging. Cautery (especially chemical) will work only in a fairly dry site. When the bleeding stopped either spontaneously or after application of vasoconstrictor solution, the site is often seen as an area of prominent vessels, overlaid by a scab or blood clot, or as a thin layer of mucosa. This is readily amenable to cautery, either chemical (silver nitrate sticks) or electrical.

Silver nitrate cautery is inactivated by moisture and requires a dry field. A way to circumvent the problem is to cauterize surrounding tissues first, in a concentric fashion, moving inward toward the bleeding site. This progressively decreases collateral flow to the bleeding site and usually allows the chemical cautery to work on the site itself. Excess silver nitrate should be removed to

avoid injuring adjacent noninvolved tissues; it can also be neutralized with sodium chloride. Topical local anesthetic should suffice before the procedure in most patients.

Electrocautery is less susceptible to moisture and is an efficient way to stop bleeding. Local submucosal anesthesia should be used. Some caution must be used with the septum. With mucosa overlying cartilage on each side, simultaneous cauterization of one location on both sides may lead to perforation and should be avoided. Unilateral cautery must not be overaggressive due to the greater depth of penetration for this type of cautery.

Initial Intervention

When active bleeding is present, several methods can be used to try to stop it initially. Pinching the nose with firm pressure for 10 minutes will control most bleeding, allowing further intervention. As described previously, injecting the tissues surrounding the bleeding site will usually stop or significantly slow down the bleeding, whether using a solution containing a vasoconstrictor or even plain saline. Local application of vasoconstrictor on cotton pledgets or neurosurgical cotton pads, left in place for 5 to 10 minutes, will also usually work, especially when combined with simultaneous nasal pinch.

Secondary Intervention: Packing

The bleeding site that persists despite these attempts requires more elaborate care. Packs of all types are then used. Anterior packing is used mainly in two cases: cautery is unable to control epistaxis, and the bleeding is coming from an anterior site, but the site itself is unreachable (e.g., behind anterior septal spur, from underside of anteroinferior turbinate). There are multiple techniques for packing and a variety of packing materials.

The classic nasal packing is the *petroleum jelly strip gauze* (½ inch × 72 inches) impregnated by antibiotic ointment. Another form is the *bismuth iodoform paraffin paste* (BIPP) on ribbon gauze, which has an unpleasant smell and taste. Telfa sponges can also be used. Placement technique is the most important element (Figure 20-2). It should be layered from the floor to the roof of the nose, using a bayonet forceps, under good visualization. In the occasional case of a very inferior bleed, the upper part of the nasal cavity may be left free, allowing some breathing above

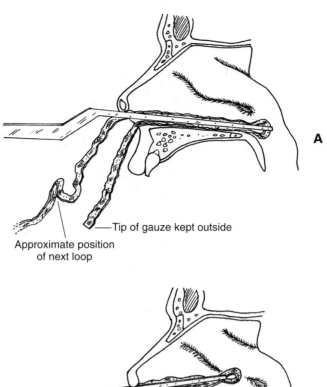

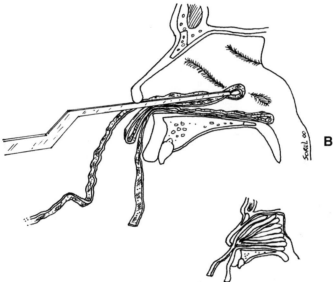

Figure 20-2. Method for packing the nose using strip gauze. **A,** Placement of the first loop, with free end left outside. **B,** Pattern for second and subsequent loops. *Inset,* Final result, with both free ends outside.

the pack. Both tails of the gauze should be outside the nose, secured to the patient's face, with only blind loops found in the posterior area of the nose (Figure 20-3). Failure to place the pack properly may bring its premature loss, may gag the patient because part of it dangles down the pharynx, and is even a risk for aspiration.

Antibiotics are used both as ointment impregnating the gauze (against odors and infection) and systematically because of increased incidence of sinusitis (the sinus ostia are often blocked) or the rare risk of staphylococcal toxic shock syndrome. An antibiotic with activity against the nasal flora and *Staphylococcus aureus* is therefore chosen (cephalosporin, amoxicillin-clavulanate).

The pack should be left in place for as short a time as practical, usually 2 to 4 days. There is some debate about packing one or both sides simultaneously. Some authors advocate packing both nasal cavities to avoid displacement of the nasal septum; others consider bilateral packing a significant cause of airway compromise that necessitates hospitalization.

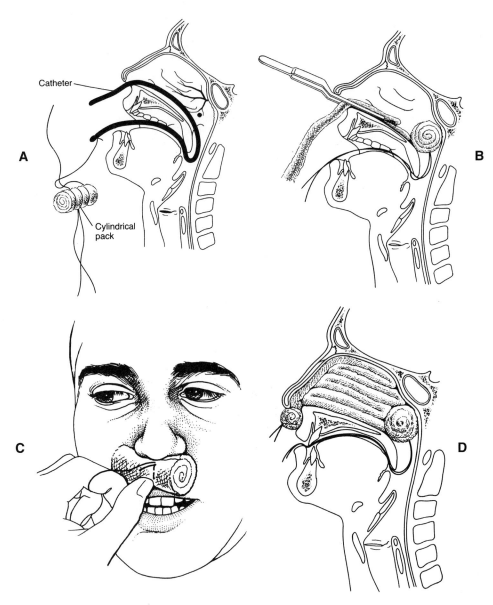

Figure 20-3. **A** to **D,** Placement of conventional posterior nasal pack. *From Parretta LJ, Denslow BL, Brown CG: Emerg Clin North Am 5(2):265-277, 1987.*

One disadvantage of petroleum jelly strip gauzes is the need to remove the pack, with the associated patient discomfort and risk of traumatic rebleeding. This has stimulated the search for a resorbable packing that would not require removal. Multiple options exist. Absorbable gelatin sponges (Gelfoam) or oxidized regenerated cellulose preparations (Oxcel, Surgicel) are popular options. These substances form an artificial clot when mixed with blood and dissolve in 2 to 3 days. *Avitene*, a microfibrillar cross-linked bovine topocollagen material, may favor platelet aggregation. Clot formation results from platelets adhering to it, having a release reaction that then brings in more platelets. Applying thrombin spray to Gelfoam or Surgicel can help the hemostatic process (see Chapter 19).

Porcine strip packing has also been used. This is a salty, fatty material originating from salt pork or fatback. It is hydrophilic and will swell when absorbing liquids, to fill the nasal cavity, taking its shape and applying pressure on the tissues.

Porcine tissue has also been shown to accelerate platelet aggregation and blood coagulation in vitro, and it possibly acts in this way in the nose. This pack can be removed, or spontaneous liquefaction occurs in a day to several days.

A more recent product becoming increasingly popular is the *Merocel nasal pack*, a compressed, dehydrated sponge (hydroxylated polyvinyl acetal) that expands to three times its normal size when rehydrated with blood or saline. Patients describe the insertion process as painless to very uncomfortable, but it takes only a few seconds. Aspiration is unlikely, but a drain string should be secured to the patient's cheek as a precaution. It has been reported that Merocel nasal packing is able to inhibit bacterial proliferation and may bring some protection against the toxic shock syndrome described previously. Another expandable packing is made of hydroxylated polyvinyl alcohol (Expandacell, Rhino Rocket).

Posterior Epistaxis

Posterior epistaxis is nose bleeding that cannot be visualized by routine intranasal examination. A more practical definition is epistaxis that cannot be treated effectively using an anterior nasal pack.

Posterior nosebleeds are in general more worrisome than anterior epistaxis. They are not easily visualized, making treatment difficult, and tend to bleed in the throat, which increases patients' distress. As with anterior bleeding, the treatment of posterior epistaxis is usually sequential. A greater palatine foramen block can be extremely useful. It will usually slow the bleeding and occasionally even stop it. Approximately 3 ml of local anesthetic is injected using a 25-gauge 2.5-cm needle introduced through the greater palatine foramen. The pterygopalatine foramen canal runs upward and backward for 2.5 to 3.0 cm, ending in the pterygopalatine fossa. The sphenopalatine and descending palatal arteries are located about 2.8 cm under the oral mucosa. The main problem is recurrence of the bleeding, and the block may need to be repeated multiple times.

In the absence of excessive bleeding, and given the availability of an endoscope, a search should be made for the bleeding site. Several authors have reported high success rates of control when using an endoscope. Flexible fiberoptic nasopharyngoscopy may be done with or without sedation in the clinic, although it will probably be required with young patients. A rigid endoscope provides better light and optics. The most

common bleeding sites have been described as the posterolateral nasal wall (just posterior to the tip of the inferior or middle turbinates) or along the posterior septum. A grounded suction cautery unit is a useful tool for these procedures. The endoscope is advanced by following the tip of the suction, and the bleeding site is cauterized under direct visualization when found. Occasionally the inferior turbinate must be fractured to produce adequate visualization of the posterolateral nasal cavity. It is recommended that direct local anesthesia and a greater palatine foramen block be provided to eliminate pain associated with procedures in that area.

Patients with posterior nasal bleeding should be referred to an ear-nose-throat specialist, and endoscopy becomes a realistic approach to the problem. In an emergency case, however, this is not always possible. Treatment modalities vary from the relatively simple (posterior nasal pack, balloon tamponade) to the highly specialized intervention (arterial ligation, embolization).

Posterior nasal packing may take the form of a conventional (classic) gauze pack, but recently, balloons of all types have become increasingly popular.

Standard Posterior Nasal Pack

Several mediums can be used, such as rolled gauze (4×4-inch gauze pad), a gauze pad filled with lamb's wool or a vaginal tampon (1-inch length, ½- to ¾-inch diameter). The chosen packing should be impregnated with an antibiotic ointment. Although multiple tying methods can be used, the one described here can be used for unilateral or bilateral packing (see Figure 20-3).

The pack is secured in the center by using one or two long silk ties (0 to 2-0) or umbilical tape, and another tie is placed laterally on each side to create a bundle. The posterior pack can be designed in a way that it will block one or both choanae (posterior nares). If unilateral packing is desired, the pack must be small enough to fit into the involved choanae, but not so long that it may obstruct both of them. A lubricated French catheter (red rubber catheter) is passed through the bleeding naris until the tip is visualized in the oropharynx. A hemostat is then used to bring it through the mouth. The two central ties are attached to it, then the catheter is pulled back through the nose, bringing the pack through the mouth all the way to the nasopharynx. A finger helps in placing it in the proper location, which is above the level of the soft palate, just posterior to the turbinates.

The soft palate must be examined after the placement; it must not be depressed by the pack, which should be replaced with any evidence of bulging. The remaining silk ties are left going through the mouth, exiting from it, and should be secured to the cheek. They will be helpful to remove the pack. The two ties in the nose are used to apply some tension on the posterior pack while anterior nasal packing is inserted. The same ties are then tied around a dental roll or a gauze pad to protect the nose base against excessive pressure.

Bilateral posterior packing is done essentially in the same way, except that a catheter is passed through each nasal cavity, and one lateral tie is then passed in the method described along each side of the septum. This effectively brings the center of the pack against the posterior septum and each side in a choana. The ties are attached in the same fashion to a dental roll or gauze pad, bridging the columella. The center ties are kept through the mouth and secured to the cheek as described previously. The pack is usually left in place 4 to 7 days, with the patient hospitalized.

Balloon Catheters

Balloons of several types can also be used, either standard urinary catheters or custom-designed for the nose. A no. 12 to 16 Foley catheter with a 30-ml catheter is usually readily available in a hospital or emergency department setting. A water-based lubricant is used to prelubricate the catheter, which is then passed through the involved nasal cavity all the way to the posterior pharynx (Figure 20-4, A). The balloon is then inflated with 10 to 20 ml of normal saline (not air, which will deflate) and is pulled back onto the nasopharynx, until it is felt to fit snugly against the choanae. As for the posterior pack, the soft palate should be examined for a downward bulge and the balloon adjusted accordingly.

Epistaxis balloons come under several names and forms. The balloon is basically a Foley catheter modified to correspond better to the inner shape of the nose and to provide a simple method for anterior and posterior nose packing (Figure 20-4, B). The *Nasostat* is a single-balloon catheter, elongated to fill the entire length of the nasal cavity, from anterior septum to the soft palate. First, 8 ml of air is instilled, and the patient is observed for further bleeding; the balloon can be inflated with up to 15 ml of air, if needed. If successful in stopping the bleeding, the air should be removed and replaced with the appropriate amount of normal saline. One disadvantage of the device is that it does not allow the placement of supplemental anterior packing.

The *Naso-blymp* is used in the same general fashion, except that it has two balloons, anterior and posterior, each with its own color-coded valve. The anterior balloon can be inflated with 10 to 25 ml of saline and the posterior (if needed after observing the effect of the anterior balloon) with 4 to 8 ml of saline.

The *Postpac* is another variation. Its design corresponds to the choanae without exerting pressure in the nasopharynx or septum. It allows continued suction along the floor of the nose and placement of an anterior pack if desired. The Postpac can be deflated and removed without disturbing the pack. Moreover, it can be used as a nasopharyngeal airway, allowing the patient to breathe through its central hollow backbone.

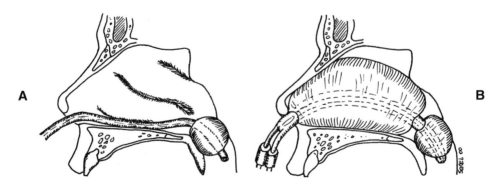

Figure 20-4. **A,** Standard urinary catheter used for emergency control of posterior epistaxis. **B,** Specially designed epistaxis balloon to facilitate control of anterior or posterior bleeding.

Complications

All patients with a posterior bleed should be seen by an otolaryngologist, and admitted to a hospital for observation. Multiple complications have been associated with posterior nasal packing. A *nasopulmonary reflex* has been described, with hypoventilation and desaturation when such packings are in place; 40% humidified oxygen supplementation is recommended. The patient should be monitored closely and vital signs taken frequently, especially in the elderly population, who have most of the posterior bleeds. Other posterior-packing-related complications include respiratory failure (often enhanced by pain medications and sedatives given to the patient because of the pack itself), sleep apnea, cardiac arrhythmias (possibly through vagal reflexes), airway obstruction (aspirated packing), or even death.

Arterial Ligation

In up to 25% of cases the previously described measures will fail to stop epistaxis. Treatment then becomes specialized surgical intervention. One definitive way of stopping bleeding from a vessel is to ligate it or embolize it. *Ligation* uses an external approach in which a vessel is exposed surgically, isolated, and then occluded by putting sutures or vascular clamps around it. Embolization entails blocking a vessel from inside, using some artificial embolus, after the vessel has been studied by angiography.

Anatomy and the surgical access dictate the targets of ligation methods. The external carotid artery ipsilateral to the bleeding nasal cavity has long been a logical target, with relatively easy access for the trained head and neck surgeon. The carotid bifurcation is found, and the external carotid artery is isolated and ligated. The main problem is the distance from the bleeding site, with substantial collateral flow from the contralateral external carotid system and from communications with the internal carotid system.

Techniques have therefore been developed to act closer to the target. The internal maxillary artery can be ligated after being surgically isolated through several possible approaches: transantrally, through a Caldwell-Luke approach, or transorally, going through the buccal mucosa, then the buccal fat pad. In some patients, ligation of the internal maxillary artery is not sufficient, and ligation of the ethmoidal arteries is recommended. An external ethmoidectomy is used for exposure, with subsequent sub-

periosteal dissection along the medial orbital wall. The anterior ethmoidal artery is usually the cause of the bleeding and is clamped with vascular clips. Persistent bleeding also requires exposure and clamping of the posterior ethmoidal artery.

Debate is ongoing in otolaryngology about ligation. Some believe that early ligation is definitive treatment, whereas others favor more traditional repeated packing methods, avoiding general anesthesia, and state that most patients will not need surgery.

Embolization

Embolization is increasingly used for refractory epistaxis. Angiography is used to locate the vessels, although active bleeding is necessary for detection. Emboli are then introduced in the involved vessel, through the catheter tip, just proximal to the bleeding site. Several substances have been used as emboli, such as Gelfoam, nonabsorbable polyvinyl alcohol particles, and coiled springs. The most common complication is a groin hematoma, but the main risk is an embolic phenomenon in the internal carotid system. The technique has been highly successful when applied by experienced angiographers.

Pharmacologic Therapy

Treatment of epistaxis by drug treatment alone is rarely done because of a general lack of effectiveness. Definitions are again important when reading the literature. Several authors refer to "medical therapy" as using packs and balloons, that is, conservative measures without surgical intervention. In this discussion, medical management is treatment by pharmacologic modality only.

Drug treatment is useful for specific cases, limited mainly to known systemic or coagulation disorders, such as uremia or hemophilia (see Chapter 19). When the defective component of the clotting cascade is known, it can be replaced with fresh frozen plasma, or vitamin K can be used to increase its production. *Desmopressin* (DDAVP) increases the circulating amount of factor VIII complex from vascular endothelial cells. The dose is 0.3 µg/kg in 50 ml of normal saline injected over 15 to 30 minutes, with a peak at 15 to 30 minutes and lasting approximately 6 hours. Although IV injection is the most effective form of administration, it can also be given intranasally or subcutaneously and repeated after 24 hours.

HEREDITARY HEMORRHAGIC TELANGIECTASIA

Osler-Weber-Rendu disease is an autosomal dominant familial disease (1 to 2 cases per 100,000 population). The disorder manifests as deficiencies in the muscular (contractile) and connective (elastic) tissue layers of the walls of small blood vessels, weakening them and predisposing them to ruptures. Once ruptured, they are also less likely to undergo vasoconstriction to stop the bleeding. Mucosal telangiectases are found through the airway and gastrointestinal tract, and the most common manifestation of the disorder is epistaxis, which tends to be recurrent and severe. The repeated epistaxis episodes present in more than 90% of the affected individuals early in life (mean age of 12 years) and worsen with age. Adults may have mean frequencies of 18 episodes a month.

Treatment of the epistaxis episodes with packing is at best a short-term relief, and cautery can worsen the bleeding by damaging the fragile mucosa. Multiple blood transfusions are the rule, and patients must be maintained on iron supplements. Systemic estrogens are of questionable benefit in decreasing the frequency of epistaxis. From a surgical standpoint, septal dermoplasty (replacing the anterior nasal mucosa with a skin graft) has proved useful. Lasers used for photocoagulation of the lesions have brought some relief to these patients. Results are variable, however, and multiple treatments are usually necessary, 4 to 6 months apart.

BLOOD DYSCRASIAS

Inherited or acquired coagulopathies may affect one or several elements of the overall hemostatic process. The patient with suspected coagulopathy should be evaluated by a hematologist, if the patient is not already known to one. These patients need special handling from the practitioner. Cautery is contraindicated in general due to a resultant increase in bleeding, and packs that must be removed will frequently damage the mucosa, with the same result. Resorbable packs are especially appropriate for these patients, as well as topical thrombin sprayed into the nasal cavity. Medical management has a role in the treatment of certain coagulopathies, and traditional packing is useful in temporary control of bleeding in the hemodynamically compromised patient.

SUGGESTED READINGS

Abelson TI: Epistaxis. In Paparella MM, editor: *Otolaryngology,* ed 3, Philadelphia, 1991, WB Saunders.

Guarisco JL, Graham HD III: Epistaxis in children: causes, diagnosis and treatment, *Ear Nose Throat J* 68:522-538, 1989.

Jackson KR, Jackson RT: Factors associated with active, refractory epistaxis, *Arch Otolaryngol Head Neck Surg* 114:862-865, 1988.

Loftus BC, Newman JP: Epistaxis. In English GM, editor: *Otolaryngology,* vol 2, Philadelphia, 1998, Lippincott–Wilkins & Wilkins.

Manning SC, Culbertson MC Jr: Epistaxis. In Bluestone CD, Stool SE, Kenna MA, editors: *Pediatric otolaryngology,* ed 3, vol 1, Philadelphia, 1996, WB Saunders.

Padgham N: Epistaxis: anatomical and clinical correlates, *J Laryngol Otol* 104:308-311, 1990.

Parretta LJ, Denslow BL, Brown CG: Emergency evaluation and management of epistaxis, *Emerg Clin North Am* 5(2):265-277, 1987.

Pringle MB, Beasley P, Brightwell AP: The use of Merocell nasal packs in the treatment of epistaxis, *J Otolaryngol Otol* 110:543-546, 1996.

Randall DA, Freeman SB: Management of anterior and posterior epistaxis, *Am Fam Physician* 43(6):2007-2014, 1991.

Santos PM, Lepore ML: Epistaxis. In Bailey BR, editor: *Head and neck surgery–otolaryngology,* ed 2, Philadelphia, 1998, Lippincott-Raven.

Ophthalmologic Injuries and Emergencies

Bertrand Sorel

Injuries to the eyes and other ophthalmologic emergencies are fortunately rare in dental practice. These can be highly stressful events, however, and the practitioner must know the proper way to address them. Adequate intervention can eliminate the problem or attenuate the possible sequelae. Proper assessment and recognition of the need to refer are also very important.

Two main types of ophthalmologic emergencies may occur in an outpatient treatment setting: medical emergencies from preexisting conditions, such as glaucoma, and traumatic events, such as exposure of the eye to caustic fluids or direct injuries by blunt or sharp objects. This chapter reviews the emergencies most likely to occur in a dental office and supports the validity of having the patient wear glasses or other protective eye device during treatment.

ANATOMY OF EXTERNAL EYE

The external and superficial parts of the eye are most likely to be traumatized in the dental office. The ability to describe the various parts of the eye is the first step in evaluating the degree and importance of an injury (Figure 21-1). The upper and lower lids meet laterally to form the lateral palpebral commissure (canthus) and medially to form the medial canthus, where the lacrimal caruncle is also found.

A *punctum lacrimale* is found on each lid, slightly lateral to the medial commissure. It leads to the lacrimal ducts, then the lacrimal sac, and is important in draining the tears from the eye. The puncta (on the surface) and the ducts are the only superficial parts of the lacrimal system likely to become injured outside of a major trauma.

The inner side of both lids and the globe itself are entirely covered with conjunctiva, except for the cornea, with the palpebral conjunctiva on the inner side of the eyelids and the bulbar conjunctiva where it covers the sclera. The zones of transition form a deep recess, the superior fornix for the upper lid and inferior fornix for the lower one. In the medial commissure area the conjunctiva forms a fold called the *plica semilunaris*.

The junction of the bulbar conjunctiva with the cornea is the limbus. The palpebral fissure is the elliptic opening found between the eyelids when the eye is open.

Eyelids

The eyelid consists of four basic layers: skin, muscle, tarsus, and conjunctiva. The skin covering these layers is the thinnest of the body but very well vascularized. The skin is tightly attached to the periosteum at the orbital margins. The skin goes over the lid margin to become conjunctiva at the posterior border.

The muscle layer consists of the *orbicularis* muscle, a sheet of elliptic striated muscle fibers innervated by the seventh nerve. It encircles the palpebral fissure and acts as a sphincter, closing the eye when contracted. Another important muscle found in the upper eyelid is the *levator palpebrae superioris*, responsible for support and elevation of the upper lid. It inserts into the superior border of the tarsal plate and also sends fibers into the subcutaneous tissue of the upper lid. Müller's (*orbitalis*) muscle is a nonstriated, sympathetically innerved accessory muscle found under the conjunctiva of the upper lid, also attaching to the tarsal plate.

The *tarsal plates* are made of a dense matrix of connective tissue, as well as some elastic tissue. They give the firm structural support found in the part of the lid close to the palpebral fissure. Meibomian glands run into the larger upper lid tarsal plate and into the lower one.

The *conjunctiva* is a mucous membrane covering the entire inside of the palpebral fissure except for the cornea. The palpebral portion is

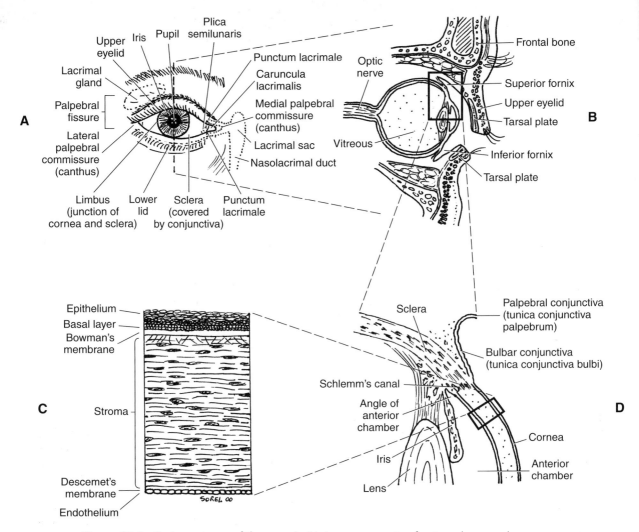

Figure 21-1. Basic anatomy of the eye. **A,** Main components of external eye and surrounding structures. **B,** Median sagittal cut of one eye, with orbital and periorbital structures. **C** shows more detail of boxed area. **C,** Anatomy of anterosuperior part of globe. **D,** Microscopic view of layers of the cornea.

firmly attached to the palpebral plates but loose and areolar over other areas. It is extremely thin in its bulbar portion, allowing the visibility of the sclera through its transparency. The bulbar conjunctiva is easily movable except at the limbus, where the corneoscleral junction occurs.

Eyeball

The most anterior part of the eye is the cornea, surrounded by the conjunctiva-covered sclera. The aqueous compartment of the eye is found behind the cornea, divided into anterior and posterior chambers by the iris diaphragm. Behind the iris is the lens, then the larger part of the eye, the posterior chamber (vitreous compartment), which is filled with a substance called the vitreous; the walls are covered with the light-sensitive retina. The *cornea* consists of six layers: (1) a tear film, made of three different layers of water and lipids from various glands; (2) epithelium; (3) Bowman's membrane; (4) stroma; (5) Descemet's membrane; and (6) endothelium. Importantly, lesions that do not involve tissues deeper than Bowman's membrane usually heal without scarring.

The *sclera* is basically a tough, three-layered envelope made of abundant collagen and elastic tissue. It supports and protects the inner structures of the eye. The *iris* is the diaphragm that adjusts the aperture of the eye (*pupil*); it is a thin and delicate tissue wearing pigments. The *lens* is composed of a highly elastic capsule containing the crystalline lens, a transparent biconvex body.

The *vitreous* is composed of a complex combination of hyaluronic acid and collagen, the latter forming a delicate skeleton attaching the vitreous to the internal membrane of the retina. The walls of the posterior chamber, besides the external sclera, present two important layers: the *choroid*, basically a plexus of blood channels feeding the outer layers of the retina, and the *retina* itself. The retina is the thin, transparent sheet of tissue made of cells that respond to light stimuli. It is made of at least 10 layers, found between the innermost internal limiting membrane and the outermost pigment epithelium. Interestingly, in retinal detachments, the separation occurs on the inner side of the pigment epithelium (within the retina itself), *not* on its outer surface that remains attached to the choroid. Finally, the ganglion cells in the retina send fibers toward the optic disc, forming the nerve fiber layer of the retina, and converge to eventually form the optic nerve.

TRAUMATIC CONTACTS
Exposure to Fluids

Caustic fluids can cause burns on the eye structures, and are usually divided into acid burns or alkali burns. As a general rule, alkalis tend to create more severe damage due to deeper penetration.

General Treatment

Regardless of the fluid to which the eye is exposed, the shorter the contact, the less is the eventual effect. Squirting a 1% solution of local anesthetic (e.g., lidocaine) in the eye is unlikely to create a significant problem, but nothing is gained by not intervening.

The most important treatment in most patients is copious irrigation of the eye with water. Tap water is adequate in an emergency, ideally followed by normal saline (NS) or lactated Ringer's (LR) solution. More caustic compounds require longer treatment. The pH of the eye should be tested periodically with litmus paper and irrigation continued until a normal of 7 is reached and remains at that level for 15 minutes after irrigation. In general, 10 to 15 minutes of irrigation is usually sufficient. The fornices of the conjunctiva should be swept with wet cotton applicators, and the eyelids should be everted and washed.

Acid Burns

Irrigation should be continued until the litmus paper indicates neutrality when touched to the fornix. Continuous irrigation of the conjunctival sac can be accomplished by an intravenous (IV) delivery system. Both the upper and the lower fornices should be irrigated, and eversion of the upper eyelid should be done whenever possible.

Alkali Injuries

Abundant irrigation is needed, and irrigation with LR or other IV solution should continue for at least 2 hours or until the conjunctival cul-de-sac is returned to neutrality.

In the dental office, judgment is needed to determine whether hospital admission or referral to an ophthalmologist is necessary. Exposure to a local anesthetic or topical spray solution should be benign except in the case of a rare allergic reaction. Other substances can be more hazardous, such as etching solutions, bonding agents, fluoride solutions, monomers for acrylics, and cement mixes. When ocular contact occurs, all these substances should be irrigated immediately as described and warrant referral to a specialist for evaluation. Whenever the eyes are concerned, the dentist cannot be overly careful.

Corneal Abrasions and Foreign Bodies

Minor traumas often result in superficial abrasions of the cornea. Although usually a minor injury, it can bring significant distress to the patient. The response varies greatly; some patients note slight discomfort, whereas others report severe pain, photophobia, increased lacrimation, and occasionally blepharospasms. A typical complaint is the sensation of a foreign body or "sand in the eye," which the patient wrongly believes to be present in the upper lid.

Examination should be performed using a topical anesthetic agent when warranted by significant discomfort. A fluorescent dye (fluorescein) will stain exposed basement membrane when examined under the blue light of a Wood's lamp or a slit lamp. The borders of abrasions are usually sharp. The examiner should look for signs of aqueous leakage (e.g., positive Seidel's test for evidence of penetrating wound) or patterns (e.g., vertical scratches indicating a foreign body on the inner side of the upper lid repeatedly scratching the cornea). In all patients, meticulous examination of the eye should be performed to rule out the presence of a foreign body.

Routine treatment of *corneal abrasions* consists of use of a broad-spectrum antibiotic ointment for infection prophylaxis, used for 1 week, and a cycloplegic agent (e.g., 5% homatropine) for patient comfort, to relieve ciliary spasm. A pressure patch is generally used to protect the cornea as it heals, keeping the eyelids from moving. Oral pain medications can be prescribed during the healing. Topical anesthetic agents should never be prescribed, since they can compromise epithelial wound healing and mask further problems that should be addressed. Topical corticosteroids can also delay wound healing and allow opportunistic fungal or bacterial infections. Daily monitoring is recommended until reepithelialization has occurred and infection is no longer a risk. Cultures should be made if infection is suspected.

Foreign bodies in general should be removed by irrigation with a bulb-type syringe or a hypodermic syringe without a needle. Much debris is removed atraumatically, but persistent particles must be removed by more precise methods.

On the *cornea*, cotton tips are avoided because of the normal epithelium it removes around the foreign body. A magnifying device should be used to improve visualization, and a sharp instrument (specially designed spud or if unavailable a 25- or 27-gauge hypodermic needle) used to gently elevate the foreign body. Once there is no more corneal foreign body, an antibiotic solution (not an ointment) such as sulfacetamide or gentamicin should be instilled in the eye. A patch is used for comfort but is removed if it worsens the situation. The eye should be examined every day as described previously. Scars do not happen with damage restricted to the corneal epithelium but do occur when Bowman's membrane is damaged.

In the *conjunctiva*, foreign bodies can be removed with irrigation, a spud, or even a cotton-tipped applicator. The upper lid may need to be everted. The conjunctiva generally heals extremely well.

Lacerations

Lacerations of any part of the eye can occur in the dental office, caused by sharp objects (e.g., scalpel blade, curette) or a rotating bur. Treatment requires immediate specialized care and is beyond the scope of the general dentist. The eye should be covered with a plain gauze soaked in NS solution to prevent dryness of the wound, and the patient brought immediately to specialized care. This section briefly reviews the type of treatment expected.

Lacerations of the *cornea* vary in depth. A partial-thickness laceration with well-apposed edges may be simply covered with an ultrathin bandage contact lens and left to heal. Deeper corneal lacerations require suturing under a microscope. Interrupted 10-0 silk or nylon sutures are used. Lacerations severe enough to cause eye prolapse necessitate complex surgical repair.

Lacerations of the *bulbar conjunctiva* that do not involve the globe rarely require surgical closure, unless they are very severe. Laceration of the sclera is a greater concern because of the association with severe damage to the inner components of the eye, as well as prolapse through the wound. A thorough assessment of the involvement and degree of damage to each structure will be needed at surgical exploration, with complex repairs performed by the specialist.

Lacerations of the *eyelid* can present in multiple forms. All these injuries should be referred immediately to the specialist, regardless of how benign they may appear. Most lacerations of the eyelids do not involve avulsion (loss of tissue) and should be repaired in a primary manner after careful irrigation. The skin in that area of the body heals extremely well; therefore debridement of apparently devitalized tissue should be minimized. The direction and depth of the laceration will influence treatment and subsequent healing. Superficial lacerations will likely heal without problem, after reapproximation with fine sutures (e.g., 6-0 nylon or silk, fast-resorbing catgut). Deeper lacerations will vary in complexity depending on their direction. Injuries parallel to the eyelid margin can usually simply be reapproximated, hopefully healing with an inconspicuous scar that runs parallel to the natural skin lines.

Full-thickness lacerations through the lid margin present a more complex challenge. The ciliary margin must be carefully reapproximated to avoid any notching; this relies first on visual alignment of anatomic markers, such as the gray line of the eyelid and the lash line. Once alignment is obtained, closure in layers is performed; the tarsal plate can be reapproximated with catgut and the skin in the usual fashion. If a full-thickness laceration is present within the inner one sixth of the eyelid, it will likely involve the lacrimal canaliculi leading to the lacrimal sac and require stenting of the canaliculi to preserve it. Loss of the lacrimal sac may result in chronic tearing (epiphora).

Prevention in the Dental Office

Traumatic events can be effectively prevented in the dental office by having the patient wear protective glasses before starting any procedure. The use of sharp or rotating instruments or manipulation of caustic products close to the eyes, especially in a conscious patient with eyes open, warrants use of protective devices, with minimal discomfort to the patient.

OTHER OPHTHALMOLOGIC EMERGENCIES

The dentist should recognize a few conditions to allow intervention or at least timely referral to the ophthalmologist.

Central Retinal Artery Occlusion

The patient reports a sudden, painless unilateral blindness. The occlusion may be caused by an embolus or thrombosis in a sclerotic central artery. Temporal arteritis may also be a cause. On examination, the pupil is semidilated. It will respond poorly to direct light, but the consensual response is normal. When this type of emergency is recognized, speed is of the essence, since retinal ischemia will rapidly lead to irreversible loss of vision. The first 30 minutes is critical to save the patient's sight.

Specialized assistance should be called immediately. In the meantime, certain minor interventions may be tried. The patient should be instructed to breathe and rebreathe in a paper bag. The hope here is to dilate the central retinal artery by increasing carbon dioxide content of the blood, allowing an eventual embolus to drift in a smaller arteriole that will compromise a smaller portion of the retina. The patient can also massage the involved globe with two fingers for several seconds, then abruptly release the pressure. This repeated action will decrease intraocular pressure, which might provide the same result as the previously described maneuver. Other interventions are performed by the specialist, who should be involved as soon as possible.

Retinal Detachment

The patient with a detached retina typically reports changes in vision, such as light flashes, black dots or "floaters," blurred vision, or a "curtain effect" as the detachment progresses. There is no associated pain. The phenomenon may be spontaneous or associated to recent trauma. The problem is a separation of the neural retina from the underlying retinal pigment epithelium. The detachment may be localized initially, with minimal visual symptoms; untreated, it may progress and involve the whole retina, creating the veil or curtain effect, and central visual acuity can decrease significantly if the macula is involved.

The patient should be referred immediately to an ophthalmologist if retinal detachment is diagnosed or suspected. The patient should be instructed to lie still, avoiding any sudden movement or use of the eye (e.g., reading).

Acute Angle-Closure Glaucoma

Also called *acute congestive glaucoma*, angle-closure glaucoma results from blockage by the iris of the drainage of aqueous humor through the trabecular space at the canal of Schlemm, in the anterior chamber. The intraocular pressure becomes greatly elevated.

Angle-closure glaucoma is the first condition to rule out when the patient has a sudden loss of vision accompanied by pain. It is usually unilateral, with marked blurred vision, halos around objects, mild photophobia. Common symptoms include frontal headache and severe pain radiating along the sensory distribution of the fifth cranial nerve. The patient may also have systemic symptoms (e.g., nausea, vomiting) that mimic an "acute abdomen."

Physical examination may show upper lid edema, lacrimation, a cloudy or "steamy" cornea secondary to edema, chemosis of the bulbar conjunctiva, and a half-dilated pupil that is nonreactive or "sluggish." The globe is stony hard on palpation because of the greatly elevated intraocular pressure, and the anterior chamber may appear shallow on examination.

Acute angle-closure glaucoma can occur spontaneously, usually at night or in a darkened room. Cases have been reported after sneezing and during labor in pregnancy. Glaucoma can also be precipitated by some medications, including topical mydriatics and rarely miotics. Systemic drugs as a cause of acute angle-closure glaucoma are much more vaguely defined, and much of the literature appears to represent rare isolated cases with poor demonstration of a direct causal effect of the drug involved. However, any agent that has anticholinergic effect (e.g., atropine-like drugs, antihistamines, antipsychotics, tricyclic antidepressants) or produces mydriasis may theoretically be involved. Implicated agents include topical intranasal cocaine, paroxetine and possibly other serotoninergic drugs, tamoxifen, inhaled ipratropium bromide taken with a β-agonist inhaler for asthma, oral imipramine, botulism toxin injected around the eyelids, oral drops containing belladonna for nasal allergy, and a patch of transdermal scopolamine delivery system. Anesthetic agents include parenteral atropine, scopolamine, ephedrine, and succinylcholine, which causes contraction of the extraocular muscles. Involvement of benzodiazepines is doubtful.

Immediate referral to an ophthalmologist is necessary because specialized care is needed. If available, a typical treatment regimen follows:

1. Topical β-blocker (e.g., levobundolol 0.5% or timolol 0.5%) in one dose.
2. Topical steroid (e.g., prednisolone 1%) every 15 to 30 minutes for four doses, then hourly.
3. Carbonic anhydrase inhibitor (e.g., acetazolamide, 250 to 500 mg intravenously or two 250-mg tablets orally, in one dose) to decrease production of aqueous humor.
4. Oral hyperosmotic agents, such as glycerin (Osmoglyn, 1.0 to 1.5 g/kg, given as a 50% solution) or isosorbide (Ismotic, 1 to 3 g/kg), to reduce the size of the vitreous. If this is not effective, an IV agent is administered, such as mannitol (Osmitrol), 1 to 2 g/kg intravenously over 45 minutes (a 500-ml bag of mannitol 20% contains 100 g of mannitol).

5. Topical apraclonidine 0.1% for one dose.
6. Pilocarpine 1% to 4% drops every 15 minutes for 1 hour, then hourly. This common intervention is usually effective when the intraocular pressure is 40 mm Hg or less, but the general dentist is usually unable to determine this measure.

Once again, acute angle-closure glaucoma is an ophthalmologic emergency. The ophthalmologist will consider surgical intervention such as a paracentesis to release the aqueous directly, and laser iridectomy to try to prevent recurrence of the problem.

SUGGESTED READINGS

Albert DM, Jacobiec FA: *Principles and practice of ophthalmology,* vol 5, Philadelphia, 1994, WB Saunders.

Bosniak S: *Principles and practice of ophthalmic plastic and reconstructive surgery,* Philadelphia, 1995, WB Saunders.

Clark RB, Farber JM, Sher NA: Eye emergencies and urgencies, *Patient Care* 23(1):24-42, 1989.

Deutsch TA, Feller DB: *Paton and Goldberg's management of ocular injuries,* ed 2, Philadelphia, 1985, WB Saunders.

Fraunfelder FT, Roy FH: *Current ocular therapy,* Philadelphia, 1995, WB Saunders.

Newell FW: *Ophthalmology: principles and concepts,* ed 8, St Louis, 1996, Mosby.

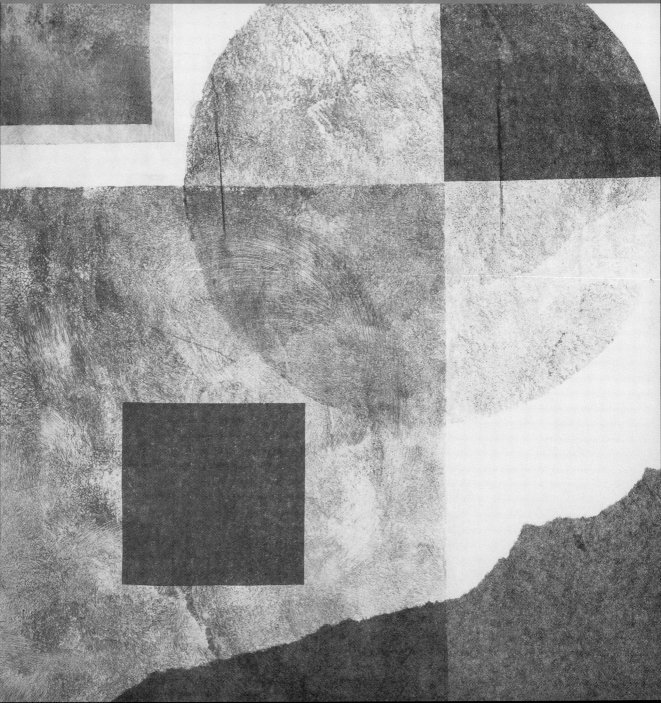

System-Based Assessment

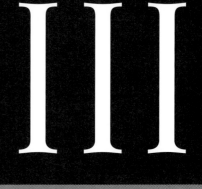

Cardiovascular Disease

Marc S. Rosenthal
Lorraine A. Rosenthal
Michael J. Buckley

A significant number of patients present to the dental office with underlying cardiovascular problems that can affect the delivery of dental care. If not recognized, these conditions can exacerbate these patients' health problems.

Understanding cardiac physiology and pathophysiology can help a dentist avoid situations that could develop into an acute medical emergency. Many patients with cardiovascular disease are treated routinely as outpatients and seek dental care in their communities. Many dentists are likely to be consulted by the patient's medical team before critical surgeries, such as cardiac valve replacement and transplantation. These patients must be free of any potential source of infection, especially pulpal and periodontal diseases, before surgery.

This chapter reviews the major cardiovascular diseases that dentists are likely to encounter and outlines the treatment and management of medical emergencies of cardiac origin in the dental office. Box 22-1 presents a functional classification of heart disease.

ATHEROSCLEROTIC DISEASE

Coronary artery disease (CAD) is the leading cause of death of people over age 45 in the United States, with an estimated 5 million people affected and more than 500,000 deaths each year.[1] Often associated with the aging process because of its insidious and potentially quiet early stages, CAD arises from atherosclerotic plaques that form in small arteries, such as the coronary vessels. The accumulation of the byproducts of cholesterol, along with low-grade vascular injuries, causes damage to the vessel's walls, resulting in narrowing and occlusion. In its final stages, CAD results in the rupture and fissuring of the intimal lining. This exposes the thrombogenic inner surface of the vessels and, along with the body's repair efforts, a thrombus forms, occluding the artery and reducing blood flow distally.[2-5] The affected myocardium, now underperfused, becomes ischemic, and if severe the ischemia will result in necrosis (Box 22-2).

Angina Pectoris

Angina pectoris is the most common symptom of coronary atherosclerotic disease and is characterized by a crushing substernal or precordial pain.[1,4,6,7] Angina is typically classified as stable or unstable. *Stable angina*, also known as *classic angina*, is initiated by exertion or stress and is typically relieved by rest and treatment with nitroglycerin. Patients with stable angina are usually aware of their symptoms and therefore manage the acute pain and activities that induce this pain.

Unstable angina involves chest pain at rest or during sleep and is unpredictable in symptomatology and timing. Unstable angina is unrelated to exercise or exertion and is typically not relieved with rest.[1,4,7,8] Therefore these patients are unable to predict levels of activity or halt attacks. Patients often wear nitroglycerin transdermal patches to provide a constant low-dose release of medication. Angina can also be classified as unstable if the symptoms are increased in duration or intensity from baseline levels.[7]

Typical symptoms of angina include a squeezing, burning, or crushing sensation in the chest and substernal area. This pain often radiates to the mandible or left arm and causes significant shortness of breath. These patients may have diaphoresis, nausea and vomiting, orthostatic hypotension, lightheadedness, and dizziness.[9] Angina pain often develops during sleep or early in the morning. The pain may occur at the same time each day for several days (Box 22-3).

Box 22-1	New York Heart Association Functional Classification of Patients with Heart Disease
CLASSIFICATION	**CHARACTERISTICS**
Class I	Patients with cardiac disease but without the resulting limitations in physical activity, dyspnea, or anginal pain.
Class II	Patients with heart disease resulting in slight limitations of physical activity. Such individuals are comfortable at rest. Ordinary physical activity results in fatigue, palpitations, dyspnea, or anginal pain.
Class III	Patients with cardiac disease resulting in marked limitation of physical activity. They are comfortable at rest. Less than ordinary physical activity causes fatigue, palpitations, dyspnea, or anginal pain.
Class IV	Patients with cardiac disease resulting in inability to perform any physical activity without discomfort. The symptoms of cardiac insufficiency or anginal syndrome may be present even at rest. If any physical activity is undertaken, discomfort increases.

Box 22-2 Risk Factors for Coronary Vascular Disease

- History of coronary artery disease (personal, familial)
- Male gender
- Older age
- Tobacco use
- Illicit drug use, especially stimulants, cocaine, and crack
- Diabetes mellitus
- Hypertension (chronic, acute crisis)
- Hypercholesterolemia, elevated low-density lipoprotein (LDL)
- Decreased high-density lipoprotein (HDL)
- Obesity
- Sedentary lifestyle

Box 22-3 Signs and Symptoms of Angina

- Squeezing, burning, crushing sensation in chest and substernal area
- Sensations radiating to mandible or left arm
- Shortness of breath
- Diaphoresis
- Nausea/vomiting
- Orthostasis
- Lightheadedness
- Dizziness
- Pulmonary edema
- Hypotension

Angina may develop in some patients with normal coronary arteries and may be secondary to ventricular hypertrophy, left ventricular outflow obstruction, severe aortic valvular regurgitation or stenosis, cardiac myopathy, and dilated ventricles.

Myocardial Infarction

If the ischemia that causes the angina pectoris (or decreased blood flow to the myocardium) continues or increases in severity, a myocardial infarction (MI) can occur. Also referred to as a "heart attack," MI is a severe imbalance of oxygen supply and demand to the heart for longer than 20 minutes, causing cardiac muscle fibers to die and never regain normal contractility. Time is crucial in the diagnosis and treatment of myocardial ischemia; after 20 minutes to 2 hours, the infarct may be only partial thickness of a wall, but after more than 2 hours, the infarct may become fully transmural (Figure 22-1).[9]

Risk factors for MI are family history of coronary valvular disease, gender (male), diabetes mellitus, hypertension, and hyperlipidemia, essentially the same risk factors as for angina. Patients who are obese, use tobacco products, and who live a sedentary lifestyle are also more prone to develop cardiovascular disease.[1-3,8]

Necrosis of the tissue of the myocardium starts at the subendocardial layer and progresses to the outer wall. The location and the extent of that damage may lead to other cardiac problems, including heart failure and arrhythmias. The signs and symptoms of acute MI are similar to those of angina. The key distinction

Changes in Anatomy

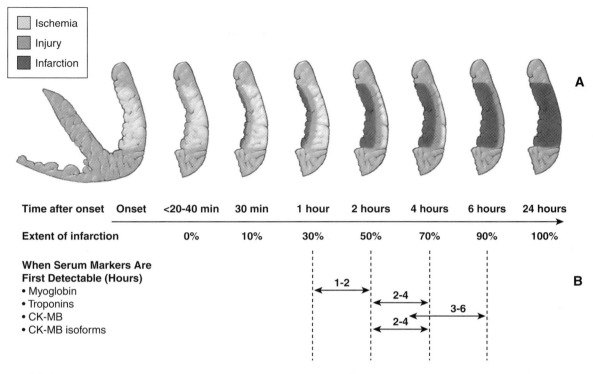

Time after onset	Onset	<20-40 min	30 min	1 hour	2 hours	4 hours	6 hours	24 hours
Extent of infarction	0%	10%	30%	50%	70%	90%	100%

When Serum Markers Are First Detectable (Hours)
- Myoglobin
- Troponins
- CK-MB
- CK-MB isoforms

1-2   2-4   3-6   2-4

A

B

ECG Changes

Ischemia (<20 minutes)
- Peaked T waves
- Inverted T waves
- ST-segment depression

Injury (20-40 minutes)
- ST-segment elevation

Infarction (>1-2 hours)
- Abnormal Q waves
- ≥2 mm wide or
- ≥25% height of R wave in that lead

C

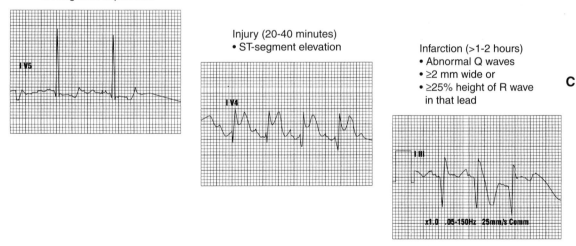

Figure 22-1 **A,** Changes in anatomy. **B,** Serum markers. **C,** ECG changes over time: ischemia, injury, and infarction. *From American Heart Association: ACLS, Dallas, 1997-1999, The Association.*

between the two, however, is that although similar symptoms may be seen initially, angina pain is transient, lasts usually less than 30 seconds, and can be relieved by sublingual nitroglycerin, whereas MI pain is unrelenting.[2,4]

The definitive diagnosis of MI is determined through electrocardiogram (ECG) findings and elevations of cardiac enzymes in the blood during progression of an MI. The primary tests used to diagnose MI are creatine kinase (CK) in the first 24 hours and serum aspartate transaminase (AST, formerly SGOT) and lactic dehydrogenase (LDH) within 3 days.[2,4,8,10] The usual pattern of ECG changes is early ST-segment elevation with subsequent T-wave inversion and Q-wave formation; a Q wave usually indicates transmural infarction and can help localize the region of the myocardial necrosis.[4] From 20% to 30% of ECGs normalize after MIs and make retrospective diagnosis difficult at times.

The diagnosis of MI is complex and requires sensitive medical tests and expertise not found in dental offices. Unless proved otherwise, chest pain unrelieved by nitroglycerin is a MI in the dental office and must be treated as such.

Percutaneous Transluminal Coronary Angioplasty

Percutaneous transluminal coronary angioplasty (PTCA) was introduced in 1977. Under fluoroscopy, a catheter is inserted through the femoral artery and maneuvered into the stenotic segment of the coronary vessel. A small inflatable balloon on the catheter tip dilates the segment and increases perfusion. After PTCA, patients are usually observed for 24 to 48 hours and take aspirin. A stress test is frequently performed between 2 to 10 days after a PTCA to assess the patient's condition and establish a baseline for further evaluation.

The indications for angioplasty are increasing. More than 400,000 percutaneous revascularization procedures are performed each year. The number of angioplasty procedures exceeds the number of coronary artery bypass surgeries.[11]

Limitations of balloon dilation have resulted in the development of alternative nonsurgical techniques, such as laser angioplasty. However, angioplasty is successful in about 90% of appropriate candidates. One third of vessels will undergo restenosis within 6 months and require a second procedure. Stress testing is frequently repeated at 3- to 6-month intervals for the first 2 years to assess the recurrence of late

stenosis. Ischemic symptoms recur in PTCA patients mainly during the first year, and long-term morbidity depends on the rapidity of the atherosclerotic disease. Reported rates of survival at 1, 5, and 10 years are 97%, 88% to 97%, and 78% to 90%, respectively. Rates of being free from subsequent MIs or coronary bypass surgery are somewhat less favorable, from 81% to 90% at 1 year, 79% at 5 years, and 65% at 10 years.[8]

Coronary Artery Bypass Graft Surgery

Coronary artery bypass graft (CABG) surgery is a component of the management of the patient with ischemic heart disease. It entails grafting portions of the host blood vessel to the coronary arteries to bypass obstructions. It is effective in controlling symptoms and improving long-term survival in certain patients, particularly those with greater than 50% stenosis in the left main coronary artery.[8] Long-term survival for patients with chronic angina after CABG is 90% and 80% for 5 and 10 years, respectively. Of these patients, 70% at 5 years and 50% at 10 years have been shown to be free of ischemic events.

Either the saphenous vein or the internal mammary artery can be used for CABG. The *saphenous vein* is taken from above or below the knee, the vein below the knee generally is preferred because it is close in diameter to the size of the coronary artery. The vein is removed from the incision made along the inner leg. The obstruction in the coronary artery is bypassed by connecting one end of the vein graft to the aorta (*proximal anastomosis*) and the other end to the coronary artery just past the obstruction (*distal anastomosis*). The long-term efficacy of the graft depends on its patency. From 10% to 30% of saphenous veins are occluded at 1 year and 50% to 60% at 10 years. Three main processes account for saphenous vein failure: thrombosis, fibrointimal hyperplasia, and atherosclerosis.[3]

The *internal mammary artery* (IMA) is an alternative to the saphenous vein for myocardial revascularization. The IMA is the second branch of the subclavian artery and descends down the anterior chest wall immediately lateral to the sternum behind the costochondral cartilage. Grafts of IMA have less atherosclerosis over time, as well as superior early and later patency rates compared with saphenous vein grafts. In one study, 90% of IMA grafts were patent 10 years postoperatively.[3]

Box 22-4	Medical Considerations in Dental Management of the Patient with Coronary Atherosclerotic Disease

1. The incidence of peritreatment myocardial infarction (MI) decreases 3 months after an MI. However, the incidence of peritreatment MI does not stabilize until 6 months after MI. Elective dental treatment should not be done within 6 months of an MI because of the risk of the complications, including sudden death and arrhythmias.
2. Patients who have successfully undergone percutaneous transluminal coronary angioplasty (PTCA) are usually in optimal condition for dental treatment shortly after the procedure. Aspirin, which is usually prescribed, should not be discontinued.
3. Elective treatment should be deferred for 6 months in the patient who has had a coronary artery bypass graft (CABG).
4. Maneuvers to minimize oxygen supply/demand imbalance will minimize the risk of cardiac complications.
   a. Supplemental oxygen
   b. Use of aspiration technique to avoid intravascular injection of vasoconstrictor
   c. Anxiolytic medication (oral premedication, nitrous oxide)

Box 22-4 lists the medical issues that should be considered in the dental management of the patient with coronary atherosclerotic disease.

CONGESTIVE HEART FAILURE

Congestive heart failure (CHF) is the inability of the heart to pump blood at a rate that meets the metabolic demands of the body. An estimated 500,000 individuals are newly diagnosed annually.[12] The heart is essentially a muscle that pumps blood with enough force to flow against the vascular resistance found in the peripheral and organ circulation. Its function can be explained by the following three factors:

- *Preload*: Volume of blood that has filled the ventricles before ejection or systole; also known as *end-diastolic volume*.
- *Afterload*: Resistance against which the heart contracts; reflected in systolic blood pressure.
- *Contractility*: Stroke work that the heart will generate during any given preload; amount of force or shortening of the heart muscles; used to describe the functional state of the myocardium.[2,8]

The most common cause of CHF found in the United States is CAD, accounting for up to 75% of all cases.[12] Other risk factors include hypertension, valvular heart disease, and previous MIs with cardiac damage.[2] Cardiomyopathies result in intrinsic damage to the muscles of the heart and can also cause CHF. Systemic diseases, such as thyrotoxicosis, can mimic signs and symptoms of failure.[4]

Signs and Symptoms

The practitioner can best determine a patient's health status through observation and a complete health history. Questions examining energy levels and exercise tolerance (e.g., distance able to walk before short of breath, ability to function on stairs) and sleep disturbances (e.g., number of pillows needed to sleep, awakening during the night with shortness of breath) provides an indication of functional reserve. The patient's fingers and ankles should be checked for edema. Resting tachycardia and peripheral vasoconstriction (skin pallor) indicate that the body needs help in maintaining an adequate blood pressure. Even though patients may be retaining greater amounts of water than usual and report a sudden increase in weight, bloating, or swelling of the lower extremities, the blood circulating is actually decreased from the normal amount[1,2,4,7,13] (Box 22-5).

Because heart function and fluid overload can be restored by medications, the dentist should always inquire not only about the medication history but also about a patient's compliance with medications. The dentist with any questions or concerns should postpone treatment until he or she has consulted with the patient's physician.

Etiology

CHF occurs when the heart's ability to pump becomes impaired. A predisposing factor is usually present, causing the heart muscle to become weak, including MI, hypertension, or cardiomyopathy. Excessive workloads on the heart from hypermetabolic states, valvular incompetence, and renal or liver failure—all of which cause volume overload—can also precipitate CHF.[1-4,7,13,14]

Box 22-5 Signs and Symptoms of Congestive Heart Failure

GENERAL
- Shortness of breath
- Sleep disturbances
- Edema
- Tachycardia
- Sudden weight gain
- Swelling of ankles and feet
- Peripheral vasoconstriction

RIGHT SIDED
- Increased jugular venous pressure
- Pitting edema around ankles
- Enlarged liver (evident on clinical examination)

LEFT SIDED
- Pulmonary venous congestion (shortness of breath)
- Fatigability
- Renal failure (under-perfusion of kidneys)
- Decreased mental status (poor circulation to brain)
- Water and sodium retention

Box 22-6 Risk Factors for Congestive Heart Failure

- Hypertension
- Coronary artery disease (e.g., massive or multiple myocardial infarction)
- Valvular heart disease (e.g., aortic stenosis, mitral regurgitation)
- Pericardial diseases
- Cardiomyopathies
- Systemic disease (e.g., thyrotoxicosis)

Box 22-7 Causes of Congestive Heart Failure

- Ischemic heart disease (e.g., coronary artery disease)
- Dilated cardiomyopathy of unknown cause, idiopathic cardiomyopathy
- Cardiomyopathy caused by toxin, virus, parasite, hypertension, valvular stenosis/regurgitation, with or without ventricular dysfunction
- Hypertrophic or restrictive cardiomyopathy
- Pericardial disease
- Pulmonary hypertension
- Congenital heart disease
- High-output states

In the early stages of failure the heart enlarges to compensate for the greater amounts of fluid and decreased cardiac output. Eventually the compensatory mechanisms are no longer effective. The hypertrophic heart subsequently adds an increased oxygen demand to an already-overworked muscle, exacerbating the patient's deteriorating condition.[5,15] The heart muscles can be compared to broken rubber bands stretched beyond the limit of elasticity, unable to contract adequately. This causes a decrease in cardiac output and backup of blood distally, further stressing the heart. With CHF, blood volumes can increase 15% to 20%, and extracellular fluid may increase 200% or more.[3] Minimal relationship may exist between the severity of the clinical signs of CHF and the patient's degree of functional disability.[9]

The heart, although one organ, has four entities or chambers (left and right atria, left and right ventricles) working in concert. It is unlikely that all four chambers will fail together. Usually either the left side or right side will fail first, eventually causing stress on the other side, the end result being total failure.

Left-sided heart failure is most often caused by coronary heart disease, aortic and mitral valvular diseases, and hypertension. Left-sided heart failure usually affects the lungs but can extend to the brain and kidneys (Box 22-6).

Right-sided heart failure is usually a result of left-sided failure. Pure right-sided failure most often occurs with a right ventricular strain produced by an increased resistance within the pulmonary circuit that overburdens the right ventricle. Less common causes include MI of the right ventricle and diffuse myocarditis, which appears to affect the right ventricle more often than the left ventricle. Rarely, tricuspid or pulmonic valvular lesions cause right-sided failure. Clinically, constrictive pericarditis simulates right-sided failure by damming the blood back into the systemic venous system, although the right ventricle itself may be normal.[5,8,10,14]

The major morphologic and clinical effect of right-sided failure that differs from left-sided failure is minimal pulmonary congestion, but with engorgement of the systemic and portal systems[4,8] (see Box 22-5). In both conditions, however, the twin problems of systemic venous congestion and impaired cardiac output remain qualitatively the same. The major sites affected by right-sided heart failure are the liver, spleen, kidneys, subcutaneous tissues, brain, and the entire portal area of venous drainage (Box 22-7).

Diagnosis

Many tests are available to diagnose CHF, but a good history and physical examination are the most efficient methods. A good indicator of the pumping efficiency of the heart is the *ejection fraction*, which is the amount of blood leaving the heart in systole that was present in diastole. Normal ejection fraction is approximately 55; patients with ejection fraction below 35 warrant further discussion between the dentist and the patient's physician.

Tests that confirm the diagnosis of CHF include *pulmonary wedge pressure* (PWP), which many physicians believe is the most important hemodynamic determinant in exercise capacity in a patient with heart failure. PWP relates to the amount of pressure in the left ventricle during diastole. A high value indicates that a high pressure gradient is needed for blood to enter the left ventricle. Any prolonged increase in the left atrial pressures leads to a dilation of the left atrium and dysfunction of the barrier reflex arcs originating within this atrium. This increases neural activity, altering vascular activity and causing the body to restrict the amount of blood flowing into the heart, with pooling in the lung and systemic vasculature. This further taxes the heart muscle and worsens the patient's condition.[5,15]

ECG findings may indicate atrial or ventricular hypertrophy, underlying disorders of cardiac rhythm, or conduction abnormalities such as right or left bundle branch block. Chest radiographs provide information about the size and shape of the heart and pulmonary vasculature. X-ray films also can indicate the relative severity of CHF by revealing if pulmonary edema is predominantly vascular, interstitial, or advanced to the alveolar and bronchial stages. Echocardiographic studies are used to reveal the size and function of cardiac valvular structures and the size and motion of both ventricles. Radionuclide angiography and cardiac catheterization are other diagnostic tests used to describe the underlying causes of CHF, such as heart defects and cardiomyopathy. Because other health problems contribute to CHF, primary medical diagnostic methods are used to detect conditions such as anemia, thyroid dysfunction, and kidney disease.[2,4,11]

Treatment and Management

Dental procedures create stress in the patient with CHF. Generally, a fully ambulatory patient without cardiac or respiratory symptoms who can come to the dental office is suitable for outpatient care. Management of dental problems in patients with cardiovascular disease requires close cooperation between the physician and dentist. The physician must be aware of the patient's dental problems, and in turn the dentist should know the patient's medical problems and resultant limitations.

CARDIOMYOPATHIES

Cardiomyopathies refer to diseases of unknown etiology involving heart muscle. Cardiomyopathies are classified into three types: dilated, hypertrophic, and restrictive. Of the three types, dilated cardiomyopathies account for more than 90% of cases.[3]

Dilated cardiomyopathy (DCM) is characterized by increased ventricular size, parasystolic function, and CHF. The clinical course is usually marked by progressive dilation of the heart chambers. As ventricular dilation increases, mitral and tricuspid insufficiencies occur as the valve leaflets are stretched and separated. Arrhythmias, such as ventricular tachycardia and fibrillation, can make management of this condition difficult and life threatening.

Hypertrophic cardiomyopathy (HCM), which rarely occurs, is distinguished by excessive myocardial hypertrophy, usually involving the septal walls. The most characteristic feature of HCM is diastolic dysfunction. The heart is able to contract but not relax and remains abnormally stiff during diastole. Death occurs in the young CHF patient usually from a ventricular dysrhythmia.[3]

The least common of the three types of cardiomyopathy in the United States is *restrictive cardiomyopathy* (RCM). Myocardial hypertrophy, fibrosis, or infiltration of the muscle may be the underlying pathologic process.

Clinical findings depend on the type of cardiomyopathy and the extent of the disease. Management of these patients is the same as for those with CHF, checking their reserves and ability to be subjected to strenuous medical treatment and consult with their physician before any dental treatment.

ARRHYTHMIAS (DYSRHYTHMIAS)

The heart consists of specialized tissue, and each part has an intrinsic ability to initiate an impulse. Any condition that interferes with cardiac electrical conduction may cause an aberrant rhythm that may become clinically important.

The *sinoatrial* (SA) *node* has the shortest refractory period and is the origin of the normal elec-

---

Box 22-8	Mechanisms of Action in Bradycardia*

CARDIAC DYSFUNCTION
Impulse formation
Impulse conduction

SYSTEMIC CONDITIONS
- Hypoxia
- Increased intracranial pressure
- Hypothermia
- Hypothyroidism

INTRACARDIAC DISEASES
- Sarcoidosis
- Amyloidosis
- Degenerative diseases of cardiac conduction system
- Ischemic heart disease
- Lyme disease
- Rheumatic heart disease

MEDICATIONS
- β-Blockers
- Calcium channel blockers
- Digoxin

From New York Heart Association: *Diseases of the heart and blood vessels: nomenclature and criteria for diagnosis,* ed 6, Boston, 1964, Little, Brown.
*History and physical examination are essential in all patients to determine current health status. Patients with newly diagnosed bradycardia or poorly controlled bradyarrhythmias are at greatest risk for problems during treatment. They should have medical clearance and medications updated before the appointment.

Box 22-9	Treatment of Bradycardia

- Obtain serial blood pressure measurements, and follow pressure trends.
- Place in Trendelenburg position, with head lower than feet.
- Administer oxygen, at least 3 to 7 L, through nasal canal.
- Terminate procedure.
- Obtain 12-lead electrocardiogram, if possible.
- Stay with and reassure patient.
- Administer 0.4 mg of atropine intramuscularly or intravenously.
- Refer to hospital or physician to investigate cause and definitive treatment.

---

trical impulse. The sinus node normally produces 60 to 100 impulses per minute. This rate may be affected by increasing or decreasing the sympathetic stimulation to the heart. After initiation of an electrical impulse from the SA node, the impulse travels through the right atrium via three internodal tracts to the left atrium. The atrium contracts in response to this stimulus, aiding the flow of blood into the ventricles. A small, rounded waveform called the P *wave* represents atrial depolarization on the ECG. The impulse then travels to the atrioventricular junction at the base of the right atrium in the junction between the atria and ventricles.

The *atrioventricular* (AV) *node* is the secondary pacemaker, with a rate of 40 to 60 beats/min. The AV node delays conduction of the impulse, permitting the atria to finish filling the ventricles. This activity is partially represented by the PR interval on the ECG. From the AV node the impulse continues into the ventricles via the bun-

dle of His and the right and left bundle branches. The contraction is represented by the QRS complex on an ECG. The ventricles also have pacemaker cells that initiate an impulse, firing only when the heart rate has decreased below 40 beats/min.[2,4,6-9]

Bradycardia and Bradyarrhythmias

Bradycardia is defined as an abnormally slow heart rate, less than 60 beats/min, with P waves and QRS complexes. This may not be a pathologic finding in many young patients or well-conditioned athletes. Their cardiovascular systems are often very efficient, contracting less frequently because more blood is pumped per stroke. However, other patients with low heart rate may feel symptomatic (e.g., lightheaded); when values are decreased from baseline, the practitioner should seek medical consultation before treatment (Box 22-8).[2,4,8]

Bradyarrhythmias are treated symptomatically with patient positioning and by the administration of oxygen. Patients should be placed in the Trendelenburg position, feet above the head, and serial blood pressure readings should be obtained. Venous access should be secured and atropine administered intravenously if there is a corresponding severe fall in blood pressure. The patient should be observed for possible degeneration of the arrhythmia and transferred immediately to a tertiary care facility (Box 22-9).

Sinus Tachycardia

Sinus tachycardia is an acceleration of the sinus node to more than 100 beats/min. Sinus tachycardia usually is caused by factors relating to an

Box 22-10	Mechanisms of Action in Tachycardia

- Stress
- Exercise
- Stimulants (e.g., caffeine, nicotine)
- Fever
- Anemia
- Hyperthyroidism
- Hypoxemia
- Congestive heart failure
- Shock
- Drugs
  Atropine
  Catecholamines (e.g., isoproterenol, epinephrine, dopamine)

increase in sympathetic tone, such as stress, exercise, and stimulants (e.g., caffeine, nicotine). Sinus tachycardia is also associated with such clinical problems as fever, anemia, hyperthyroidism, hypoxemia, CHF, and shock (Box 22-10).

More important than sinus tachycardia is the underlying case of the dysrhythmia. Tachycardia is often a sign of a serious underlying problem. The dentist must always investigate the potential causes of tachycardia before any dental procedures. The increase in workload on the myocardium causes an increase in oxygen demand. Patients with preexisting cardiac conditions are particularly at risk. A simple technique of carotid massage or the Valsalva maneuver stimulates the vagal nerve and produces a parasympathetic impulse to the heart, slowing the heart rate.

Atrial Fibrillation and Flutter

Atrial fibrillation or flutter is an ectopic rhythm in which the atria fires rapidly. Fibrillation produces a heart rate of 250 to 350 beats/min and a flutter rate of 350 to 500. With atrial flutter the P waves are less defined and usually appear as small, quivering bumps. The pulse is clinically evident and described as "irregularly irregular." Some patients tolerate this rhythm, and with the physician's approval, dental treatments are safe.[2-4,8,14] Most patients with atrial fibrillation take coumadin, which affects coagulation. If a patient converts to an atrial dysrhythmia during a dental visit, immediate action should be taken to place the patient in the Trendelenburg position and administer oxygen. The patient may describe feelings of lightheadedness and should be transferred to a medical facility.

Ventricular Tachycardia

Ventricular tachycardia (VT) is diagnosed by a wide, bizarre, QRS complex that has a fairly regular rhythm on the ECG at a rate greater than 100 beats/min. P waves are usually not seen. VT is a common early complication of MI and requires immediate intervention. All dental procedures should immediately be terminated. Some patients may be able to sustain adequate perfusion. In many cases, however, VT is a medical emergency, and the physician should immediately institute at a minimum the airway, breathing, and circulation guidelines (ABCs) of basic cardiopulmonary resuscitation (CPR).

VALVULAR HEART DISEASE

Cardiac valves—tricuspid, pulmonic, mitral, and aortic—maintain the unidirectional flow of blood. Structural changes resulting from disease can impair function. *Pulmonic valve* changes usually result from congenital abnormalities. *Tricuspid valve* disease may be caused by endocarditis, rheumatic fever, or left-sided heart failure. Because of the low pressure of the right side of the heart, the hemodynamic effects of tricuspid abnormalities are usually less significant than those of left-sided valve disease. *Mitral valve* and *aortic valve* abnormalities are more common than tricuspid and pulmonic conditions and produce profound hemodynamic changes.

Mitral Regurgitation

Mitral valve regurgitation occurs when the mitral valve leaflets connecting the left atrium to the left ventricle are forced back and up into the atrium during systole. This produces a systolic sound and may be associated with a regurgitative murmur heard with auscultation.[2,4,7] Mitral valve disease occurs in 1% to 6% of the population and is a significant finding with Graves' disease, muscular dystrophy, sickle cell anemia, Marfan's syndrome, and rheumatic heart disease.[2,8,12]

Symptomatic patients usually complain of fatigue, dizziness, orthostatic hypotension, palpitations, or non-anginal chest pain. Such patients are also at increased risk for emboli, especially to the brain, and often are taking anticoagulation medication, which must be taken into consideration before they undergo dental treatment.[1,2,4,8,13]

Symptomatic patients with mitral valve regurgitation should be treated with agents that act to reduce the size of the regurgitant orifice area. This can be achieved by the use of drugs that increase contractility (e.g., digitalis) and reduce

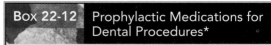

| Box 22-11 | Guidelines for Prevention of Bacterial (Infective) Endocarditis |

HIGH-RISK CONDITIONS
- Prosthetic cardiac valves, including bioprosthetic and homograft valves
- Previous bacterial endocarditis
- Complex congenital heart disease

MODERATE-RISK CONDITIONS
- Most other congenital cardiac malformations
- Acquired valvular dysfunction
- Mitral valve prolapse with valve regurgitation or thickened leaflets
- Hypertrophic cardiomyopathy

CONDITIONS THAT DO NOT WARRANT PROPHYLAXIS
- Physiologic, functional, or otherwise benign heart murmurs
- Mitral valve prolapse without valvular regurgitation
- Previous rheumatic fever without valve damage
- Previous coronary artery bypass graft surgery
- Cardiac pacemakers
- Surgical repair of atrial or ventricular septal defect (> 6 months postoperatively)

| Box 22-12 | Prophylactic Medications for Dental Procedures* |

STANDARD PROPHYLAXIS
Amoxicillin
　Adults: 2.0 g
　Children: 50 mg/kg†

PENICILLIN-ALLERGIC PATIENTS
Clindamycin
　Adults: 600 mg
　Children: 20 g/kg†
or
Azithromycin or clarithromycin
　Adults: 500 mg
　Children: 15 mg/kg†
or
Cephalexin or cefadroxil‡
　Adults: 2.0 g
　Children: 50 mg/kg†

*Administered 1 hour before treatment; no follow-up dose recommended.
†Total children's dose should not exceed adult dose.
‡Cephalosporins should not be used in patients with immediate-type hypersensitivity reactions (urticaria, angiodema, anaphylaxis) to penicillins.

ventricular preload and afterload (e.g., diuretics, vasodilators). Patients with severe mitral regurgitation who remain symptomatic despite medical therapy should be considered for surgical repair or replacement of the mitral valve.

These and other patients with valvular disease must have antibiotic prophylaxis to prevent bacterial endocarditis (Boxes 22-11 and 22-12).

Mitral Stenosis

Mitral stenosis is an obstruction of blood flow between the left atrium and left ventricle through a narrowed lumen. The mitral valve does not open all the way, secondary to possible calcification, therefore causing turbulent blood flow through a fixed stenotic opening. Rheumatic fever is usually a precursor to mitral stenosis.

Subjective signs of mitral stenosis include exertional dyspnea and fatigue. Pulmonary edema occurs when increased left atrial pressure causes blood to back up into the lungs. These patients are also at increased risk for emboli. Median sur-

vival is usually 7 years after diagnosis if left untreated; much depends on the surface area of the valve affected. Another symptom is *Wortner's syndrome*, or paralysis of the left vocal cord. The patient will have a husky voice due to injury of the left recurrent laryngeal nerve, caused by a compressed left atrium against a dilated pulmonary artery. Patients with Wortner's syndrome may also present with a plum-colored malar flush called *mitral facies*, a condition seen with low cardiac output and severe pulmonary hypertension.

Auscultation reveals an opening "snap," heard loudest at the apex of the left lower sternal border, but only when the mitral valve is still mobile. The snap comes from the high pressure generated to force open the mitral valve. The snap is usually followed by a low-frequency murmur across the stenotic valve. Again, these patients must be treated prophylactically using the guidelines for subacute bacterial endocarditis (see later discussion), even if they are not asymptomatic.[1,3,4,8]

Anticoagulation Therapy

Anticoagulation therapy is mandatory for all patients with mitral stenosis who have a history of atrial fibrillation or have experienced an embolic event. Anticoagulants are recommended to prevent the risk of emboli for all patients with mitral stenosis who have symptoms of CHF. Anticoagulation therapy should also be considered for all patients with previous CHF, especially if the left atrium is enlarged.

Aortic Regurgitation

Aortic regurgitation occurs when blood flows from the aortic arch back to the left ventricle through an incompetent aortic valve. It is usually precipitated by rheumatic heart disease, infective endocarditis, or trauma. A bicuspid valve, instead of the normal tricuspid aortic valve, is often involved.

Patients with aortic regurgitation may present with severe hypertension. They may be symptom free for many years until their reserves are depleted, when they present with deepens on exertion, apnea, or paroxysmal nocturnal deepens (PND). They may also develop palpitations because the left ventricle increases in size to pump out the excess blood. On examination these patients have a rapidly increased and slapping-type pulse described as a *water-hammer pulse* or *collapsing pulse*. Auscultation reveals a pandiastolic decrescendo murmur, heard best over the sternum of the left border.

Symptomatic patients with severe aortic regurgitation are treated with digitalis, diuretics, and vasodilators until their condition improves enough to consider valvular replacement surgery. Vasodilator drugs play an important role in therapy. Definitive treatment is aortic valve replacement; patients also must receive prophylaxis against endocarditis. As with any valve replacement, patients may be taking anticoagulants.[10,13,14]

Aortic Stenosis

Aortic stenosis is a narrowing of the aortic outflow caused by valve obstruction from the left ventricle to the ascending aorta, producing higher pressure in the left ventricle. Aortic stenosis usually results from congenital or idiopathic degenerative calcification of the aortic cusp and less often from rheumatic fever. Patients have a higher incidence of hemolysis and gastrointestinal bleeding from the right colon and aortic dissection caused by the pressure increases. The classic triad of symptoms is syncope, angina, and deepens on exertion.

As in other valve diseases, patients with aortic stenosis require prophylaxis against endocarditis and ultimately valve replacement.[1,2,4,7] Patients should be advised against vigorous activity. Comorbidity with atrial arrhythmias should be treated aggressively to avoid the loss of atrial transport function. Surgery is recommended for symptomatic patients with severe aortic stenosis.

INFECTIVE ENDOCARDITIS

Infective endocarditis is a microbial infection of the endocardium caused by turbulent blood flow through pathologically altered valves, usually on the left side of the heart. The patient experiences fever, murmurs, petechiae, anemia, embolisms, and endocardial vegetations, which can damage valves, cause obstruction or abscess in the myocardium, or create a mycotic aneurysm. Men are usually affected twice as often as women; the age of onset is usually over 50. A high incidence of right-sided endocarditis is associated with intravenous (IV) drug abuse. Invasive endocardial surgery may also cause endocarditis.[8,12,15]

Subacute Bacterial Endocarditis

Subacute bacterial endocarditis (SBE) is usually caused by oral α-hemolytic streptococci (*Streptococcus viridans*), microaerophilic or anerobic streptococci, and less often *Staphylococcus epidermidis* and *Haemophilus*. SBE develops on abnormal valves and is usually caused by normal flora from the peridontium or gastrointestinal or genitourinary tracts. Acute infective endocarditis is usually caused by *Staphylococcus aureus* or group A hemolytic streptococci, as well as by pneumococci, gonococci, or less virulent streptococcal organisms. Susceptible normal valves are occasionally infected.

SBE most often affects the mitral valve, followed by the aortic valve, both mitral and aortic valves, then the tricuspid valve, and finally the pulmonic valve. Patients with congenital coronary defects or rheumatic valvular diseases as children are at higher risk of developing SBE. The condition has a very insidious onset, with low-grade fever of 39° C. Patients complain of night sweats, fatigability, malaise, chills, arthralgias, and weight loss. Examination reveals valvular insufficiency. Patients also may have emboli-induced stroke, MI, hematuria, flank or abdominal pain, and arterial insufficiency in the arms and legs. On physical examination they may appear normal, may have pallor and fever, or may demonstrate a change in a preexisting murmur (e.g., regurgitative murmur where none existed). They may also be tachycardic or may have petechiae on the upper trunk and distal extremities, painful red subcutaneous nodules on the tips of the digits (*Osler's nodes*), split hemorrhages under the nails, and hemorrhagic retinal lesions with a small, white, round or oval center.

Prosthetic Valve

Prosthetic valve endocarditis develops in about 2% of patients approximately 1 year after replacement. The incidence is less thereafter. It occurs more often in artificial aortic and mitral valves and is less common in porcine valves. Causative microorganisms include S. *epidermidis*, diphtheroids, coliform bacteria, *Candida*, and *Aspergillus* fungi. Infection usually develops when microorganisms are carried in turbulent blood flow through the valves and adhere to fibroid platelet vegetations, enabling them to colonize. The colonies are usually covered with a layer of fibrin, which conceals them from the circulating white blood cells. Prolonged endocarditis may cause clubbing of the fingers and toes. Hematuria and proteinuria may be seen as a result of embolic infarction of the kidneys. Eventually, prosthetic valve endocarditis may lead to transient ischemic attacks and encephalopathies secondary to brain abscesses.[1-5,7,8,12,14]

Right-Sided Acute Bacterial Endocarditis

Right-sided acute bacterial endocarditis is similar to SBE but has a more rapid course, higher fever, more toxic appearance, and greater destruction of the valves. Septic phlebitis, fever, pleurisy, septic pulmonary infarction, and tricuspid regurgitation usually accompany right-sided endocarditis. Untreated, all types of infective endocarditis are fatal.[1,2,4,8]

PREVENTION

Most cardiac patients should be aware of their health status and be able to produce a list of their medications before the appointment. This helps identify medical problems and directs further investigations of cardiac conditions. The cardiologist or primary care physician should be consulted for patients with known cardiac disease before they undergo dental procedures.

Before dental care, patients must be instructed on how their cardiac medications might affect the proposed treatment. Aspirin and other nonsteroidal antiinflammatory drugs (NSAIDs), which interfere with platelet function, should be stopped 7 to 10 days before any significant surgical interventions. Similarly, patients should be instructed to follow normal medication regimens after treatment to ensure maintenance of the schedules, unless otherwise instructed.

Patients with thromboembolic disease and those taking coumadin or a heparin-related drug should have prothrombin time (PT) and partial thromboplastin time (PTT) checked before any oral surgery. The coumadin anticoagulants (warfarin, dicumarol) are vitamin K antagonists and depress clotting factors II, V, VII, IX, and X. Heparin-related drugs affect the intrinsic clotting pathway, including factors III, IV, VI, VII, VIII, and X, and are followed with the PTT. The PT level also varies depending on the type of activator used; normal levels are usually 10 to 15 seconds. PT results are also given as the international normalized ratio (INR); standard levels are about 1.0, with INR values of 2.0 to 3.0 being appropriate for management of acute MI, atrial fibrillation, and deep vein thrombosis, as well as for prevention of systemic embolism. Many oral surgical procedures can be safely performed with INRs under 3.0, if appropriate cautionary measures are taken.

MANAGEMENT

The first step in treatment of a patient in a cardiac crisis is to apply the ABCs of CPR, as well as defibrillation, as part of advanced cardiac life support (ACLS) ABCDs (see Chapter 1).

Every dentist and staff should be current at a minimum in basic CPR certification. Early diagnosis and treatment are crucial when dealing with acute cardiac events. Prompt therapy helps to preserve ventricular function, relieve pain and anxiety, reduce oxygen demand, increase oxygen supply, improve and restore myocardial perfusion, and finally, reduce risks of postischemic arrhythmias and other complications. Whenever a patient appears to be experiencing a cardiac problem, the dental procedure should immediately be stopped and the basic ABCs implemented. The dentist immediately determines the patient's level of consciousness, checks the airway and ensures adequacy of ventilation, and delivers oxygen via face mask. The patient is placed in the Trendelenburg position to increase blood return to the heart and blood flow to the brain. After ventilation is assessed and corrective measures initiated, cardiac status can be evaluated by determination of the heart rate and blood pressure.

For acute chest pain, nitroglycerin and oxygen are the drugs of choice and should be immediately available in every dental office. *Nitroglycerin* may be administered sublingually or through a metered-spray device. Complications include headache, intracranial hypertension, respiratory distress syndrome, and hypotension. If the patient is experiencing angina, nitroglycerin should alleviate the symptoms. If the patient becomes hypotensive (systolic blood pressure less than 90 mm Hg), nitroglycerin is stopped. If the pain is not relieved by nitroglycerin, acute MI should be suspected, and the patient should be transported immediately to a hospital.

The first 30 to 60 minutes of an MI are crucial. If the dentist is trained in venipuncture or ACLS, an IV catheter can be inserted for delivery of resuscitative drugs. Other therapies include administration of *morphine sulfate*, 1 to 4 mg every 5 minutes, to reduce pain. Morphine may also produce favorable hemodynamics by decreasing venous load. The conscious patient can immediately chew a regular-strength *aspirin* (160 to 325 mg) to decrease the risk of emboli formation after MI. An *automatic external defibrillator* (AED) interprets arrhythmias and automatically delivers an electrical shock to patients in ventricular fibrillation. This is the most effective resuscitative intervention to improve survival. It is crucial to defibrillate immediately.

Drugs for Advanced CPR

Practitioners who have taken ACLS courses from the American Heart Association may want to equip their offices with the IV drugs listed in the various algorithms. Dentists who administer deep sedation or general anesthesia must have this advanced training to deliver safe treatment for their patients.

REFERENCES

1. Rose LF, Kaye D: *Internal medicine for dentistry*, ed 2, St Louis, 1990, Mosby.
2. Beer MH, Berkow R: *The Merck manual*, ed 7, Whitehouse Station, NJ, 1999, Merck Research Laboratories.
3. Hudak CM, Gallo BM, Morton PG: *Critical care nursing: a holistic approach*, ed 7, Philadelphia, 1998, Lippincott.
4. Isselbacher KJ, Braunwald E, Wilson JD, et al: *Harrison's principles of internal medicine*, ed 3, New York, 1994, McGraw-Hill.
5. Robbins SL, Kumar V: *Basic pathology*, ed 4, Philadelphia, 1987, WB Saunders.
6. American Heart Association: *Advanced cardiac life support*, Dallas, 1998, The Association.
7. Bates BA: *Guide to physical examination and history taking*, ed 5, Philadelphia, 1991, Lippincott.
8. Lilly LS, editor: *Pathophysiology of heart disease*, Philadelphia, 1993, Lea & Febiger.
9. Willerson JT et al: *Treatment of heart diseases*, New York, 1992, Gower.
10. Chernecky CC, Berger BJ: *Laboratory tests and diagnostic procedures*, ed 2, Philadelphia, 1997, WB Saunders.
11. Braunwald E, editor: *Heart diseases: a textbook of cardiovascular medicine*, Philadelphia, 1997, WB Saunders.
12. Young VB et al: *Blueprints in medicine*, Mulden, Mass, 1998, Blackwell Science.
13. Lynch MA, Brightman VJ, Greenberg MS: *Burket's oral medicine: diagnosis and treatment*, ed 8, Philadelphia, 1984, Lippincott.
14. Manrino PL: *The ICU book*, ed 2, Baltimore, 1998, Williams & Wilkins.
15. Schneider AS, Szanto PA: *Pathology*, Philadelphia, 1993, Harwal.

Neuromuscular Disorders

Joseph F. Piecuch
Stuart E. Lieblich

A number of relatively uncommon but significant neuromuscular conditions may affect dental treatment, particularly in elderly patients. Inability to carry out proper oral hygiene may result in an increased caries rate and greater incidence and severity of periodontal disease, causing these patients to seek dental care for chronic and acute disorders. Consideration of the medications used to treat these disorders and an understanding of disease pathophysiology provide the scientific basis for dealing with the clinical implications of neuromuscular disorders.

CENTRAL NERVOUS SYSTEM DISORDERS: PRIMARY DEMENTIAS

Although considered to be a normal attribute of the aging process, a progressive decrease in long-term and short-term memory may become pronounced in about 10% of the population over age 70.[1] The most common cause is Alzheimer's disease, which affects more than half these patients. The primary dementias may begin with minor episodes of forgetfulness, followed by a gradually deteriorating clinical course that may last for 8 to 10 years (Huntington's disease) or up to 25 years or more (Alzheimer's disease). The differential diagnosis includes stroke, brain tumor, chronic subdural hematoma, depression, drug or medication intoxication, vitamin deficiency, and Parkinson's disease, in which 30% of patients develop dementia.

Alzheimer's Disease

Alzheimer's disease (AD) was first described by Dr. Alois Alzheimer in 1905 in a middle-aged German woman with progressive loss of memory and other cognitive functions. AD is now one of the most common disorders of aging, affecting 20% to 40% of the population over age 85. Currently, an estimated 4 million Americans are affected. With the ever-increasing aging population, some estimate a prevalence of 14 million by the year 2050.

AD results from the formation of neuritic plaques that contain amyloid, proteoglycans, and other proteins, causing progressive and irreversible neuronal injury and cortical atrophy. Diagnosis is typically made using clinical criteria developed by the National Institute of Neurological and Communicative Disorders (NINCD) and the Alzheimer's Disease and Related Disorders Association (ADRDA) (Box 23-1).[2] Loss of intellectual function typically involves more than two cognitive domains, including recent memory, speech and language usage, visual-spatial function, higher cognition, and mood and personality.[3] In some patients, clinical diagnosis can be confirmed by neuroimaging, including magnetic resonance imaging (MRI) and computed tomography (CT), which show a diffuse cortical atrophy with ventricular enlargement.

Risk factors for development of AD include old age, family history, and previous head trauma. Environmental factors are undergoing exhaustive research. The development of AD has not been significantly related to cerebrovascular disease. Recent studies have suggested that the use of nonsteroidal antiinflammatory drugs (NSAIDs) may reduce the incidence of AD; however, no recommendations have yet been made for the use of NSAIDs as prophylaxis.

The clinical course of AD is a slow, unrelenting process of memory loss, inability to learn new tasks, and difficulty in problem solving, eventually progressing to an inability to perform self-care. Mild depression is common in the early stages as the patient realizes the nature of the condition. Other noncognitive behavioral changes include emotional lability, apathy, and psychosis. Depression may also be present in family members, who may become extremely fatigued caring for the patient.

Box 23-1	Criteria and Supporting Factors in Diagnosis of Alzheimer's Disease

CRITERIA
1. Dementia, established by clinical examination, mental status testing, and neuropsychiatric testing
2. Deficits in at least two cognitive domains
3. Progressive cognitive decline, including memory
4. Normal level of consciousness
5. Onset between ages 40 and 70
6. No other possible medical explanation

SUPPORTING FACTORS
1. Progressive aphasia, apraxia, or agnosia
2. Impaired activities of daily living
3. Family history
4. Brain atrophy on neuroimaging
5. Normal cerebrospinal fluid and electroencephalogram

Modified from Caselli R, Boeve B: The degenerative dementias. In Goetz C, Pappert E, editors: *Textbook of clinical neurology*, Philadelphia, 1999, WB Saunders.

Pharmacologic Therapy

No known cure exists for AD.[4-7] Several amino acridines have been developed that seem to increase memory function but fail to slow disease progression. Tacrine, 80 to 160 mg/day, appears to benefit 10% to 20% of patients, particularly in early stages of AD. Tacrine acts as a cholinesterase inhibitor to increase cerebral levels of acetylcholine. Because it may adversely affect hepatic function, liver enzymes must be monitored. Tacrine has no benefit in advanced cases. Several similar drugs (donepezil, rivastigmine, metrifonate) are being introduced and have the advantages of once-daily dosing, no effect on the liver, and fewer drug interactions.

Patients with AD may also be taking antioxidants (e.g., vitamin E), antipsychotics (e.g., haloperidol, clozapine, risperidone), monoamine oxidase (MAO) inhibitors, tricyclic antidepressants for depression, selective serotonin reuptake inhibitors (SSRIs), and anxiolytics (e.g., lorazepam, haloperidol) for agitation or insomnia. Occasionally, AD patients may have associated seizure disorders and are treated with phenytoin or carbamazepine.

Dental implications. The dental practitioner must be aware of the medications prescribed for AD, their side effects, and cumulative effects in elderly patients. AD patients will present to the dental office with acute emergencies and more often with severe periodontal disease, caries, and other therapeutic needs that reflect their inability to provide adequate oral hygiene.[8]

As in all geriatric patients, pharmacokinetic changes in absorption, distribution, and elimination of various drugs can occur.[9] In the absence of gastrointestinal pathology, absorption generally remains the same as in younger individuals, but it can be delayed by anticholinergic medications as well as by antacids, which decrease gastric emptying. Distribution can be affected by alterations in body fat and lean muscle mass. An increase in body fat, ranging from 18% in young men to 36% in elderly men and up to 48% in elderly women, increases the volume of distribution of lipid-soluble drugs, such as psychotropic medications. These drugs therefore accumulate and have a longer duration of activity in the elderly patient. Water-soluble drugs, however, have a decreased volume of distribution due to decreases in lean muscle mass and in body water. Serum concentrations therefore increase, and effects may be greater with normal doses. Decreased protein binding secondary to decreases in circulating serum albumin may increase the percentage of the unbound (active) form of medications and thus the drug's effects.

Elimination of most drugs is through hepatic metabolic processes. Liver blood flow decreases 40% to 45% between ages 25 and 65. Therefore a significant decrease in first-pass hepatic metabolism is often seen. Drugs that remain active for much longer periods include phenytoin, diazepam, alprazolam, and amitriptyline, all of which have active metabolites. Drugs that are generally unaffected include lorazepam, oxazepam, and triazolam. Therefore, when ordering sedatives for elderly patients, the physician should choose medications that are not affected by the patient's age.

Vascular Dementias

AD-like symptoms may be the result of severe cerebrovascular disease and multiple infarcts leading to the loss of functional tissue. Severity is related directly to the total amount of damaged cortex and can be documented on MRI as multiple infarcts without the cerebral atrophy seen in AD. Treatment is related to the underlying disease, and patients may be taking various cardiac medications, antihypertensives, and anticoagulants (e.g., warfarin).

Before planning surgical procedures, the dentist should specifically ask patients with cardiovascular or cerebrovascular disease and elderly patients if they are taking aspirin daily.

Huntington's Disease

Caused by a mutation on the fourth chromosome, Huntington's disease is a progressive autosomal dominant condition with a frequency of 10 per 100,000 population. Although the frequent, sudden, irregular jerky movements (chorea) are the hallmarks of this disease, memory losses and other AD-like symptoms of dementia also are often present, particularly late in the disease process. Likewise, delusions, depression, and obsessive-compulsive behavior may accompany Huntington's disease. These patients may be taking similar medications as AD patients.

Onset of Huntington's disease is usually in the fourth and fifth decades, although a small percentage of patients are affected before age 20. Males and females are equally affected. Mild personality changes may be the first manifestations, followed by choreiform movements and dementia. Patients with chorea may respond to benzodiazepines, phenothiazines, or haloperidol.

Death usually occurs 10 to 30 years after onset, often from complications of cachexia and aspiration pneumonia. Family members can now undergo DNA testing to confirm or rule out the diagnosis early. No specific treatments exist for Huntington's disease. Current research focuses on the decline in neurotransmitters (e.g., GABA, acetylcholine).

Dental patients with Huntington's disease may have difficulty swallowing, with risk of aspiration in advanced cases. Anesthetic drugs (e.g., barbiturates) should be avoided because prolonged apnea (up to 1 hour) after induction with thiopental has been reported.[10] Propofol is considered safe. Reports are conflicting on the possibility of a similar prolonged response to succinylcholine. Glycopyrrolate may be used to control excessive saliva because its anticholinergic effects do not act centrally, although choreiform movements may worsen.

EXTRAPYRAMIDAL DISORDERS
Parkinson's Disease

Described as "shaking palsy" by Parkinson in 1817, Parkinson's disease (PD) is manifested by chronic, progressive combinations of resting tremor, cogwheel rigidity, and bradykinesia (slowness of voluntary movement).[11] Initial symptoms may be mild and unilateral. As PD progresses, manifestations include a characteristic shuffling gait, postural instability, sleep disorders, constipation, dysphagia, depression (one third of patients), and dementia (20% of patients). Patients with severe PD may have drooling and involuntary eye closing.

Despite considerable research, no specific cause has been found for PD. A variety of environmental and hereditary factors have been considered, but none has been proven. PD starts in middle or late life and leads to progressive disability. It affects about 100 per 100,000 population but increases significantly after age 65 and affects an estimated half of the population over 85. The specific lesion involves neuronal loss of dopaminergic cells in the substantia nigra. An estimated 65% to 85% of the neurons must be lost before symptoms occur.

About 75% of patients with PD-like symptoms have true Parkinson's disease. Such symptoms may also be present in patients with depression, Huntington's disease, Wilson's disease, and benign essential tremor (see following discussion).[12] Drug-induced symptoms may be seen with use of calcium channel blockers, methyldopa (Aldomet), haloperidol (Haldol), phenothiazines, and metoclopramide (Reglan).

The diagnosis of PD is made through the history and clinical examination. MRI is not diagnostic but can rule out other disorders. Some diagnostic benefit has been seen with positron emission tomography (PET) and single-photon emission computed tomography (SPECT) scans, but these modalities are not in common use.

Pharmacologic Therapy

Medical management of patients with PD must include education about the disorder, exercise therapy to maintain strength, and proper nutrition (Box 23-2). Early diagnosis is important because symptoms can be controlled for 4 to 6 years before deterioration becomes noticeable.[13]

Pharmacologic treatment can be classified as "protective" (preventive) or "symptomatic." Selegiline (Eldepryl), a selective MAO-B inhibitor, blocks oxidative metabolism of dopamine and is thought to decrease progressive neuronal degeneration, thus delaying the need for symptomatic treatment. Selegiline has been used in low does (<10 mg/day) with some preventive effect. Current research focuses on developing drugs to prevent neuronal degeneration and creating new neurons through fetal transplantation or gene

<table>
</table>

Box 23-2 Summary of Management for Patients with Parkinson's Disease

I. *All patients:* education, exercise therapy, nutrition program
II. *Patients with no clinically significant disability:* selegiline regimen
III. *Patients with clinically significant disablility:*
   A. Job security threatened: levodopa, controlled release
   B. Job security *not* threatened:
      1. *Young patients with tremor:* anticholinergic drugs or amantadine
      2. *Older patients:* amantadine, dopamine agonists
      3. *Elderly patients:* levodopa
IV. *Patients with progressive disability:* levodopa plus selegiline
V. *Patients with specific complications:*
   A. Motor fluctuations with levodopa therapy: carbidopa-levodopa (Sinemet), selegiline, catechol
   B. O-methyltransferase inhibitors
   C. Hallucinations: reduced dosages of medications, except Sinemet, clozapine, or neuroleptics

Modified from Jancovic J, Stacy M: Movement disorders. In Goetz CG. Pappert E, editors: *Textbook of clinical neurology,* Philadelphia, 1999, WB Saunders.

Box 23-3 Medications for Patients with Parkinson's Disease

DOPAMINERGIC DRUGS
Amino acid precursors: levodopa, carbidopa-levodopa (Sinemet, controlled release)
Dopamine agonists: bromocriptine (Parlodel), pergolide (Permax), pramipexole (Mirapex), ropinirole (ReQuip)
Monoamine oxidase B inhibitor: selegiline (Deprenyl)
Indirect agonist: amantadine (Symmetrel)
Catechol O-methyltransferase inhibitors: tolcopone, entacopone

OTHER DRUG CLASSES
Anticholinergics: trihexyphenidyl (Artane), benztropine (Cogentin)
Neuroleptic: clozapine (Clozaril)
Antidepressant: amitriptyline (Elavil)

therapy. Such treatments currently are only experimental. Symptomatic treatment involves numerous agents (Box 23-3).

The mainstay of therapy for PD is levodopa, which is converted in the brain into dopamine by dopa-decarboxylase. Dopamine itself cannot cross the blood-brain barrier. Levodopa (L-dopa) is probably the most efficient treatment for PD, especially for the rigidity and bradykinesia. Problems with its use include poor absorption due to peripheral decarboxylation, fluctuation in effect ("wearing-off" phenomenon), and dyskinesia in 50% of patients after 5 years of use. The combination of levodopa with the dopa-decarboxylase inhibitor carbidopa, which does not cross the blood-brain barrier, prevents peripheral effects while allowing maximum delivery to brain tissue. The controlled-release form of levodopa-carbidopa (Sinemet) helps to decrease fluctuations in effect.

Dopamine receptor agonists (e.g., bromocriptine, pergolide) have been available for two decades and provide benefit by direct stimulation of dopamine receptors, thus moderating the effects of levodopa.[14] Pramipexole and ropinirole, both introduced in 1997, are more effective than earlier dopamine agonists and can be used alone without levodopa. Catechol O-methyltransferase (COMT) inhibitors decrease dopamine metabolism, thereby increasing bioavailability.[15] Tolcapone, introduced in 1998, increases the length of activity of Sinemet and decreases the "wearing-off" phenomenon; unfortunately, it also elevates liver enzyme levels. Entacapone, a newer and similar agent, does not appear to increase liver enzymes.

Anticholinergics (e.g., benztropin, trihexyphenidyl) may be used to reduce parkinsonian tremor, particularly in patients whose only problem is tremor early in the disease. Side effects include dry mouth, nausea, and blurred vision. Amantadine, an antiviral agent, has mild dopaminergic activity as well as anticholinergic action, but it also has significant side effects. Other drugs used in advanced cases include antipsychotics (e.g., clozapine) for visual hallucinations and antidepressants (e.g., amitriptyline) for depression and insomnia.[16]

Dental implications. The dental practitioner should be aware of the pathophysiology and symptoms of PD as well as the mechanism of action and potential side effects of therapeutic drugs. When general anesthesia is required, abrupt discontinuation of levodopa may result in skeletal rigidity and difficult ventilation.[17] Since it can only be taken orally and has a short half-life (1 to 3 hours), levodopa should be continued despite NPO status. Anesthetic agents that sensitize the myocardium to catecholamines (e.g., halothane) must be avoided in patients taking levodopa. Muscle relaxants (e.g., succinylcholine) and propofol are safe, but opioids linked to rigidity should be avoided.

Because of autonomic dysfunction, hypotension may be a problem postoperatively. Patients with PD should be monitored closely and oral drug therapy resumed as soon as possible.

Benign Essential Tremor

Benign essential tremor may be a familial disorder. Its only manifestation is the tremor, which may involve the head and voice, unlike PD. Although some consider benign essential tremor to be a risk factor for PD, this has not been proven. Typically the disorder is nonprogressive. A single dose of propranolol is often used to decrease symptoms during significant events (e.g., lecturing, public performance).

Tardive Dyskinesia

As a result of long-term antipsychotic treatment with dopamine antagonists, a patient may develop abnormal movements involving localized areas such as hands ("pill rolling") or face ("lip smacking"). Particularly if the latter is involved, such dyskinesias can be socially inhibiting. Unfortunately, withdrawal of the predisposing drug does not eliminate the symptoms in most patients. Very few drugs affect these movements. Reserpine may decrease the intensity of the movements.

NUTRITIONAL AND METABOLIC DISORDERS
Vitamin B$_{12}$ Deficiency

Subacute combined degeneration of the spinal cord is caused by vitamin B$_{12}$ deficiency, with demyelinization of the dorsal and lateral columns and occasionally of the cranial nerves, particularly the optic nerve, and cerebral white matter. This abnormality can cause permanent disability.[18]

Cyanocobalamin and other cobalamins are collectively known as vitamin B$_{12}$. The typical Western diet contains sufficient amounts to meet dietary requirements. Therefore a deficiency implies an intestinal absorption problem. Body stores are so high that this disorder takes 2 to 5 years to develop. Factors necessary for absorption of viamin B$_{12}$ include an intact gastric mucosa, intrinsic factor, pancreatic enzymes, and normal function of the terminal ileum. In the stomach, acids and pepsin release free vitamin B$_{12}$ from dietary protein. The vitamin then binds immediately with R protein in the stomach and is carried into the proximal small intestine, where pancreatic enzymes degrade the R protein, releasing free B$_{12}$, which combines with intrinsic factor, a glycoprotein secreted by gastric parietal cells. The vitamin B$_{12}$–intrinsic factor complex attaches to specific membrane receptors in the terminal ileum and is absorbed. Vitamin B$_{12}$ is stored in protein-bound form in the liver. Gastric mucosal conditions, pancreatic disease, ileal disease, lack of intrinsic factor due to nonfunctional parietal cells (pernicious anemia), and liver disease all can contribute to defects in vitamin B$_{12}$ absorption.

Although vitamin B$_{12}$ deficiency is associated most strongly with a macrocytic anemia, up to one fourth of patients can develop significant neurologic disease in the absence of anemia. Therefore a screening test for mean cell volume or hematocrit is not sufficient to rule out this disorder. Specific measurement of serum vitamin B$_{12}$ level is indicated.[19]

Neurologic manifestations may initially present as generalized weakness of the extremities and paresthesias ("pins and needles" sensation). In later stages, depression, confusion, cognitive impairment, memory loss, hallucinations (especially with optic nerve involvement), ataxia, and abnormal gait are prominent.

Treatment generally consists of intramuscular doses of cobalamin, which usually need to be maintained for life.[20] Complete regression of symptoms usually occurs if the disease is treated immediately on diagnosis. However, late cases do not respond well, and restoration of normal B$_{12}$ levels may only prevent further progression.

Vitamin B$_{12}$ deficiency is important in dentistry mainly because of its association with nitrous oxide toxicity (see later discussion).

Alcoholic Cerebellar Degeneration

Cerebellar degeneration occurs frequently in chronic alcohol abusers. It is progressive once symptoms begin and involves primarily the lower extremities. It is characterized clinically by a classic wide-based gait. In advanced cases, nystagmus and incoordination may occur. In most patients, abstinence from alcohol and replenishment of nutrition result in gradual resolution of symptoms as the neuropathy resolves.

Hypoglycemic Encephalopathy

Hypoglycemia in the diabetic patient is a medical emergency. The patient who skips breakfast before a dental appointment because of anxiety and an upset stomach but injects the normal daily dose of insulin will likely become hypoglycemic. Mild hypoglycemia may result in restlessness, agitation, tachycardia, and confusion. This condition must be recognized and treated with oral sugar, or the patient will rapidly deteriorate to unconsciousness and seizures. Continued hypoglycemia (25 mg%) can lead to irreversible neuronal damage. If the patient becomes unconscious, definitive treatment is required (see Chapter 24).

Although severe hyperglycemia can also produce diabetic coma, this usually occurs very slowly and is not typically associated with treatment in a dental office.

Wernicke's Encephalopathy

Caused by a deficiency of thiamine, Wernicke's encephalopathy is found primarily in severe alcoholics but can also present in other malnourished individuals, such as cancer, renal failure, and elderly patients. A recent study showed that up to 40% of hospitalized elderly patients exhibited thiamine deficiency.[21] The classic triad of ophthalmoplegia (especially lateral rectus palsy), ataxia, and confusion and a history of alcohol abuse are usually sufficient to make the diagnosis.[22]

Some patients exhibit severe mental abnormalities, including inattention, loss of memory, and confabulation, termed *Korsakoff's psychosis*. The brain is unable to utilize cerebral glucose because of an absent or diminished thiamine level. Irreversible damage and even death can occur rapidly. Administration of glucose-containing intravenous fluids can precipitate the encephalopathy. Therefore it is common practice in hospital admissions to administer thiamine to all alcoholics, regardless of signs of encephalopathy on admission.

Implications for dental practice are few, although Wernicke's encephalopathy can account for the disorientation and lack of compliance seen in some patients.

MOTOR NEURON AND DEMYELINATING DISEASES
Amyotrophic Lateral Sclerosis

Commonly known as "Lou Gehrig's disease," amyotrophic lateral sclerosis (ALS) is an idiopathic disease involving progressive degeneration of upper and lower motor neurons with no treatment or cure.[23] Patients eventually die of respiratory failure, with a mean survival after diagnosis of 3 to 5 years. The specific lesion within the brain involves degeneration of cortical, bulbar, and medullary motor neurons that affect voluntary motor function. This leads to muscle denervation, manifesting initially as weakness, then wasting, atrophy, and fasciculation. An estimated one third of motor neurons in a given tract must be destroyed before significant symptoms occur; therefore the time until diagnosis after presentation of the earliest symptoms is approximately 16 to 18 months.

The incidence of ALS is 1 to 3 per 100,000 population, with a current prevalence in the United States of approximately 30,000 patients. The onset is usually between ages 50 and 70. The etiology is unknown. Many theories exist regarding toxins, autoimmune disease, and inherent enzymatic defects.[24] A family history is present in about 10% of ALS patients, with a small percentage being autosomal dominant.

The initial presentation of ALS usually involves a single lower extremity with weakness and incoordination.[25] Difficulty may occur initially with fine motor function (e.g., buttoning clothes, turning keys). If bulbar neurons are involved, hoarseness in speech may be the first symptom. Subsequently, muscle atrophy becomes apparent, with cramping pain on movement, immobility, spasticity, difficulty swallowing, emotional changes, depression, cachexia, and respiratory failure. The stages of ALS are mild, moderate, severe, and terminal.[26] Throughout its progression, cognitive function is spared, and patients remain fully aware of their deteriorating condition.

Pharmacologic Therapy

Treatment is mostly symptomatic, although one newer drug, riluzole, has been shown to delay the progression of symptoms in mild and moderate stages. Its use remains controversial, however, because Riluzole can have significant side effects, and survival is extended only 3 to 6 months.[27] Medications for ALS symptoms include baclofen for spasticity, diazepam or lorazepam for vesiculations, NSAIDs for joint pain and contractures, and tricyclic antidepressants for depression and sleep disorders. Many patients with ALS exhibit greater cachexia than would be expected because gastrointestinal function remains normal.

Because difficulty swallowing and fear of choking may be associated with ALS, percutaneous endoscopic gastrostomy (PEG) may help to prolong survival. Caloric requirements typically increase due to difficulty with ventilation. A variety of noninvasive, mechanical ventilation support methods have also been developed. Invasive ventilatory support involving tracheostomy is frequently used in the United States but is less common in other countries.

Dental implications. Although ALS is rare, the unusual patient who has hoarseness or difficulty speaking or swallowing should be referred for evaluation. Any patient with swallowing disorders should receive particular attention regarding small instruments and materials during dental treatment.

Anesthetic considerations include avoidance of succinylcholine because a hyperkalemic response may occur. Most anesthetic techniques and agents are safe for these patients. Intraoperative and postoperative ventilatory support is often necessary due to respiratory muscle weakness.

Multiple Sclerosis

Multiple sclerosis (MS) is characterized by inflammation and destruction of myelin in the central nervous system with gliosis (scarring). Peripheral nerves are generally spared, with exception of the optic nerve, which is involved in a large percentage of cases.

MS is a disease of temperate climates with varied incidence in different parts of the world, ranging from 2 per 100,000 population in Japan to more than 250 in 100,000 in the islands of northern Scotland. An estimated 350,000 to 400,000 persons in the United States have MS, affecting females twice as often as males. MS can occur at any age, but the peak incidence is between ages 15 and 50, with a decreased incidence later in life.

The specific etiology is unknown, but many consider MS to be an autoimmune disorder directed against myelin, possibly from environmental factors (e.g., toxins, viral infection) in a genetically susceptible host. MS is much more common in families of affected persons and in whites of European origin. Virtually unknown in the African black population, MS occurs in African Americans but considerably less than in the white population. There is some evidence of increased incidence in migrant populations settling in endemic areas.[28]

Specific lesions involve demyelinated plaques, ranging from several millimeters to several centimeters in size, in several locations within the brain and spinal cord. The extent of damage does not always correlate with clinical manifestations. Demyelination has two opposite effects: a slowing of conduction through nerve fibers and the generation of ectopic impulses, which may fire alternately from one nerve to the next, creating spastic movements.

Early symptoms of MS characteristically involve sensory or motor deprivation of a single limb spreading centrally. In about 15% to 20% of patients the first manifestation is visual blurring or diplopia caused by optic neuritis. As symptoms progress, the patient may develop paresthesias, leading to persistent sensory loss, ataxia, pain, decreased visual acuity, facial palsy, trigeminal neuralgia, vertigo, bladder urgency, spasticity, and loss of dexterity. Some believe that the most common cause of trigeminal neuralgia in patients under age 40 is MS. Patients with advanced disease typically have memory loss, decreased cognitive function, and fatigue. The most advanced cases involve complete inability to walk. Despite its severity, MS usually does not decrease life expectancy, except in patients with extremely advanced disease.[29]

Clinical diagnosis of MS is very difficult. The presence of widespread abnormal symptoms and signs without specific focal deficits may prevent early diagnosis. However, two separate attacks of the disorder with at least two proven central nervous system lesions would define a clinically definite diagnosis. Laboratory diagnosis assists primarily in ruling out other possible causes of the patient's symptoms. Cerebrospinal fluid evaluation may show an increase in mononuclear cells and an increase in total immunoglobulins, especially IgG. MRI shows multiple hyperdense areas on T2-weighted sequences, which reflect increased water content of areas containing demyelinated plaques. The presence of more than three lesions greater than 6 mm in size, particularly in paraventricular regions, supports the diagnosis.[30] Differential diagnosis includes systemic lupus erythematosus, human immunodeficiency virus, sarcoid, Lyme disease, and acute disseminated encephalitis.

Patients with MS have a variable clinical course that may be characterized by repeated attacks of severe symptoms, many of which may resolve over time, followed by a gradual progression.[29] This categorization, however, is not linked definitively to prognosis or to severity (Box 23-4).

Box 23-4	Types of Multiple Sclerosis

Relapsing remitting
Secondary progressive
Primary progressive
Progressive relapsing

Relapsing remitting MS is characterized by unpredictable attacks lasting 1 to 2 weeks, followed by partial or complete recovery lasting 4 to 8 weeks or longer, without significant progression between attacks. Attacks typically occur at a rate of one or two per year. Most patients return to their preattack baseline state after recovery. Secondary progressive MS starts as relapsing and remitting, then slowly progresses, with an increase in symptoms between attacks. Primary progressive MS is characterized by a gradual progression of disability, without severe attacks, recovery periods, or periods of stability. Progressive relapsing MS appears similar to the primary progressive form but has occasional superimposed relapses.

Regardless of type, the clinical course of MS is highly variable, with no significant association between frequency of attacks and severity of symptoms. Fifteen years after diagnosis, up to 20% of patients have no significant functional disability, but 75% are unemployed, and 70% require assistance with activities of daily living.

Pharmacologic Therapy

There is no available prevention or cure for MS. Therapy involves two general goals: stop the progression of the disease and manage the symptoms.[31,32] Current therapeutic trials include use of interferon (INF), particularly INF-β_{1b} (Betaseron) and INF-β_{1a} (Avonex), which have been shown to decrease frequency of relapses. Glatiramer (Copaxone), a synthetic polypeptide mimicking the basic protein of myelin, has been shown to forestall the relapse rate for up to 3 years. Recent MRI data showed a 35% reduction in gadolinium-enhancing lesions after 9 months of glatiramer therapy, with a 33% decrease in relapse rate.[33] Intravenous (IV) immune globulin may also show similar benefit, although adverse effects (e.g., headache, nausea, skin reactions) occurred in 58% of patients. Acute relapses have been modified by use of high-dose IV methylprednisolone, followed by oral prednisone. This is used particularly for patients with symptoms of optic neuritis. Numerous immunosuppressive medications have been used, including methotrexate, azathioprine, and cyclophosphamide.

Therapy to manage MS symptoms includes baclofen, diazepam, and cyclobenzaprine for spasticity; phenytoin, carbamazepine, and amitriptyline for trigeminal neuralgia; and clonazepam and primidone for tremor. Bladder urgency and dysfunction are treated with anticholinergics, and urinary retention is often treated with the cholinergic agent bethanechol. A variety of treatments for depression and fatigue are available.

Dental implications. Similar to other diseases discussed, the direct implications of MS for dentistry are minimal other than awareness and management of the patient's medications. Patients receiving long-term steroid therapy should have their dose supplemented with major surgery. Review of anesthetic agents shows no adverse effects on MS. However, hyperpyrexia in the perioperative period may exacerbate symptoms. Severely debilitated patients are at risk for succinylcholine-induced hyperkalemia, but nondepolarizing muscle relaxants are safe.

Nitrous Oxide Toxicity

Nitrous oxide toxicity results from inactivation of methionine synthase, an enzyme dependent on vitamin B_{12}. It results in defective synthesis of myelin. The symptoms are typically numbness, paresthesia, and ataxia, which can become extremely severe, leading to inability to walk. Nitrous oxide toxicity may resolve over time if exposure is discontinued, but recovery may be prolonged and incomplete.[34]

Two types of patients develop the myeloneuropathy associated with nitrous oxide. Patients with the first type have a clinical or subclinical cobalamin (vitamin B_{12}) deficiency, caused by either a decrease in ileal absorption or a deficiency of intrinsic factor. This deficiency affects between 7% and 21% of elderly people.[35] Symptoms in this patient population may develop after a single use or after repeated use of nitrous oxide in general anesthesia or in dentistry.

Patients with the second type of nitrous oxide toxicity have normal serum cobalamin levels but repeated and prolonged exposure, often for recreational use. In 1978, Layzer reported on 15 patients (14 dentists and one hospital technician) who had severe symptoms from constant exposure to nitrous oxide.[36] The initial symptoms on presentation included numbness and tingling of the hands, loss of balance, and loss of finger dexterity. Eventually, all these patients had distal numbness of their legs, and many were unable to walk. Thirteen of these patients (12 dentists and one technician) practiced self-administration almost daily for 3 months and up to 5 years. The other two cases were oral surgeons whose condition was purely occupational exposure before implementation of "scavenging" systems. All 15 patients exhibited slow improvement on discontinuation of use or on implementation of scavenging. However, none of the patients recovered fully, but all were eventually able to walk.

Dental professionals must be aware of the possibility of demyelination in the elderly patient after nitrous oxide administration. The dentist should obtain a nutritional history and should consult with the patient's physician regarding laboratory testing, as appropriate. All dentists also must be aware of the necessity for scavenging systems.

PERIPHERAL NERVOUS SYSTEM DISORDERS: NEUROPATHIES AND NEUROJUNCTIONAL DISTURBANCES
Guillain-Barré Syndrome

Characterized by the rapid onset of weakness and paralysis, and generally by the absence of cranial nerve involvement, Guillain-Barré syndrome (GBS) is an acute motor neuropathy thought to be related to certain bacterial and viral infections. The incidence of GBS is 1 to 2 per 100,000 population. Approximately two thirds of cases occur 1 to 3 weeks after a viral infection. Gastrointestinal illnesses with certain predominant bacteria have also been implicated (Box 23-5). Although GBS can occur at any age, elderly persons are at greater risk.

Initial presentation of GBS typically involves paresthesias of the feet and hands, rarely the

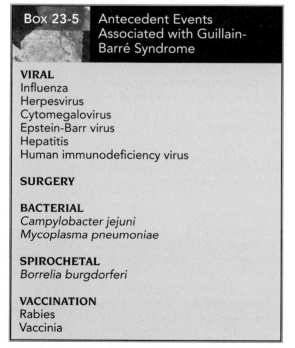

| Box 23-5 | Antecedent Events Associated with Guillain-Barré Syndrome |

VIRAL
Influenza
Herpesvirus
Cytomegalovirus
Epstein-Barr virus
Hepatitis
Human immunodeficiency virus

SURGERY

BACTERIAL
Campylobacter jejuni
Mycoplasma pneumoniae

SPIROCHETAL
Borrelia burgdorferi

VACCINATION
Rabies
Vaccinia

Modified from Sheilds RW, Wilbourn AJ: Demyelinating disorders of the peripheral nervous system. In Goetz C, Pappert E, editors: *Textbook of clinical neurology*, Philadelphia, 1999, WB Saunders.

perioral area, followed by weakness several days later, which is progressive for up to 3 to 4 weeks. Some patients develop a motor paralysis, with absence of reflexes and with or without sensory abnormalities. Up to 35% require ventilatory support. Although the mortality is approximately 5%, 75% of patients affected with GBS make a complete recovery in 6 to 12 months. Nevertheless, 10% to 15% have permanent sequelae.

The diagnosis of GBS is typically made by clinical examination. Supportive laboratory testing includes examination of the cerebrospinal fluid, which shows an increase in protein with a normal cell count. Nerve conduction studies will show slowing of conduction and in some cases a blockade.

Treatment of GBS generally involves hospitalization as soon as the diagnosis is made, since some patients undergo extremely rapid deterioration.[37] If the patient has paralysis, low-dose heparin and pneumatic compression devices to prevent pulmonary embolus are important. Ventilatory support, usually without tracheostomy, is often indicated. The course of GBS can be shortened by plasmapheresis if done in the first 2 weeks, as well as by use of high-dose IV immune globulins. High-dose corticosteroids have been used, but their effectiveness in shortening the course of the disease has been questioned.

Dental patients requiring general anesthesia who have respiratory and autonomic compromise are susceptible to depolarizing agent–induced hyperkalemia and variations in blood pressure. Direct intraarterial blood pressure monitoring has been suggested. Anesthetic agents are safe; however, assisted ventilation may be required postoperatively if respiratory depressants (e.g., narcotics) are used.

Myasthenia Gravis

Myasthenia gravis (MG) is an immune-mediated disorder characterized by fatigue and weakness of skeletal muscle without disturbances of reflexes, sensory innervation, or coordination abnormalities. It often begins with the ocular muscles, which may exhibit either diplopia or ptosis. Within 6 months, 50% of patients develop generalized weakness, and in 1 year, 75% exhibit generalized MG. Progression includes symptoms of dysphagia, articular difficulties, and peripheral weakness. Only 15% of ocular MG patients remain free of systemic symptoms long-term.[38]

Although MG can occur at any age, the most significant initial presentation is in the second and third decades in women, whereas in males it occurs in the fifth and sixth decades. Overall prevalence is estimated at 1 in 25,000 people. Differential diagnosis includes botulism and Lambert-Eaton myasthenic syndrome, associated with oat cell carcinoma of the lung.

Pathophysiology of MG includes the development of antibodies to acetylcholine receptors, which bind to the receptors, decreasing their efficiency and leading to their destruction. Definitive diagnosis of MG is through detection of acetylcholine receptor antibodies in serum by radioimmunoassay. This test is sensitive in 50% for ocular myasthenia and in 80% for generalized MG. The classic edrophonium (Tensilon) test produces improvement in 2 minutes after IV injection. A thymoma or thymic hyperplasia may be seen on CT or MRI in up to 90% of patients.

Classification of MG typically relates to the degree of severity: (1) isolated ocular MG; (2) mild-to-moderate generalized weakness; (3) severe generalized weakness; and (4) myasthenic "crisis" accompanied by respiratory failure. Approximately 2.5% of MG patients experience a myasthenic crisis in any given year, and up to 25% of patients eventually have a crisis over the course of the disease. Before the discovery of the immunologic basis of this disease and institution of modern therapeutic methods, up to 80% of patients undergoing myasthenic crisis died.[39] Current mortality rate for crisis is less than 5% and overall for MG extremely low.[40]

Pharmacologic Therapy

Therapy for MG can be subdivided into two general concepts.[41] The first is rapid, short-term improvement in strength, which is typically provided by acetylcholinesterase inhibitors, plasmapheresis, or IV immune globulin. Pyridostigmine and neostigmine provide short-term relief. Side effects may include gastrointestinal hypermotility and increased production of oral and respiratory secretions, which may often be well controlled with atropine or glycopyrrolate. Plasma exchange often produces improvement, with five to six treatments on alternate days for about 10 weeks. Side effects may include hypotension and depletion of clotting factors. Expense is a consideration. IV immunoglobulins for 5 days results in a short-term success rate similar to plasmapheresis.

Long-term immunosuppressive therapy is the mainstay of treatment for generalized MS. Thymectomy through a sternal approach is at least partially successful in up to 85% to 90% of patients and produces a stable complete remission in 15% to 60%. Such treatment is reserved for younger healthy patients without other medical compromise. Corticosteroids, 40 to 60 mg/day, produce a positive response in more than 70% of patients within the first several weeks of treatment. Once success occurs, the steroids may be tapered while azathioprine, 2 to 3 mg/kg/day, is instituted. Azathioprine is particularly useful for patients who have an inadequate response to steroid treatment and thymectomy or who are poor surgical candidates. The positive effect from azathioprine often takes more than a year to develop fully. Alternative immunosuppressive medications for patients refractory to these agents include cyclophosphamide and cyclosporine. These drugs typically produce an initial improvement in 2 to 4 weeks, with maximum improvement over 3 to 4 months.

Dental implications. Myasthenic crisis rarely occurs suddenly, and patients with crisis typically do not present for dental treatment. For routine dental care, awareness of immunosuppressive medications and the potential for increased respiratory and oral secretions is mandatory, with appropriate dose modification in those rare cases when extensive surgical procedures must be performed. Many antibiotics, including erythromycin,[42,43] clarithromycin,[44] imipenem,[45] and fluoroquinolones,[46] may worsen MG. These agents should be avoided.

Ester local anesthetics may be hydrolyzed more slowly and thus may be more toxic. Small doses are not contraindicated. Most general anesthetic agents are safe.[47,48] Mechanical ventilatory support may be required during recovery. Anticholinesterase agents may increase the duration of effect of narcotics. MG patients are also very sensitive to the nondepolarizing muscle relaxants.

DISORDERS OF MUSCLE
Muscular Dystrophy

Although often included in discussions of neurologic disorders, muscular dystrophy is technically a myopathy, a disorder of the skeletal muscle fiber. Muscular dystrophy is a congenital myopathy presenting with muscle weakness and wasting. It is differentiated from neurogenic disorders by the location. The weakness in muscular dystrophy is proximal, in contrast to the distal weakness of neurogenic origin.

Muscular dystrophy encompases a variety of inherited myopathies presenting as progressive muscular weakness.[49] Muscles degenerate and are replaced by fibrous and fatty connective tissue. The muscular dystrophies traditionally were classified by age of onset and inheritance pattern. Contemporary identification of abnormal gene products and locations of genetic mutation has lead to newer classification systems.

The initial presentation of patients with muscular dystrophy involves nonepisodic progressive muscle weakness and wasting, in contrast to the episodic weakness of disorders such as MG. Laboratory confirmation is obtained by serum muscle enzymes, electromyography, and muscle biopsy.

The two most common forms of muscular dystrophy, Duchenne's and Becker's, are caused by a defect in the production of dystrophin. Dystrophin provides support to the muscle membrane during contraction. The gene defect is found on the X chromosome, so these dystrophies have an X-linked recessive transmission pattern.

The frequency of Duchenne's muscular dystrophy is 1 in 3500 male births, with 30% to 40% arising from a new mutation. Female carriers will transmit the disease to 50% of their male children, and 50% of their female children will be carriers. Female carriers are usually asymptomatic but may demonstrate moderate limb girdle weakness.

Duchenne's muscular dystrophy presents as early as 2 to 3 years of age and is progressive until complete disability and death, usually in the 20s. Death is usually caused by respiratory complications. The progression is marked by frequent falls at age 5 to 6, wheelchair bound by age 12, and frequent hospitalizations due to pneumonia during the later teens. Compromised respiratory function is present early in life, and by age 10 a reduction in vital capacity may be noted on pulmonary function tests. Cardiac muscle is involved, and congestive heart failure and arrhythmias are found.[50]

Abnormal ECG findings include tall right precordial R waves and deep left precordial Q waves (due to scarring). Central nervous system involvement presents as intellectual impairment, possibly from lack of dystrophin at brain synapses. A significant laboratory finding is the marked (20 to 100 times normal) elevation of the serum creatine kinase (CK), which is present from birth. The CK level tends to decrease as muscle wasting occurs over the years. Female carriers will also tend to have an elevated CK level. Patients with Duchenne's dystrophy do not have an increased susceptibility to malignant hyperthermia as occasionally reported. Confusion between this disorder and central core my-

opathy has led to this misinformation (see following discussion).

A milder defect in dystrophin production causes Becker's muscular dystrophy. It is less common than Duchenne's type but presents with a similar pattern of progressive muscle weakness. Since Becker's type is less severe, onset is often detected later, at 5 to 15 years of age. Calf hypertrophy is often present, and early complaints of exercise-induced calf pain are common. Patients usually remain ambulatory until age 20 and are wheelchair bound after age 30. Continued progression of respiratory and cardiac complications lead to death, usually by age 40.

Mild respiratory infections in both forms of muscular dystrophy are potentially fatal and are treated aggressively with antibiotics. Once forced vital capacity falls below 1.2 liters, permanent ventilatory support is needed. No treatment exists, but long-term corticosteroids are often used and seem to decrease the rate of muscle loss.

Dental Considerations

Patients with muscular dystrophy can often have conventional care in a dental office that is wheelchair accessible, but some treatment modifications are necessary (Box 23-6). As with any wheelchair-bound patient, care in transferring the individual is mandatory to avoid injury to the patient and the staff. Many staff back injuries have occurred while attempting to transfer a patient with inadequate assistance. It is appropriate to ask the caregiver of the patient how the patient is transferred from wheelchair to bed, as well as use the person's assistance with the patient's physical movement. Depending on the patient's size, three or four people are needed, with one person solely in charge of ensuring that the head and cervical region are supported.

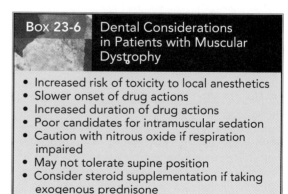

Box 23-6 Dental Considerations in Patients with Muscular Dystrophy

- Increased risk of toxicity to local anesthetics
- Slower onset of drug actions
- Increased duration of drug actions
- Poor candidates for intramuscular sedation
- Caution with nitrous oxide if respiration impaired
- May not tolerate supine position
- Consider steroid supplementation if taking exogenous prednisone

Once placed in the dental chair, the patient's tolerance to being reclined must be determined. As pulmonary reserves are lost, the patient may not tolerate a fully supine position. The patient also may not tolerate impediments to normal respiration, such as the use of a rubber dam.

Other concerns relate to the reduction of cardiac output. As it decreases, the ability to metabolize and clear drugs decreases proportionately. Toxicity may occur at lower-than-expected levels, and total drug dose reductions of 25% to 50% are indicated. The potential for cardiac arrhythmia would indicate limiting the dose of epinephrine to that of a cardiac-compromised patient (0.04 mg in a full-size adult). Longer onset of action and increased effect of medications should be expected.

Patients taking long-term exogenous corticosteroids may need supplementation before a stressful procedure such as complicated extractions. These patients have an increased risk of infection, and prophylactic antibiotics before the surgical procedure may be considered.

The patient with diminished respiratory reserve depends on low levels of oxygen to maintain respiratory drive. Although not specifically contraindicated, the higher oxygen concentrations associated with nitrous oxide administration could interfere with spontaneous respiration. The practitioner should monitor the patient carefully and be able to assist respiration with positive pressure if needed.

Numerous cases of cardiac arrest during or after general anesthesia have been reported. A specific cause has not been identified, but it may be related to hyperkalemia. However, general anesthesia, when necessary, is usually safe.

Central Core Myopathy

It is important to distinguish the congenital myopathies, specifically central core myopathy, from the muscular dystrophies. Most congenital myopathies are present at birth and are relatively nonprogressive. Clinical findings include reduced muscle bulk, long narrow face with skeletal abnormalities (high-arched palate, pectus excavatum, dislocated hips) and limb girdle weakness. Individuals with central core myopathy have a defect on the same gene as individuals with malignant hyperthermia (ryanodine receptor gene). Both disorders are transmitted through autosomal dominance inheritance. Many patients with central core myopathy are susceptible to malignant hyperthermia and therefore require standard anesthetic precautions.

Myotonic Dystrophy

Myotonic dystrophy is a muscle disease transmitted by autosomal dominance affecting 5 per 100,000 population. It is an extremely slowly progressive disease, with involved muscles becoming atrophic and weak. Myotonic dystrophy is characterized by myotonia, which is sustained muscle contraction after the cessation of a voluntary effort. The primarily distal distribution affects the muscles of the hands, forearms, distal limbs, neck, tongue, and face.[51] However, cardiac abnormalities, including mitral valve prolapse and syncopal attacks, are common. Cardiac involvement affects the conduction system in the heart, predisposing to arrhythmias. Severe cardiac fibrosis can lead to sudden death.

The respiratory and cardiac involvement requires close observation and monitoring of the patient during dental procedures. Frequency of arrhythmias is greater than with muscular dystrophy, and the dentist should limit or eliminate epinephrine in local anesthesia injections for patients with myotonic dystrophy. The high incidence of valvular defects should lead to consideration of antibiotic prophylaxis unless a normal cardiac evaluation is documented.

Chronic Fatigue Syndrome

Chronic fatigue syndrome (CFS) is a debilitating disorder that affects approximately 500,000 individuals in the United States. Encompassing a constellation of symptoms, CFS has a varied presentation.[52] Although abnormal laboratory values may occur, no specific test exists for CFS. Instead, patients present with prolonged idiopathic fatigue and four or more of the symptoms listed in Box 23-7 for at least 6 months.

Contemporary research into the treatment of patients with CFS has focused on neuroendocrinology. Early studies showed a low cortisol level, suggesting that the defect is in the hypo-

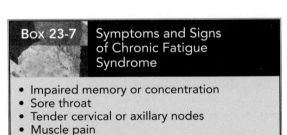

Box 23-7	Symptoms and Signs of Chronic Fatigue Syndrome

- Impaired memory or concentration
- Sore throat
- Tender cervical or axillary nodes
- Muscle pain
- Multiple-joint pain
- New-onset headaches
- Nonrefreshing sleep
- Postexertional malaise

thalamic-pituitary-adrenal axis. Many patients also present with neurally mediated hypotension.

The management of patients with CFS is primarily symptomatic, with medications for sleep disorders, pain, and depression. Cognitive-behavioral therapy may help the patient cope. A carefully monitored and graded exercise program may also be beneficial.[53]

Dental Considerations

Dental practitioners can safely treat patients with CFS. A detailed history including medications must be obtained. Patients may have had significant interaction with the health care system in trying to alleviate or "cure" their problem. The dentist must be aware of the psychological impact of a disease that has no outwardly objective signs but still may have a profound impact on a patient's life. A callous or nonbelieving attitude may lead to "secondary wounding" of the patient.

Although conventional care can be given to these patients, it is important to involve them in all decision making. Shorter appointments should be the norm, with continuous inquiry as to whether the procedure is becoming too stressful. Patients with CFS require the dentist's willingness to listen and consider their views seriously. The dentist must also be willing to let the patients take credit for any success in their care. Smaller amounts of medication may have a more profound effect, so lower doses, titrated to effect, are preferred. Some patients report increased fatigue after emotional or physical stress, and they may require weeks to return to their baseline state. Finally, the temptation to provide an extensive treatment to manage a constellation of vague symptoms, such as "full-mouth reconstruction" to hopefully alleviate headaches and facial, neck, and back pain, should not be attempted.

REFERENCES

1. Kupman D: Initial recognition of dementia, Am J Med 104(4A):2S-12S, 1998.
2. Caselli R., Boeve B: The degenerative dementias. In Goetz C, Pappert E, editors: Textbook of clinical neurology, Philadelphia, 1999, WB Saunders.
3. Adair JC: Is it Alzheimer's? Hosp Pract 33:35-38, 1998.
4. Small G: Treatment of Alzheimer's disease: current approaches and promising developments, Am J Med 104(4A):32S-38S, 1998.
5. Rivas-Vazquez RA, Carranzana EJ, Rey GJ, et al: Alzheimer's disease: pharmacological treatment and management, Clin Neuropsychol 14(1):93-109, 2000.
6. Parnetti L: Therapeutic options in dementia, J Neurol 247(3):163-169, 2000.
7. Elmilien G, Beyreuther K, Masters CL, Maloteaux JM: Prospects for pharmacological intervention in Alzheimer's disease, Arch Neurol 57(4):454-459, 2000.
8. Henry RG, Wekstein DR: Providing dental care for patients diagnosed with Alzheimer's disease, Dent Clin North Am 41(4):915-943, 1997.
9. Kompoliti K, Goetz C: Neuropharmacology in the elderly, Neurol Clin 16(3):599-610, 1998.
10. Cangemi CF, Miller RJ: Huntington's disease: review and anesthetic case management, Anesth Prog 45(4):150-153, 1998.
11. Colcher A, Simuni T: Clinical manifestations of Parkinson's disease, Med Clin North Am 83(2):327-348, 1999.
12. Adler CH: Differential diagnosis of Parkinson's disease, Med Clin North Am 83(2):349-368, 1999.
13. Hauser RA, Zesiewicz TA: Management of early Parkinson's disease, Med Clin North Am 83(2):393-414, 1999.
14. Factor S: Dopamine agonists, Med Clin North Am 83(2):415-444, 1999.
15. Siderowf A, Kurlan R: Monoamine oxidase and catechol-O-methyltransferase inhibitors, Med Clin North Am 83(2):445-468, 1999.
16. Stacy M: Managing late complications of Parkinson's disease, Med Clin North Am 83(2):469-482, 1999.
17. Mason LJ, Cojocaru TT, Cole DJ: Surgical intervention and anesthetic management of the patient with Parkinson's, Int Anesthesiol Clin 34(4):133-150, 1996.
18. Baik HW, Russell RM: Vitamin B_{12} deficiency in the elderly, Ann Rev Nutr 19l:357-377, 1999.
19. Snow CF: Laboratory diagnosis of vitamin B_{12} and folate deficiency: a guide for the primary care physician, Arch Intern Med 159:1289-1298, 1999.
20. Stabler SP: Vitamin B_{12} deficiency in older people: improving diagnosis and preventing disability, J Am Geriatr Soc 46:1317-1319, 1998.
21. Pepersack T: Clinical relevance of thiamine status amongst hospitalized elderly patients, Gerontology 45(2): 96-101, 1999.
22. Cook C, Hallwood P, Thomson AB: Vitamin deficiency and neuropsychiatric syndromes in alcohol misuse, Alcohol 33:317-336, 1998.
23. Walling AD: Amyotrophic lateral sclerosis: Lou Gehrig's disease, Am Fam Physician 59:1489-1496, 1999.
24. Milonas I: Amyotrophic lateral sclerosis: an introduction, J Neurol 245(suppl 2):S1-S3, 1998.
25. Brooks BR: Earlier is better: the benefits of early diagnosis, Neurology 53 (suppl 5):S53-S54, 1999.
26. Riviere M: An analysis of extended survival in patients with amyotrophic lateral sclerosis treated with Riluzole, Arch Neurol 55:526-528, 1998.
27. Ludolph AC, Riepe MW: Do the benefits of currently available treatments justify early diagnosis and treatment of amyotrophic lateral sclerosis? An argument against, Neurology 53(suppl 5):S46-S49, 1999.
28. Sadovnick AD, Ebers G: Genetics of multiple sclerosis, Neurol Clin 13(1):99-118, 1995.
29. Weinshenker BG: The natural history of multiple sclerosis, Neurol Clin 13(1):119-146, 1995.
30. Francis GS, Evans AC, Arnold DL: Neuroimaging and multiple sclerosis, Neurol Clin 13(1):147-172, 1995.
31. Weiner H, Hohol M, Khoury S: Therapy for multiple sclerosis, Neurol Clin 13(1):173-196, 1995.
32. Weinstock-Guttman B, Jacobs LD: What is new in the treatment of multiple sclerosis? Drugs 59(3):401-410, 2000.
33. Corvi G, Filippi M: The Copaxone MRI Study Group, Neurology 52:A289, 1999.

34. Kinsella IJ, Green R: Anesthesia paresthetica: nitrous oxide induced cobalamin deficiency, *Neurology* 45:1608-1610, 1995.

35. Pennypacker L: High prevalence of cobalamin deficiency in elderly outpatients, *J Am Geriatr Soc* 40:1197-1204, 1992.

36. Layzer RB. Myelomyopathy after prolonged exposure to nitrous oxide, *Lancet* II:1227-1230, 1978.

37. Visser IH, Dutch Guillain-Barré Study Group: Risk factors for treatment related clinical fluctuations in Guillain-Barré syndrome, *J Neurol Neurosurg Psychiatry* 64:242-244, 1998.

38. Boonyapisit K, Kaminski HJ, Ruff RL: Disorders of neuromuscular junction ion channels, *Am J Med* 106:97-113, 1999.

39. Berrouschot J: Baumann I, Kalischewski P, et al: Therapy of myasthenia gravis, *Crit Care Med* 25(7):1228-1235, 1997.

40. Bedlack RS, Sanders DB: How to handle myasthenic crisis: essential steps in patient care, *Postgrad Med* 107(4):211-214, 220-222, 2000.

41. Kokontis L, Gutman NL: Current treatment of neuromuscular diseases, *Arch Neurol* 57:939-943, 2000.

42. Absher JR, Bale JF: Aggravation of myasthenia gravis by erythromycin, *J Pediatr* 119(1):155-156, 1991.

43. May EF, Calvert PC: Aggravation of myasthenia gravis by erythromycin, *Ann Neurol* 28(4):577-579, 1990.

44. Pijpers E, van Rijswijk RE, Takx-Kohlen B, Schrey GA: Clarithromycin-induced myasthenic syndrome, *Clin Infect Dis* 22(1):175-l76, 1996.

45. O'Riordan J, Javed M, Doherty C, Hutchinson M: Worsening of myasthenia gravis on treatment with imipenem/cilastatin, *J Neurol Neurosurg Psychiatry* 57(3): 383, 1994.

46. Sieb JP: Fluoroquinolone antibiotics block neuromuscular transmission, *Neurology* 50(3):804-807, 1998.

47. Krucylak PE, Naunheim KS: Preoperative preparation and anesthetic management of patients with myasthenia gravis, *Semin Thorac Cardiovasc Surg* 11(1):47-53, 1999.

48. Lorimer M, Hall R: Remifentanil and propofol total intravenous anaesthesia for thymectomy in myasthenia gravis, *Anaesth Intensive Care* 26(2):210-212, 1998.

49. Leyten QH, Gabreels FJ, Renier WO, ter Laak HJ: Congenital muscular dystrophy: a review of the literature, *Clin Neurol Neurosurg* 98(4):267-280, 1996.

50. Munoz J, Sanjuan R, Moraell JS, Ibanez M: Ventricular tachycardia in Duchenne's muscular dystrophy, *Int J Cardiol* 54(3):259-262, 1996.

51. Killiardis S, Katsaros C: The effects of myotonic dystrophy and Duchenne muscular dystrophy on the orofacial muscles and dentofacial morphology, *Acta Odontol Scand* 56(6):369-374, 1998.

52. Levine PH: What we know about chronic fatigue syndrome and its relevance to the practicing physician, *Am J Med* 105(3A):100S-103S, 1998.

53. Demitrack M: Chronic fatigue syndrome and fibromyalgia, *Psychiatr Clin North Am* 21(3):671-692, 1998.

Diabetes Mellitus

Daniel S. Sarasin
K. Jeff Westlund

Diabetes mellitus (DM) is an endocrine disease characterized by carbohydrate, protein, and fat metabolic abnormalities. DM is caused by a deficient action of insulin on target tissue resulting from a lack of insulin, insulin insensitivity, or both. DM is frequently diagnosed by high blood glucose (hyperglycemia). Diabetes alters the metabolism of all the body's energy nutrients, and its complications affect most organ systems.

Advances in the understanding and management of diabetes have improved patients' quality of life and slowed the onset of long-term complications. Acute metabolic complications, especially hypoglycemia, are frequently seen in the dental office. Dental professionals must be knowledgeable about DM in order to provide safe care for the patient population. This chapter focuses on type 1 and 2 DM. Three common acute metabolic complications seen in diabetic patients will be reviewed: hypoglycemia, diabetic ketoacidosis, and nonketotic hypertonicity.

PANCREATIC PHYSIOLOGY

The pancreas is a large, elongated gland approximately 20 cm (8 inches) in length. The long axis lies transversely between the spleen and duodenum, behind the stomach. Two major tissue types make up the pancreas: *acini* are involved in external secretion, which uses various digestive enzymes, and the *islets of Langerhans* provide internal secretion (endocrine pancreas). The islets are groups of cells dispersed throughout the pancreas. The pancreatic islet cells make up 1% of the pancreas and produce several peptide hormones, including insulin, glucagon, and somatostatin. *Insulin* is produced by *beta cells* (B cells) in the core of the islets of Langerhans. The beta cells constitute 60% to 80% of all the cells in the islets. The other three cell types are the *alpha cells*, which produce glucagon; the *delta cells*, which produce somatostatin; and the F *cells*, which produce pancreatic polypeptides. These cells lie in the mantle around the edges of the islets and are bathed by insulin-rich venous blood from the core beta cells. Hormones produced by the mantle cells bypass the beta cells and go directly to the liver and on to the tissues.

Insulin is produced as the primary biosynthetic product *preproinsulin*. This peptide is rapidly converted to *proinsulin*. Within the B-cell secretory granules, proinsulin is converted to insulin and C *peptide* after proteolytic cleavage. Final B-cell secretory product is 95% insulin and C peptide, along with 5% unconverted proinsulin. Granules release their contents into the bloodstream by exocytosis. The regulation of insulin release is influenced by various factors and is extremely complex. However, *glucose* is the most important stimulus for insulin secretion. After a circulating time of 4 to 8 minutes, insulin interacts with target tissues to exert its regulatory effects. At the target cell, insulin binds to specific cell surface insulin receptors. Once formation of the insulin receptor complex occurs, a signal pathway triggers a variety of cellular effector systems to produce the ultimate biologic effects. After secretion, insulin is rapidly removed from the blood and degraded, mainly by the liver.

The anabolic effects of insulin regulate protein and fat metabolism. In skeletal muscle, insulin (1) induces protein synthesis by increasing amino acid uptake and (2) reduces muscle breakdown by decreasing release of amino acids. Insulin also prevents fat breakdown and induces lipid formation by increasing the amount of stored fats as triglycerides. Additionally, *somatomedin* secretion is stimulated by insulin, which appears to play a role in growth.

Tight regulation of blood glucose, between 70 and 120 mg/dl, is essential to maintenance of the internal milieu despite wide variations in physiologic conditions; the body is able to adjust to nutritional intake, exercise, and stress.

The *absorptive* (*fed*) *state* occurs after ingestion of a meal and is characterized by utilization and

Table 24-1	Cellular Substrates Released and Metabolized in Fed and Fasting States			
	FED STATE		**FASTING STATE**	
Cell Type	**Primary Substrate Metabolized**	**Primary Byproduct Released**	**Primary Substrate Metabolized**	**Primary Byproduct Released**
Brain	Glucose	CO_2	Glucose	CO_2
Liver	Glucose	CO_2	Amino acids	Glucose
	Amino acids		Fatty acids	Ketones
Muscle	Glucose	CO_2	Fatty acids	CO_2
	Amino acids		Ketones	Amino acids
Fat	Glucose	—	—	Fatty acids
	Triglycerides			

storage of ingested nutrients. Glucose from the meal provides the primary energy source. A rise in blood glucose and the presence of various gastrointestinal hormones stimulates an increase in plasma insulin levels through secretion and synthesis. The presence of insulin, which binds to insulin receptors, thereby activating glucose transporters, stimulates the diffusion of glucose into adipose and muscle cells. Plasma insulin inhibits the production of glucose by the liver. After glucose diffuses into cells, it may be oxidized for energy needs (*glycolysis*) or converted to glycogen by the liver and muscle cells (*glycogenesis*).

In the *postabsorptive* (*fasting*) state, plasma insulin levels fall to a basal rate, and glucagon levels increase, causing a catabolic effect. Glucose is released from stored glycogen in the liver and muscles (*glycogenolysis*) and produced from amino acids and other substrates in the liver (*gluconeogenesis*). In the fasting state, up to 75% of glucose is produced by glucagon-stimulated glycogenolysis and gluconeogenesis. The primary energy source for muscle is *free fatty acids*, produced by the breakdown of fat from adipose tissue (*lipolysis*) resulting from the reduction in insulin. Neural tissue preferentially uses glucose (Table 24-1).

Glucoregulatory hormones also play a role in glucose metabolism. They are produced by the pituitary (adrenocorticotropic hormone, growth hormone), adrenal cortex (cortisol), and adrenal medulla (epinephrine, norepinephrine). These counterregulatory hormones are produced in response to exercise and stress and are involved with glucose homeostasis in the fasting state. Corticosteroids interfere with the action of insulin and stimulate gluconeogenesis. Growth hormone increases peripheral insulin resistance, and prevents the reduction of hepatic glucose production by insulin. Epinephrine and norepinephrine increase glucose production by stimulating gluconeogenesis and glycogenolysis.

CLASSIFICATION

The development of new diagnostic criteria and classification systems for DM by the World Health Organization and National Diabetes Data Group has clarified a chaotic situation.[1,2] Historically, enormous variations in nomenclature and diagnostic criteria have been the main causes for the confusion. The revised classification encompasses both clinical descriptive criteria and a complementary etiologic classification of DM. The clinical staging reflects that diabetes progresses through several clinical stages (i.e., various degrees of hyperglycemia) during its natural history, regardless of etiology. The disease process may be present but may not have progressed sufficiently to cause elevated blood glucose levels. The classification of etiologic type is a result of improved understanding of the cause of diabetes. The defect or disease process, which can progress to diabetes, may be identifiable at any clinical stage, even normoglycemia. The terms "insulin-dependent diabetes mellitus" (IDDM) and "non-insulin-dependent diabetes mellitus" (NIDDM) have been eliminated because they classified patients on the basis of treatment rather than pathophysiology.

Box 24-1 summarizes the revised etiologic classification of DM. Clinical diabetes may be divided into four general categories: (1) *type* 1, caused by pancreatic islet B-cell destruction and characterized by absolute insulin deficiency; (2) *type* 2, caused by relative insulin deficiency and insulin resistance; (3) other *specific types* of diabetes, associated with various identifiable clinical conditions or syndromes; and (4) *gestational*

Box 24-1   Classification of Glucose Metabolism Disorders

I. Type 1 diabetes mellitus
   A. Immune mediated
   B. Idiopathic
II. Type 2 diabetes mellitus
III. Other specific types of diabetes
   A. Genetic defects of beta cell function
   B. Genetic defects in insulin action
      1. Type A insulin resistance
      2. Leprechaunism
      3. Rabson-Mendenhall syndrome
      4. Lipoatrophic diabetes
   C. Diseases of exocrine pancreas
      1. Pancreatitis
      2. Pancreatectomy secondary to trauma
      3. Neoplasia
      4. Cystic fibrosis
      5. Hemochromatosis
      6. Fibrocalculous pancreatopathy
   D. Endocrinopathies
      1. Acromegaly
      2. Cushing's syndrome
      3. Glucagonoma
      4. Pheochromocytoma
      5. Hyperthyroidism
      6. Somatostatinoma
      7. Aldosteronoma
   E. Drug or chemical induced
      1. β-Adrenergic agonists
      2. Diazoxide
      3. Glucocorticoid steroids
      4. Interferon-α
      5. Nictotinic acid
      6. Pentamidine
      7. Phenytoin
      8. Thiazide
      9. Thyroid hormone
      10. Vacor
   F. Infections
      1. Congenital rubella
      2. Cytomegalovirus
   G. Uncommon forms of immune-mediated diabetes
      1. Stiff-man syndrome
      2. Anti–insulin receptor antibodies
IV. Gestational diabetes

OTHER GENETIC SYNDROMES ASSOCIATED WITH DIABETES
   1. Down syndrome
   2. Klinefelter's syndrome
   3. Turner's syndrome
   4. Friedreich's disease
   5. Huntington's chorea
   6. Laurence-Moon (Bardet-Biedel) syndrome
   7. Myotonic dystrophy
   8. Porphyria
   9. Prader-Willi syndrome

STATISTICAL RISK OF TYPE 2 DM
   1. Impaired glucose tolerance
   2. Impaired fasting glucose

Modified from American Diabetes Association: *Diabetes Care* 20(7):1183-1197, 1997.

---

diabetes. In addition to these four clinical subgroups, *impaired glucose tolerance* (IGT) and *impaired fasting glucose* (IFG) refer to an intermediate metabolic state between normal glucose homeostasis and overt diabetes. IGT is classified as a stage of impaired glucose regulation, since it can be observed in any hyperglycemic disorder but is not itself diabetes. IFG is a clinical stage for individuals who have fasting glucose values greater than the normal range but less than the diagnostic levels for diabetes. IGT and IFG are conditions that may significantly increase the later risk of developing DM and macrovascular disease.

Type 1

Type I DM, previously termed type I diabetes, IDDM, or juvenile-onset diabetes, results from an interplay of genetic, environmental, and autoimmune factors that selectively destroy beta cells. The rate of destruction varies. The rapidly progressive destruction form is usually seen in previously healthy nonobese children and young adults but may occur in older adults. These individuals may present with ketoacidosis as the first manifestation of the disease. Others have modest fasting hyperglycemia that can progress to severe hyperglycemia and ketoacidosis in the presence of infection or stress.

The slowly progressive form generally occurs in adults. These people may retain residual beta cell function sufficient to prevent ketoacidosis. Approximately 80% of cases of type I DM are characterized by the presence of islet cell or insulin antibodies, which identify the autoimmune processes that lead to beta cell destruction. Patients have little to no insulin secretory capacity and depend on exogenous insulin to prevent metabolic decompensation (ketoacidosis), coma, and death. Some patients with this clinical form of diabetes have no evidence of an autoimmune process and are classified as having type 1 idiopathic DM.

Type 2

Type 2 DM previously encompassed NIDDM, or adult-onset diabetes. It is characterized by disorders of insulin action and insulin secretion, either of which may be the predominant feature. People with this type of diabetes have a relative insulin deficiency. Ketoacidosis is infrequently found; when seen, it usually arises in association with the stress of another illness. Hyperglycemia in type 2 DM results from undefined genetic defects, the expression of which is modified by environmental factors.

Several different mechanisms probably result in type 2 DM. The number of patients in this category likely will decrease in the future as identification of specific pathogenetic processes and genetic defects permit better differentiation. Although the specific etiologies of type 2 diabetes are unknown, by definition, autoimmune destruction of the beta islet cells does not occur.

Gestational

Gestational diabetes describes pregnant women with IGT, which usually appears in the second or third trimester. Gestational diabetes closely resembles type 2 diabetes, although the pathogenesis is unknown. In the pregnant patient, tissue insulin resistance is present secondary to weight gain and placental hormones. During a normal pregnancy, women require two to three times as much insulin as they do in a nonpregnant state. In gestational diabetes, women are unable to produce enough insulin to meet their needs in pregnancy.

EPIDEMIOLOGY

Prevalence of diabetes in adults worldwide was estimated at 4.0% (135 million) in 1995 and will rise to an estimated 5.4% (300 million) by the year 2025. The rate is higher in developing countries.[3] In the United States, 15.7 million people, or 5.9% of the population, have DM (Box 24-2). More than one third of these individuals with diabetes (5.4 million people) are unaware that they have the disease. Each day, approximately 2200 individuals are diagnosed with diabetes. Type 1 DM is diagnosed in 5% to 10% of the cases, and type 2 DM accounts for 90% to 95%. Prevalence rates for type 1 and 2 diabetes are significantly different among different ethnic

---

| Box 24-2 | Epidemiology of Diabetes Mellitus in the United States |

Incidence of diabetes in the United States:
  15.7 million, or 5.9% of population
Incidence of undiagnosed diabetes:
  5.4 million, or 34% of diabetic population

TYPE 1
Diabetic patients affected: 5%-10%
Prevalence in population: ~0.3%-0.4 %
Prevalence in people under 20 years of
  age: 1.7%

TYPE 2
Diabetic patients affected: 90%-95%
Prevalence in population: ~6%
Prevalence in people over 50 years of age:
  ~10%-15%
Incidence in American Caucasians: 7.8%
Incidence in African Americans: 10.8%
Incidence in Hispanic Americans: 10.6%
Incidence in Native Americans: 12.2%

TESTING/FASTING
Prevalence of impaired glucose
  testing/impaired fasting glucose: ~6%-8%

---

groups living in the same geographic region. These differences are likely caused by variation in susceptibility secondary to genetic makeup.

Type 1

The estimated U.S. prevalence rate for type 1 DM is 0.3% to 0.4%. Because type 1 DM patients usually become symptomatic, prevalence rates are relatively accurate. The prevalence of type 1 diabetes is much higher in Finland, Scandinavia, and Scotland. In Southern Europe, the Middle East, and a number of Asian countries the prevalence rate is lower. The incidence of type 1 DM has risen in the last half century. From infancy through adolescence the incidence of type 1 diabetes rises, then declines; the low rate continues for many decades. The prevalence is 1.7 per 1000 individuals younger than 20 years. The Caucasian populations have a higher incidence of type 1 diabetes than African-American, Asian, Hispanic, or Native-American populations. There is little gender difference in incidence of type 1 DM.[4,5]

Type 2

The prevalence rate for type 2 DM is imprecise; many type 2 diabetics are asymptomatic, and their disease is undiagnosed. In the United States the prevalence rate is approximately 6%, increasing to 10% to 15% in individuals older than 50 years of age.[4] Nonwhite populations have a greater incidence. The incidence of type 2 diabetes for American Caucasians is 7.8%, 10.8% in African Americans, 10.6% in Hispanic Americans, and 12.2% in Native Americans (Box 24-2). In some Native-American tribes, 50% of the population have diabetes. Besides being more common in these minority populations, type 2 diabetes occurs at an earlier age. Type 2 DM prevalence rates vary worldwide, with a high propensity for Asiatic Indians, Australian Aborigines, and Polynesians, who are adapting to the behavioral patterns of westernization.[6]

The incidence of type 2 diabetes is higher in women. Increased age, reduced physical activity, and obesity promote disease expression in individuals with genetic susceptibility. Type 2 DM is more common in obese individuals with one or two parents with this condition. In women with a history of gestation diabetes, 30% to 40% will develop type 2 diabetes within 5 to 10 years.

Gestational

Gestational diabetes occurs in 2% to 5% of pregnancies. Risk factors include obesity, family history of type 2 diabetes, age greater than 40 years, previous history of gestational diabetes, and offspring weighing more than 4 kg (9 pounds) at birth.

Impaired Glucose

The prevalence of impaired glucose testing and impaired fasting glucose in the United States is estimated at 6% to 8%, but precise statistical data are lacking. Approximately 25% to 30% of these patients will eventually develop type 2 diabetes.

DIAGNOSIS

The diagnosis of DM should be well established. The requirements for diagnostic confirmation for an individual presenting with symptoms of hyperglycemia differ from the person that is asymptomatic with elevated blood glucose laboratory values. Urine glucose testing may strongly suggest diabetes but should never be used exclusively; low renal threshold for glucose can give misleading information.

The diagnosis of DM is usually straightforward when classic symptoms of hyperglycemia

are present (polydipsia, polyuria, fatigue, weight loss). All that is required to confirm a diagnosis of diabetes when symptoms are present is a random plasma glucose level that is 200 mg/dl or greater if acute infection or physiologic stress is not present. Further diagnostic testing for diabetes can delay treatment and is unwarranted.

The diagnosis of diabetes in an asymptomatic subject requires more laboratory testing. A single elevated blood glucose value does not indicate an asymptomatic individual has diabetes. At least one additional serum/blood glucose test result with a value that is elevated in the diabetic range is essential, either through fasting or the oral glucose tolerance test. The *fasting plasma glucose test* is preferred because it is less variable from day to day and is more resistant to nonspecific factors affecting glucose metabolism. The diagnosis is established if fasting serum glucose level is 126 mg/dl; the subject may have IFG. Further testing is needed to determine if the individual with IFG has severe postprandial hyperglycemia.

The *oral glucose tolerance test* (OGTT) is used to evaluate the postprandial glucose level. After ingestion of 75 g of glucose, the plasma glucose concentration is measured 2 hours later. A glucose level of 200 mg/dl or greater is diagnostic for diabetes. If the 2-hour OGTT level is 140 to 200 mg/dl, the subject is classified as having IGT.[1,2] The disadvantage of OGTT is that the test may lead to overdiagnosis of DM because of factors that can cause erroneous elevation of glucose levels.

Screening for type 2 diabetes is recommended due to the high prevalence of undiagnosed cases. All adults over 45 years of age should be screened every 3 years. Individuals with risk factors (e.g., obesity, family history, history of gestational diabetes, previous IGT or IFG) should be evaluated more frequently. Routine screening for type 1 DM is not recommended unless signs or symptoms of hyperglycemia are present. All dental patients should be regularly questioned about symptoms of hyperglycemia.

PATHOPHYSIOLOGY
Type 1

In type 1 DM, with little or no insulin secreted, uptake of glucose and conversion into glycogen in the liver is limited or does not occur. Portal insulin deficiency is present, and hepatic glucose production is consistently elevated. Insulin deficiency leads to hypersecretion of glucagon and growth hormone (GH), which further increases

Table 24-2	Pathophysiology of Energy Metabolism in Types 1 and 2 Diabetes Mellitus	
Organ/Tissue	Type 1	Type 2
Gastrointestinal tract	Glucose	Glucose
Liver	Free fatty acids out*	—
	Ketoacids	—
	Glucose (glycogenolysis)	Glucose (glycogenolysis)
	Glucose (gluconeogenesis)	Glucose (gluconeogenesis)
Pancreas	Glucagon	Glucagon
	—	Insulin
Muscle tissue	Free fatty acids out*	Glucose out*(insulin resistance)
	Ketoacids out*	
Adipose tissue	Free fatty acids	—
Neural tissue	Glucose out*	Glucose out*
	Ketoacids out*	

*Substrates in blood unless noted as out of bloodstream.

glucose production. Gluconeogenesis accelerates and increases glucose production. Loss of the insulin-regulating effect on alpha cells leads to a relative increase in portal glucagons. In the liver, therefore, uptake and conversion of glycogenic substrates to glucose increase. Glucose uptake by the peripheral tissues is impaired by the lack of insulin and the development of insulin resistance secondary to chronic insulin deprivation, leading to the toxic effects of chronic hyperglycemia. The end result is further elevation of blood glucose, only partially compensated by renal glycosuria.

If absolute insulin deficiency is present, excessive release of a variety of counterregulatory hormones causes further increases in gluconeogenesis and blocks compensatory increases in glucose disposal. Patients with hyperglycemia are susceptible to electrolyte disturbances and volume depletion from osmotic diuresis. In addition, fasting levels of free fatty acids (FFAs) are frequently elevated because of accelerated mobilization of fat stores. The mobilized FFAs are readily converted into ketone bodies. The insulin deficiency combined with the presence of glucagon suppresses fat synthesis in the liver. Ketone turnover decreases, enhancing the magnitude of ketosis for any given level of ketone production. The rise in glucagon accelerates hepatic ketogenesis. Lipolysis and delivery of FFAs to the liver increase because of elevated levels of catecholamines, GH, and cortisol[6] (Table 24-2).

Type 2

In type 2 DM, fasting hyperglycemia is accompanied by an inappropriate increase in hepatic glu-

cose production. Glucagon and GH levels are increased. Elevated levels of FFAs occur in the presence of normal or increased insulin. FFAs are not directly converted to glucose but provide the liver with energy to support gluconeogenesis. In addition, they interfere with glucose uptake by reducing glucose transport and utilization in muscle. Endogenous insulin secretion is sufficient to prevent hepatic conversion of FFAs to ketones. The effects of delayed insulin secretion and hepatic insulin resistance prevent the liver from converting glucose into glycogen and inhibit suppression of hepatic glucose production. Hyperglycemia is present, although insulin levels may be elevated because insulin resistance reduces the capacity of muscle to remove and store the excess glucose.[6] Patients with type 2 DM may have electrolyte disturbances and volume depletion secondary to osmotic diuresis during hyperglycemia (Table 24-2).

CLINICAL FEATURES

Table 24-3 summarizes clinical features of types 1 and 2 DM.

Type 1

Type 1 DM typically appears abruptly in previously healthy non-obese children or young adults, with a peak onset at age 14. The typical patient is extremely sick and has classic signs and symptoms of hyperglycemia: *polyuria* (excessive secretion of urine), *polydipsia* (excessive thirst), *polyphagia* (excessive hunger), and *weight loss*. Polyuria is caused by the osmotic diuretic effect of elevated serum glucose levels in the re-

Table 24-3	Distinguishing Features Between Types 1 and 2 Diabetes Mellitus	
Factor	Type 1 DM	Type 2 DM
Frequency	5%-10%	90%-95%
Age of onset	<40 years, peak 14 years	>40 years
Body habitus	Normal to thin	Obese
Plasma insulin	Low to absent	Low to elevated
Rate of onset	Rapid	Slow
Acute complication	Ketoacidosis	Nonketotic hypertonicity
Autoimmune reaction	Yes	No
Insulin therapy	Responsive	Responsive to resistant
Sulfonylurea therapy	Unresponsive	Responsive

Modified from Foster DW: In Fauci AS et al, editors: *Harrison's principles of internal medicine*, ed 14, New York, 1998, McGraw-Hill.

nal tubules. Polydipsia follows secondary to the developing dehydration. Polyphagia and weight loss are caused by the body's failure to utilize glucose. Ketoacidosis, when present, can be a life-threatening acute metabolic complication.

Type 2

Type 2 DM usually appears in adults after age 40, with an insidious onset of symptoms. The classic symptoms of this disorder are more mild (fatigue, weakness, dizziness, blurred vision, other nonspecific complaints). Nonketotic hypertonicity is a serious acute metabolic complication. Ketoacidosis is rare.

TREATMENT
Nonpharmacologic Therapy

The treatment of DM involves diabetic education, lifestyle changes, and pharmacologic intervention to achieve short-term and long-term goals. The short-term goals include restoration of near-normal or normal metabolic homeostasis and improvement in the patient's sense of well-being. The long-term goals in diabetes treatment are to delay or eliminate chronic diabetic complications, including accelerated atherosclerosis, renal and retinal microangiopathy, and both peripheral and autonomic neuropathy.

Education

Diabetes education is essential for diabetic patients and their families. In type 1 DM the primary focus is to replace insulin deficiency; lifestyle changes (e.g., diet, exercise) are important to optimize insulin therapy and improve

overall health. In type 2 DM, lifestyle changes (e.g., diet, weight reduction) are essential, especially in the early stages. A variety of skills must be learned and mastered to optimize glucose control and reduce acute and chronic complications. Daily tasks include (1) performing blood glucose testing, (2) recording and interpreting test results, (3) administering medications (insulin, oral hypoglycemic agents), (4) identifying and treating medication side effects, and (5) complying with dietary plans. Diabetics are a diverse group with wide variation in age, ethnic background, education, intellectual ability, and motivation. Therefore, diabetic education must be tailored to individual's needs.

Nutrition

Nutrition plays a key role in diabetes management. Balancing the intake of carbohydrates, fats, and proteins with insulin or oral glucose-lowering agents is essential. Changing the composition, patterns, and timing of meals as well as caloric consumption is frequently necessary to improve glycemic control. Current recommendations by the American Diabetes Association are for an individual's diet to contain 60% to 70% of the dietary calories distributed between monounsaturated fats and carbohydrates. The diet should be composed of no more than 10% of calories from saturated fat as well as polyunsaturated fats. Lower fat diets are appropriate for patients attempting to reduce weight.[7] A dietitian is usually involved with the development of a food plan and implementation of the diet. Dietary compliance is improved when the diabetic is motivated in controlling glucose levels and is able to have a variety of food choices.

Exercise

Regular exercise can play a significant role in health maintenance. Exercise is important to reduce cardiovascular risk factors by reducing hypertension, dyslipidemia, and obesity. Dyslipidemia is prevented by improving the ratio of low-density lipoprotein to high-density lipoprotein (LDL/HDL) triglycerides. Although exercise reduces insulin requirements by improving insulin sensitivity in type 1 DM, there is little evidence that it improves glycemic control. In some patients with type 2 DM, exercise may reduce and even eliminate the need for pharmacologic agents. Safeguards must be built into exercise programs to avoid the exacerbation of diabetic complications, including hypoglycemia, especially in type 1 diabetics.

Glucose Monitoring

Patient *blood glucose monitoring* (BGM) is a vital step in diabetes management and has improved glycemic control in patients. BGM allows for rapid treatment adjustments and is crucial for daily management of pharmacologic and diet therapy.

Self-monitoring of blood glucose is only of value if it is routinely performed. For type 1 DM, daily monitoring at least before meals and at bedtime is indicated. No clear guidelines have been established for the frequency of testing of blood glucose in type 2 diabetics, although individuals taking insulin should conduct daily self-monitoring before breakfast, before dinner, and at bedtime. In diabetics taking oral glucose-lowering agents, BGM depends on the duration of therapy and metabolic control achieved. Glucose testing should be done more frequently at the beginning of treatment and when metabolic control is deteriorating.

Current monitors are accurate and many have computerized memories, which aid in record keeping. Testing for ketonuria is indicated during acute illness or stress, when blood glucose levels are greater than 300 mg/dl, and when symptoms of diabetic ketoacidosis are present. Urine glucose tests provide a rough estimate of current blood glucose levels but provide no information about blood glucose levels below renal threshold, which is 180 mg/dl for most patients.[8]

Pharmacologic Therapy
Oral Glucose-Lowering Medications

In type 2 DM an oral glucose-lowering medication is frequently used when diet and exercise have failed to control hyperglycemia. Several classes of antidiabetic drugs are now available, with a variety of mechanisms of action to improve blood glucose control (Box 24-3). These drugs are used alone or in combinations to control blood glucose.[9] Oral agents tend to be the first-line therapy if hyperglycemia is mild, the patient is older, and obesity is present. When severe hyperglycemia is present, insulin is generally used in the initial treatment phase to reduce glucose levels. After the glucose level has normalized, the patient is changed to an oral agent. Oral antidiabetic agents are contraindicated in cases of absolute or severe insulin deficiency and pregnancy.

Sulfonylureas. Sulfonylurea drugs have been used for more than 40 years and are the most common agents used to treat type 2 diabetes. Sulfonylureas were the only oral class of agents available in the United States before 1995. They act by enhancing insulin secretion. These drugs are highly protein bound and are prone to displacement by other protein-bound drugs.

The sulfonylureas differ in duration of action, effective dosing, metabolism, relative potency, and side effects. The *short-acting* drugs, which are metabolized by the liver, have advantages in el-

---

Box 24-3 Oral Antidiabetic Medications

SULFONYLUREAS (INCREASE INSULIN SECRETION)
Tolbutamide, acetohexamide, tolazamide, chlorpropamide, glipizide, glyburide, glimepiride

BENZOIC ACID DERIVATIVE (INCREASE INSULIN SECRETION)
Repaglinide

BIGUANIDE
Increase skeletal muscle uptake of glucose; decrease gluconeogenesis; decrease glucose absorption
Metformin

THIAZOLIDINEDIONE
Reduce insulin resistance; stimulate peripheral glucose metabolism
Pioglitazone
Rosiglitazone

α-GLUCOSIDASE INHIBITOR (DELAY DIGESTION OF COMPLEX CARBOHYDRATES)
Acarbose
Meglitolare

derly patients with impaired renal function because they are more vulnerable to hypoglycemia. *Long-acting* sulfonylurea drugs are used once a day, and therefore compliance is improved. The risk of hypoglycemia is high, especially if a meal is missed.

Primary drug failure, a term used to describe the lack of blood glucose reduction, occurs in about 15% to 20% of type 2 diabetic patients. *Secondary drug failure*, occurring at a rate of 5% to 10% per year, is caused by progression of beta cell destruction, drug intolerance, failure to maintain diet and exercise regimen, and superimposition of other medical conditions or drugs. Another class of oral glucose-lowering drugs is often added or insulin therapy may be instituted if secondary drug failure does not resolve (improved glucose control) with dietary and exercise adjustments.[6,10]

Benzoic acid derivatives.   Benzoic acid derivatives represent the newest class of oral antidiabetic drugs. *Repaglinide* is a nonsulfonylurea that stimulates insulin secretion. It has a rapid onset and duration of action. Repaglinide requires frequent daily dosing and is taken at the beginning of each meal. It may reduce the risk of hypoglycemia.[11]

Biguanides   *Metformin*, a biguanide drug, is another type of oral hypoglycemic agent. It acts to decrease blood glucose by increasing skeletal muscle uptake, decrease gluconeogenesis, and decrease the absorption of glucose. Unlike sulfonylureas, metformin does not enhance insulin secretion and normally does not produce hypoglycemia except in cases of prolonged fasting. It may induce mild weight loss and is particularly useful in obese patients either as monotherapy or as combined therapy with other oral glucose-lowering drugs. Lactic acidosis is a rare but potentially fatal side effect of metformin, occurring predominantly in patients with underlying renal failure.[12,13]

Thiazolidinediones.   *Pioglitazone* and *rosiglitazone* are new thiazolidinedione antidiabetic agents. They have replaced troglitazone, which was removed from the market by the U.S. Food and Drug Administration. These drugs decrease insulin resistance by improving insulin-mediated glucose disposal and reduce plasma insulin concentrations. Their biologic effect is mediated through stimulation of peripheral glucose metabolism, with little effect on hepatic glucose production. Use of the thiazolidinediones is contraindicated in patients with liver function abnormalities; liver function should be routinely checked, and pioglitazone or rosiglitazone should be discontinued if liver enzymes are elevated. Hy-

poglycemia can occur when these agents are used with insulin or a sulfonylurea.[14,15]

α-Glucosidase inhibitors.   The fifth class of oral glucose-lowering agents includes *acarbose* and *meglitolare*. The α-glucosidase inhibitors delay the digestion of complex carbohydrates and subsequent absorption of starch, sucrose, and maltose in the small intestine, by reversible inhibition of the digestive enzymes (α-glucosidase). These drugs do not affect the absorption of monosaccharides (glucose). α-Glucosidase inhibitors do not cause hypoglycemia by themselves. If these drugs are used in combination with other antidiabetic medications that can cause hypoglycemia, the treatment of hypoglycemic events can be complicated; sucrose should not be administered because of drug-induced delay in absorption.[16,17] Glucose-containing products need to be given to treat low blood glucose levels rapidly.

Insulin

Insulin has been the cornerstone of diabetes treatment since its initial administration to humans in 1922. The therapeutic goals in type 1 DM have evolved from the maintenance of life to approximating physiologic insulin secretion (intensive insulin therapy) to restore normal plasma glucose concentrations and reduce complications. The exact range of acceptable glucose control is tailored to the patient's personal situations. Two general insulin strategies are implemented, conventional or standard therapy and intensive therapy. *Conventional therapy* uses one or two daily injections of intermediate-acting insulins. *Intensive therapy* consists of either multiple daily injections or short-acting insulin administered by a continuous subcutaneous (SC) insulin infusion. Insulin therapy for type 2 diabetics varies greatly. Insulin therapy is used in all individuals with type 1 DM and approximately one third of individuals with type 2 DM.

In the United States and other industrialized countries, only a variety of highly purified bioengineered human insulin preparations are available; they differ mainly in their time of onset and duration. These insulins result in fewer problems related to insulin antigenicity compared with animal insulin preparations, such as allergy, resistance, and lipoatrophy. Insulin antibodies, which are more common with the use of beef and pork insulins, result in a delay in insulin absorption and action. Insulin is usually administered by SC injections, although

Table 24-4	Classification of Insulin Preparations			
Action	**Type of Insulin**	**Onset (hr)**	**Peak (hr)**	**Duration (hr)**
Rapid	Lispro	0.25-0.5	1-2	3-5
	Aspart	0.25-0.5	1-2	3-5
Short	Regular	0.5-1.0	2-4	6-8
Intermediate	NPH	2-4	5-7	13-18
Long	Ultralente	4-6	8-12	18-30
	Glargine	4	None	30+

new methods of delivery are evolving, including intranasal, intrapulmonary, and oral routes.

Three classes of insulin, which vary in their onset and duration, are typically used in combinations to improve glucose control[18] (Table 24-4). The *rapid-acting* insulins blunt the elevation in glucose levels after meals secondary to their fast onset and effects. Regular insulin, which has served as the prototype of rapidly acting insulins for almost the entire history of insulin therapy, begins to act in about 30 minutes after SC injection.

Lispro insulin is a *short-acting* insulin analog that is absorbed faster than regular insulin and may reduce hypoglycemic events. Serum concentrations of lispro insulin peak more than two times higher and in half the time than human regular insulin. A*spart* insulin is the newest short-acting insulin analog and has similar pharmacokinetic properties to lispro insulin.[19]

Intermediate/long-acting insulin preparations are modified to delay absorption at the injection site, so their action is prolonged. They are usually administered twice a day. *Ultralente* is a long-acting insulin with a peak action of 8 to 10 hours. It was believed to be the most optimal basal insulin available for intensive insulin therapy before the development of glargine. The long-acting insulin analog *glargine* has recently been approved and released for use. Studies of this insulin analog suggest that they may have better basal characteristics, with a more constant, peakless delivery of insulin over 24 hours.[19]

Premixed insulin preparations, using a combination of rapid-acting and intermediate-acting insulins, are available and may be a convenient form of therapy for some patients, particularly those with type 2 DM.

ASSESSMENT OF GLYCEMIC CONTROL

Clinicians use several methods to determine glycemic control of their diabetic patients.

Glycosylated Hemoglobin (Hemoglobin A₁c)

The most common laboratory test used in the United States to evaluate glycemic control is the measurement of glycosylated hemoglobin (hemoglobin A$_{1c}$). HbA$_{1c}$ is formed at a rate dependent on the glucose concentration to which the erythrocyte is exposed. It reflects the overall degree of glycemic control over the previous 6 to 8 weeks. Glycosylation of hemoglobin occurs throughout the 120-day lifetime of the red blood cell. All ages of erythrocytes are exposed to recent levels of glycemia, whereas only the oldest cells have been exposed to glucose levels from 4 months previously. Therefore the more recent the period of glycemia, the greater the influence will be on the glycosylated Hb values. Half the HbA$_{1c}$ value may be attributable to changes in glucose levels over the preceding month, another quarter to changes from the month before that, and the remaining quarter a reflection of previous months 3 and 4.

HbA$_{1c}$ values of less than 7% are considered desirable. An HbA$_{1c}$ value greater than 8% indicates a need for changes in the therapeutic regimen. Factors influencing measurements include (1) lack of standardization among laboratories; (2) underestimation secondary to hemoglobinopathies, impaired hemoglobin synthesis, and reduced erythrocyte survival; and (3) overestimation secondary to elevated fetal hemoglobin, uremia, high-dose aspirin therapy, and increased age.[20]

Fructosamine

Serum fructosamine measurement is another method to monitor glucose control. It is a useful indicator of glycemic control over the previous 1 to 2 weeks. Fructosamine level should not be considered equivalent to measurement of glycosylated hemoglobin, since fructosamine only indicates glycemic control over a short time. The assay measures a variety of serum proteins that form *ketoamines* after glycosylation, generically called fructosamines, which are able to act as reducing agents in alkaline solution. The ketoamine level can be measured by spectrophotometer instruments. This test can be performed at most laboratories. Factors influencing serum fructosamine levels include (1) lack of standardization and (2) underestimation secondary to pathologic changes in serum proteins and elevated body mass index.[20]

Home Monitoring

Review of home blood glucose records is an important method of assessing glycemic control. It is useful in evaluating daily fluctuations in glucose levels. The success of glucose test strips and monitors has seen the measurement of blood glucose move away from laboratories and into the hands of diabetic patients and health care workers. Inaccurate blood glucose measurements result from user and analytic errors. An important source of user error, which should be kept in mind when reviewing glucose records, is falsification of results by patients. Despite the possible errors in home blood glucose diaries, they are a helpful adjunct with HbA_{1c} and fructosamine levels to determine glycemic control.[20]

CHRONIC COMPLICATIONS

Chronic complications are generally grouped into two categories, vascular and neuropathic. Vascular complications are divided into microvascular component (i.e., damage to the capillaries) and macrovascular component (i.e., damage to larger blood vessels in the cardiovascular tree).

The onset of chronic complications varies among diabetic patients; the average time for development of these complications after overt hyperglycemia is 15 to 20 years. Glycemic control is related to the incidence and progression of chronic complications associated with diabetes. Tight control of blood glucose levels (HbA_{1c}, 6% to 7%) in type I DM has a marked reduction of retinal, renal, and neuropathic complications.[21] Similar findings regarding glycemic control and chronic complications have been shown in type 2 DM.[22,23]

The pathogenesis of chronic complications of diabetes is poorly understood but likely involves several mechanisms. Two mechanisms involved in the pathogenesis of microvascular and neuropathic complications are (1) nonspecific protein glycosylation and (2) formation of sorbitol. Proteins are glycosylated in direct proportion to the blood glucose level. The nonenzymatic glycosylation process affects hemoglobin as well as serum and basement proteins, LDLs, peripheral nerve proteins, and secretory proteins. Advanced glycosylated end products of long-lived proteins (e.g., collagen, laminin) accumulate in blood vessels and kidneys. The other biochemical mechanism that may impair cell function is the polyol pathway, where glucose is reduced to sorbitol by aldose reductase. Sorbitol may function as a tissue toxin.

Vascular complications result from atherosclerosis and microangiopathy. Atherosclerotic lesions appear to be initiated by the oxidation of LDL. Glycosylated LDL has a longer plasma half-life than normal LDL and is not recognized by normal LDL receptors. Therefore it may contribute to the low HDL/LDL ratio by slowing LDL turnover and increasing circulating LDL available to be oxidized. Microangiopathic changes in patients with diabetes include thickening of the intima, endothelial proliferation, lipid deposition, and accumulation of periodic acid–Schiff (PAS)–positive material. These changes create functional problems, with increased capillary permeability resulting in increased vascular pressure, vascular stasis, and decreased oxygen tension (tissue hypoxia). Altered cellular metabolism, decreased collagen synthesis, and impaired leukocyte function may result from the tissue hypoxia.

Increase in platelet adhesiveness is an important factor in the formation of vascular complications. Hyperglycemia increases endothelin-1, a vasoconstrictor, while decreasing nitric oxide production. Nitric oxide inhibits platelet aggregation, and with reduced nitric oxide levels, platelet aggregation is elevated. In addition, poorly controlled diabetes favors coagulation with fibrinolysis impairment, secondary to an elevation in levels of tissue plasminogen activator inhibitors.[6]

Cardiovascular Disease

Coronary artery disease, hypertension, and cerebrovascular accidents (CVAs, strokes) are commonly seen in diabetes.[24] Adults with diabetes are two to four times more likely to have heart disease, which is the leading cause of diabetic-related deaths (75%). The risk of CVA is also two to four times higher in diabetics. Hypertension affects 60% to 65% of patients with DM. Atherosclerosis produces numerous medical disorders in a variety of sites, ranging from peripheral vascular disease to impotency.

Retinopathy

Diabetic retinopathy is the leading cause of blindness in adults 20 to 40 years of age. Blindness occurs 20 times more frequently in diabetic patients. Approximately 10% to 15% of type 1 diabetics become legally blind, whereas in type 2 diabetics the risk is less than half that value. The lesions in the retina are classified as either nonproliferative or proliferative. Approximately 85% of diabetics develop retinopathy. Proliferative retinopathy is more common in type 1 DM.[25]

Nephropathy

Diabetes is the leading cause of *end-stage renal disease* (ESRD) in the United States and Europe. Diabetic nephropathy accounts for approximately one third of all cases of ESRD. In 1995, almost 100,000 people with diabetes underwent dialysis or kidney transplantation. Type 1 diabetics are more likely to develop ESRD (20% to 30%). A larger number of individuals with type 2 diabetes have ESRD; they are frequently found to have microalbuminuria and overt nephropathy shortly after diagnosis, because the diabetes is present for many years before diagnosis is made. Without specific intervention, approximately 80% of type 1 diabetics and 30% to 40% of type 2 patients with microalbuminuria progress to overt nephropathy. ESRD develops in 50% of type 1 patients with overt nephropathy in 10 years and in more than 75% by 20 years. Only 20% of type 2 diabetics with overt nephropathy for 20 years after onset will progress to ESRD.[26]

Neuropathy

Symptomatic, potentially disabling nerve damage caused by diabetic neuropathy affects 60% to 70% of diabetic patients. Neuropathic complications are divided into autonomic dysfunction and sensory dysfunction.[27] *Diabetic autonomic neuropathy* (DAN), a common finding affecting the sympathetic and parasympathetic nervous systems, is present in 20% to 40% of all diabetic patients. DAN may be more severely manifested in one organ system than another. Patients with DAN have a poor long-term prognosis, with greater than 50% mortality 5 years after diagnosis.[28] Autonomic complications include cardiovascular dysfunction (e.g., orthostatic hypotension, bradycardia or tachycardia, significant blood pressure liability, silent myocardial ischemia/infarction, sudden death) gastrointestinal disturbances (e.g., gastroparesis), bladder dysfunction, and sexual dysfunction. Sensory disturbances include dysesthesias (severe pain), paresthesias, or lack of sensation in the extremities, especially the feet.[27] Neuropathy is largely responsible for the increased risk of serious foot problems. The risk of leg amputation is 15 to 40 times greater for the patient with diabetes.

ACUTE METABOLIC COMPLICATIONS
Hypoglycemia

Hypoglycemia is the most common endocrine medical emergency because of the large number of diabetics who are at risk of developing a blood glucose level below 70 mg/dl as a result of pharmacologic therapy. Risk factors for hypoglycemia in DM are extensive (Box 24-4). The incidence of hypoglycemia varies, estimated at 20% for type 2 diabetics treated with sulfonylureas and at 100% for type 1 diabetics. Severe hypoglycemia affects 10% to 25% of type 1 patients at least once a year. Severe hypoglycemia can vary greatly, from requiring the help of another person to emergency medical assistance. Individuals who do not have diabetes can develop hypoglycemia (Box 24-5). Hypoglycemia is defined as an emergency because significant risk for cognitive dysfunction results from the deprivation of glucose to the brain without emergent treatment.

Pathophysiology

Glucose is the principal fuel for normal brain function. The continuous glucose requirement of the neural tissue is primarily supplied by hepatic gluconeogenesis and glycogenolysis. Approximately 50% of basal glucose production is metabolized by the brain. Elevated glucagon levels are responsible for stimulating gluconeogenesis and glycogenolysis in the liver. From 2 to 5 years after the onset of type 1 DM, glucagon secretion during hypoglycemia is diminished or absent. Glucose metabolism is closely linked to oxygen consumption in the brain. A decrease in blood glucose is associated with corresponding reduction in cerebral oxygen consumption. Glucose transport proteins transfer glucose across the blood-brain barrier. Certain areas of the brain are more susceptible to hypoglycemia, and extremely low blood glucose levels appear to cause impairment of event-related brain-evoked potentials and cognitive function.

The risk of prolonged or permanent neurologic injury is related to the severity and duration of hypoglycemia. Neurologic manifestations of hypoglycemia include confusion, hemiparesis, convulsions, decortication, decerebration,

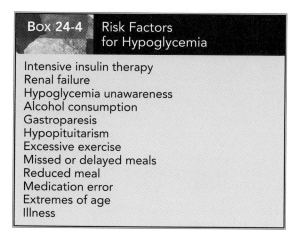

Box 24-4 Risk Factors for Hypoglycemia

Intensive insulin therapy
Renal failure
Hypoglycemia unawareness
Alcohol consumption
Gastroparesis
Hypopituitarism
Excessive exercise
Missed or delayed meals
Reduced meal
Medication error
Extremes of age
Illness

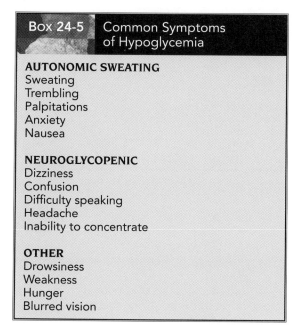

Box 24-5 Common Symptoms of Hypoglycemia

AUTONOMIC SWEATING
Sweating
Trembling
Palpitations
Anxiety
Nausea

NEUROGLYCOPENIC
Dizziness
Confusion
Difficulty speaking
Headache
Inability to concentrate

OTHER
Drowsiness
Weakness
Hunger
Blurred vision

ataxia, and coma. Permanent neurologic deficit is rare. It is unclear if neurologic damage occurs with milder episodes of hypoglycemia. Pathologic alterations secondary to hypoglycemia are in the middle layer of the cerebral cortex, especially in the temporal region.[29,30]

Clinical Features

Symptoms of hypoglycemia are divided into two groups, autonomic and neuroglycopenic, although some symptoms cannot be segregated into either category (Box 24-6). The autonomic symptoms are often the earliest subjective warning signs of hypoglycemia and include sweating, tremor, and palpitations. These symptoms are seen when blood glucose is 60 to 70 mg/dl. Symptoms and signs of central nervous system glucose deficiency, called *neuroglycopenia*, include diplopia, oral paresthesia, slurred speech, and behavioral disturbances (e.g., irritability, confusion). Drugs that can blunt the symptoms or the perception of hypoglycemia include ethanol, sedatives, and β-adrenergic blockers. Complete unconsciousness with or without tonic or clonic muscular movement may occur if hypoglycemia progresses. A rapid thready pulse, hypotension, and hypothermia may be present.

Nearly half of type 1 patients with DM more than 10 years will undergo a stimulus-specific decrease in their epinephrine response to hypoglycemia. The recognition of the autonomic symptoms may be lost, a condition termed hypoglycemic unawareness. The mechanism underlying the lowering of plasma glucose for release of epinephrine and other counterregulatory hormones has not been established. Patients with hypoglycemic unawareness are prone to the sudden onset of severe neuroglycemic symptoms. Loss of awareness of symptoms is more likely in patients with long-standing diabetes or when patients are switched to intensive insulin regimens. Hypoglycemic unawareness is likely caused by iatrogenic hypoglycemia. Some type 2 diabetics may also be affected.[29,30]

Treatment

If symptoms of hypoglycemia are present, the blood glucose should be checked by the dentist to confirm a hypoglycemic event is occurring. Emergency treatment should not be delayed if blood glucose level cannot be readily assessed. If the blood sugar level is below 65 mg/dl and no symptoms are evident, hypoglycemia should still be treated. Dental treatment should be stopped, and the patient should immediately consume a simple-carbohydrate product. Glucose tablets or gels are easily ingested; the amount should be at least 15 g of carbohydrates initially. If these products are not available, good alternatives for treatment of hypoglycemia include 4 teaspoons of sugar dissolved in water or 5 ounces of a regular (not diet) soft drink. Symptoms usually subside in 10 to 15 minutes. The blood glucose level should be rechecked. If the blood glucose level is still less than 65 mg/dl, a second carbohydrate dose of 15 g is given. Candy containing chocolate should not be used because chocolate is slowly broken down. As mentioned earlier, glucose products should be administered to

Box 24-6	Clinical Classification of Hypoglycemic Disorders

PATIENT APPEARS HEALTHY
No Coexisting Disease
Drugs
Ethanol
Salicylates
Quinine
Haloperidol
Conditions
Insulinoma
Islet hyperplasia/nesidoblastosis
Severe exercise
Ketotic hypoglycemia
Compensated Coexisting Disease
Drugs
Dispensing error
Disopyramide
β-Adrenergic blocking agents
Conditions
Autoimmune insulin syndrome with sulfhydryl-
  or thiol- containing drugs
Consumption of unripe ackee fruit

PATIENT APPEARS ILL
Drugs
Pentamidine: *Pneumocystis pneumoniae*
Sulfamethoxazole-trimethoprim: renal failure
Propoxyphene: renal failure
Topical salicylates: renal failure
Quinine: malaria
Predisposing illness
Glycogen storage disease
Defects in amino acid and fatty acid metabolism
Reye's syndrome
Hypopituitarism
Isolated growth hormone deficiency
Isolated ACTH deficiency
Addison's disease
Galactosemia
Hereditary fructose intolerance
Carnitine deficiency
Defective type 1 glucose transporter in brain
Acquired severe liver disease
Large non–beta cell tumor
Sepsis
Renal failure
Congestive heart failure
Lactic acidosis
Starvation
Anorexia nervosa
Insulin receptor antibody hypoglycemia

Modified from Rizza RA, Service FJ: In Goldman JC et al, editors: *Cecil textbook of medicine*, ed 21, Philadelphia, 2000, WB Saunders.

patients taking α-glucosidase inhibitors, since complex sugar breakdown is delayed.

The local emergency medical services (EMS) system should be activated. In patients with severe hypoglycemic reactions, intravenous (IV) access is established, and a bolus of one ampule of IV glucose (50 ml of 50% glucose solution) is administered.

The use of intramuscular glucagon (1 mg) is indicated for patients who are extremely uncooperative, combative, or unconscious and those in whom IV access cannot be established. Glucagon must be mixed just before administration. It is strongly recommended to include an ampule of 50% glucose and glucagon in medical emergency kits. Type 2 diabetics taking long-acting sulfonylureas (e.g., chlorpropamide, glyburide) who develop a severe hypoglycemic reaction should be hospitalized. Hypoglycemia may recur several times after initial, seemingly successful treatment, so close monitoring is required (Figure 24-1).

In patients with acute neurologic conditions (e.g., seizures, coma) and suspected hypoglycemia, blood should be drawn for glucose determination using laboratory and office glucose monitors. One ampule of 50% glucose should be administered. In suspected alcoholic patients, 25 to 50 mg of thiamine is given to prevent an acute episode of Wernicke-Korsakoff syndrome. Coma caused by hypoglycemia that does not reverse after glucose administration requires complicated medical management. Blood sugar should be maintained at about 140 mg/dl. Dexamethasone and mannitol are used to treat cerebral edema. Further work-up is warranted to look for other causes.

Diabetic Ketoacidosis

Diabetic ketoacidosis (DKA) is a serious acute metabolic complication. DKA occurs most frequently in type 1 DM, but type 2 diabetics are susceptible under certain conditions. Before the

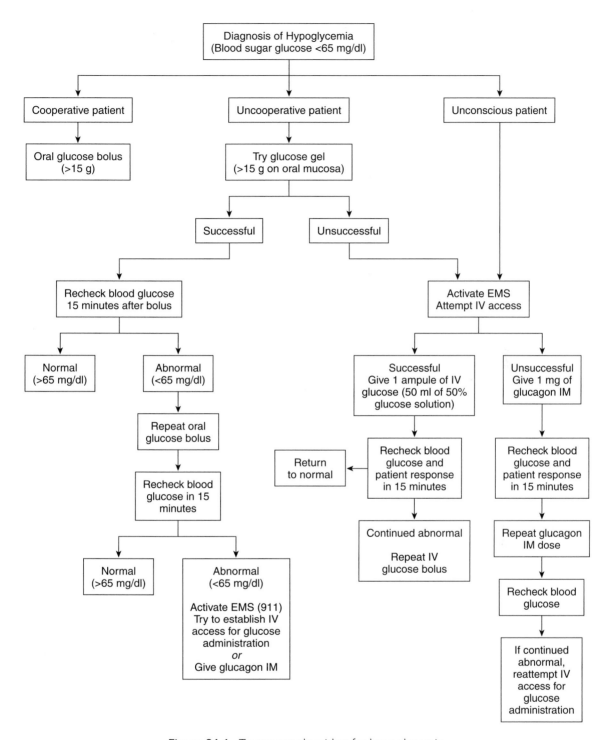

Figure 24-1. Treatment algorithm for hypoglycemia.

discovery of insulin in 1922, the mortality rate of this complication was almost 100%. The mortality rate from DKA has been reduced to less than 5% with current understanding of the condition and treatment. DKA is a metabolic derangement consisting of three concurrent abnormalities: hyperglycemia, high levels of ketone bodies, and metabolic acidosis.[31] Common precipitating factors leading to DKA include infection, omission of or inadequate use of insulin, new-onset type 1 DM, and miscellaneous events. In the past, SC insulin infusion pumps have been associated with an increased incidence of DKA.

Pathophysiology

DKA is characterized by severe alterations in the metabolism of carbohydrates, protein, and lipids, mainly as a result of a lack or ineffectiveness of insulin with concomitant elevations of counterregulatory hormones. Insulin-sensitive tissues alter their intermediary metabolism from a carbohydrate-metabolizing system to a fat-metabolizing system. Hyperglycemia and lipolysis play key roles in the genesis of the metabolic decompensation. Catecholamines, in the absence of insulin, cause triglyceride breakdown (lipolysis) to FFAs and glycerol. Glycerol provides the carbon skeleton, and FFAs are used for gluconeogenesis. As mentioned earlier, hyperglycemia occurs primarily through an increase in gluconeogenesis, but it is also accelerated by glycogen breakdown (glycogenolysis) and by inadequate utilization of glucose by the muscle and fat secondary to insulin deficiency. Circulating catecholamines further reduce the utilization of glucose peripherally. Ketone bodies increase due to the beta oxidation of accumulated FFAs. In the liver, FFAs are also converted into very-low-density lipoprotein (VLDL). Ketogenesis is further enhanced by reduction in malonyl coenzyme A levels, which subsequently increases carnitine palmitoyl transferase, the rate-limiting enzyme in ketogenesis.

The major cause of fluid loss in DKA is *osmotic diuresis*, caused by excessive secretion of glucose in the urine. Large amounts of sodium chloride (NaCl) and potassium are excreted in the urine, accompanied by severe water loss, approximately 100 ml/kg body weight. During the development of DKA, glucose is restricted to the extracellular space, so water is driven from the intracellular to extracellular compartment. Initially, intracellular fluid volume is depleted. Expansion of the extracellular space results in dilution of plasma sodium concentration. The excess fluid in the extracellular space is excreted by osmotic diuresis in the urine along with NaCl. Water loss exceeds NaCl loss. Although there is an overall deficit of sodium of 7 to 10 mEq/kg, plasma sodium concentrations are normal or low because of the osmotic water shift, despite extensive water loss. In DKA, total body potassium is depleted, approximately 5 mEq/kg, although plasma potassium concentrations appear normal or slightly elevated because of three factors: (1) a shift of water and potassium from the intracellular to the extracellular space, (2) acidosis resulting from the breakdown of intracellular proteins, and (3) reduced potassium entry into the cell due to insulinopenia. Intracellular potassium is greatly depleted. Excessive amounts of potassium are excreted by the kidney, largely from the effects of osmotic diuresis and secondary hyperaldosteronism.

The mechanism for acidosis in DKA is a buffer deficit secondary to increased production of ketoacids. Metabolic acidosis is caused by excessive hydrogen ions (ketoacids) being buffered by both extracellular (essentially bicarbonate) and intracellular buffers. An increase in the plasma anion gap occurs as a result of retained ketoanions. The increase in anion gap correlates closely with the bicarbonate deficit in most patients with DKA.[31-35]

Clinical and Diagnostic Features

Patients with DKA have a history of rapid deterioration in health over days with symptoms of increasing hyperglycemia. Constant periumbilical abdominal pain, anorexia, nausea, and vomiting may be present. Physical findings of DKA result from dehydration and acidosis and include dry skin, tachycardia, orthostatic hypotension, reduction in mental status, and Kussmaul respiration (deep, rapid). Dental findings include xerostomia (recent onset) and sweet, fruity breath odor.

In most patients, diagnosis of DKA is straightforward using (1) a concise history, (2) rapid clinical assessment, (3) rapid determination of a high blood glucose level (250 to 1000 mg/dl, determined by a blood glucose monitor), and (4) urine ketone test. Dentists should be able to perform the first three diagnostic components in their dental office, with emergency referral or work-up if DKA is suspected. The clinical examination must evaluate airway patency (e.g, difficulty breathing), mental status, cardiovascular and renal status, source of infection, and state of hydration.

Diagnosis of DKA is confirmed by (1) hyperglycemia (equal to or greater than 250 mg/dl), (2) low bicarbonate level (≤15 mEq/L), (3) low pH (<7.3), and (4) ketonemia and moderate ketonuria. A white blood count is usually elevated, with a left shift if infection is present. Initial laboratory work-up should include blood chemistries, glucose by finger-stick and laboratory evaluation, serum and urine ketones, complete blood cell count with differential, arterial blood gas (ABG) and pH, and urinalysis (Table 24-5).[31-35] A definitive diagnosis of DKA must be verified with an ABG determination that shows metabolic acidosis (e.g., low arterial pH, low calculated bicarbonate concentration). An IV infusion should be started with 1 L of 0.9% NaCl while other medical tests, including electrocardiogram (ECG), are initiated.

Treatment

The most important aspect of successful treatment of DKA is frequent monitoring of the patient by competent and concerned health care providers, with careful scrutiny for precipitating factors.

Restoration of fluids and electrolytes is the first priority because patients are dehydrated and NaCl depleted. Early rehydration reduces mortality (0.5%). Initial fluid therapy with isotonic saline (1 L) rapidly expands the extracellular space and corrects plasma volume. Subsequent fluid therapy is administered as hypotonic saline (0.45% NaCl) at 200 to 1000 ml/hr, depending on the state of hydration, to replace gradually both intracellular and extracellular spaces. Treatment of DKA is safer and more efficacious with initial hydration before initiation of insulin therapy.

In the conscious patient the initial dose of insulin should be based on body weight, with 0.3 to 0.4 unit of regular insulin/kg. Half should be given as an IV bolus and the other half subcutaneously. If the blood glucose does not decrease by 10% in the first hour, the initial dose should be repeated. In the comatose patient the initial insulin dose is 7 to 10 units by continuous IV infusion. Subsequent insulin therapy depends on the location of the patient and the resources available. If the patient is in the emergency department or in an intensive care unit, IV infusion of 7 units every hour is indicated, with close monitoring of glucose levels. If the patient is on a general hospital floor, hourly SC injections are recommended so that the nursing staff can evaluate the patient at least every hour. If blood glucose levels are 200 mg/dl or lower, the IV solution should be changed to 5% dextrose, 0.45% NaCl solutions.

Treatment of DKA with hydration and insulin results in a rapid decline in plasma potassium concentration. The major lowering effect is insulin-mediated reentry of potassium into the intracellular compartment. Also, extracellular volume expands, with resolution of acidemia. Developing *hypokalemia* is potentially the most life-threatening event during treatment of DKA. In most patients with potassium levels less that 5.5 mEq/L and the kidneys are producing urine, 20 to 30 mEq of potassium is added to each liter of IV NaCl solution. The potassium level should be checked initially every 1 to 2 hours. The goal is to maintain potassium levels between 4 and 5 mEq/L while the total body potassium deficit is corrected (Figure 24-2).[31-35]

Most endocrinologists do not recommend the routine use of sodium bicarbonate therapy in the treatment of DKA. Bicarbonate results in no significant difference in the decline of glucose and ketoanion concentrations or in the rate of increase in pH or bicarbonate concentrations. It may be of some benefit when pH is less than 6.9.[36]

Complications of therapy for DKA include cerebral edema, adult respiratory distress syndrome, hypercholemic acidosis, hypokalemia, and hypoglycemia. Close monitoring and careful treatment by a knowledgeable health care team are essential to reduce morbidity and mortality.

Table 24-5	Laboratory Characteristics of Diabetic Ketoacidosis (DKA) and Nonketotic Hypertonicity (NKH)		
Laboratory Test	**DKA**	**NKH**	
Blood glucose (mg/dl)	>250	>600	
Arterial pH	<7.3	>7.3	
Urine/serum ketone level	Elevated	Normal or slightly elevated	
Serum osmolarity	Variable	>320 mOsm/L	
Serum Na+ (mEq/L)	130-140	>145	

Modified from Kitabchi AE, Wall BM: *Med Clin North Am* 79(1):10, 1995.

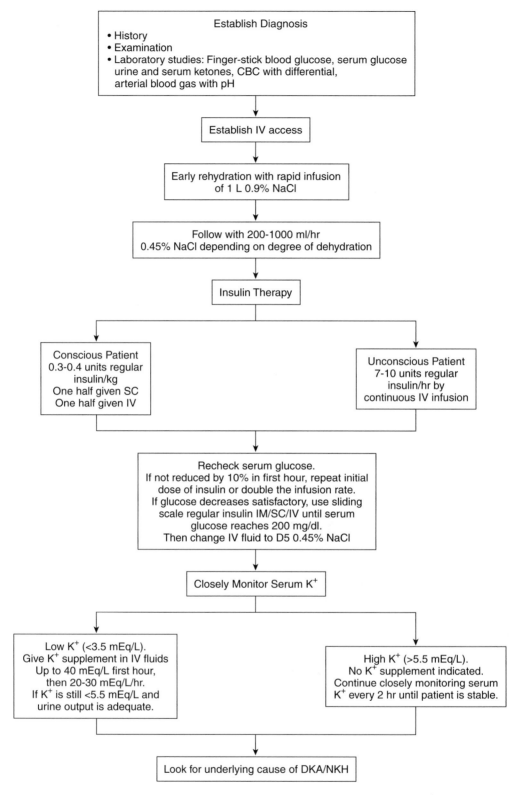

Figure 24-2. Treatment algorithm for diabetic ketoacidosis (DKA) and nonketotic hypertonicity (NKH). *CBC,* Complete blood count; *SC,* subcutaneous.

Nonketotic Hypertonicity

Nonketotic hypertonicity (NKH) is a metabolic disorder with a high mortality rate in patients with DM. Terms used to describe NKH include *hyperglycemic hyperosmolar nonketotic coma, nonketotic hyperosmolar diabetic coma,* and *nonketotic hyperosmolar state.* The first two terms have fallen into disfavor because coma occurs in less than 10% of patients with NKH. In the past decade, mortality rates have dropped but are still alarmingly high at 10% to 17%. Extreme hypertonicity is associated with increased mortality. NKH is more prevalent than previously believed and occurs more frequently in type 2 DM, usually in elderly patients. The syndrome is characterized by dehydration, hyperglycemia (>600 mg/dl), and increased effective osmolarity (>320 mOsm/L) without significant ketoacidosis. Common precipitating factors include impaired thirst recognition, polypharmacy, dementia, infection, and undiagnosed diabetes.[31,34,37]

Pathophysiology

Under normal circumstances, intracellular and extracellular osmolarity are equal, and no net water flux occurs across the cell membrane. Osmotically active substances are present in each compartment. These substances include those that can freely pass through the cell membrane in the body fluids (e.g., urea, alcohol) and those that are relatively impermeable (e.g., glucose, sodium, potassium). If permeable agents are added to the extracellular fluid (ECF), they flow into the intracellular fluid (ICF) until equilibrium occurs. No net osmotic gradient occurs, but serum osmolarity increases. There is no water flow between spaces. *Effective osmolarity* (tonicity) is a more useful term than "total osmolarity" because it describes the net influx of water between compartments. If impermeable molecules are added to the ECF, they cannot cross the cell membrane, so water flows out of the ICF (i.e., effective osmolarity occurs). The loss of hypotonic solution from ECF also causes hypertonicity from development of an osmotic gradient. Effective osmolarity can be determined by using the following calculation:

$$\text{Effective osmolarity (mOsm/L)} = 2(Na + K) + \text{Plasma glucose (mg/dl)}/18$$

The level of consciousness generally correlates to the duration and severity of hypertonicity.

Uncontrolled diabetes with abnormal metabolism of a major impermeable solute (glucose) represents a mixed hypertonicity: (1) addition of glucose into ECF and (2) hypotonic diuresis from glycosuria. Water crosses the cell membrane from the ICF space, so the ECF space is expanded. Subsequent hypotonic osmotic diuresis decreases all body water compartments. Metabolic decompensation may present with ketone body formation (ketoacidosis) or marked hyperglycemia and increased effective osmolarity. In NKH, the ICF space is contracted more due to ECF hypotonic fluid loss and circulating glucose. Glucose in the ECF is diminished, and water flows back into the ICF when insulin is administered. In patients with severe dehydration, vascular collapse occurs if the patient is not adequately rehydrated.

In decompensated diabetics with NKH, glucose concentrations are high but insufficient to cause significant hypertonicity because the osmotic contribution of glucose is only 5 mOsm/L for every 90-mg/dl increase in glucose. The loss of hypotonic fluid from the ECF is the major contributor to the hypertonicity. In the hydrated diabetic patient, filtered glucose in the renal tubules is fully resorbed if the tubular fluid glucose levels are below the renal glucose threshold, about 180 mg/dl. When glucose levels are above the renal threshold, glucose remains in the tubular fluid, causing the induction of hypotonic osmotic diuresis. The urine produced is hypotonic, containing 50 to 70 mEq of sodium. Osmotic contribution of sodium is high, 2 mOsm/L for 1-mEq increase in sodium in the ECF. As sodium and water loss continues, the total fluid volume contracts, causing a reduction of glomerular filtration of glucose; the result is an increase in hyperglycemia and NKH.

Adequate fluid intake and replacement of urinary losses can prevent severe hypertonicity. Most cases of NKH are associated with restricted access to water. A number of medical interventions can cause or exacerbate NKH (Box 24-7).[31,34,37] Patients with NKH do not have significant ketosis because of a combination of physiologic factors, including lower counterregulatory hormone levels, decreased lipolysis, and higher levels of intraportal insulin.

Clinical Features

In the development of NKH there is a slow progression of increasing polyuria and polydipsia. Manifestations of NKH include profound dehydration (e.g., xerostomia, absent axillary sweat, poor skin turgor). Tachycardia and low-grade fever are also present. Cardiovascular and respiratory examinations are normal, unless pneumonia is

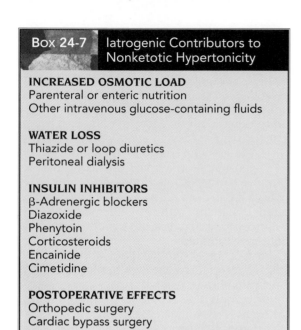

Modified from Lorber D: *Med Clin North Am* 79(1):43, 1995.

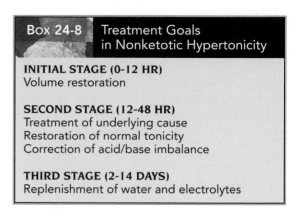

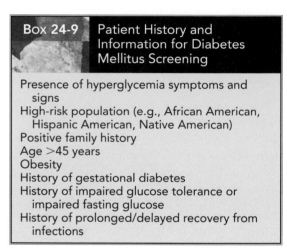

present (50% of patients with infections). Kussmaul respiration is absent. Abdominal examination may show evidence of gastroparesis (distention, pain, nausea, vomiting). Common neurologic signs are found in every level of the brain and range from focal findings to coma. Lethargy and disorientation are frequently seen. Coma is usually associated with marked hypertonicity (≥350 mOsm/L).

Other neurologic conditions associated with NKH include grand mal or focal seizures, aphasia, hemisensory or motor deficits, and exacerbation of preexisting organic mental disorders. Patients with NKH are often admitted to the hospital with the diagnosis of a CVA, but the focal deficits usually resolve completely with correction of the hypertonicity.[31,37]

Diagnosis

The accepted diagnostic criteria for NKH are severe hyperglycemia (glucose concentration ≥600 mg/dl), serum osmolarity above 320 mOsm/L, and serum ketone level low or absent. The diagnosis of NKH can be unsuspected until a marked elevation of blood glucose is found, despite high serum sodium levels. Laboratory tests for NKH work-up should include serum electrolytes, blood glucose determination, complete blood cell count with differential, ABGs, serum/urine ketone determination, and a liver panel.

Treatment

The goals of NKH treatment are volume rehydration, treatment of the underlying cause, restoration of normal tonicity, correction of acid-base imbalance, and replenishment of water and electrolytes. The goals of therapy can be divided into three stages (Box 24-8). Treatment of NKH is the same as for DKA (see Figure 24-2).[31,34,37]

PREVENTION OF ACUTE DIABETIC EMERGENCIES

A thorough medical history and physical evaluation are extremely important in known diabetic and nondiabetic patients alike, since many patients have undiagnosed DM. Screening of nondiabetic patients is directed toward risk factors that may predispose them to developing diabetes, as well as symptoms of hyperglycemia (Box 24-9). Patients with suspected undiagnosed DM should be sent for medical work-up.

Careful evaluation of the known diabetic patient focuses on glycemic control, pharmacologic and nonpharmacologic therapies, and existing chronic complications. Every dental office should have a blood glucose monitor to assess current blood glucose levels before initiating treatment. Monitors are inexpensive and easy to use. Contacting the patient's physician is recommended to obtain an accurate history, including the patient's motivation and compliance with treatment.

Appointments should be kept short; scheduling of the patient with diabetes should be favorable to the patient's diabetic management. The dentist should inquire about dietary intake before the dental appointment. If a dental procedure will result in dietary restrictions (e.g., multiple extractions, periodontal surgery), consultation with the patient's physician or dietitian is warranted. The dentist should avoid altering pharmacologic regimens without consulting the patient's physician. The dentist and staff should be familiar with the signs and symptoms of hypoglycemia and hyperglycemia; early identification and prompt management of acute complications are necessary to reduce morbidity.

SUMMARY

Patients with diabetes are frequently seen in the dental office. The dental professional must have a working knowledge about diabetes in order to provide safe care for this patient population. Acute complications of diabetes must be identified early and treated appropriately in the dental office or other health care setting. Complications in the diabetic patient can be prevented with careful planning.

REFERENCES

1. American Diabetes Association: Report of the Expert Committee on the Diagnosis and Classification of Diabetes Mellitus, *Diabetes Care* 20:1183-1197, 1997.
2. Alberti KGMM, Zimmet PZ: Definition, diagnosis, and classification of diabetes mellitus and its complications. Part 1. Diagnosis and classification of diabetes mellitus. Provisional report of a WHO consultation, *Diabet Med* 15:539-553, 1998.
3. King H, Aubert RE, Herman WH: Global burden of diabetes, 1995-2025: prevalence, numerical estimates, and projections, *Diabetes Care* 21:1414-1431, 1998.
4. *Diabetes: 1996 vital statistics*, Alexandria, Va, 1996, American Diabetes Association.
5. National Diabetes Information Clearinghouse: *Diabetes statistics*, NIH Pub No 96-3926, Bethesda, Md, 1996, US Department of Health and Human Services, Public Health Service, National Institutes of Health.
6. Sherwin RS: Diabetes mellitus. In Goldman L, Bennett JC, editors: *Cecil textbook of medicine*, ed 21, Philadelphia, 2000, WB Saunders.
7. American Diabetes Association: Nutritional recommendations and principles for patients with diabetes mellitus, *Diabetes Care* 22(suppl 1): S42-S45, 1999.
8. Goldstein DE, Little RR: Monitoring glycemia control in diabetes: short-term assessment, *Endocrinol Metab Clin North Am* 26:475-486, 1997.
9. Feinglos MN, Bethel MA: Oral agent therapy in the treatment of type 2 diabetes, *Diabetes Care* 22(suppl 3):C61-C64, 1999.
10. Zimmerman BR: Sulfonylureas, *Endocrinol Metab Clin North Am* 26:511-522, 1997.
11. Malaisse WJ: Mechanism of action of a new class of insulin secretagogues, *Exp Clin Endocrinol Diabetes* 107 (suppl 4): S140-S143, 1999.
12. Davidson MB, Peters AL: An overview of metformin in the treatment of type 2 diabetes mellitus, *Am J Med* 102:99-110, 1997.
13. Bell PM, Hadden DR: Metformin, *Endocrinol Metab Clin North Am* 26:523-537, 1997.
14. Nattrass MM, Bailey CJ: New agents for type 2 diabetes, *Baillieres Clin Endocrinol Metab* 13(2):309-329, 1999.
15. Balfour JA, Plosker GL: Rosiglitazone, *Drugs* 57(6):921-930, 1999.
16. Lebovitz HE: Alpha-glucosidase inhibitors, *Endocrinol Metab Clin North Am* 26:539-551, 1997.
17. Scott LJ, Spencer CM: Miglitol: a review of its therapeutic potential in type 2 diabetes mellitus, *Drugs* 59(3):521-549, 2000.
18. Burge MR, Schade DS: Insulins, *Endocrinol Metab Clin North Am* 26:575-598, 1997.
19. Bolli GB, DiMarchi RD, Pack GD, et al: Insulin analogues and their potential in the management of diabetes mellitus, *Diabetologia* 42:1151-1167, 1999.
20. Kilpatrick ES: Problems in the assessment of glycaemic control in diabetes mellitus, *Diabet Med* 14:819-831, 1997.
21. Diabetes Control and Complication Trial research group: The effect of intensive diabetes treatment on the development and progression of long-term complications in insulin-dependent diabetes mellitus, *N Engl J Med* 329:977-986, 1993.
22. Ohkubo Y, Kishikawa H, Araki E, et al: Intensive insulin therapy prevents the progression of diabetic microvascular complications in Japanese patients with non-insulin-dependent diabetes mellitus: a randomized prospective 6-year study, *Diabetes Res Clin Pract* 28:103-117, 1995.
23. UK Prospective Diabetes Study Group: Intensive blood-glucose control with sulfonylureas or insulin compared with conventional treatment and risk of complications in patients with type 2 diabetes (UKPDS33), *Lancet* 352:837-853, 1998.
24. Sowers JR, Lester MA: Diabetes and cardiovascular disease, *Diabetes Care* 22(suppl 3):C14-C20, 1999.
25. Aiello LP, Gardner TW, King GL, et al: Diabetes retinopathy, *Diabetes Care* 21:143-156, 1998.
26. American Diabetes Association: Diabetes nephropathy, *Diabetes Care* 22(suppl 1):S66-S69, 1999.
27. Dejgaard A: Pathophysiology and treatment of diabetic neuropathy, *Diabet Med* 15:97-112, 1998.
28. Ewing DJ, Campbell IW, Clarke BF: The natural history of diabetic autonomic neuropathy, *Quarterly J Med* 49(193):95-108, 1980.
29. Cryer PE, Fisher JN, Shamoon H: Hypoglycemia, *Diabetes Care* 17:734-755, 1994.

30. Service FJ: Hypoglycemia, *Med Clin North Am* 79:1-8, 1995.
31. Kitabchi AE, Fisher JN, Murphy MB, et al: Diabetic ketoacidosis and the hyperglycemic hyperosmolar nonketotic state. In Kahn CR, Weir GC, editors: *Joslin's diabetes mellitus*, ed 13, Philadelphia, 1994, Lea & Febiger.
32. Cefalu WT: Diabetic ketoacidosis, *Crit Care Clin* 7:89-108, 1991.
33. Fleckman AM: Diabetic ketoacidosis, *Endocrinol Metab Clin North Am* 22:181-207, 1993.
34. Umpierrez GE, Khajavi M, Kitabchi AE: Review: diabetic ketoacidosis and hyperglycemic hyperosmolar nonketotic syndrome, *Am J Med Sci* 311:225-233, 1996.
35. Kitabchi AE, Wall BM: Diabetic ketoacidosis, *Med Clin North Am* 79:9-37, 1995.
36. Viallon A, Zeni F, Lafond P, et al: Does bicarbonate therapy improve the management of severe diabetic ketoacidosis? *Crit Care Med* 27: 2690-2693, 1999.
37. Lorber D: Nonketotic hypertonicity in diabetes mellitus, *Med Clin North Am* 79:39-52, 1995.

Thyroid Disorders

Patrick J. Vezeau

T he thyroid is an endocrine gland that is infrequently considered in the day-to-day practice of dentistry. Thyroid pathology rarely manifests clinical concerns in dental practice because of the safety of dental procedures, the early detection of thyroid disorders in medical practice, and the uncommon nature of devastating thyroid disease. However, occult thyroid disorders are surprisingly common and, if treated casually, may result in a significant morbidity or even mortality. The inherently stressful environment that patients perceive in the dental office and the administration of medications that may interact with thyroid hormones (e.g., vasoconstrictor local anesthetics) may precipitate an emergency situation if thyroid physiology and pathology are not fully appreciated.

ANATOMY AND PHYSIOLOGY

The thyroid gland originates as an outpouching of the embryonic pharyngeal epithelium and descends from its original position at the junction of the anterior two thirds and posterior one third of the tongue, the area of the foramen cecum. The thyroid's path of descent along the deep midline of the tongue and anterior neck forms an embryonic thyroglossal duct, the remnants of which may give rise to cysts and tumors in the adult.[1] In the rare occurrence of congenital absence of the thyroid gland, remnants of thyroid tissue in the tongue may function in the adult as an accessory thyroid gland (lingual thyroid).[2] In the adult the thyroid gland is a bilobed structure that lies on either side of the trachea below the cricoid cartilage. Often the lobes are attached by a narrow isthmus of thyroid tissue.

Thyroid Hormones

The thyroid gland is composed of many follicles lined by cuboidal epithelial cells, which are filled with colloid containing the protein *thyroglobulin*. The thyroglobulin molecules bind with iodide ions, acting as a reservoir of iodine.[3] Iodinated thyroglobulin molecules undergo enzymatic proteolytic cleavage to form two active thyroid hormones: *triiodothyronine* (T_3) and tetraiodothyronine (T_4), or *thyroxine* (Figure 25-1). Proteolytic cleavage of active thyroid hormone is a slow process, and the supply of iodinated thyroglobulin is sufficient to last several months in cases of low dietary iodine intake.[4]

The hormones released from the thyroid gland are composed of more than 90% T_4 and less than 10% T_3. After release into the circulation, T_4 is predominantly bound to several serum proteins, including *thyroxine-binding globulin* (TBG), *transthyretin* (TTR), and *albumin*.[5] TBG affinity for T_3 binding is only ⅟₂₀th that shown for thyroxine. T_3 does not bind to albumin. However, only the portion of serum T_3 and T_4 not bound to plasma proteins is metabolically active. Therefore the actual physiologic effect of T_3, which is less protein bound and more metabolically active than T_4, is greater than suggested by the total plasma T_3/T_4 ratio.[6] T_3 is approximately four times more potent than T_4 and has a more rapid onset in target tissues. Thyroxine has a longer duration of action because of its greater affinity for target tissue proteins and its intracellular metabolism by iodide ion removal into the more metabolically active T_3 molecule.[7] Metabolism of these thyroid hormones occurs as iodide ions are stripped from the molecule, followed by elimination of the core protein. T_3 and T_4 may also be metabolized in the liver by one of several metabolic routes.[8]

The thyroid gland is also the site of another cell population, *parafollicular cells*, or C cells, which are responsible for production of the hormone calcitonin. *Calcitonin* decreases serum levels of calcium by inhibiting osteoclastic bony turnover and is involved in calcium regulation of the blood and bone.[9] Greatly increased calcitonin levels, however, such as occur with medullary thyroid carcinoma, do not cause severe hypocalcemia. Similarly, low or absent serum calcitonin levels, such as may occur after total thyroidectomy, do not cause significant hypocalcemia.[9] Therefore dysfunction of thyroid C cells is unlikely to be involved in a medical emergency.

Mechanisms of Action

T_3 and T_4 bind to specific cellular receptor sites, which in turn influence sites on various chromosomes that regulate genetic expression. This genetic expression is not immediate, as demonstrated by the considerable lag time between exogenous thyroid hormone administration and clinical evidence of altered metabolism.[10] The effects of T_3 and T_4 on genome expression and mitochondrial regulation alter many physiologic events, leading to generalized increases in overall metabolic rate, with the following consequences:

- Increases in basal metabolic rate and the metabolism of carbohydrates and fats
- Increases in cardiac output, blood pressure, and blood volume
- Central nervous system (CNS) excitation
- Muscle tonus gains
- Overall increases in appetite and gastrointestinal food turnover
- Input into normal libido and menstruation
- Promotion of growth in children and adolescents

As with any regulatory hormone, a delicate balance is needed to avoid excessive thyroid hormone, with injurious levels of cellular metabolism, and deficient hormone, with depressed levels of metabolism.[11]

Hormone Regulation

The release of thyroid hormones is through a negative feedback loop involving the hypothalamus, anterior pituitary, and thyroid gland (Figure 25-2). The hypothalamus secretes minute amounts of *thyrotropin-releasing hormone* (TRH), which is then transported through the hypothalamic-pituitary portal venous system to the anterior pituitary gland. TRH secretion is modulated by the CNS neurotransmitters *somatostatin* and *dopamine*.[12] At the anterior pituitary, TRH stimulates basophilic cells to secrete *thyroid-stimulating hormone* (TSH). TSH, in turn, is secreted into the general circulation and delivered to the cuboidal epithelial cells of the thyroid gland, where it stimulates the production of thyroglobulin and the proteolytic cleavage and release of T_3 and T_4.

The negative feedback is provided by systemic levels of T_3, which inhibit the action of TRH in the pituitary gland, thereby decreasing the release of TSH. T_3 inhibition of TRH begins to occur when free T_3 levels in the blood are approximately 1.5 to 2 times above normal levels.[13] Estrogens increase the response of the anterior pituitary to TRH, resulting in the thyroid hormone–mediated metabolic increases of pregnancy,[14] whereas increased serum glucocorticoid levels decrease TRH stimulation of thyroid hormone release.[15] Also, intraglandular regulation of thyroid hormone production plays a significant role, but the details of this autoregulation are incompletely understood.

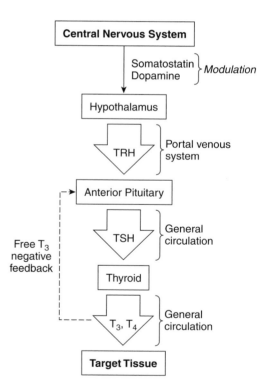

Figure 25-2. Regulation of thyroid function. *TRH,* Thyrotropin-releasing hormone; *TSH,* thyroid-stimulating hormone.

Figure 25-1. Triiodothyronine (T_3). *Thyroxine (tetraiodothyronine, T_4) has an iodide moiety at the cyclic position.

Regulation of thyroid hormone release may be disrupted, leading to overproduction or underproduction of these important substances. The clinical ramifications of either state are important and may influence treatment in the dental practice setting. Indeed, thyroid dysfunction may be initially detected by the dental professional through a comprehensive health history and a thorough head and neck examination.

THYROID EXAMINATION AND PATIENT HISTORY

In the adult the two lateral lobes of the normal thyroid gland lie on either side of the trachea, inferior to the thyroid cartilages (Figure 25-3.) The lobes are about 2 cm thick and about 4 cm in height and may be palpated medial to the sternocleidomastoid muscle.[16] The paired lobes are connected by the thyroid isthmus, which usually lies anterior to the second and third tracheal rings. Palpation may be aided by displacing the trachea toward the side to be palpated. Each lobe should be identified, and excessive size should be noted (Figure 25-4). Palpable nodules or significant asymmetries between sides may be appreciated. The lobes should be "rubbery," and palpation should cause no discomfort. Excessively hard lobes or pain to palpation should be noted. The gland should move up and down with the trachea during swallowing. The isthmus may not be palpable; if it is, it normally lies just below the cricoid cartilage.

Unusual glandular enlargements, especially if found beneath the sternocleidomastoid muscle, may be significant. Extremely enlarged thyroid glands, especially if extending beneath the sternum, can compress deeper structures. In such cases, raising the arms above the head may cause compression of the jugular veins and engorgement of the neck vasculature, difficulty with breathing, and giddiness or syncope (Pemberton's sign).[17] Sudden hoarseness caused by tracheal compression or recurrent laryngeal nerve pressure may suggest a neoplasm. In some areas of the world with low dietary iodine, endemic enlargement of the thyroid gland (*goiter*) is common, although this is rare in the United States.

Thyroid Function Tests

A number of thyroid function tests are available to the practitioner (Table 25-1). *Radioactive iodine uptake* tests the ability of the thyroid gland to store iodine and is useful in the diagnosis of diffuse glandular hyperthyroidism or focal nodular hyperthyroidism. Direct assessment of total serum T_3 and T_4 levels by highly specific and sensitive *radioimmunoassay* can be used to gain indirect measurement of free (unbound to plasma protein) T_3 and T_4 levels. The affinity of T_4 for the plasma proteins TBG, TTR, and albumin can be assessed and compared with plasma levels of these proteins in order to evaluate serum protein binding qualities. Levels of serum TSH can be compared to T_3 and T_4 levels to determine if abnormal thyroid hormone levels are caused by thyroid or pituitary dysfunction.

Ultrasonography of the thyroid gland can detail nodules, cysts, and other pathologic changes in gland structure while sparing the patient ex-

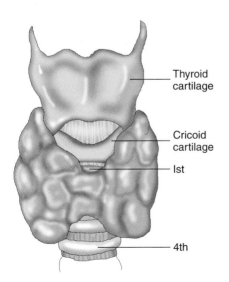

Figure 25-3. The thyroid gland. *1st, 4th,* Tracheal rings (cartilages).

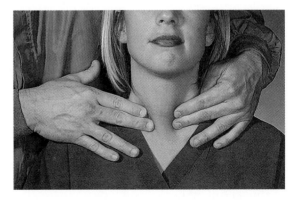

Figure 25-4. Clinical palpation of the thyroid gland.

Table 25-1	Common Thyroid Function Tests		
State	Thyroid-Stimulating Hormone	Thyroxine (T_4)	^{131}I Uptake
Euthyroid	0.3-3.0 mU/L	5-12 μg/dl	20%-30% of administered dose located in thyroid gland after 24 hours
Hyperthyroid	Elevated in *pituitary origin* hyperthyroidism Decreased in *thyroid origin* hyperthyroidism	Elevated	Elevated uptake in *thyroid origin* hypothyroidism Decreased uptake in *factitious* hyperthyroidism (with elevated T_4)
Hypothyroid	Elevated in *thyroid origin* hypothyroidism Decreased in *pituitary origin* hypothyroidism	Decreased	Decreased uptake (with decreased T_4)

Table 25-2	Medical History Correlations with Thyroid Dysfunction States		
Condition	Symptoms	Medications	Medications Avoided
Hyperthyroidism	Palpitations/rapid heartbeat Increased appetite Weight loss Nervousness, irritability Tremors Diarrhea Sweating/heat intolerance Muscular weakness	PTU Iodide Glucocorticoids (e.g., prednisone) Propranolol Radioactive iodine (^{131}I)	Caffeine (coffee, colas) Vasoconstrictor local anesthetics Bronchodilators (β-adrenergic)
Hypothyroidism	Lethargy Decreased appetite Confusion Constipation Muscle stiffness	Liothyronine (T_3) Levothyroxine (T_4) Liotrix (T_4/T_3)	Central nervous system depressants (benzodiazepines, narcotics, antihistamines, alcohol, barbiturates)

PTU, Propylthiouracil.

posure to radiation.[18] Computed tomography (CT) and magnetic resonance imaging (MRI) are used less often for thyroid gland study, although thoracic CT scans may be useful in the detection of thyroid tumor metastases.

Since many thyroid diseases are autoimmune in nature, assay of various antibody levels to thyroid cuboidal cells, T_3, T_4, TSH, and other substances can help identify a specific etiology for a dysfunctional thyroid state.[19]

Medical History

A thoughtful and detailed medical history can yield clues suggestive of thyrotoxicosis or hypothyroid states. These details are combined with clinical findings indicative of dysfunctional thyroid states (Table 25-2). Pertinent points from the patient history can alert the practitioner to the possibility of a thyroid disorder, especially since subtle clinical manifestations may be easily overlooked by the patient's physician. Subjective symptoms or even medications mentioned on a health history form may be indicative of hyperthyroid or hypothyroid disorders.

Symptoms associated with thyroid *hyperfunctioning* may include palpitations (rapid heartbeat), increased appetite and food intake (especially with weight loss), unexplained nervousness or irritability, tremors, diarrhea or gastrointestinal irritability, sweating and intolerance of heat or exercise, and muscular weakness.

Table 25-3	General Clinical Findings in Thyroid Dysfunction	
System	**Thyrotoxicosis**	**Hypothyroidism**
Cardiovascular	Tachycardia (>100 resting) Rhythm disturbances • Atrial fibrillation • Premature atrial/ventricular contractions (myxedema) Increased systolic blood pressure (>170) Increased pulse pressure (little effect on diastolic blood pressure) Angina	Cardiac enlargement Bradycardia (myxedema) Profound hypotension (end-stage myxedema)
Pulmonary	Increased respiratory rate (>20/min) Dyspnea, especially exertional	Decreased respiratory rate and depth (end-stage myxedema) Obstructive sleep apnea
Gastrointestinal	Increased appetite and food intake Weight loss Diarrhea, frequent stools, cramping	Decreased appetite Weight gain Constipation
Thermoregulatory	Increased temperature (>99° F/39° C) Heat intolerance	Decreased temperature Cold intolerance
Dermatologic	Flushed, warm, moist skin, sweating	Skin dry, coarse, cool Hair dry, sparse Periorbital puffiness
Nervous	Agitation, emotional lability Sleep disturbances, insomnia Tremulousness Hyperreflexia	Lethargy Hypersomnolence, fatigue Ataxia Hyporeflexia
Musculoskeletal	Muscular weakness (often proximal limb muscles affected first)	Muscle stiffness and cramping

Medications associated with the active treatment of hyperthyroidism, especially if recently prescribed, include propylthiouracil, glucocorticoids (e.g., prednisone), supplemental iodides, β-adrenergic blockers (e.g., propranolol), and radioactive iodine (^{131}I). Additionally, medications listed under "allergies" or mentioned as "avoided" include caffeine, coffee, and colas; "novocaine," specifically vasoconstrictor anesthetics; and bronchodilators, such as albuterol.

Symptoms associated with thyroid *hypofunctioning* are often the inverse of those associated with hyperthyroidism, including lethargy, loss of appetite (especially with weight gain,) confusion, and constipation. Medications associated with the treatment of hypothyroidism are the thyroid hormones (T_3/liothyronine, T_4/levothyroxine, T_3 and T_4/Liotrix). Medications that may cause "reactions" include the CNS depressants: benzodiazepines, narcotics, antihistamines, alcohol, and barbiturates.

The dentist should query the patient about subjective symptoms, such as onset, severity, and quantification, to help establish the seriousness of the suspected disorder.

Thyroid Dysfunctional States

The action of thyroid hormones may be either excessive or insufficient. The general terms for these states are *thyrotoxicosis* (usually from hyperthyroidism) and *hypothyroidism*, respectively (Table 25-3). Generalized enlargement of the thyroid gland (goiter) may accompany either of these states or may be asymptomatic. Also, a number of cystic or neoplastic processes may affect the size or function of the thyroid gland.

THYROTOXICOSIS AND HYPERTHYROIDISM

The physiologic overproduction of thyroid hormone action may result from excessive function of the thyroid gland (hyperthyroidism) or from other causes (Box 25-1). Regardless of the cause, however, disorders with excess secretion of thyroid hormone show similar clinical presentations and may have similar adverse effects.

With all thyrotoxic diseases, excessive metabolism leads to most symptoms (see Table 25-3). Tachycardia, fine tremulousness, fatigue, weight loss (often accompanied by increased

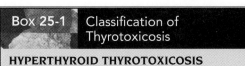

| Box 25-1 | Classification of Thyrotoxicosis |

HYPERTHYROID THYROTOXICOSIS
Graves' disease
Thyroid adenoma/adenocarcinoma
Toxic multinodular goiter
Tumors secreting thyroid-stimulating
  substances

NONHYPERTHYROID THYROTOXICOSIS
Factitious thyrotoxicosis
Ectopic thyroid hormone–producing tissue
Acute release of preformed thyroid hormone
  (thyroid inflammatory toxicosis)

appetite and food intake), warm flushed skin, and heat intolerance are common findings.[20] Increases in pulse pressure (difference between systolic and diastolic blood pressure) and disturbances in cardiac rhythm (most often atrial fibrillation but also premature atrial or ventricular beats) may occur. Elderly patients and those with cardiovascular disease may have high-output cardiac failure and angina. Increased resting respiratory rate, exertional dyspnea, menstrual irregularities, muscle wasting, and a widened stare with infrequent blinking are common. Enlargement (sometimes asymmetric) of the thyroid gland is often seen in hyperthyroidism and may vary depending on the etiology of thyroid hyperfunction (see following discussion). Differentiation between thyrotoxicosis and other hypermetabolic disorders (e.g., adrenal tumors) often requires laboratory analysis. Graves' disease and toxic multinodular goiter are the most common thyrotoxic syndromes.

Graves' Disease

Graves' disease is autoimmune in nature and may exhibit thyrotoxic, ophthalmologic, and dermatologic symptoms.[21]
Etiology.   The thyrotoxic aspect of Graves' disease is caused by autoantibodies that directly stimulate thyroid cuboidal cells, increasing release of T_3 and T_4 independent of pituitary TSH control. Graves' disease often coexists with other endocrine autoantibody disorders. The thyroid gland is infiltrated by inflammatory cells, and the thyroid cuboidal cells undergo hyperplasia. Ophthalmologic findings result from inflammatory cell infiltration to the soft tissues of the orbit outside the globe. This infiltrate leads to enlargement and fibrosis of the extraocular muscles and orbital fat. Inflammatory cell infiltration also causes dermal thickening and mucopolysaccharide deposition.
Epidemiology.   Graves' disease most often develops in patients in their 20s and 30s. A marked female preponderance exists, with several distinct genetic subtypes more common in various racial and ethnic groups.
Clinical features.   When hyperthyroidism is present, clinical symptoms are similar to those of other thyrotoxicoses (see Table 25-3). The thyroid gland itself is uniformly enlarged, soft, and nontender. *Exophthalmos* (forward displacement of the optic globe) may be present, resulting in excessive exposure of the sclera and an "excited" or "frightened" stare. Exophthalmos may initially be unilateral, with progression to bilateral involvement if not treated. Increasing exophthalmos can lead to corneal dryness and scarring because of the inability to close the eye, as well as damage to the optic nerve. Damage to the extraocular muscles may limit eye movements. Dermatologic manifestations include a raised, thickened appearance in the anterior calf and dorsum of the foot. Ophthalmologic and dermatologic symptoms may develop independently of endocrine involvement. However, the presence of ophthalmologic and thyrotoxic symptoms is often pathognomonic for Graves' disease.

Toxic Multinodular Goiter

Toxic multinodular goiter typically arises as hyperfunctioning of a previously asymptomatic enlarged thyroid gland, usually later in life (see Goitrous Hypothyroidism).[22]
Etiology.   Nodular areas in the thyroid begin to secrete T_3 and T_4 relatively independently of TSH control. Often there is a gradual transition from nontoxic to toxic goiter. Glandular hyperfunctioning may be caused by chronic iodine deficiency in the diet, but the exact pathogenesis is still unclear.
Epidemiology.   The incidence of toxic multinodular goiter is highly variable but generally much more common in areas of relative iodine deficiency. Since it often develops gradually over years in previously asymptomatic goitrous glands, the typical patient is over age 60. No gender predilection appears to exist.
Clinical features.   The clinical presentation of toxic goiter is similar to other thyrotoxic diseases, with cardiovascular symptoms predominating in this older patient population, including palpitations, chest pain, breathlessness, and widened pulse pressure. The thyroid is often

considerably enlarged and may be nodular and firm. In the presence of established cardiac or coronary artery disease, the extra demands placed on the heart by toxic multinodular goiter may cause cardiac decompensation, especially when the patient is placed under stressful situations. The onset may be insidious, however, and symptoms subtle. Generally, thyrotoxic symptoms are often less pronounced than those seen with Graves' disease.

Thyroid Adenoma

Occasionally a focus of thyroid cuboidal cells begins to undergo neoplastic change, secreting T_3 and T_4 independently of feedback loop control.[23]
Etiology. The slowly developing autonomy of the nodule from the TSH axis is incompletely understood.
Epidemiology. Solitary nodular adenomas may develop in as many as 50% of elderly adults by the time of demise. The slow development of thyroid adenomas makes them more common in elderly patients. There is no gender predilection.
Clinical features. Often the solitary thyroid adenoma forms a nodule or cyst. These usually reach greater than 1 cm in size before being clinically palpable. These may be viewed on ultrasound or visualized by intense focal uptake of a radioactive tracer (scintigraphy). Often an adenoma is located in an enlarged, goitrous gland. Symptoms of thyrotoxicosis may ensue, depending on the functional state of the adenoma.

Thyroid Carcinoma

Malignant neoplasms of thyroid cuboidal cells may cause thyrotoxic symptoms.[24]
Etiology. Uncontrolled malignant growth of thyroid epithelial cells may have several histologic types. Radiation to the thyroid or neck during childhood has been identified as a contributing factor to thyroid follicular cell cancer.
Epidemiology. Most follicular epithelial carcinomas of the thyroid occur later in life (age 60 and older), although *papillary thyroid carcinoma* also occurs frequently in the second and third decades. No gender predilection is known for these disorders.
Clinical features. Physical findings typical of thyrotoxicosis are often present. Firm, asymmetric, and rapidly developing thyroid enlargements may be detected on physical examination. Metastatic cervical lymphadenopathy may be present.

Thyroid Inflammatory Toxicosis

Thyroid inflammatory toxicosis causes increased release of presynthesized thyroid hormone byproducts but not increases in actual hormone production.
Etiology. Immune-mediated mechanisms are common to most inflammatory thyroiditic conditions. In *subacute thyroiditis* a viral infection of the gland, often after an upper respiratory infection, initiates a transient, painful inflammation.[25] *Silent thyroiditis* or *painless thyroiditis*, also known as *Hashimoto's thyroiditis*, is an autoimmune-mediated glandular disorder that causes a transient, painless increase in thyroid size with an increase in thyroid hormone release.[26] This is normally followed by a period of hypothyroidism, then a return to a euthyroid or hypothyroid state. *Postpartum thyroiditis* shares many traits of silent thyroiditis. It occurs 3 to 12 months after pregnancy and does not normally recur.[27]

In most forms of thyroid inflammatory toxicosis, TSH levels fall due to increases in serum thyroid hormone. Duration of increase in serum thyroid hormone levels is self-limiting to the inflammatory event or lasts until presynthesized glandular stores are exhausted.
Epidemiology. Subacute thyroiditis occurs equally in both genders and at all ages. Postpartum thyroiditis occurs in women of childbearing age, whereas silent thyroiditis is more common in middle-aged women.
Clinical features. Thyroid appearance and palpation may be variable, depending on the degree of inflammation. Subacute thyroiditis often produces a tender thyroid to palpation. Silent thyroiditis is usually goitrous. Severity of thyrotoxic symptoms depends on thyroid hormone levels. Often, chronic inflammation may lead to eventual decreases in functional thyroid tissue mass, ending in hypothyroidism.

Extrinsic Thyroid Hormone Ingestion

Symptomatic increases in thyroid hormone levels may occur in *factitious thyrotoxicosis* (thyrotoxicosis factitia, self-administration of supratherapeutic doses of thyroid hormone) or with ingestion of undercooked meat products containing thyroid tissue ("hamburger thyrotoxicosis").

Pituitary Hormone–Secreting Tumors

Rare cases of thyrotoxicosis may arise from TSH-secreting pituitary tumors. Other tumors may elaborate hormones, such as human chorionic gonadotropin, that cross-react with TSH receptors in thyroid tissue.

Thyrotoxic Crisis

An acute exacerbation of hypermetabolic symptoms, thyrotoxic crisis may occur in the patient with thyrotoxicosis.[28]

Etiology.   Formerly, thyrotoxic crises were most often caused by thyroid hormone liberation during thyroidectomy of a hyperfunctioning gland. However, medical treatment of thyroid hyperfunction before gland removal has largely eliminated this source of crisis. Currently, the most common type of *thyroid storm* is the "thyroid medical storm," in which a hypermetabolic crisis is precipitated in an untreated or poorly treated hyperthyroid patient; often by (emergency) surgery, stress, parturition, or sepsis. Thyroid medical storm does not represent a further increase in total thyroid hormone levels but may result from a relatively sudden shift from protein-bound to free (and metabolically active) thyroid hormone by mechanisms that are still poorly defined.

Epidemiology.   The incidence of thyroid storm has decreased with improved medical diagnosis and management. The rare storm occurs almost exclusively in the untreated, poorly controlled thyrotoxic patient. Precipitating factors (e.g., stress, sepsis) may be present in the dental office setting.

Clinical features.   The thyroid medical storm syndrome may be manifested by fever, often higher than 41° C; tachycardia, often more than 140 beats per minute; severe hypotension, with systolic pressure less than 90 mm Hg; restlessness; delirium or coma; and prostration. Cardiac complications include ectopy, pulmonary edema, and high-output heart failure.

Even with contemporary medical care, acute thyrotoxic crisis carries a significantly high mortality. The treatment focus for dental patients is to avoid the problem, that is, identify susceptible individuals in the medical history and clinical examination and refer them for medical management.

Clinical Differential Diagnosis

The symptoms of thyrotoxicosis just outlined are similar to those elicited in adrenal tumors (e.g., pheochromocytoma), cocaine or amphetamine overdose, cardiac tachydysrhythmias, extreme anxiety, and aggressive psychiatric disorders. Increased systolic blood pressure may be found in a number of other disorders, including essential hypertension. Widened pulse pressures typical of thyrotoxicosis also suggest aortic valvular abnormalities or significant hypovolemia and dehydration. Inadvertent intravascular administration of vasoconstrictor-containing local anesthetic solutions may simulate or exacerbate these symptoms. Nodular thyroid swelling with symptoms similar to those of hyperthyroidism may also represent the rare multiple endocrine neoplasia syndrome type II (MEN-II), which is characterized by pheochromocytoma and thyroid swelling from medullary thyroid (parafollicular, or C-cell) carcinoma. The similarity of the physical findings among these pathologic states often mandates the use of laboratory testing to determine a diagnosis.

Laboratory Tests

A number of laboratory tests may be involved in the diagnosis of subtle thyroid disorders (see Table 25-1). The rate of radioactive iodine uptake by the gland is elevated in hyperthyroid states, in which the gland synthesizes thyroid hormone at a level above normal physiologic needs. However, glandular uptake is not elevated when thyrotoxicosis results from causes other than hyperfunctioning of the thyroid gland, such as thyrotoxicosis factitia, hamburger toxicosis, thyroid inflammatory toxicosis, and metastatic thyroid follicular carcinoma. Levels of T_3 and T_4 can be compared with TSH to establish the location of thyroid dysfunction and deliver appropriate therapy (see Figure 25-2). For example, in many thyrotoxic states, such as Graves' disease, toxic multinodular goiter, and thyroid adenoma, thyroid hormone levels are elevated, whereas TSH is depressed; this represents suprametabolic thyroid gland secretion relatively independent of the feedback mechanism involving TSH. Often the hypermetabolic state affects other hormonal systems, with alterations in serum cortisol and insulin levels. Extensive laboratory testing is indicated to assess the full impact of increased thyroid hormone on the patient.

Dental Management

The identification of individuals who may be thyrotoxic often begins with the medical history. The medical questionnaire may include queries concerning rapid heartbeat or palpitations, weight loss, mental changes, and "nerve disorders," which may be caused by tremulousness or CNS excitation. A history of therapeutic radia-

Table 25-4	Physical Parameter Guidelines for Suspected Hyperthyroid Patients			
Parameter	Routine Dental Care	Medical Consult Before Routine Dental Care	Palliative Care/ Timely Medical Referral*	Immediate Medical Attention†
Systolic blood pressure (mm Hg)	<140	140-170	170-200	>200
Diastolic blood pressure (mm Hg)	<90	90-105	105-140	>140
Respirations (per minute)	8-14	15-20	21-24	>25
Pulse	<80 and regular	80-100 or 1-2 irregularities/min	100-130 or 3-8 irregularities/ min	>130 or >8 irregularities/ min
Anxiety	None	Mild to moderate	Marked	Severe

*Consider directing referral to see patient within 2 days.
†Consider immediate referral or emergency transport to an acute care facility; emergency dental care in acute care setting (i.e., operating room with anesthesia monitoring).

tion to the neck may increase susceptibility for thyroid adenocarcinoma. Medical history findings should be correlated with the clinical examination and vital signs (Table 25-4).

The differential diagnosis of conditions with symptoms typical of thyrotoxicosis includes disorders that may also make elective dental treatment problematic, such as uncontrolled essential hypertension, adrenergic tumor, CNS dysfunction, and drug abuse. The correlation of an enlarged or tender thyroid gland with appropriate clinical symptoms may indicate a thyroid origin, which then must be confirmed by imaging and laboratory testing.

Dental management risk is greatest in the patient with a suspicious medical history and clinical findings but who has had no recent medical work-up. For the patient exhibiting significant physical findings, all except palliative treatments should be avoided until a definitive diagnosis and medical-surgical management is complete. Stressful situations must be avoided in the patient with suspected or diagnosed thyrotoxicosis. The judicious use of nitrous oxide may aid in anxiolysis while causing minimal respiratory depression for a potentially compromised airway in the goitrous patient. The use of β-adrenergic vasoconstrictors, such as in local anesthetics or gingival retraction cord, should be minimized.[29] Dental emergencies should be managed in consultation with the patient's physician and may require treatment in the hospital setting.[30]

The rare (and often avoidable) occurrence of thyrotoxic crisis is a true medical emergency. Marked fever (>41° C), severe tachycardia (>140 beats/min), severe hypotension (systolic pressure <90 mm Hg), and prostration should lead to an immediate presumptive diagnosis. Dental office intervention should include immediate cessation of all dental procedures, supplemental oxygen by nasal cannula (3 L/min) or face mask (>5 L/min), a comfortable position for the patient, constant monitoring and reassurance, and frequent vital sign and temperature assessment. For those offices equipped for intravenous (IV) access, starting an IV line (at least 18 gauge) and an infusion of 5% dextrose in 0.45% saline or lactated Ringer's solution at a moderate rate (1.5 ml/kg/hr) may prevent dehydration. Slow administration of 4 mg of dexamethasone (over 5 minutes) is helpful in these patients, who have increased glucocorticoid demand and often exhibit depletion of adrenal reserve. Cardiac nitrates (e.g., sublingual nitroglycerin) for anginal symptoms may be needed in the patient with cardiac vascular disease, and prompt cardiopulmonary support (CPR) must be immediately available.

Most importantly, the emergency medical services (EMS) system must be immediately activated for patient transport to an emergency department or other facility. The mnemonic "SAVING" summarizes the dental office management of thyrotoxic crisis (Box 25-2).

Box 25-2 Dental Office Management of Thyrotoxic Crisis

DIAGNOSIS
Fever (>41° C/105° F)
Tachycardia (>140 beats/min)
Hypotension (<90 mm Hg)
Severe fatigue, exhaustion, confusion

MANAGEMENT
S   Stop dental procedures.
A   Administer oxygen.
     Assume comfortable position for patient.
V   Vital signs frequently (blood pressure,
     pulse, temperature every 5 minutes)
I   Intravenous access (D5, LR, or NS with
     dexamethasone, 4 mg slowly)
N   Nitroglycerin tablet, 0.4 mg ready for
     sublingual use
G   "Get help;" activate EMS system
     immediately (call 911).

D5, Dextrose 5%; *LR,* lactated Ringer's solution; *NS,* normal saline; *EMS,* emergency medical services.

Medical Management

Thyrotoxicosis management may be either medical or surgical and is directed to the specific cause of increased thyroid hormone levels.

Pharmacologic Therapy

Chemical suppression.   Suppressive drugs may be used alone when thyrotoxic states are not severe and physical decompensation has not occurred. *Propylthiouracil* (PTU) and *methimazole* decrease the amount of thyroxine released by the gland. PTU also decreases the peripheral conversion of T_4 to T_3. Thyroid suppression only lasts as long as the suppressive medication is administered. These drugs may cause leukopenia and an intolerable increase in size of a goitrous thyroid. Therefore suppressive drugs are used primarily in patients in whom ablation of thyroid tissue may not be desired, such as children, adolescents, and pregnant women.

Iodide may be administered to suppress *transiently* the release of intraglandular presynthesized thyroid hormones, which explains its use in pending thyrotoxic crisis. Iodide must be used with another suppressive drug, however, or iodine stores in the gland will increase and worsen chronic hyperthyroidism.[31]

Glucocorticoid therapy is used to (1) decrease thyroid inflammatory states and thus inhibit release of presynthesized thyroxine, (2) supplement the depleted reserve capacity of the adrenal gland to make cortisol, (3) decrease the peripheral conversion of T_4 to T_3, and (4) blunt the effect of TRH on pituitary release. *Dexamethasone* is the drug of choice for steroid supplementation.

Chemical ablation.   Ablation of thyroid tissue by administration of radioactive iodine is often used for older patients, who often have goitrous hyperplastic thyroid tissue, or in those for whom surgery is contraindicated.[32] Radioactive iodine treatment is not done in the pregnant hyperthyroid patient to avoid ablation of fetal thyroid tissue. Radioactive iodine therapy causes a gradual decrease in thyroid functioning. A major drawback is that often hypothyroidism eventually occurs, necessitating lifetime exogenous supplemental thyroid hormone administration. Also, a transient radiation-induced thyroiditis may temporarily increase release of preformed thyroid hormone, necessitating chemical suppressive therapy before chemical ablation. In the elderly patient with cardiac disease, β-adrenergic blockade and glucocorticoid support typical of treatment for acute thyrotoxic crisis may also be necessary.

Surgical Ablation

Gland removal is indicated in younger patients who do not respond to thyroid suppressive drug therapy. The hyperthyroid state is first and temporarily controlled by chemical suppression to decrease the release of preformed thyroxine that results from surgical manipulation of the thyroid gland. After gland removal, the resulting hypothyroid state is treated by lifetime exogenous thyroid hormone therapy. The small multiple parathyroid glands, which synthesize parathyroid hormone (PTH, the major control mechanism of serum calcium homeostasis), may be removed with thyroid tissue, resulting in hypocalcemia (low serum calcium). This requires ongoing treatment with calcium and vitamin D supplements.

Other Interventions

The cardiostimulative and adrenergic effects of thyroid hormone are often treated by a β-adrenergic blocker, usually *propranolol.* β-Blockers must be given with caution and with full monitoring, especially in elderly patients who may have heart failure. Cardiac glycosides (e.g., digitalis derivatives) or antiarrhythmic agents (e.g., procainamide) may be necessary to control ectopic

Box 25-3	Classification of Hypothyroid States

TYPE	LOCATION/CAUSES
Trophoprivic	*Hypothalamus*
	Neoplasm (benign or malignant)
	Congenital hypothalamic defect
	Infection
	Infiltrative (sarcoidosis or other chronic inflammatory disorder)
	Pituitary
	Granular (TSH-secreting cell) defect
	Panhypopituitarism (congenital, hypophysectomy)
Thyroprivic	*Thyroid*
	Ablative (surgical or medical thyroidectomy)
	Congenital lack of thyroid
	Idiopathic
	Radiation induced
Goitrous	*Thyroid*
	Endemic (iodine deficiency)
	Drug or dietary induced
	Silent (Hashimoto's) thyroiditis
	Hormone synthesis defect(s)
Other	*Thyroid*
	Postpartum (transient)
	Recovery from thyroid inflammatory toxicosis (transient)

activity of the heart; concurrent antihypertensive medication may be indicated. Often, thyrotoxic states cause excessive metabolism of endogenous glucocorticoids (cortisol) and insulin; both of which may need supplementation while the thyroid hormone levels are brought under control. Thyrotoxicosis in pregnancy must be handled especially carefully to avoid thyroid suppression in the embryo or fetus. In pregnant patients, thyroid suppressive drugs are titrated in minimal doses, and radioactive iodine is contraindicated. The services of an experienced internist or endocrinologist are essential.

Thyrotoxic crisis management often delivers interventions simultaneously. The most severe thyrotoxic cases usually involve untreated patients with another medical condition (e.g., emergency surgery, sepsis) that contributes to the acute nature of the thyroid storm. Treatment is aimed at providing supportive therapy to preserve affected organ systems while alleviating the thyrotoxic state. Rehydration is begun by IV fluids. Nutritional support and high-dose dexamethasone supplements are uniformly used. High temperature (hyperpyrexia) is treated with cooling blankets and humidified oxygen. β-Adrenergic blockade is often necessary to decrease cardiac response to hypermetabolism. An-

tiarrhythmic therapy may be indicated. Immediate thyroid suppressive therapy (PTU and temporary iodate) is used to decrease thyroxine release.

After hypermetabolism is controlled, plans for thyroid control can be undertaken. Laboratory indices and the clinical presentation of the patient are used to guide therapy. As with many other disorders, the dental professional, through the medical history and the head and neck examination, may be the first health care provider to notice thyrotoxicosis and refer the patient for timely management.

HYPOTHYROIDISM

Hypothyroidism is the syndrome of insufficient synthesis of thyroid hormones (Box 25-3). More than 95% of hypothyroid states arise at the level of the thyroid gland, and less than 5% arise in the hypothalamus or pituitary gland.

The clinical manifestations of the hypothyroid state vary considerably depending on severity of disease and age at onset (see Table 25-3). Developmental abnormalities resulting from congenitally low thyroid titers are termed *cretinism*, and symptoms of severe hypothyroidism in the adult is *myxedema*. Although hypothyroidism occurs in 1 of 5000 live births in the United States, cretinism is rare due to the routine assay of neonatal thyroid hormone levels. In the infant, jaundice, constipation, and somnolence are early signs. If not treated, growth and intellectual developmental delays ensue, with classic cretin features that include coarse hair, macroglossia, abdominal protrusion, flat nasal bridge, hypertelorism, and delays in tooth eruption. The older child who develops hypothyroidism will display fewer overt physical and mental developmental effects.[33]

Adult hypothyroidism may not be noticed in its early stages. Early signs may include lethargic feelings, fatigue, and cold intolerance, symptoms that may otherwise be common in elderly patients. More severe decreases in thyroid hormone levels eventually lead to dry skin, increased somnolence, weight gain even with appetite suppression, and decreased mental acuity and activity.[34] Increases in intercellular proteoglycan deposition lead to increased tissue fluid retention, nonpitting edema (especially of the face), and periorbital swelling. Pericardial effusion may be present, and respiratory depression with increased carbon dioxide retention may occur. Advanced stages may lead to stuporous coma and death, usually by respiratory mechanisms. Blood pressure may be decreased if hypothyroidism is acute or may be elevated with symptoms of atherosclerotic vascular disease, which is common in the chronically hypothyroid patient. Hypothyroid goiter may be present, with potential venous or airway obstruction.

Trophoprivic Hypothyroidism

Trophoprivic hypothyroidism describes hypothyroid states that originate in the hypothalamus or the anterior pituitary gland (adenohypophysis).
Etiology. Low secretion of TSH by the anterior pituitary may be part of a total pituitary hypofunction syndrome, often after pituitary gland surgery, or as an isolated congenital granular cell deficiency of the adenohypophysis.[35] A number of problems at the level of the hypothalamus can decrease TRH secretion, including neoplasia, infection, congenital defects, and sarcoidosis. TRH deficiency in turn decreases stimulation of TSH release, resulting in a hypothyroid state.[36]
Epidemiology. Congenital pituitary hypoplasia or hypothalamic causes of hypothyroidism lead to cretinism, which is manifest by several months of age. Hypothalamic and hypophyseal causes of hypothyroidism are rare.
Clinical features. Often, congenital hypothalamic problems are accompanied by other neurologic deficits, sometimes profound. The lack of function of hypothalamic or hypophyseal tissue often leads to a lack of other hypophyseal factors, such as adrenocorticotropic hormone (ACTH), causing hypoadrenalism; follicle-stimulating and luteinizing hormones (FSH, LH), causing lack of sexual maturation; and growth hormone (GH), causing profound growth retardation.

Thyroprivic Hypothyroidism

Thyroprivic hypothyroidism denotes a lack of sufficient functional thyroid tissue.
Etiology. The most common cause of this loss is by ablation (radioiodide or surgical) for hyperthyroidism.[37] Primary idiopathic hypothyroidism may involve an autoimmune process against thyroid cuboidal cells or against the TSH receptor on the cell surface. Either disorder often coexists with other autoimmune diseases, such as lupus erythematosus, diabetes mellitus, rheumatoid arthritis, or Sjögren's syndrome.[38] Primary agenesis or hypogenesis of the thyroid gland is the most common factor for cretinism. A transient hypothyroid state, sometimes with a preceding hyperthyroid period, is common after pregnancy. Transient hypothyroidism may also occur after resolution of the inflammation accompanying the hyperthyroidism of acute thyroiditis (see previous discussion).
Epidemiology. Mild thyroprivic hypothyroidism affects more than 10% of adults over 50 years of age. More severe forms are much less common, primarily because of early diagnosis and treatment.
Clinical features. The onset of thyroprivic hypothyroidism is often quite slow, taking years to manifest clinically. General symptoms of lethargy, weight gain, fatigue, and slowed mentation are common findings. Palpation of the thyroid gland usually yields no enlargement or nodules. Increased vascular resistance by atherosclerosis may cause hypertension.

Goitrous Hypothyroidism

Goitrous hypothyroidism denotes hypothyroidism accompanied by thyroid gland hyperplasia.
Etiology. Initial inadequate secretion of thyroid hormones leads to increased TSH secretion, which may increase the size of the thyroid gland (goiter). In many cases, hyperplasia of functional thyroid tissue may allow normal thyroid hormone levels to be maintained. However, if the enlarged thyroid gland cannot produce normal thyroid

hormone levels even with this increase in TSH, goitrous hypothyroidism occurs. Goitrous hypothyroid states may be caused by chronically inadequate iodide intake, but this is rare in the American diet. *Silent (Hashimoto's) thyroiditis* is the most common goitrous hypothyroid etiology in the U.S. population.[39] Certain medications, most notably lithium and large doses of iodine, can interfere with thyroid hormone synthesis. Drugs that can precipitate goitrous hypothyroidism include phenylbutazone, aminosalicylic acid, and thionamides. Causative foodstuffs include cabbage and turnips.[40]

Epidemiology.   Endemic areas of iodine deficiency can cause universal goiter and possible hypothyroid states locally. Generally, goitrous hypothyroidism affects adults over age 40 in the United States, since the chronic process of autoimmune thyroid gland inflammation and destruction often takes years to yield insufficient thyroid hormone levels.

Clinical features.   Together with typical hypothyroid and hypometabolic findings, goiter that is usually painless may be present. The goiter may become large enough to cause respiratory difficulties.

Acute Hypothyroid Crisis

The nature of hypothyroidism makes acute critical episodes very rare. Postablational hypothyroidism is generally rendered euthyroid by monitored thyroid replacement therapy. Also, the hypometabolic state of myxedema does not usually present the physiologic catastrophe seen in hyperthyroid crisis.

Etiology.   Generally, acute hypothyroid crisis, usually the coma of myxedema, is caused by an acute physical challenge (e.g., infection, emergency surgery) in a poorly controlled hypothyroid patient. Insufficient thyroid hormone reserves are available to support the increased metabolic demands of the initiating event. However, the possibility of thyroid supplement noncompliance in a formerly hyperthyroid patient after thyroid ablation may cause a more rapid onset of symptoms.

Epidemiology.   Although no data are available, acute hypothyroid *crises* are rare.

Clinical features.   The patient presents with the usual signs of myxedema but may be stuporous to unconscious, often with slowed respirations (< 6/min) and partial airway obstruction from fat, goiter, or an enlarged tongue, with sonorous breathing (see Table 25-3). Blood pressure may be low or normal. Hypoxia and hypercarbia may lead to cardiac dysrhythmias and an irregular pulse.

Clinical Differential Diagnosis

The puffy facial appearance of the myxedemic patient is similar to that of the nephrotic syndrome (chronic loss of plasma proteins in the urine). Myxedematous edema is nonpitting, however, unlike edema of the nephrotic syndrome. Sluggishness, mental confusion, and ataxia in the elderly patient may be incorrectly attributed to advanced age, Parkinson's syndrome, stroke, or Alzheimer's disease. Acute deterioration in the dental office with increased mental lethargy may be mistaken for cerebrovascular accident, acute hypoglycemia/insulin shock, or myocardial infarction.

Laboratory Tests

Patients with thyroprivic or goitrous hypothyroidism often have decreased levels of T_3 and T_4, with elevated TSH. Patients with trophoprivic states often have decreased levels of TSH or TRH, depending on the location of the primary disease. Radioactive iodine uptake may be decreased by 75%. Also, significantly increased lipid levels, especially low-density lipoproteins and cholesterol, are typical of adult hypothyroid patients. Atherosclerosis is common.

Dental Management

In the adult, hypothyroidism does not present the risks of acute metabolic catastrophe as does hyperthyroidism (thyrotoxicosis). However, hypothyroid symptoms may become exacerbated in the nonmanaged patient under the physiologic stress of the dental office. Advanced cardiovascular disease in this patient population, combined with carbon dioxide retention, may predispose to cardiac rhythm disturbances, especially under stress or excessive administration of adrenergic agonists (e.g., vasoconstrictors). Symptoms of cardiac ischemia (e.g., chest pain, nausea, profuse cold sweating) should be treated as possible angina or myocardial infarction (see Chapters 7 and 22). Because the noncorrected hypothyroid patient is extremely sensitive to CNS depressants, oral or parenteral sedatives should be used with caution, if at all.[41]

The hypothyroid patient who has been returned to a physiologically normal (*euthyroid*) state by intake of exogenous thyroid hormone has no contraindication to routine dental care,

| Box 25-4 | Dental Office Management of Acute Hypothyroid Crisis |

DIAGNOSIS
Cool, pale, dry skin
Cold intolerance
Confusion, stupor, unresponsiveness
Hypopnea, sonorous breathing
Suspicious history (ablated thyroid, myxedema facies)

MANAGEMENT
S   Stop dental procedures.
H   Heat (blankets, warm room) for patient
A   Airway; be sure patient is not obstructing with enlarged tongue (protrude tongue for patient).
     Administer oxygen.
K   Know vital signs (blood pressure, pulse, temperature every 5 minutes).
I   Intravenous access, if available (D5, LR, NS)
N   Noxious stimulation (shaking or chest rub)
G   "Get help;" activate EMS system immediately (call 911).

including sedation techniques. If the hypothyroid patient has other endocrine problems, especially hypoadrenalism (see following discussion), additional management steps may be necessary in concert with the endocrinologist.

In the patient with a suspicious history, especially if accompanied by a myxedematous appearance who experiences marked lethargy, stupor, or cold intolerance, acute hypothyroid crisis must be suspected. Dental procedures must be stopped. The patient is kept warm by blankets and by warming the room. The airway may tend to obstruct, and the lower jaw or tongue may need to be protracted or a nasal trumpet airway inserted (if available) to allow air exchange. Oxygen is administered (preferably by face mask at 5 L/min.) Vital signs (blood pressure, pulse, temperature) are taken at 5-minute intervals. For offices so equipped, IV access with at least an 18-gauge catheter with an infusion of 5% dextrose in 0.45% saline or lactated Ringer's solution at minimal flow (10 ml/hr) would allow rapid medication administration by responding emergency personnel. A trial of a noxious stimulus (e.g., chest rubbing, smelling salts) may arouse the patient enough to maintain respiration. The EMS system must be activated for transport of the patient to an acute care facility. The mnemonic "SHAKING" summarizes dental office management of hypothyroid patients (Box 25-4).

Medical Management

With all hypothyroid states, the common goal of treatment is to establish normal thyroid hormone levels by administration of exogenous thyroid hormone supplements. Prompt medical correction of neonatal or childhood hypothyroid states is critical to avoid developmental delays associated with cretinism. First, however, the source of the congenital hypothyroid disorder must be ascertained. For example, in the case of panhypopituitarism (lack of activity in entire pituitary) a lack of pituitary ACTH may result in adrenal gland suppression with low levels of serum cortisol. The increased metabolic demands caused by administering exogenous supplemental thyroid hormone must be accompanied by administration of cortisol substitutes to avoid an adrenal crisis, characterized by profound shock.[33] Other important hormones (GH, FSH, LH) must be provided to allow normal growth and sexual development.

In the adult, gradual correction of a hypothyroid state will allow time for the body to produce physiologic adjustments of cardiovascular, endocrine, and other organ systems. However, the patient with myxedematous coma requires rapid administration of IV thyroxine, often with supplemental corticosteroids and β-blockers to protect the cardiovascular system from sudden increases in metabolic demand. The most common oral thyroid supplement is *levothyroxine* (L-thyroxine), which allows a gradual normalization of T_3 levels by tissue conversion of levothyroxine to T_3.

SIMPLE (NONTOXIC) GOITER

A generalized enlargement of the thyroid gland may occur when levels of T_3 and T_4 are normal. This may represent a hyperplasia of the gland in response to low iodine intake or the ingestion of thyroid suppressive drugs or foods. In the United States, however, goiter usually occurs spontaneously as a result of defective or insufficient T_3 and T_4 synthesis by idiopathic mechanisms, in which TSH-mediated hyperplasia of the gland enables sufficient thyroid hormone synthesis to allow attainment of normal thyroid hormone serum levels.[42] With time, however, gradual thyroid failure often ensues, leading to goitrous hypothyroidism.

A major sequela of goiter may be compression of surrounding structures, leading to venous congestion, airway compromise, and dysfunction of the recurrent laryngeal nerve. The role of the dentist in routinely performing a thorough neck examination may be key to early detection of an enlarged thyroid.

OTHER DYSFUNCTIONAL STATES

The biosynthesis and regulation of thyroid hormones involve a multistep process, and any step may be affected by disease. The sequential addition of iodine to the thyroglobulin molecule may be defective, as may the deiodinization of T_4 to the more active T_3 in the peripheral tissues. Plasma or tissue protein binding by thyroid hormone may be inadequate, as may specific tissue responses to thyroid hormone stimulation. Any step in the hypothalamic or pituitary regulation of the thyroid gland may be deranged, leading to subtle or significant clinical evidence of disease. A host of sophisticated tests are available to the endocrinologist to aid in the diagnosis and treatment of these uncommon disease states.[17]

SUMMARY

Thyroid dysfunction may lead to metabolic disturbances that can cause emergency situations in the dental office. A thorough medical history and clinical examination may aid the practitioner in intercepting undiagnosed states of thyroid dysfunction and avoiding a potentially catastrophic medical emergency. Caution must be exercised with the suspected thyrotoxic patient, especially if a stressful procedure or the use of β-adrenergic medications is anticipated. Less often the stresses of dental treatment may exacerbate an untreated chronic hypothyroid state, especially in the elderly patient.

As with all medical emergencies, astute examination, cautious differential diagnosis, timely referral, and preplanned emergency procedures (which should be written and regularly rehearsed with office staff) are crucial in the avoidance or recognition and treatment of urgent or emergent thyroid dysfunctional states.

REFERENCES

1. Ericson LE, Friderickson G: Phylogeny and ontogeny of the thyroid gland. In Greer MA, editor: *The thyroid gland: comprehensive endocrinology*, New York, 1990, Raven.
2. Hollinshead WH: *Anatomy for surgeons: the head and neck*, ed 2, New York, 1968, Hoever Medical.
3. Fisher DA, Klein AH: Thyroid development and disorders of thyroid function in the newborn, N Engl J Med 304:702-704, 1981.
4. Gershengorn MC, Wolff J, Larsen PR: Thyroid-pituitary feedback during iodine repletion, J Clin Endocrinol 43:601-605, 1976.
5. Bartalena L: Thyroid hormone-binding proteins: update 1994, Endocr Rev 13:140-142, 1994.
6. Pardridge WM: Plasma protein–mediated transport of steroid and thyroid hormones, Am J Physiol 252:E158-E164, 1987.
7. Larsen PR, Silva JE, Kaplan MM: Relationships between circulating and intracellular thyroid hormones: physiological and clinical implications, Endocr Rec 2:87-102, 1981.
8. Berry MJ, Larsen PJ: Selenocysteine and the structure, function, and regulation of iodothyronine deiodination: update 1994, Endocr Rev 3:265-269, 1994.
9. Potts JT: Chemistry of the calcitonins, Bone Miner 16:169-173, 1992.
10. Hennemann G, Docter R: Plasma transport proteins and their role in tissue delivery of thyroid hormone. In Greer MA, editor: *The thyroid gland: comprehensive endocrinology*, New York, 1990, Raven.
11. Guyton AC: The thyroid hormones. In *Textbook of medical physiology*, ed 6, Philadelphia, 1981, WB Saunders.
12. Beck-Peccoz P, Mariotti S, Guillausseau PJ: Treatment of hyperthyroidism due to inappropriate secretion of thyrotropin with somatostatin analogue SMS-201-995, J Clin Endocrinol Metab 68:208-214, 1989.
13. Larsen PJ, Silva JE, Kaplan MM: Relationships between circulating and intracellular thyroid hormones: physiological and clinical implications, Endocr Rev 2:87-102, 1981.
14. Burrow GN: Thyroid function and hyperfunction during gestation, Endocr Rev 14:194-202, 1993.
15. Nicoloff JT, Fisher DA, Applemen MD: The role of glucocorticoids in the regulation of thyroid function in man, J Clin Invest 49:1922-1935, 1970.
16. Bates B: A *guide to physical examination*, ed 2, Philadelphia, 1979, Lippincott.
17. Larsen P, Davies T, Hay I: The thyroid gland. In Wilson J, Foster D, Kronenberh H, et al, editors: *Williams textbook of endocrinology*, ed 9, Philadelphia, 1998, WB Saunders.
18. James EM, Charboneau JW, Hay ID: The thyroid. In Rumack CM, Wilson SR, Charboneau JW, editors: *Diagnostic ultrasound*, St Louis, 1991, Mosby.
19. Salvi M, Fukazawa H, Bernard N, et al: Rate of autoantibodies in the pathogenesis and association of endocrine autoimmune disorders, Endocr Rev 9:450-462, 1988.
20. Landsberg L: Catecholamines and hyperthyroidism, Clin Endocrinol Metab 6:697-718, 1977.
21. McDougal IR: Graves disease: current concepts, Med Clin North Am 19:685-696, 1990.
22. Sawin CT, Geller A, Herschmann JM, et al: The aging thyroid, JAMA 261:2653-2655, 1989.
23. Goldstein R, Hart IA: Follow-up of solitary autonomous thyroid nodules treated with ^{131}I, N Engl J Med 109:1473-1476, 1983.
24. Mazzaferrin EL: Papillary thyroid carcinoma: factors prognosis and current therapy, Semin Oncol 14:315-327, 1987.
25. Stancek D, Stancekova-Gressnerova M, Janotka M, et al: Isolation and some serological and epidemiological data on the viruses recovered from patients with subacute thyroiditis, Med Microbiol Immunol 161:133-144, 1975.
26. Papapetrou PD, Jackson IMD: Thyrotoxicosis due to silent thyroiditis, Lancet 311:363-365, 1975.
27. Jansson R, Bernander S, Karlsson A, et al: Autoimmune thyroid dysfunction in the postpartum period, J Clin Endocrinol Metab 58:681-687, 1984.
28. Burch HB, Wartofsky L: Life-threatening thyrotoxicosis: thyroid storm, Endocrinol Metab Clin North Am 16:235-242, 1995.

29. Malamed S: *Handbook of local anesthesia*, ed 4, St Louis, 1997, Mosby.

30. Sincer PA, Cooper DS, Levy E, et al: Treatment guidelines for patient with hyperthyroidism and hypothyroidism, *JAMA* 273:808-812, 1995.

31. Wolff J: Iodide goiter and the pharmacologic effects of excess iodide, *Am J Med* 47:101-124, 1969.

32. Wise H, Ahmad A, Burnet RB, et al: Intentional radioiodine ablation for Graves disease, *Lancet* 2:1231-1233, 1975.

33. Klein AH, Foley TP Jr, Larsen PR, et al: Neonatal thyroid function in congenital hypothyroidism, *J Pediatr* 89:545-549, 1976.

34. De Groot LJ, Larsen PR, Hennemann G, editors: *The thyroid and its diseases*, ed 6, New York, 1996, Churchill-Livingstone.

35. Bateman A, Singh A, Kral T, et al: The immune-hypothalamic-pituitary-adrenal axis, *Endocr Rev* 10:92-112, 1989.

36. Lechan RM: Neuroendocrinology of pituitary hormone regulation, *Endocrinol Metab Clin North Am* 16:475-501, 1987.

37. Taft AD, Irvine WJ, McIntosh D, et al: Temporary hypothyroidism after surgical treatment of thyrotoxicosis, *Lancet* 2:817-819, 1976.

38. Rees-Smith B, McLachlan SM, Furmaniak J: Autoantibodies to the thyrotropin receptor, *Endocr Rev* 9:102-121, 1988.

39. Nokolai TF, Coombs GJ, McKenzie AK: Lymphocytic thyroiditis with spontaneously resolving hyperthyroidism and subacute thyroiditis, *Arch Intern Med* 141:1455-1458, 1981.

40. Surks MI, Sievert R: Drugs and thyroid function, *N Engl J Med* 333:1688-1694, 1994.

41. Donatello S: Endocrine physiology and function. In Weinberg GL, editor: *Basic science review of anesthesiology*, New York, 1997, McGraw-Hill.

42. Wartofsky L: Diseases of the thyroid. In Isselbacher KJ, Braunwald E, Wilson JD, et al, editors: *Harrison's principles of internal medicine*, ed 13, New York, 1994, McGraw-Hill.

Adrenal Insufficiency

Samuel J. McKenna

The adrenal gland plays an essential role in the regulation of carbohydrate, fat and protein metabolism, fluid balance, and immune regulation. The adrenal gland is crucial to the maintenance of homeostasis under periods of physiologic stress such as illness, trauma, and surgery. The understanding and clinical management of adrenal insufficiency is one of the great achievements of modern medicine. Applied to the practice of dentistry, this knowledge provides for the safe management of the medically compromised patient with adrenal insufficiency from any cause.

NORMAL ADRENAL CORTICAL FUNCTION

The adrenal or "suprarenal" gland is a paired organ located retroperitoneally at the upper pole of each kidney. Weighing approximately 4 g, each gland functions as two distinct endocrine organs. The inner portion, or medulla, comprises about 10% of the gland and functions as part of the autonomic nervous system. The medulla secretes the catecholamines epinephrine, norepinephrine, and dopamine. The cortex, the bulk of the gland, is divided into three functionally distinct zones: the outer, glomerulosa; middle, fasciculata; and inner, reticularis. The glomerulosa secretes the major adrenal mineralocorticoid, aldosterone. The fasciculata secretes corticosteroid precursors and cortisol. The reticularis is the site of androgen hormone synthesis and minute quantities of estrogen precursor hormones. The synthesis of all adrenal hormones begins with LDL cholesterol and, to a lesser extent, acetate. Cortisol, the principal glucocorticoid produced by the adrenal cortex, promotes hepatic glycogenolysis, ketogenesis, and gluconeogenesis. Other effects of cortisol include suppression of bone and cartilage formation, attenuation of the inflammatory response, inhibition of growth hormone secretion, and enhancement of the vasoactive effects of catecholamines.

Aldosterone, the other important adrenal product, is the predominant mineralocorticoid. Aldosterone serves a key role in body fluid homeostasis by promoting sodium conservation. As a result, aldosterone has important effects on blood volume, osmolarity, and blood pressure.

Weak androgens produced by the adrenal cortex serve as precursors for the formation of the potent androgen testosterone. Similarly, the androgen androstenedione is converted to the estrogen estrone. However, in contrast to gonadal production, the adrenal cortex is not a quantitatively important source of androgens and estrogens. Only in states of adrenal hyperfunction is the adrenal production of such sex steroids of clinical importance.

Regulation of Adrenal Cortical Products

Approximately 13 to 20 mg ($7.5/M^2$) of cortisol is secreted daily by the adrenal cortex.[1,2] Corticotropin (adrenocorticotropic hormone [ACTH]) released into the circulation by the anterior pituitary is the principal regulator of cortisol production. In turn, corticotropin release is controlled by corticotropin-releasing hormone (CRH) and arginine vasopressin, produced by the paraventricular nucleus of the hypothalamus and posterior pituitary, respectively. Importantly, cortisol provides feedback inhibition both at the level of the hypothalamus and pituitary. This hierarchy of hypothalamic, pituitary, and adrenal function is referred to as the *hypothalamic-pituitary-adrenal* (HPA) *axis* (Figure 26-1). Amplification occurs at each level of the HPA axis so that picogram/milliliter concentrations of CRH and corticotropin result in microgram/milliliter concentrations of released cortisol.

Aldosterone production is under the control of the renin-angiotensin system. Renin is released by the juxtaglomerular cells of the kidney in response to decreased blood volume or through sympathetic nervous system stimulation. Under the influence of renin, angiotensinogen is converted to angiotensin. In turn, angiotensin promotes aldosterone release by the adrenal cortex (Figure 26-2). Aldosterone promotes sodium and water retention and potassium excretion.

To maintain physiologic homeostasis, cortisol is released continuously in a series of pulses. A diurnal variation in corticotropin secretion leads to higher cortisol levels in the morning between 2 AM and 8 PM.[3] In addition to the diurnal variation in cortisol production, corticotropin release is triggered by physiologic stressors such

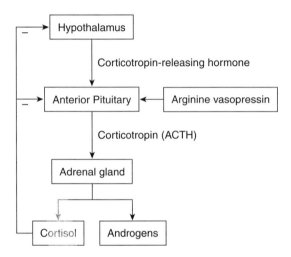

Figure 26-1. HPA axis. – Denotes negative feedback. *ACTH*, Adrenocorticotropic hormone.

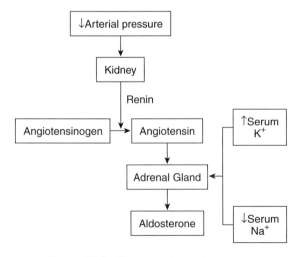

Figure 26-2. Renin-angiotensin system.

as pain, fever, hypoglycemia, and hypotension. Preoperative emotional factors such as fear and insomnia begin the cascade of increased cortisol production around the time of surgery. The rise in cortisol production is proportionate to the magnitude of the surgical procedure. Barring postoperative complications, cortisol production returns to baseline within 24 hours of surgery.[4,5] Failure of the HPA axis to meet the periodic requirement for increased cortisol production can lead to circulatory collapse and death.

Laboratory Evaluation of Adrenal Function

Unstimulated cortisol levels are approximately 10 to 25 µg/dl in the morning and 2 to 10 µg/dl in the evening.[1] A morning plasma cortisol concentration of at least 19 µg/dl is consistent with normal adrenal function. Of greater clinical importance than unstimulated cortisol levels is the response of the adrenal cortex to exogenous administration of corticotropin, the corticotropin stimulation test. In this test 250 µg of synthetic corticotropin (cosyntropin) is administered intravenously. Plasma cortisol is measured just before the injection and 60 minutes after the injection. A twofold increase in serum cortisol above baseline or a serum cortisol concentration of at least 20 µg/dl reflects normal adrenal function. Other tests of HPA axis function include serum ACTH level, dexamethasone suppression test, metyrapone test, and insulin tolerance test. The selective application of these tests can identify the location of specific HPA axis defects. The literature contains good discussions on the topic of laboratory assessment of HPA axis function.[1,3,6]

Pathophysiology of Adrenal Insufficiency

Adrenal insufficiency (AI) is the condition in which adrenal cortex output is insufficient to meet physiologic demand for cortisol through a number of possible HPA axis abnormalities. Primary AI (Addison's disease) is caused by destruction of the adrenal gland. At least 70% to 80% of the adrenal glands must be destroyed before the clinical picture of AI emerges.[2] Primary AI usually involves the entire cortex, which results in a deficiency of cortisol, aldosterone, and adrenal androgens. The adrenal medulla is often spared in primary AI. Granulomatous infection from tuberculosis or histoplasmosis, once the most common cause of primary AI, now accounts for a minority of cases. Autoimmune adrenal destruction by antiadrenal cortex antibodies is the most important cause of primary AI.[3] This condition also may be associated with other autoimmune endocrine deficiencies such as hypothyroidism (polyendocrine deficiency syndrome). Primary AI also can occur in the setting of adrenomyeloneuropathy, a hereditary disorder marked by progressive myelin degeneration in the brainstem or spinal cord.[7] Primary AI can complicate acquired immunodeficiency syndrome (AIDS) with adrenal destruction by a variety of opportunistic infections or infiltration by Kaposi's sarcoma. Finally, infiltration of the adrenal gland by metastatic disease (lung, breast, colon, stomach, pancreas, skin) may result in acute AI.

Secondary AI arises from abnormalities of the hypothalamus or pituitary that result in decreased corticotropin production. Because mineralocorticoid release is controlled by the renin-angiotensin system, aldosterone production is unaffected in secondary AI. Causes of secondary AI are listed in Box 26-1. Patients with AI secondary to hypothalamic or pituitary disorders, especially intracranial space-occupying lesions (e.g., pituitary tumor) often demonstrate other hormonal deficiencies along with neurologic or ophthalmologic abnormalities. An important cause of secondary AI is the therapeutic administration of supraphysiologic doses of corticosteroids. Feedback inhibition of both CRH and corticotropin release from supraphysiologic doses of exogenous corticosteroid results in adrenal cortical atrophy. Corticosteroids are used extensively in clinical medicine for management of a variety of inflammatory and immunologic diseases. Therefore the dentist periodically will be confronted with the patient who is currently taking or who has taken supraphysiologic doses of corticosteroids.

Cortisone is the original therapeutic corticosteroid. Subsequently a number of synthetic analogues of cortisol have been used therapeutically. These drugs can be compared to naturally occurring cortisol by corticosteroid potency (Table 26-1). Corticosteroids may be administered systemically or topically. Although the topical administration of corticosteroid agents produces less HPA axis suppression, any formulation in prolonged and sufficient doses can produce secondary AI.[8,9] In general, corticosteroids with greater potency and duration of action produce greater HPA axis suppression. However, high dose and/or prolonged corticosteroid therapy does not invariably correlate with the degree of HPA axis suppression.[10,11,12] Compared to daily dosing, alternate-day administration can provide both a sufficient quantity of corticosteroid to suppress the condition for which the corticosteroid has been prescribed and produce less adrenal suppression.[8,13] It is difficult to predict on the basis of corticosteroid dose, frequency, and duration, which patient will have clinically important HPA axis suppression after corticosteroid therapy is discontinued.[14] At one

Box 26-1	Causes of Secondary Adrenal Insufficiency

Long-term corticosteroid administration
Pituitary or metastatic tumor
Hypothalamic tumor
Pituitary surgery or radiation
Postpartum pituitary necrosis
Head trauma

Table 26-1	Comparison of Corticosteroid Preparations	
Duration/Preparation	**Corticosteroid Potency**	**Equivalent Dose (mg)**
SHORT-ACTING		
Hydrocortisone (cortisol)	1	20
Cortisone	0.8	25
INTERMEDIATE-ACTING		
Prednisone	4	5
Prednisolone	4	5
Methylprednisolone (Medrol)	5	4
LONG-ACTING		
Dexamethasone (Decadron)	30	0.75
Betamethasone (Celestone)	25	0.60

extreme, HPA axis suppression should be suspected with the administration of the equivalent of prednisone 20 to 30 mg over a period as short as 1 to 2 weeks.[15] Higher doses (prednisone 25 mg twice a day) administered for 5 days produce short-term AI.[16] At the other dose extreme, it is unlikely that long-term daily doses as low as 2.5 to 5.0 mg of prednisone are associated with significant adrenal suppression. LaRochelle and colleagues showed no HPA axis suppression with a long-term daily dose of prednisone less than 5 mg for rheumatologic disease.[17] Intuitively, this is reasonable, as 5 mg of prednisone is equivalent to normal unstressed daily cortisol production. In contrast, patients receiving more than 5 mg had a widely varied response to corticotropin stimulation testing.[17] Long-term daily doses between 5.0 to 7.5 mg have been shown to produce HPA axis suppression in 50% of patients, whereas daily doses of 10 mg or more produce HPA axis suppression in 96% of patients.[18] However, even with daily corticosteroid equivalent doses in excess of 7.5 mg of prednisone, adrenal reserve may be adequate to satisfy cortisol requirements during periods of clinical stress.[19] In an animal model, adrenalectomized monkeys undergoing cholecystectomy experienced postoperative cardiovascular instability only when provided one-tenth the physiologic replacement dose of corticosteroid. Adrenalectomized animals receiving physiologic replacement doses of corticosteroid had no more complications related to AI than a group of animals that received ten times the physiologic replacement dose.[20] Notwithstanding the variability in HPA axis suppression from corticosteroid administration, it is apparent that factors other than the integrity of the HPA axis are involved in the physiologic response to stress.[11,21]

The time to recovery of HPA axis function after discontinuation of corticosteroids is also controversial. Two imprecisely understood and interacting factors are corticosteroid dose and duration. Graber and colleagues noted that after discontinuation of 1 year of daily supraphysiologic doses of corticosteroid, approximately 9 to 12 months were required for the return of adrenal cortex responsiveness to corticotropin.[22] Hypothalamic and pituitary function returned sooner, in 5 to 9 months. In contrast, HPA axis response to stress returns to normal within a week of discontinuing short-duration (<5 days), high-dose prednisone.[16] An estimate of adrenal gland recovery can be made from the observation that changes in corticosteroid dose more

than 7 months before HPA axis testing do not affect test results.[17] Based on a review of the literature, Glick concluded that HPA axis response to clinical stress can occur much earlier, in 14 to 30 days.[23] However, studies supporting his conclusion involved short-term corticosteroid administration in children. Even with long-term administration, HPA axis recovery may occur earlier in children.[24] With regard to the effect of daily prednisone dose, Livanou and colleagues noted that HPA axis recovery occurs sooner in patients receiving 7.5 mg or less than in those receiving 10 mg.[12]

Although the corticosteroid dose and duration threshold necessary to produce clinically significant AI is unclear, a conservative estimate is that a corticosteroid equivalent dose greater than 5 mg of prednisone taken for at least 2 weeks may cause AI. After discontinuation of the corticosteroid, adrenal cortex function may recover in as few as 2 to 4 weeks but may take as long as a year. For the clinician faced with the uncertain risk of clinically significant AI, the response to provocative adrenal cortex testing is the safest method to estimate the degree of adrenal cortical recovery. Without such objective measure of adrenal cortex recovery, it is prudent to assume that adrenal response to stress will be compromised for 6 months after discontinuation of exogenous corticosteroid.[8]

Clinical Manifestations of Adrenal Insufficiency

The symptoms of primary and secondary AI are similar and are caused by deficient cortisol production (Box 26-2). Chronic AI presents insidiously, with fatigue, weakness, anorexia, weight loss, apathy, and lightheadedness when assuming an upright posture (orthostatic hypoten-

Box 26-2	Signs and Symptoms of Adrenal Insufficiency
CHRONIC	**ACUTE**
Fatigue	Abdominal cramping
Weakness	Nausea and vomiting
Anorexia, weight loss	Diarrhea
Apathy	Hypotension
Hyperpigmentation skin, mucosa	Mental status changes
Orthostatic hypotension	Depressed consciousness
Salt craving	Loss of consciousness

sion). Orthostatic hypotension is more pronounced in primary AI because of aldosterone deficiency. Some patients may manifest more acute symptoms: abdominal cramping, vomiting, and diarrhea. The most specific sign of primary AI is hyperpigmentation of skin and mucosal surfaces due to the chronic elevation of corticotropin. In contrast, hyperpigmentation is not seen in secondary AI as corticotropin levels are decreased. A specific symptom of primary AI is salt craving as a result of impaired aldosterone production. Manifestations of other hormonal deficiency may be seen in secondary AI as a result of impaired hypothalamic or pituitary function. Symptoms of secondary AI from ongoing chronic therapeutic corticosteroid administration may be masked by adequate, albeit supraphysiologic, doses of corticosteroid. In fact, signs of corticosteroid excess (truncal obesity, moon facies, cutaneous striae, and so on) may alert the astute clinician to the risk of impaired adrenal reserve if corticosteroid administration is abruptly discontinued.

Evaluation of Suspected Adrenal Insufficiency

The evaluation of suspected AI is straightforward. With impending adrenal collapse, routine laboratory tests may reveal hyponatremia (low serum sodium), hyperkalemia (elevated serum potassium), and elevated blood urea nitrogen. If measured, serum corticotropin levels will be elevated in primary AI and depressed or undetectable in secondary AI. The definitive diagnosis of AI can be established with the corticotropin stimulation test, as previously described. Other provocative tests may be required to isolate the location of HPA axis disease.

Acute Adrenal Insufficiency (Adrenal Crisis)

Acute adrenal insufficiency, or adrenal crisis, is a rare, life-threatening condition that usually develops in association with severe illness. The most common cause is massive hemorrhagic adrenal infarction occurring in the setting of acute illness such as sepsis or cardiac disease, with anticoagulation, postoperatively or in hypercoagulable states. Of greater practical importance in dentistry is the occurrence of acute AI in the patient with known chronic AI, or relative AI. *Relative* AI refers to the clinical situation in which endogenous cortisol production or exogenous corticosteroid administration, although sufficient to meet the needs of the unstressed indi-

vidual, is insufficient to support homeostatic functions in the clinically stressed individual.[25]

The presentation of acute AI varies from the gradual onset of symptoms over several days in the unstressed individual, to the precipitous development of hypotension brought on by clinical stress. Factors causally related to the appearance of acute AI in the susceptible patient include fever, dehydration, illness, injury, surgery, and anesthesia. The extent to which routine dental care is likely to precipitate adrenal crisis in the patient with chronic AI is uncertain. Unless blood pressure is continuously monitored, clinically important hypotension first may be recognized by the abrupt onset of mental status changes, possibly progressing to the loss of consciousness. Hypotension may be accompanied by pallor, diaphoresis (profuse perspiration), nausea, and compensatory tachycardia. Importantly, in the patient with underlying coronary artery disease, hypotension may cause myocardial ischemia and angina. Clinically important hypotension may be precipitated by moving the supine or semirecumbent dental patient into an upright position (orthostatic hypotension). Conversely, positioning the hypotensive patient in the supine or Trendelenburg (supine, 30-degree, head-down tilt) position may afford some protection from the development of symptomatic hypotension. In the monitored patient, progressive, symptomatic hypotension is clinically more important than an isolated blood pressure measurement.

Management of Adrenal Insufficiency

Individuals with symptomatic chronic AI require life-long corticosteroid replacement therapy. Usually the equivalent of 20 to 30 mg of hydrocortisone divided into two unequal daily doses (2/3 AM, 1/3 PM) is sufficient replacement in the setting of Addison's disease. The dose is adjusted to eliminate symptoms and signs of cortisol deficiency. Daily mineralocorticoid supplement is also necessary, satisfied by fludrocortisone (Florinef) 0.05 to 0.3 mg. This dose is adjusted to maintain blood pressure (both supine and standing) and serum potassium within the normal range. In the patient receiving chronic supraphysiologic doses of corticosteroids, symptomatic AI is minimized by dose tapering before discontinuing therapy.

Adrenal crisis is a life-threatening condition that requires immediate treatment with adequate doses of parenteral corticosteroid and fluid resuscitation. Therapy for suspected acute

Box 26-3 Patients at Risk for Adrenal Crisis

HISTORY OF TREATMENT FOR ADRENAL INSUFFICIENCY
Inadequate replacement therapy/symptoms of AI
Noncompliance with maintenance therapy
Concurrent illness (fever and so on)
History of long-term supraphysiologic dose corticosteroid administration
Recent abrupt discontinuation of corticosteroid
Concurrent illness (fever and so on)

Box 26-4 Management of Adrenal Crises

Terminate dental procedure
Evaluate/monitor blood pressure
Trendelenburg position if blood pressure <90/60 or symptomatic
Activate emergency medical system: Call 911
Dexamethasone (Decadron) 4 mg IV or IM*
Fluid resuscitation: Normal saline with 5% dextrose rapid IV infusion for hypotension

*Alternatively hydrocortisone 100 mg IV or IM.

AI should never be delayed or withheld while awaiting the results of confirmatory laboratory tests, although in the hospital setting an initial blood sample to evaluate serum cortisol, aldosterone, sodium, potassium, glucose, and corticotropin can be collected.

The first role of the dentist in the office management of adrenal crisis is to identify the patient at risk for adrenal crisis. This is accomplished with a thoughtful evaluation of the past medical history, including medication use (Box 26-3). The diagnosis of impending adrenal crisis should not be difficult for the dentist who is aware of a patient's history of chronic AI and knowledgeable of the signs and symptoms of acute AI. There are two circumstances where the dentist may encounter adrenal crisis. In one situation, a patient is receiving maintenance corticosteroid for chronic AI. The other more likely circumstance is the patient who is receiving or has received supraphysiologic doses of corticosteroids. Blood pressure should be evaluated before and after particularly stressful procedures (extractions, surgery, general anesthesia) in the patient at risk for acute AI. Blood pressure should be evaluated every 5 to 10 minutes during the procedure if sedatives or general anesthesia have been administered, as these agents mask early mental status changes variably associated with hypotension. Hypotension should alert the astute clinician to impending adrenal crisis. When adrenal crisis is suspected, dexamethasone 4 mg should be administered intravenously (Box 26-4). Alternatively, hydrocortisone 100 mg may be administered, but if the diagnosis of AI must be confirmed, serum cortisol will be falsely elevated with the corticotropin stimulation test. In the acute situation where the dentist does not have the capability to adminis-

ter intravenous (IV) medication, dexamethasone may be administered by the intramuscular (IM) route. However, especially in the setting of impending shock, the IM route may not provide sufficient circulating drug for a successful resuscitation. Dental treatment in progress should be terminated, and hypotension may be temporarily managed by placing the patient in the Trendelenburg position.

IV fluid resuscitation may begin in the dental office if the clinician has the necessary training and equipment to provide this service. Due to associated aldosterone deficiency, primary AI is associated with profound fluid depletion. Fluid replacement should mirror the composition of extracellular fluid. Therefore the fluid of choice in this situation is normal saline. Additionally, due to the effect of corticosteroid on hepatic gluconeogenesis and glycogenolysis, hypoglycemia often accompanies acute AI. Therefore replacement fluids should contain dextrose. Generally, at least 1 L normal saline with dextrose may be rapidly infused safely.

Oral replacement of fluid and glucose is not sufficient in the setting of acute AI. Simultaneously, local emergency services (911) should be activated for patient transfer to a hospital. Subsequent hospital care consists of additional corticosteroid administration, aggressive fluid resuscitation, and confirmation of the diagnosis of AI in the previously undiagnosed patient. Additionally, drugs to support blood pressure such as dopamine may be required briefly for the management of hypotension.

Prevention of Acute Adrenal Insufficiency

For the patient with chronic AI, adrenal crisis is prevented with maintenance corticosteroid replacement (Box 26-5). Maintenance doses should be increased during times of increased physio-

| Box 26-5 | Recommendations: Prevention of Acute Adrenal Insufficiency |

ROUTINE RESTORATIVE PROCEDURES WITH LOCAL ANESTHESIA
Excellent anesthesia/pain control.
Consider conscious sedation in anxious patient.
No supplemental corticosteroid required.*

EXTRACTIONS, PERIODONTAL SURGERY, GENERAL ANESTHESIA
Excellent anesthesia/pain control.
Consider conscious sedation in anxious patient.
Equivalent of hydrocortisone 50 mg before procedure and daily postoperatively for exceptional pain or complications.

ODONTOGENIC INFECTION WITH PAIN, FACIAL SWELLING, FEVER
Treat offending tooth.
Surgical drainage of anatomic space(s).
Hydration
Equivalent of hydrocortisone 50-100 mg/day until clinical improvement (usually 24-48 hours).

*This recommendation assumes proper dose tapering in patient who has discontinued corticosteroids in past 6 months to 1 year, or adequate maintenance replacement therapy. If taking corticosteroids, usual daily dose administered.

logic stress such as severe illness, injury, surgery, and general anesthesia. It is generally recommended that for illness not otherwise requiring medical attention (upper respiratory tract infection, and so on), the daily maintenance dose of corticosteroid should be doubled until the illness has resolved.[3] This standing recommendation does not necessarily take into account the magnitude of the stress and an estimate of "stress" cortisol requirement. A somewhat different situation exists in the patient with secondary AI from long-term administration of supraphysiologic doses of corticosteroid. In contrast to the patient with Addison's disease, the patient may still have some functioning adrenal cortex. Acute AI is prevented by avoiding rapid corticosteroid withdrawal and by the administration of supplemental corticosteroid for those situations associated with clinical stress.

In 1953, Lewis and colleagues described a patient on chronic cortisone therapy who died from AI several hours after orthopedic surgery.[26] Long-term suprapyhsiologic dose cortisone had been discontinued the day before surgery. This case resulted in recommendations for a prophylactic fourfold increase in corticosteroid dose before surgery. Although still controversial, recommendations for perioperative corticosteroid administration have been refined since this early description of adrenal crisis. For example, Salem and colleagues recommended that perioperative corticosteroids be replaced only in amounts equivalent to the normal physiologic adrenal response to surgical/anesthetic stress.[5] Therefore an understanding of the normal adrenal gland response to different clinical stressors has been a valuable addition to the knowledge base. Using data on daily cortisol secretion Salem et al concluded that the HPA axis response to minor surgery (short-duration procedure under local anesthesia) is probably minimal, and they recommend a daily equivalent corticosteroid target dose of hydrocortisone 25 mg.[5] If a patient is already receiving a daily corticosteroid dose that matches or exceeds the estimated stress requirement, additional doses are unnecessary. For example, if a patient's usual corticosteroid dose is prednisone 5 mg (equivalent to hydrocortisone 25 mg), no additional dose is required before minor surgery.

The magnitude of HPA axis stimulation and the normal production of "stress" cortisol with different dental procedures are unclear. However, based on the measurement of salivary cortisol concentration, Miller and colleagues demonstrated no significant elevation in salivary cortisol after dental examination, root canal therapy, and routine restorative treatments.[27] In fact, salivary cortisol levels decreased in these groups during the course of the procedure. In contrast, 30% of patients undergoing dental prophylaxis and 80% of those undergoing extraction experienced a statistically insignificant increase in salivary cortisol concentration. One hour after extraction, cortisol levels remained elevated, in contrast to the patients undergoing prophylaxis only. The authors speculate that these results were clinically significant because of the frequency of cortisol elevation with extraction. Although direct comparison between even minor surgical procedures and routine dental procedures is difficult, more complete data are available regarding the normal adrenal response to different levels of surgical and anesthetic stress.[4,5,28]

Most dental patients with chronic AI undergoing routine treatments are probably subjected to minimal clinical stress and require no supplemental corticosteroids in excess of daily maintenance doses. Likewise, the patient who has recently discontinued long-term corticosteroid use and is free of any corticosteroid withdrawal symptoms does not require supplemental doses for routine dental procedures. However, if supraphysiologic corticosteroid doses have been decreased or stopped abruptly, relative AI may occur. In this situation, the last regular daily dose of corticosteroid may be administered before the planned dental treatment. In general, the dentist should confer with a patient's primary physician to establish a safe and reasonable supplemental corticosteroid regimen for planned treatments in the setting of AI.

With regard to greater clinical stress, Kehlet estimated that adults secrete 50 mg of cortisol a day in response to "minor" surgery (minor orthopedic procedure) and 75 to 150 mg a day in response to "major" surgery (major abdominal, thoracic procedure).[28] For the patient subjected to "moderate" surgical stress (appendectomy, joint replacement, and so forth), Salem and colleagues recommend a supplemental daily equivalent corticosteroid dose of 50 to 75 mg of hydrocortisone for 1 to 2 days—a recommendation based on natural cortisol production.[5] Patients undergoing extractions, dentoalveolar surgery, periodontal surgery, and general anesthesia may be subject to "moderate" clinical stress. For the patient receiving corticosteroids, published recommendations to empirically double the daily dose in preparation for extractions, surgery, or similar stressful events fail to take into account estimates of normal stress cortisol production and the maintenance dose of corticosteroid.[29,30,31] For example, if a patient is taking a daily dose of 10 mg prednisone for systemic lupus erythematosus, doubling the maintenance dose in preparation for extractions provides the equivalent of 100 mg cortisol. If one assumes that the natural stress cortisol production with extractions is 25 to 50 mg, this supplemental prednisone dose is far in excess of the amount required to match natural stress cortisol production. In contrast to the patient receiving chronic supraphysiologic doses of corticosteroid, the patient with Addison's disease generally receives an unstressed daily maintenance dose of corticosteroid. Doubling the maintenance dose in preparation for extractions or a similar procedure is reasonable, as this dose approximates normal stress cortisol production for procedures associated with minor-to-moderate stress.

Depending on the severity of the infection, patients with odontogenic infection may also be subject to moderate clinical stress. Fever and decreased oral intake associated with significant infection may precipitate dehydration and adrenal crisis in the individual with compromised adrenal reserve. Consideration for in-hospital care to satisfy critical requirements for supplemental corticosteroid and fluid management must be considered in the treatment of the infected patient with AI.

Although unlikely to occur in the routine dental patient, major clinical stress (cardiac surgery, major abdominal surgery) should be matched with a corticosteroid dose equivalent of 100 to 150 mg of hydrocortisone for each day that the patient is subjected to the stress. Regardless of the cause of AI, there is little justification to ever exceed the equivalent of 200 to 300 mg of cortisol in the first 24 hours after surgery.[5]

Recent discussion regarding supplemental perioperative corticosteroid use has even questioned the necessity of matching normal "stress" adrenal cortisol production in the major surgical patient. Citing a number of studies demonstrating cardiovascular stability in patients receiving long-term corticosteroid therapy with either no or low-dose perioperative corticosteroid supplements, Henriques and Lebovic recommend limiting perioperative corticosteroid administration to those at risk, with risk determined by preoperative corticotropin stimulation test.[32-34]

In addition to these considerations, the dentist should effectively manage pain and anxiety in the dental patient at risk for AI. Adequate local anesthesia and careful postoperative pain management minimizes clinical stress in the patient with AI. Regardless of the cause of AI, the astute clinician must be sensitive to the development of signs or symptoms of impending adrenal crisis. Especially in the sedated patient, where the level of consciousness will be depressed pharmacologically, continuous blood pressure monitoring is important.

SUMMARY

Adrenal insufficiency is one of many medical conditions that may impact on the care of the dental patient. Through careful evaluation of each patient's past medical history, including medication history, the patient at risk for acute AI can be identified. In consultation with the primary physician, the dental clinician can design a management strategy that minimizes clinical stress and ensures adequate exogenous corticosteroids in advance of the dental procedure(s). If, in spite of these preventive efforts, adrenal crisis is precipitated, the knowledgeable clinician can provide life-saving treatment while awaiting advanced medical support.

REFERENCES

1. Federman DD: The adrenal. In Rubenstein E, Federman DD, editors: Scientific American medicine, *Sci Am* 3:IV, 1997.
2. August GP: Treatment of adrenocortical insufficiency, *Pediatr Rev* 18:59-62, 1997.
3. Werbel SS, Ober KP: Acute adrenal insufficiency, *Endocrinol Metab Clin North Am* 22:303-328, 1993.
4. Naito Y, Fakate J, Tamai S, et al: Biphasic changes in hypothalamo-pituitary-adrenal function during the early recovery period after major abdominal surgery, *J Clin Endocrinol Metab* 73:111-117, 1991.
5. Salem M, Tainish RE, Bromberg J, et al: Perioperative glucocorticoid coverage. A reassessment 42 years after emergence of a problem, *Ann Surg* 219:416-425, 1994.
6. Grinspoon SK, Biller BMK: Clinical review 62: laboratory assessment of adrenal insufficiency, *J Clin Endocrinol Metab* 79:923-931, 1994.
7. Kannan CR: Diseases of the adrenal cortex, *Disease-a-Month* 34:606-674, 1998.
8. Holland EG, Taylor AT: Glucocorticoids in clinical practice, *J Fam Prac* 32:512-519, 1991.
9. Kountz DS, Clark CL: Safely withdrawing patients from chronic glucocorticoid therapy, *Am Fam Phys* 55:521-525, 1997.
10. Treadwell BLJ, Savage O, Sever ED, et al: Pituitary-adrenal function during corticosteroid therapy, *Lancet* 1:355-358, 1963.
11. Jasani MK, Boyle J, Greig WR, et al: Corticosteroid-induced suppression of the hypothalamo-pituitary-adrenal axis: observations on patients given oral corticosteroids for rheumatoid arthritis, *QJM* 143:261-276, 1967.
12. Livanou T, Ferriman D, James VHT: Recovery of hypothalamo-pituitary-adrenal function after corticosteroid therapy, *Lancet* 2:856-859, 1967.
13. Ackerman GL, Nolen CM: Adrenocorticoid responsiveness after alternate-day corticosteroid therapy, *N Engl J Med* 278:405-409, 1968.
14. Schlaghecke R, Kornely E, Santen RT, et al: The effect of long-term glucocorticoid therapy on pituitary-adrenal responses to exogenous corticotropin-releasing hormone, *N Engl J Med* 326:226-230, 1992.
15. Axelrod L: Glucocorticoid therapy, *Medicine* 55:39-63, 1976.
16. Streck WF, Lockwood DH: Pituitary adrenal recovery following short-term suppression with corticosteroids, *Am J Med* 66:910-914, 1979.
17. LaRochelle GE, LaRochelle AG, Ratner RE, et al: Recovery of the hypothalamic-pituitary-adrenal (HPA) axis in patients with rheumatic diseases receiving low-dose prednisone, *Am J Med* 95:258-264, 1993.
18. Wood JB, Frankland AW, James VHT, et al: A rapid test of adrenocortical function, *Lancet* 1:243-245, 1965.
19. Glowniak JV, Loriaux DL: A double-blind study of perioperative steroid requirements in secondary adrenal insufficiency, *Surgery* 121:123-129, 1997.
20. Udelsman R, Ramp J, Gallucci WT, et al: Adaptation during surgical stress: a re-evaluation of the role of glucocorticoids, *J Clin Invest* 77:1377-1381, 1986.
21. Christy NP: Pituitary-adrenal function during corticosteroid therapy. Learning to live with uncertainty, *N Engl J Med* 326:266-267, 1992.
22. Graber AL, Ney RL, Nicholson WE, et al: Natural history of pituitary-adrenal recovery following long-term suppression with corticosteroids, *J Clin Endocrinol Metab* 25:11-16, 1965.
23. Glick M: Glucocorticoid replacement therapy: a literature review and suggested replacement therapy, *Oral Surg Oral Med Oral Pathol Oral Radiol Endod* 67:614-620, 1989.
24. Morris HG, Jorgensen JR: Recovery of endogenous pituitary-adrenal function in corticosteroid-treated children, *J Pediatr* 79:480-488, 1971.
25. Lamberts SWJ, Bruining HA, DeJong FH: Corticosteroid therapy in severe illness, *N Engl J Med* 337:1285-1292, 1997.
26. Lewis L, Robinson RF, Yee J, et al: Fatal adrenal corticoid insufficiency precipitated by surgery during prolonged continuous cortisone treatment, *Ann Intern Med* 39:116-125, 1953.
27. Miller CS, Dembo JB, Falace DA, Kaplan AL: Salivary cortical response to dental treatment of varying stress, *Oral Surg Oral Med Oral Pathol Oral Radiol Endod* 79:436-441, 1995.
28. Kehlet H: A rational approach to dosage and preparation of parenteral glucocorticoid substitution therapy during surgical procedures, *Acta Anesthiol Scand* 19:260-264, 1975.
29. Bahn SL: Glucocorticoids in dentistry, *J Am Dent Assoc* 105:476-481, 1982.
30. Kalkwarf KL, Hinrichs JE, Shaw DH: Management of the dental patient receiving corticosteroid medications, *Oral Surg* 54:396-400, 1982.
31. Little JW, Falace DA, Miller CS, et al: *Dental management of the medically compromised patient*, St. Louis, 1997, Mosby.
32. Kehlet H, Binder C: Adrenocortical function and clinical course during and after surgery in unsupplemented glucocorticoid treated patients, *Br J Anaesth* 45:1043-1048, 1973.
33. Symreng T, Karlberg BE, Kagedal B, et al: Physiological cortisol substitution of long-term steroid-treated patients undergoing major surgery, *Br J Anaesth* 53:949-953, 1981.
34. Henriques HF, Lebovic D: Defining and focusing perioperative steroid supplementation, *Am Surg* 61:809-813, 1995.

Hematologic Disorders

Thomas B. Dodson

The dentist plays an important role in the diagnosis and management of patients with hematologic disorders. Red blood cell (RBC) and white blood cell (WBC) disorders and human immunodeficiency virus (HIV) infections are common medical conditions. In addition, patients are living longer with their diseases in remission. Therefore individuals with hematologic disorders are likely to present to the dental office for treatment. Typically these patients can receive conventional dental treatment with minimal to no modifications in usual practice.

Hematologic disorders frequently have oral manifestations. As such, the dentist has the opportunity to diagnose and refer patients with hematologic disorders for early, appropriate care. For patients undergoing chemotherapy to manage their WBC disorders, the dentist plays a critical role in pretreatment evaluation. Since immunosuppressed patients may develop life-threatening infections, the dentist must identify and eliminate oral sources of infection before induction therapy.

RED BLOOD CELL DISORDERS
Anemia

Anemia is a common and frequently asymptomatic disorder that may go undiagnosed until the patient has a routine physical examination. Anemia is defined as a decrease in the number of circulating RBCs, decrease in hemoglobin, or decrease in the hematocrit. No single laboratory test, however, unambiguously defines anemia. The diagnosis of anemia is based on a combination of the history, physical findings, and laboratory data. For example, a pregnant woman will have a decreased hematocrit, RBC count, and hemoglobin concentration due to an increase in plasma volume during the third trimester, but anemia is not present. Conversely, a trauma patient who loses 1 liter of blood manifests signs of shock, but the usual RBC indices are within normal limits.

The major consequence of anemia is the reduction in oxygen-carrying capacity of the blood and associated tissue hypoxia. Although often symptomatic, symptoms may begin to appear as the hematocrit drops below 30%. Common but nonspecific complaints of anemic patients include fatigue, shortness of breath, headache, weakness, and dizziness. Clinical examination findings suggestive of anemia include pallor of the skin, increased heart rate at rest (tachycardia), or changes in blood pressure based on position (orthostatic hypotension). In patients with significant cardiac disease, anemia may present as chest pain due to cardiac ischemia or congestive heart failure. The differential diagnosis of anemia is based on RBC morphologic classifications—normochromic, hypochromic, and macrocytic or microcytic—and on kinetic analyses—blood loss, hemolytic disorders, or production defects (Box 27-1).

Kinetic analyses are useful in discriminating between blood loss and impaired RBC production as the major cause of anemia. If these major causes of anemia can be ruled out, then hemolytic causes of anemia should be considered. The major causes of anemia due to blood loss are gastrointestinal (GI) bleeding and excessive menstrual bleeding. Serum sampling of more than 300 ml of blood each week or frequent blood donations also can result in anemia.

Laboratory tests to assess RBC production include RBC count, reticulocyte count, hematocrit, and assessment of red cell morphology (Box 27-2). The clinical findings, laboratory data, and morphologic studies help to establish an initial differential diagnosis.

Acute Blood Loss

Acute blood loss and its source are usually obvious. In some cases, however, the cause is more subtle, with acute blood loss possibly resulting from retroperitoneal bleeding following iliac crest bone graft harvesting, or from bleeding into the soft tissues of the thigh or pelvis following a femur or pelvic fracture.[1] Persistent postoperative bleeding following dental extractions or periodontal surgery can necessitate additional treatment to achieve hemostasis and manage the symptomatic hypovolemia. The absence of an obvious bleeding source should prompt the clinician to initiate a work-up for an underlying coagulopathy. Presenting symptoms include hypotension, resting tachycardia, and low central venous pressure (CVP). Acute blood loss greater than 1 L will manifest as acute shock, and death can follow. Physiologic mechanisms for restoring blood volume operate slowly. The hematocrit

may not reach its new level until 3 days after the acute blood loss.[2] Immediate management of acute blood loss is replacement of volume with crystalloid (normal saline or lactated Ringer's), colloid (albumin solution). or blood transfusion. Crystalloids are administered in a 3:1 ratio (3 ml of crystalloid for each 1 ml of blood loss).

Iron Deficiency Anemia

Epidemiology and pathophysiology. From a public health perspective, iron deficiency anemia is a serious problem affecting an estimated 15% of the world population.[3] Common causes of iron deficiency anemia are chronic blood loss from the GI or genital tracts and diversion of iron from mother to child during pregnancy and lactation. Other causes can include dietary deficiency or iron malabsorption, though these are rare in developed countries.

As blood is lost, somatic iron stores are gradually depleted. As iron deficiency progresses, hemoglobin synthesis is compromised and anemia develops.[4] The absolute reticulocyte count is low or normal and a bone marrow biopsy reveals minimal erythroid hyperplasia, suggesting a severe production defect. To compensate, the body increases iron absorption. From a normal, unsupplemented diet, only 2 to 4 mg of iron per day is available for absorption.[5]

Box 27-1	Red Cell Morphology and Associated Types of Anemia
RBC MORPHOLOGY	**ANEMIA**
Microcytic, hypochromic	Iron deficiency Thalassemias
Macrocytic anemia	Vitamin B$_{12}$ deficiency Folate deficiency
Normochromic, normocytic	Anemia of chronic disease Acute blood loss Early iron deficiency

Box 27-2	Normal Hematologic Parameters
HEMATOLOGIC PARAMETER	**NORMAL RANGE**
White blood cell (WBC) count	4.5–11.0 K/mm^3
Hematocrit (Hct)	36%-46%
Hemoglobin (Hb)	12-16 g/dl
Red blood cell (RBC) count	4.0-5.2 million/mm^3
Platelet count	150-350 K/mm^3
Mean corpuscular volume (MCV)	80-100 μm^3
Mean corpuscular hemoglobin (MCH)	26-34 pg/RBC
Mean corpuscular hemoglobin concentration (MCHC)	31-37 g/dl
WBC DIFFERENTIAL	
Polymorphonucleocytes (PMNs)	40%-70%
Lymphocytes	22%-44%
Monocytes	4%-11%
Eosinophils	0-8%
Basophils	0-3%
Absolute neutrophil count	1.8-7.7 K/mm^3
Absolute lymphocyte count	1.0-4.8 K/mm^3
Absolute monocyte count	0.2-0.4 K/mm^3
Absolute eosinophil count	0.1-0.3 K/mm^3
Absolute basophil count	0.0-0.3 K/mm^3

K, Thousand cells.

Systemic symptoms of iron deficiency anemia include poor exercise tolerance, breathlessness, and fatigue. Iron deficiency during pregnancy is associated with increased risk for premature birth and perinatal mortality.[6] Iron deficiency can contribute to impaired motor and mental function in both children and adults.[3,6] Severe iron deficiency increases the risk for enteritis, chronic mucocutaneous candidiasis, and recurrent herpes simplex infection.[3,7] Other signs and symptoms of iron deficiency include cold intolerance, blue sclera, thrombocytosis, nail changes, GI mucosal atrophy (including oral mucosa), gastric achlorhyria, and pica.[8,9]

Diagnosis. Hypochromic and microcytic changes of erythrocytes seen on peripheral blood smears suggest iron deficiency anemia. Two common conditions that produce similar findings on blood smears are thalassemia trait, and anemia of chronic disease. Rare conditions confused with iron deficiency anemia include unstable hemoglobinopathies and sideroblastic anemias. In the United States, most cases of iron deficiency anemia are mild, with hemoglobin values ranging from 9 to 12 g/dl with near-normal RBC indices and morphology.[10] Typical RBC changes associated with iron deficiency anemia do not appear until severe iron deficiency develops. Borderline cases are difficult to diagnose, but low serum iron and iron-binding capacity (<15%) support a diagnosis of iron deficiency anemia. A good response to dietary iron supplementation—increase in hemoglobin of 2 g/dl in 3 weeks, or restoration of hemoglobin concentration to normal in 6 weeks—supports the diagnosis of iron deficiency anemia.[10]

Treatment. Iron replacement therapy is controversial and often ineffective due to the patient's intolerance of side effects. Although commonly prescribed, compound iron preparations, both slow release and enteric coated, are expensive and absorbed variably.[11,12] To avoid the issue of variable disintegration rates of the solid preparations, the practitioner should prescribe a liquid preparation ingested in a fasting state.[10] A recommended schedule for treatment is 5 ml of ferrous sulfate once a day, taken 30 minutes before a meal, for 1 week. During the second week the frequency is increased to two times per day, and in the third week to three times per day. This schedule results in the absorption of about 20 mg of iron per day and should be continued for 2 months.[10] Reasons for failure to respond to treatment include (1) an incorrect diagnosis, (2) continued GI or vaginal bleeding, (3) a concurrent inflammatory disorder that is blocking RBC

production, (4) a concomitant cobalamin or folic acid deficiency, (5) patient noncompliance with therapy, and (6) food, phosphates, or antacids inhibiting absorption.[10]

Hemolytic Anemia

Regardless of diagnosis, the final common denominator in all hemolytic anemias is an alteration of the erythrocyte cell membrane resulting in cell lysis or removal of damaged cells from the circulation by the reticuloendothelial macrophages. The severity of anemia is a function of the rate of RBC destruction and erythrocyte production. If erythrocyte production is not compromised, RBC survival time may be reduced as much as one-sixth normal without inducing anemia or jaundice.[13] There is a marked reticulocytosis. If a patient develops a systemic stress compromising erythrocyte production, hemoglobin levels drop dramatically, triggering an aplastic crisis.

Cell Membrane Defects

Disorders of salt and water metabolism are uncommon causes of hemolytic anemia. Examples include hereditary stomatocytosis and xerocytosis. Lipid abnormalities, such as vitamin E deficiency, contribute to hemolysis in premature infants. Hereditary protein abnormalities produce mild to severe hemolytic anemia. Individuals who have no immunologically identifiable components of the Rh antigen system develop a mild, compensated hemolytic condition.[13]

Hereditary elliptocytosis is an autosomal dominant disorder that appears to result from a lesion in the membrane cytoskeleton.[13] Prevalence estimates of this disorder range from 250 to 500 cases per million. Heterozygotes for this disorder can have abnormal peripheral blood smears characterized by the presence of elliptical erythrocytes and a mild, compensated hemolysis. Homozygotes can develop severe hemolytic anemia. Splenectomy may be indicated to manage symptoms. A variant of hereditary elliptocytosis is *hereditary pyropoikilocytosis*, an autosomal recessive trait that causes severe hemolysis in young children.[13] Peripheral blood smears demonstrate severe microcytosis and marked variation in red cell morphology. Splenectomy can reduce the hemolysis rate.

Inherited as an autosomal dominant trait, hereditary spherocytosis affects 220 people per million. Due to a decrease in the surface area of the erythrocyte, the cell assumes a microspherocytic shape and cannot deform adequately to pass through the spleen's vasculature. The spleen traps and destroys the red cells, producing hemolysis. Approximately 25% of affected patients are well compensated and manifest symptoms when physiologically stressed due to pregnancy or infection. Findings suggestive of hereditary spherocytosis include (1) predominant number of microspherocytes on peripheral smear, (2) mean corpuscular hemoglobin concentration (MCHC) above 35 g/dl, (3) reticulocytosis with mild jaundice and splenomegaly, and (4) positive family history. Treatment includes splenectomy, which controls the systemic manifestations of the disease.

Paroxysmal nocturnal hemoglobinuria (PNH) appears to be an acquired protein abnormality resulting in a hemolytic anemia. The erythrocyte defect is due to an abnormal susceptibility to complement.[13] Complement attacks the erythrocyte, producing lysis and intravascular hemolysis. The patient commonly reports the presence of blood in the urine (hemoglobinuria) on voiding after sleep.[14] Other systemic complications associated with PNH include venous occlusion and subsequent embolic episodes, and aplastic anemia.[15] Chronic hemoglobinuria may result in severe iron deficiency.[13]

Given signs of recurrent hemoglobinuria or venous thrombosis, the practitioner should consider the diagnosis of PNH. The RBCs of PNH patients do not show morphologic abnormalities. A bone marrow biopsy reveals marrow hypoplasia, which, in conjunction with hemolysis, is an important finding.[13] A reliable diagnostic modality is to measure the degree of hemolysis in acidified serum (Ham test).[16]

Treating PNH is challenging. Regular transfusions are indicated due to severe anemia. Fluoxymesterone (20 to 30 mg/day) increases hemoglobin by increasing RBC production.[17] Prednisone can decrease transfusion requirements.[18] Splenectomy is of little value. Hemolysis and venous occlusion due to stasis and trauma complicate surgical procedures. Warfarin used in the early postoperative period to induce a prophylactic anticoagulation can prevent venous occlusion and embolic events. Children and young adults are at risk for serious or fatal aplastic anemia. Allogeneic bone marrow transplants may be indicated in children and young adults as they are at risk for serious or fatal episodes of aplastic anemia.

Metabolic Defects

Reduced glutathione (GSH), NADH, and NADPH provide the RBC with reducing power. Insufficient stores of these agents result in ox-

---

Box 27-3	Drugs that Induce Hemolysis in G6PD-Deficient Patients

Antimalarials (primaquine, chloroquine)
Sulfonamides and sulfones (dapsone)
Analgesics (phenacetin, acetylsalicylic acid or aspirin)
Nitrofurans
Water-soluble vitamin K derivatives (menadiol)

---

idation of hemoglobin and membrane-bound proteins with production of Heinz bodies. Heinz bodies produce rigid RBCs that are selectively removed by the reticuloendothelial system.[13] Patients with defective GSH synthesis develop hemolysis due to oxidative attacks on the RBCs.

Glucose-6-phospate dehydrogenase (G6PD) catalyzes the conversion of NAPD+ to NADPH. Erythrocytes deficient in G6PD are susceptible to oxidation and subsequent hemolysis.[13] G6PD deficiency affects approximately 10% of African American males. After exposure to a drug or substance (fava bean) that produces oxidative stress, hemolysis may occur in the G6PD deficient patient (Box 27-3). Other stressors triggering hemolytic events are infection, diabetic ketoacidosis, or renal failure. The development of hemolytic anemia and the presence of bite cells or Heinz bodies suggest the diagnosis of G6PD deficiency. Critical to the management of G6PD deficiency is the avoidance of drugs known to produce hemolysis.

Defects in the glycolytic pathway can produce hemolysis. The most common disorder is a deficiency of pyruvate kinase (PK).[19] Hemolysis is of variable severity, and presenting signs include mild jaundice and splenomegaly. Peripheral blood smears reveal normal erythrocytes. Aplastic anemia occasionally develops, and infection due to parvovirus may be the etiologic stressor.[20] Splenectomy may be indicated for patients who require transfusions to manage PK deficiency. Other examples of defects in glycolysis producing hemolytic anemias are found in patients with hexokinase and glucophosphate isomerase deficiencies.[13]

Hemoglobinopathies

More than 100 different hemoglobinopathies have been described. Normal adult hemoglobin (hemoglobin A) is composed of two α and two β chains ($\alpha_2\beta_2$). Two α chains are required for all forms of hemoglobin. Variations in the β chains due to replacement by γ or δ chains or amino acid substitutions produce hemoglobinopathies. For example, valine substitution for the glutamate residue in the sixth position on the β chain produces hemoglobin S or sickle hemoglobin.[13]

Hemoglobinopathies are classified based on the underlying defect. Such defects include: (1) hemoglobin that tends to gel or crystallize (sickle cell anemia), (2) hemoglobin that is unstable (congenital Heinz body anemias), (3) hemoglobin that has unusual oxygen-binding properties (hemoglobin Chesapeake), or hemoglobin that readily oxidizes to methemoglobin (methemoglobinemia). Unequal rates of hemoglobin chain synthesis produce thalassemias. This discussion focuses on more common hemoglobinopathies, specifically sickle cell anemia and the thalassemias.

Sickle Cell Disease

Sickle cell anemia is inherited as an autosomal trait. In the heterozygous condition, sickle trait (HbAS) is common (affecting 8% to 10% of African Americans), and generally asymptomatic.[13] Patients who are homozygous for the condition (HbSS) have 70% to 98% of hemoglobin S type and manifest disease (sickle cell anemia).

Sickle cell disease has two primary manifestations: (1) chronic hemolysis that is debilitating but stable and (2) vaso-occlusive crises that are acute, episodic, and produce organ failure with significant morbidity and mortality. In the deoxygenated state, hemoglobin S polymerizes into long tubelike fibers which then causes erythrocyte sickling due to poor solubility of hemoglobin S.[13] Factors such as hypoxemia and acidosis promote deoxyhemoglobin S polymerization and subsequent RBC sickling. Deformed erythrocytes are removed from the circulation by the reticuloendothelial system. Hemolysis ensues with anemia of varying severity. The anemia is generally stable and well tolerated. Acute, vaso-occlusive sickle crises, however, are potentially life-threatening. Risk factors associated with sickle crises include an elevated hemoglobin level (>8.5 g/dl), pregnancy, cold weather, and a high reticulocyte count.[13] Avascular necrosis of the bone marrow is usually the source of pain.[21]

The diagnosis of sickle cell anemia is based on clinical presentation and the presence of sickled erythrocytes, holly leaf cells, and RBCs with Howell-Jolly bodies on a peripheral blood smear.[13] The clinical signs of sickle cell disease are due to a chronic, stable hemolysis producing anemia and jaundice. Common signs are

musculoskeletal pain or cholecystitis due to cholelithiasis. Liver disease is due to congestive heart failure, viral hepatitis secondary to blood transfusions, impaired liver blood flow due to sickling in the hepatic sinusoids. Acute lung complications include pneumonia and vascular occlusion of the pulmonary arterial system. Hypoxemia and pulmonary hypertension with cor pulmonale are chronic pulmonary complications. Renal failure contributes to death in up to 20% of the patients with HbSS.[13] Ocular complications include retinopathy, vitreous bleeding, and neovascularization. Patients with sickle cell disease are prone to infection due to hyposplenism and complement abnormalities. Sickle cell disease produces neurologic dysfunction due to stroke, subarachnoid hemorrhage, and focal areas of occlusion. Aplastic anemia may develop from bone marrow necrosis or viral infection.[20,22]

Medical management of sickle cell crises is primarily supportive and includes rest, hydration, and pain control. In the acidotic patient, administration of bicarbonate corrects acid-base abnormalities. Providing supplemental oxygen (2 to 5 L/min via nasal canula) also helps to decrease the concentration of HbS.[13] General anesthesia and intravenous sedation can increase the risk for a sickling crisis due to hypoxemia and vascular stasis. The risk of sickling crises and the value of prophylactic interventions is unknown.[23-25]

In contrast to sickle cell disease, patients with sickle trait are generally asymptomatic. Some reported complications include hyposthenuria and renal hematuria, bacteriuria, pyelonephritis, splenic infarction.[26,27] Management of renal hematuria includes hydration, diuretics, bicarbonate therapy, transfusion, or ε-aminocaproic acid.[13]

Thalassemias

The fundamental disorder in thalassemias is unbalanced synthesis of normal globin chains ($\alpha\beta_2$). When one of the chains is insufficiently produced, there is a relative excess of the other chain. Ineffective erythrocyte production results from the accumulation of the unpaired chain in RBC precursors and their subsequent cell death. The β-thalassemias result from diminished β-globin production and subsequent α-chain accumulation and aggregation. The intracellular α-chain aggregates precipitate and interfere with intracellular metabolism, induce cell surface abnormalities, and produce rigid, malformed cells.[28] The decrease in hemoglobin synthesis results in peripheral blood smears characterized by hypochromic target cells.

In principle, the α-thalassemias have an underlying globin synthetic defect similar to β-thalassemias, with different clinical manifestations. In α-thalassemias, patients accumulate an excess of β-globin chains, and aggregates occur in the presence of oxidative stressors such as infection. In contrast to β-thalassemias, α-thalassemias are characterized by destruction of circulating erythrocytes, not ineffective RBC production.[13]

Anemia due either to ineffective RBC production or destruction of peripheral circulating erythrocytes is the major complication of the thalassemias. β-*Thalassemia major*, also known as *Cooley's anemia*, is a homozygous condition that presents in the first year of life with jaundice, hepatosplenomegaly, erythroid marrow expansion, and increased infection risk. The anemia is severe and requires long-term transfusion therapy. The peripheral blood smear is characterized by the presence of nucleated erythrocytes and misshapen hypochromic cells with basophilic stippling.[13] Therapy focuses on maintaining adequate hemoglobin level (12 g/dl or greater) by aggressive RBC transfusions. Splenectomy may be indicated if hypersplenism results in significant pancytopenia. Bone marrow transplantation has also been used if HLA-matched sibling donors are available.[13]

β-*Thalassemia minor* is a heterozygous condition, and patients have mild or no anemia. The peripheral smear shows hypochromic, microcytic cells with basophilic stippling. Occasionally patients have enlarged spleens. Given the appearance of the peripheral smear, iron deficiency anemia needs to be considered in the differential diagnosis. Thalassemia trait patients have a relatively normal RBC count, while patients with iron deficiency anemia will have low RBC counts. It should be noted, however, that patients with thalassemia trait could also have iron deficiency anemia due to chronic blood loss.[15]

Extracorpuscular Defects

When patients present for management of hemolytic disorders and a negative history for anemia or hemolysis, the clinician should search for an extracorpuscular defect. The management of the defect depends on the diagnosis. Common diagnoses include microangiopathic hemolysis, immune (autoimmune and drug-induced) hemolysis, hypersplenism, hemolysis from toxins and physical agents, and systemic diseases such as liver or renal failure.

Although normal erythrocytes can withstand significant alteration in shape and form, supraphysiologic stresses cause cells to disintegrate, producing hemolysis.[29] Such stresses develop as blood passes through abnormal heart valves, arteriovenous shunts, ventricular septal defects, or heart valve prostheses. The diagnosis of *microangiopathic hemolysis* is suggested by the presence of hemolysis in conjunction with peripheral blood smears demonstrating the presence of oddly shaped, fragmented RBCs, such as schistocytes or helmet cells.[13] Management focuses on treating and correcting the underlying anatomic or mechanical disorder.

The development of acute, extravascular hemolysis suggests a diagnosis of *autoimmune hemolytic anemia* (AHA).[13] AHA can develop secondary to other diseases such as systemic lupus erythematosus, Hodgkin's or non-Hodgkin's lymphoma, cancer, myeloma, HIV, or chronic ulcerative colitis.[30] The spleen removes RBCs sensitized to IgG, while the liver removes cells sensitized to IgG and complement. Hemolytic severity is a function of the number and type of IgG molecules attached to the RBC surface. Asymptomatic patients are diagnosed by a positive Coombs' test when their blood is screened by a blood bank. Acute hemolytic episodes can result in change in the hematocrit from 45% to 15% in 48 hours. Patients develop jaundice and hepatosplenomegaly. Peripheral blood smears demonstrate multiple abnormal findings, including macrocytosis, polychromatophilia, spherocytosis, and autoagglutination of RBCs. The patient will have a positive direct Coombs' test.[13] Management consists of steroid therapy, splenectomy, or immunosuppressive drugs.

Immune hemolysis of varying severity and a positive direct Coombs' test may follow drug administration. Drugs such as penicillin and cephalosporins can elicit an immune response when administered in high doses.[13] Other drugs known to produce immune hemolysis include cisplatin, tolbutamide, methyldopa, levodopa, mefenamic acid, and procainamide.[13,31,32]

Hypersplenism, characterized by an enlarged spleen and hemolysis, occurs in a wide array of clinical conditions including hepatic cirrhosis, Gaucher's disease, lymphoma, connective tissue disorders, Felty's syndrome, sarcoidosis, and tuberculosis.[13] As part of normal function, the spleen removes defective RBCs from the circulation. An enlarged spleen has greater blood flow and thus exposes a larger than normal quantity of blood cells to its culling processes. If the spleen is not clinically palpable, but the diagnosis is suggestive of hypersplenism, ultrasonography or radioisotope scanning may be indicated. If an enlarged spleen is producing clinically significant symptoms and the underlying disorder cannot be corrected, splenectomy is considered.

Hemolysis may be caused by drugs, toxins, venoms, and other physical agents. Drugs such as dapsone, sulfasalazine, phenacetin, sodium perchlorate, nitroglycerin, primaquine, and vitamin K analogs can precipitate an oxidative attack on the RBCs, resulting in hemolysis and removal of the damaged cells by the reticuloendothelial system.[13] Snake venom and clostridial lecithinases attack erythrocyte membrane phospholipids producing cellular destruction with RBC fragmentation, spherocytosis, and intravascular and extravascular hemolysis. Accidental intravenous administration of sterile water causes intravascular hemolysis due to osmotic lysis.[13] While the main features of lead poisoning include colic, vomiting, constipation and peripheral neuropathy, lead exposure may produce a hemolytic, sideroblastic anemia.[13]

Hemolysis occurs in association with liver or kidney disease. The inflammatory aspect of hepatitis inhibits erythrocyte production, as does alcohol ingestion. Malnutrition may result in folate deficiency and macrocytic anemia due to ineffective erythropoiesis. Alcoholic gastritis and cirrhosis result in significant blood loss due to bleeding. Iron stores can be depleted by frequent blood donation. This is sometimes seen in derelict alcohol abusers using donation as a means of income. Splenomegaly and hypersplenic hemolysis can develop in the cirrhotic patient.[13]

Chronic renal disease can produce anemia through several different mechanisms. Erythropoiesis is impaired. Uremic colitis produces bleeding and chronic iron deficiency anemia. The diseased renal vasculature can cause microangiopathic hemolysis. An underlying inflammatory disorder can cause both renal disease and affect red cell production. Aluminum toxicity can develop in patients undergoing chronic hemodialysis, producing a hypochromic, microcytic anemia. Severe uremia is associated with hemolysis.[13] Other causes of hemolysis include hypophosphatemia, accumulation of copper, and cardiopulmonary bypass.

Cell Production Defects

Impaired erythrocyte production can cause anemia and can aggravate an ongoing anemic state produced by hemolysis or blood loss. Defects in erythrocyte production are associated with both normal and abnormal appearing bone marrow and as such bone marrow biopsy may be a useful diagnostic modality.

Anemia of chronic disease is associated with inflammatory or traumatic conditions, infections, neoplasms, alcoholic liver disease, congestive heart failure, renal disease, and diabetes mellitus. The anemia is of moderate severity and stable. Hematocrit levels range from 27% to 35%. The anemia is caused by decreased erythrocyte survival, lack of available iron due to iron being trapped in the reticuloendothelial system, and impaired erythropoiesis.

Clinically, anemia of chronic disease presents as a mild to moderate normochromic, normocytic anemia in conjunction with a chronic disease. It can, however, manifest as a hypochromic, microcytic anemia mimicking iron deficiency anemia or thalassemia trait. Diagnosing the underlying chronic disease is key to treating the anemia. Supplemental iron therapy will not help because the iron is trapped in the reticuloendothelial system. Pharmacologic doses of erythropoietin stimulate RBC production, thus avoiding transfusions.[33]

Severe renal disease can result in anemia due to poor RBC production, as well as other etiologies (see Hemolytic Anemia). Stimulation of RBC production by the use of erythropoietin is the mainstay of therapy. Poor caloric intake can affect erythrocyte production, producing anemia that can be corrected with proper nutrition. In general, elderly persons have normal RBC indices and hemoglobin levels. Aging is not necessarily associated with erythrocyte production defects. Anemia in the elderly needs appropriate work-up and should not be dismissed as a consequence of aging. Certain drugs cause production defects without associated marrow aplasia. These agents include ethanol, chloramphenicol, and arsenic. Endocrine disorders such as hypothyroidism, panhypopituitarism, and hyperparathyroidism are associated with RBC production defects and anemia. Correction of the underlying disorder is necessary.[33]

Pancytopenia or varying degrees of anemia, neutropenia, and thrombocytopenia suggest damage to the bone marrow. Bone marrow biopsies may demonstrate tumor, fat, or fibrotic connective tissue replacement of the marrow. Various drugs, agents, therapies (e.g., ionizing radiation, chemotherapy), inflammatory disorders, and premalignant or malignant conditions induce marrow aplasia. Regardless of etiology, marrow aplasia produces anemia, clotting disorders, and a significantly immunocompromised state.[33]

A paradoxical situation develops in the presence of anemia and an intense marrow hyperplasia. This clinical situation occurs when there is ineffective RBC production or hemolysis of RBCs in the marrow (*intramedullary hemolysis*). Disease states associated with impaired RBC production are megaloblastic anemias and thalassemias (see earlier).

Megaloblastic Anemia

The peripheral blood smears of megaloblastic anemias characteristically demonstrate macrocytosis, fishtail erythrocytes, hypersegmented neutrophils, and occasional nucleated erythrocytes. Bone marrow biopsies demonstrate megaloblastic erythroid hyperplasia. Cobalamin and folic acid deficiencies produce megaloblastic anemias. Exposure to nitrous oxide for as short as 6 hours may produce megaloblastosis. Chronic nitrous oxide exposure is associated with peripheral neuropathies similar to those seen with cobalamin deficiency. Neither folic acid nor cobalamin are produced in humans in adequate amounts and must be obtained from food.

Clinically, patients with *cobalamin deficiency* present with megaloblastic anemia, atrophy of the lingual papilla with glossitis, and peripheral neuropathy characterized by paresthesia, ataxia, limb weakness, and gait disturbance.[33] The diagnosis of cobalamin deficiency is confirmed by the patient's response to parenteral administration of cobalamin. Once the diagnosis is confirmed, the cause of the deficiency needs to be determined. The Schilling test is used to confirm the diagnosis of pernicious anemia due to anti–intrinsic factor antibodies.[33] If the Schilling test is negative, other causes of cobalamin deficiency, such as pancreatic insufficiency or a profound nutritional deficiency, need to be considered.[33] Management strategies focus on specific replacement of cobalamin. Transfusions may be indicated if the patient is symptomatic from the anemia.

In the absence of glossitis, peripheral neuropathies, and a negative family history of pernicious anemia, the practitioner should consider *folic acid deficiency* as the cause of megaloblastic anemia. Ethanol ingestion interferes with folate metabolism, lowers serum folate levels, and inhibits the erythrocyte response to folate administration.[26] As part of the work-up, serum should be obtained to determine folate, cobalamin, and RBC folate levels. Management consists of folate replacement (1 mg/day of folic acid).

Oral Manifestations

The oral findings in anemic patients are similar regardless of etiology. Mucosal pallor is a nonspecific finding. Glossitis and angular cheilitis suggest iron deficiency anemia but are nonspecific findings. Glossitis with lingual atrophy is associated with pernicious anemia. Spontaneous oral bleeding and evidence of opportunistic infection in association with mucosal pallor suggests an underlying pancytopenia due to marrow aplasia.

In the thalassemias and other anemias due to production defects, erythroid hyperplasia results in enlarged marrow spaces and associated radiologic findings (Figure 27-1). Generalized radiographic changes include cortical erosions, subcortical radiolucencies, and enlarged nutrient foramina or marrow spaces.[34] Changes seen on dental radiography include a generalized increase in the radiolucent appearance of the maxilla and mandible, thinning of the cortical bone (manifested as a thinning of the lamina dura), and enlarged marrow spaces and coarse trabeculations producing a chicken-wire pattern. Tooth roots may be short and the premaxilla prominent.[35] Skull films may reveal a "hair-on-end" appearance caused by cortical erosion of the skull.[34] In severe cases, pneumatization of the sinuses is delayed, or the bony enlargement obstructs the nasal cavity or middle ear.[34,36]

Complaints of glossodynia (burning tongue), although nonspecific, are reported by patients with thalassemias, iron deficiency anemia, and folic acid deficiency.[33,37,38] As such, dentists seeking to treat these oral symptoms are well positioned to make the initial diagnosis and referral. Nonspecific physical findings include atrophy of lingual papilla, an erythematous appearing tongue, mucosal ulceration, and erythematous mucosal patches.[33,37-43] Random biopsies from patients with pernicious anemia show epithelial atrophy, increased mitotic activity in the basal epithelial level, and binucleate epithelial cells in the prickle layer. These changes can be reversed with hydroxycobalamin therapy.

Dental Treatment

As most dental care is elective, treatment may be deferred pending consultation with the pa-

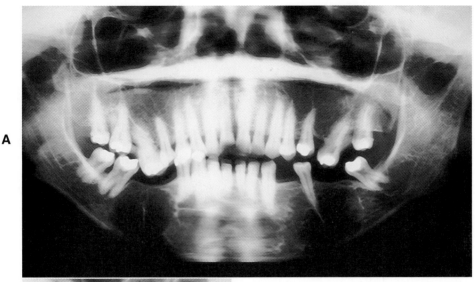

A

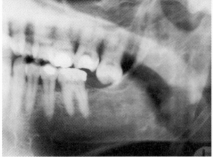

B

Figure 27-1. **A,** Honeycomb radiolucencies in the mandible and maxilla, characteristic of thalassemia. **B,** Abnormal trabecular pattern of sickle cell anemia. *From Sapp JP, Eversole LR, Wysocki GW: Contemporary oral and maxillofacial pathology, St Louis, 1997, Mosby.*

tient's primary care physician or hematologist. Most dental procedures produce minimal physiologic stress and blood loss. In many patients the anemia is chronic. The patient therefore may be well compensated for the anemic state and stable. As such, most patients with these disorders should be able to undergo routine dental treatment with little intervention or alteration in treatment due to their underlying disease.

Routine vital signs such as heart and respiratory rates or blood pressure may be valuable in making the early diagnosis of anemia. Findings such as tachycardia at rest, increased respiratory rate, or orthostatic hypotension are suggestive of anemia. The dental management of patients with anemia depends on their risk stratification. For example, low-risk patients may undergo routine dental treatment with little or no change in the planned treatment protocol. Low-risk patients include those with (1) a past history of anemia, asymptomatic, corrected, with normal hematocrit or (2) mild anemia, diagnosed, hematocrit greater than 30%, with or without

treatment. High-risk patients include those with (1) undiagnosed anemia and abnormal RBC indices, (2) hematocrit less than 30% and no identifiable cause, (3) evidence of persistent bleeding, (4) associated coagulopathy, or (5) a requirement of repeated RBC transfusions to alleviate their symptoms. For high-risk patients, routine, elective treatment should be deferred until the patient's clinical status is optimized. After the patient's clinical status is optimized, the dentist should consider shorter appointments and the use of adjunctive sedation techniques to relieve physiologic stress.

Modification of routine practice is indicated for some specific conditions. Asplenic patients may need prophylactic antibiotics because they are at increased risk for infection.[44] In some conditions, blood transfusion is the management keystone. Consequently, these patients are at risk for acquiring transfusion-associated infections, such as HIV or hepatitis. Supplemental oxygen (2 L/min via nasal canula) may be indicated when treating patients with sickle cell anemia. No treatment modifications are indicated for patients with sickle cell trait. Certain drugs precipitate the development of a hemolytic anemia for patients with G6PD deficiency and should be avoided.

WHITE BLOOD CELL DISORDERS

WBC disorders are characterized by a proliferation of an abnormal clone of hematopoietic cells. These abnormal WBCs respond poorly to normal mechanisms of regulation, tend to differentiate abnormally, and have an expanding clonal cell line that is detrimental to the normal development of other hematopoietic cells. The adverse consequences of leukemias result from the expanding cell lines that infiltrate the marrow, producing marrow aplasia and death due to infection or bleeding. The leukemic cells cause symptoms and organ failure by infiltrating the liver, spleen, lymph nodes, meninges, and gingiva.[45] The leukemias are classified based on the cell line involved and on the acuity or chronicity of the disease. Myeloid leukemias affect myeloid stem cells. Lymphocytic leukemias affect lymphoid cell lines.

The diagnosis of leukemia depends on cytologic and morphologic findings. Confirmation of the diagnosis depends on finding abnormal cells in the circulation and on the presence of abnormal cells replacing normal blood cell elements in the marrow. Treatment depends on the specific diagnosis, with goals ranging from inducing remission to producing a cure. Treatments include intense chemotherapy or bone marrow transplantation (BMT) and have significant morbidity and mortality.

Chemotherapy has various treatment phases. During the induction phase, the treatment goal is to reduce or eliminate the leukemic cell burden and induce clinical remission. Consolidation or cytoreduction therapy is the second phase, in which residual leukemic cells are destroyed. A final stage is sometimes used to destroy any residual leukemic cells by intense chemotherapy while the patient is in complete clinical remission. As a consequence of the underlying disease and the myelosuppressive aspects of chemotherapy, infection and bleeding can limit the intensity of treatment.

Bone Marrow Transplantation

BMT is used to treat acute leukemias and chronic myeloid leukemia.[45] The goal of BMT is to restore normally proliferating stem cells. The bone marrow donor may be the patient, an identical twin, or a histocompatible donor, most commonly a sibling. A more inclusive term for this treatment is *hematopoietic stem cell transplantation* because the source of stem cells can be peripheral or umbilical cord blood in addition to bone marrow.

BMT carries considerable morbidity and mortality. Early complications develop almost immediately and include nausea, vomiting, and mild skin erythema. Oral mucositis develops 5 to 7 days after transplantation. About 10 days after transplantation, alopecia and marked granulocytopenia develop.[46] In 10% to 20% of patients, veno-occlusive disease of the liver will develop, producing ascites, hepatomegaly, jaundice, and fluid retention.[47] Most pneumonias that develop are caused by microbial infection, but in 5% to 10% of cases, it is a direct result of pulmonary injury due to the chemotherapeutic agent.[48]

Late complications of BMT include impaired growth and development of secondary sex characteristics.[49] In postpubertal women and men, ovarian failure and azoospermia often develop.[50] High-dose glucocorticoid therapy can be used to treat or prevent graft-versus-host disease (GVHD), with the associated consequences of steroid therapy. Patients are at risk for developing secondary malignancies.[51,52] A major treatment complication is graft failure and loss of marrow function.

Graft-versus-Host Disease

GVHD is a consequence of transplanting allogeneic T cells that react with the genetically different host. As early as 3 months after transplantation, GVHD may present with a rash on the palms or soles, anorexia, diarrhea, and liver disease.[53] Soft tissue biopsies of the skin, liver or gastrointestinal tract confirm the diagnosis. Risk factors for GVHD are increasing age, poor tissue match, and inadequate therapy to prevent GVHD.[54] Manifestations of chronic GVHD include a malar rash, sclerodermatous changes, sicca syndrome, obliterative bronchiolitis, and arthritis.[55] In most cases the GVHD resolves, but, while being treated with immunosuppressive agents, the patients are susceptible to bacterial infections and may be receiving prophylactic antibiotics.

Early after transplantation, patients become severely granulocytopenic. Patients develop fever, with positive blood cultures in a third of the cases. These patients are treated with broad-spectrum antibiotics. Death from infection in these patients can be as high as 5%.[46] In addition to bacterial infections, the patients are at risk for infection from fungal or viral agents.

Chronic Myeloid Leukemia

Chronic myeloid leukemia (CML) has three disease stages: (1) chronic stable, (2) accelerated, and (3) blast crisis.[45] CML is characterized by the presence of the Philadelphia chromosome.[45] A hypermetabolic state and hepatosplenomegaly are the early signs of CML. Patients have a moderate anemia with nucleated RBCs seen on a peripheral smear. Platelets are large and the platelet count is very variable. The WBC count is high (50,000 to 3 million/µl), but there is orderly progression of neutrophil maturation. During the accelerated phase the spleen and liver enlarge and there is progressive thrombocytopenia and anemia. Patients develop bone pain, fever, weight loss, and night sweats. The involvement of extramedullary sites (e.g., lymph nodes, bone, soft tissues) indicates accelerated disease. The symptoms become more severe during the blast phase.

During the chronic stable phase, hyperuricemia is common and treated with allopurinol. High WBC counts can produce emboli lodging in the pulmonary, cerebral, and retinal vasculature, producing ischemic damage to the involved organs and tissues. Allogeneic BMT is the treatment of choice for otherwise healthy patients who have a fully matched sibling donor because it offers a potential for cure.[45] In the accelerated and blast crisis phase, treatment is less effective. The 5-year survival after BMT in the accelerated phase ranges from 25% to 83% and up to 15% for those in the blast crisis phase.[56]

Acute Myeloid Leukemia

Acute myeloid leukemia (AML) is an aggressive malignancy with survival ranging from 40 to 100 days if left untreated. After treatment of a different malignancy, AML may develop. For example, several years after treating Hodgkin's disease, about 5% of cases develop a subacute form of AML.[45] AML evolves slowly, with a prodrome lasting several days to weeks, characterized by fatigue, bleeding, and fever due to infection. Physical signs that develop include petechiae, sternal tenderness, adenopathy, and hepatosplenomegaly. Bone marrow biopsies reveal a myeloblastic infiltrate replacing normal marrow tissues. Due to the near total replacement of marrow elements, patients develop anemia,

thrombocytopenic bleeding, and neutropenic infection. The marrow morphologic examination is complemented by cytogenetic analyses to refine the diagnosis.[45]

Treatment carries significant risk. Induction therapy for AML averages over a month of hospitalization. During hospitalization, the patient will be aplastic for 20 to 30 days and is at risk for bacteria, fungi, and viral infection. Regular platelet and RBC transfusions are administered. Factors affecting prognosis include the patient's age, general well-being, and cytogenetic abnormalities. The treatment focus has changed from inducing a complete remission to obliteration of the residual clonal leukemic blast cells. Treatment goals are to prolong remission and the disease-free interval. Postremission therapy consists of a series of high-dose chemotherapy.[45]

Chronic Lymphocytic Leukemia

Chronic lymphocytic leukemia (CLL) involves a clonal disorder of morphologically mature B lymphocytes. Patients with CLL can develop hypo- or hypergammaglobulinemia, autoimmune hemolytic anemia, and immune thrombocytopenic purpura. The clinical presentation ranges from mild adenopathy and splenomegaly to marked pancytopenia and nodal enlargement with organomegaly and recurrent infection. The absolute mature lymphocyte count varies between 10,000 and 100,000/mm^3. The clinical course depends on the degree of marrow infiltration and replacement by tumor cells.

CLL is diagnosed by an absolute lymphocytosis of 5000 to 10,000 WBCs/µl with a B-cell clonal pattern. Lymph node or marrow biopsies reveal a diffuse, well-differentiated small cell infiltrate. Treatment consists of managing the complications of CLL including hemolytic anemia and thrombocytopenic purpura. Repeated infections require antibiotic therapy. Local disease is treated with radiation therapy.[45] Chemotherapy is indicated as patients become more symptomatic, evidenced by falling RBC and platelet counts with enlarging lymph nodes. Splenectomy is occasionally indicated if the spleen becomes painful.

Acute Lymphoblastic Leukemia

In adults, acute lymphoblastic leukemia (ALL) is less common than AML and represents about 15% of the acute leukemias. ALL is subdivided into categories based on immunologic markers.

These markers have prognostic and therapeutic value, with the B-cell variants having a poorer response. The pathophysiology and clinical manifestations of ALL are not markedly different from AML, except CNS disease is more common in ALL.[57] Poor prognostic risk factors include a peripheral blood blast count greater than 50,000/μl and patients older than 30 years. Treatment consists of an induction phase followed by sequential courses of chemotherapy to obliterate malignant cells.

ORAL MANIFESTATIONS

Patients with WBC disorders frequently have oral findings suggesting the diagnosis. As such, dentists are in a position to identify leukemic patients presenting for routine dental treatment. In one study, 13% of the patients with leukemias had the initial symptoms evaluated and a diagnosis made by a dentist.[58] General somatic complaints are fatigue, shortness of breath, and night sweats. On physical examination there may be skin and mucosal pallor, fever, skin bruising, lymphadenopathy, and hepatosplenomegaly. Oral symptoms include mouth pain due to tooth or mucosal lesions and bleeding or enlarged gingiva.[59] The tooth pain may be caused by infection but also by leukemic cells infiltrating the dental pulp.[60] Oral physical examination reveals mucosal pallor, ecchymosis, ulcerations due to viral infection (herpes simplex), or gingival, tonsillar, or submucosal leukemic infiltrates presenting as enlarged tissues.[61]

Dental Management
Pretreatment Evaluation

For patients with a newly diagnosed hematologic malignancy, a dental examination before initiating chemotherapy is mandatory. During a 3-year period, 398 patients were referred for evaluation and treatment of dental problems that developed while the patients were undergoing cytotoxic treatment for tumors, including leukemias. Most of the problems were treatable with proper medical and dental support either before or between courses of chemotherapy.[62] In related studies, Bergmann assessed the risk of fever due to oral infection for patients undergoing immunosuppressive treatment of hematologic malignancy.[63,64] In 14.1% of the episodes, acute oral infection was the only identifiable source of fever. In 25.6% of the febrile episodes, acute oral infection or an extraoral site may have

been the cause of fever. Bergmann concluded that the prevention or elimination of oral infections prior to induction therapy might reduce the morbidity of chemotherapy for leukemias.

The major goal of pretreatment dental examinations is to identify and eliminate any sources of oral infection. What is a straightforward problem in the immunocompetent patient becomes a significant management issue for the neutropenic or thrombocytopenic patient undergoing chemotherapy. Diagnosis of periodontal, pulpal, or pericoronal infections is difficult in neutropenic patients due to lack of immune response.

Since WBC disorders often affect children or young adults who may be undergoing orthodontic treatment, the fixed appliances and retainers should be removed to facilitate hygiene and eliminate mucosal irritants.[65] In the otherwise healthy patient, extraction of asymptomatic impacted teeth is controversial. For patients preparing to undergo induction chemotherapy, however, the removal of asymptomatic wisdom teeth is indicated. The rationale for this recommendation is based on (1) the increased risk for complications due to bleeding, infection, or poor wound healing if the extraction must be done after chemotherapy is initiated and (2) the probability that the management of the impacted tooth will interfere with cancer treatment. Chemotherapy may need to be interrupted to permit the marrow to recover.[66]

In addition to the oral surgical treatments, any needed restorative treatment and professional dental cleanings should be rendered in an efficient manner. It is critical to review oral hygiene, including the use of mechanical aids such as the toothbrush and floss. Trays should be prepared and used to administer fluoride after chemotherapy starts.

Chemotherapy

Leukemia treatment frequently produces profound stomatologic side effects including oral infections from gram negative enteric bacteria, viruses, and yeast; cytotoxic mucositis; and oral bleeding.[62,67-69] Up to 80% of patients receiving cytotoxic treatment for acute leukemia developed oral complications.[61,67,68] While patients are undergoing active chemotherapy, daily hygiene with mechanical aids such as the toothbrush and floss should be performed as long as the granulocyte counts are greater than 500/μl and the platelet count is greater than 40,000/μl. When the granulocyte or platelet counts drop below these levels, the patient should try to maintain hygiene using a toothette or moistened cloth. The prophylactic use of chlorhexidine mouthrinse to prevent oral complications associated with cytotoxic treatment is unclear.[68,70-74] Advocates of chlorhexidine have little data to support their claims in the face of known side effects, including staining teeth and discomfort with use. For patients who can maintain hygiene with mechanical means, there is little incremental value in using chlorhexidine.

Oral mucositis is a common, serious complication of cytotoxic treatment. It manifests as a burning sensation of the mucosa and is followed 2 to 7 days later by painful, persistent oral mucosal erosions and ulcerations. Keratinized and nonkeratinized mucosa are affected.[67] The mucositis is associated with significant pain and disability resulting in treatment modification such as suspension of treatment or implementation of parenteral nutrition.[75] In addition, the loss of oral mucosal integrity increases the risk for seeding of bacterial or yeast infections. Risk factors for the development of mucositis in the BMT patients include low marrow cell dose, prolonged aplastic episodes, herpes simplex positivity, and conditioning with total body irradiation.[76]

While maintaining good oral hygiene is important for preventing oral infections, it is not clear that aggressive oral hygiene significantly affects outcome in terms of preventing or modulating the symptoms of oral mucositis.[77] Symptomatic relief, wound care, and the use of 0.12% chlorhexidine with broad antibiotic therapy are indicated in the management of patients with oral stomatitis. Prophylactic administration of acyclovir (400 mg bid) was compared to placebo in a randomized clinical trail to determine if acyclovir reduced the risk of oral ulcers in patients treated for AML. Acute oral ulcerations developed in 25 of 37 patients in the treatment group versus 36 of 37 in the control group (relative risk, .69; 95% confidence interval, 0.55 to 0.87; $p < 0.05$). Excluding the soft palate, most oral ulcerations were caused by the herpes simplex virus.[78]

A major dental challenge is managing an odontogenic infection in the neutropenic patient. The lack of an inflammatory response makes it difficult to localize the source of infection. In addition, neutropenia produces a minimal host response to infection increasing our reliance on antibiotic therapy. Isolating the etiologic bacteria is difficult, making the antibiotic choice for therapy challenging. The best way

to avoid this clinical scenario is to identify and eliminate any potential sources of dental infection before induction therapy. However, despite best efforts, dentists will need to care for patients who are neutropenic and develop orofacial infections.[79]

Management of severe orofacial infections in the neutropenic patient is based on the concept of sequential addition of antibiotics based on response to therapy.[79] The initial antibiotic therapy used is a β-lactam/aminoglycoside combination, followed by the addition of metronidazole to intensify anaerobic coverage, and then a β-lactamase stabilizing agent. Of particular importance are the changing bacterial flora associated with oral infections in the neutropenic patient. Most often, as the WBC count drops, patients become colonized with gram-negative enteric bacteria such as *Klebsiella*, *Enterobacter*, *Pseudomonas*, and *Escherichia coli*. [80]

Remission

As treatment improves, patients will live longer and seek routine dental care. One consideration is the patient's long-term immunosuppressed state prior to initiating any invasive therapy. A consultation with the patient's hematologist or oncologist is indicated. Elective treatment, such as implants, extensive restorative care, extractions, endodontic or periodontal therapy, depends as much on the patient's desires as on their medical status. In advanced stages of disease, treatment is limited to more urgent or emergent care. Transfusion therapy may be indicated, depending on the patient's preoperative hematologic parameters. Chronic corticosteroid use increases the risk for postoperative complications such as infection or poor wound healing. For patients with hypogammaglobulinemia due to CLL, perioperative antibiotic therapy may decrease the risk of postoperative complications. In consultation with the hematologist, one can use immunoglobulin therapy to enhance immune function.[81-83] Caution is needed when treating the immunocompromised patient, but treatment should not be delayed or compromised. During active chemotherapy, elective dental care is provided between courses of treatment, when the patient's hematologic parameters have recovered and been optimized.[84]

Teeth are prone to caries due to chemotherapeutic-induced xerostomia.[85] A recent study, however, noted that children with ALL treated with chemotherapy and/or cranial radiotherapy did not have an increased risk for caries.[86] The children did, however, have higher plaque and periodontal index scores, a finding that underscores the need for aggressive oral care.

Growing children receiving radiation to the skull can develop skeletal or dental deformities.[87,88] In one study, 11 of 14 patients who had received BMT as children (mean age at diagnosis, 8 years) to treat leukemia had dental abnormalities, including agenesis, crown opacity and hypoplasia, and impaired root development.[85]

The granulocyte and platelet counts are used to guide dental treatment. If the granulocyte count is greater than 2000/µl, routine dental treatment may be provided. For lower granulocyte counts, antibiotic prophylaxis is indicated. For platelet counts greater than 40,000/µl, routine treatment can be administered. Bleeding problems become more likely as the platelet count drops below 40,000/µl. There is small likelihood of significant bleeding following dental treatment if the patient's platelet count is greater than 20,000/µl, *as long as the patient's platelets are effective*. Platelet counts under 20,000/µl usually require transfusion before tooth extraction.

Graft-versus-Host Disease

GVHD is caused by an adverse immunologic reaction between the host and transplanted tissues. In this discussion the major cause of GVHD is transplantation of bone marrow from one individual to another. By definition, acute GVHD develops within 100 days of BMT. Clinical findings include xerostomia, mucosal inflammatory lesions involving the conjunctiva, GI tract (mouth and esophagus), liver disease, and scleroderma-like skin lesions.[89] Chronic GVHD develops in 25% to 40% of long-term survivors, and 80% of affected patients have oral lesions.[55] The clinical oral findings of GVHD are not unique and diagnosis is based on history and exclusion of other disease entities. Acute oral findings include mucositis, xerostomia, pain, and bleeding. Chronic findings include mucosal atrophy and erythema, pain, and lichenoid lesions.[90]

Treatment of GVHD focuses on prevention and limiting the morbidity of the disease. Prophylactic extraction of diseased teeth and the removal of dental appliances are indicated before BMT. After BMT, topical steroids, analgesics, salivary substitutes, or stimulants should be used in conjunction with maintenance of excellent oral hygiene. There may be a role for topical cyclosporin in the management of GVHD.[91]

HUMAN IMMUNODEFICIENCY VIRUS INFECTION
Pathophysiology and Diagnosis

HIV is a ribonucleic acid (RNA) virus. The virus selectively infects macrophages and the CD4+ lymphocytes. HIV infection frequently leads to the development of HIV disease that manifests itself by varying degrees of immunosuppression. HIV infection, the cause of an incurable communicable disease (AIDS), is spread by sexual contact, by contact with infected blood, and from pregnant mother to fetus. After initial infection, the patient can manifest flulike symptoms but is commonly asymptomatic for many months. After several weeks to months, the patient develops antibodies to the HIV and becomes positive (HIV+). The progression of HIV infection ranges from asymptomatic infection to AIDS, with associated life-threatening opportunistic infections and malignancies. HIV infection is diagnosed using a screening test (ELISA) to identify antibodies to proteins expressed by HIV-infected cells. If the screening test is positive, a Western blot is performed to confirm the diagnosis.

Until recently, HIV disease was a progressive, terminal illness. Advances in management of HIV disease have changed it from a terminal to a chronic disease. As such, dentists will be seeing more patients with HIV infection. Dentists should be prepared to recognize and manage the oral manifestations of HIV disease. In addition, some of the oral manifestations are important in terms of staging HIV disease.

Oral Manifestations

HIV infection produces multiple oral manifestations that are often symptomatic, require intervention, and are important for diagnostic or classification purposes. A common oral mucosal lesion is *candidiasis*.[92-94] A patient with a transient oral candidiasis in association with an acute viral syndrome should be screened for HIV infection if other common causes (diabetes, chronic antibiotic use) can be ruled out.[95] Risk factors for the development of oral candidiasis include xerostomia, decreased CD4+ counts, and age. Symptoms of candidiasis include oral burning or discomfort and dysguesia. Oral pain can be so severe, especially in conjunction with esophageal candidiasis, that oral intake is compromised. Clinical findings include either pseudomembranous (white or creamy colonies) or erythematous lesions on the oral mucosa or angular cheilitis (Figure 27-2).

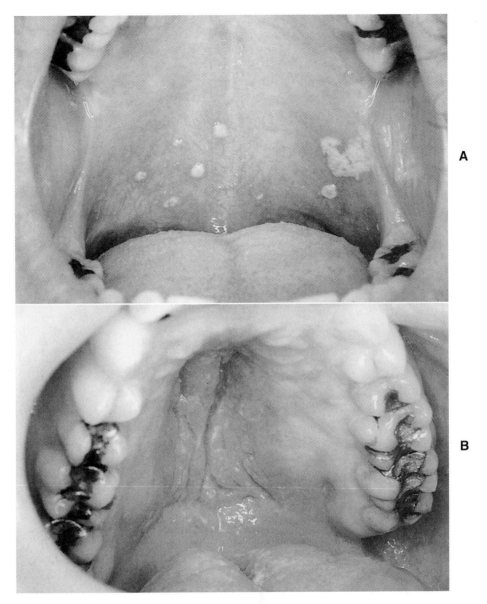

Figure 27-2. Two forms of candidiasis typically found in AIDS patients: **A,** pseudomem-branous; **B,** erythematous. *From Silverman S: Color atlas of oral manifestations of AIDS, ed 2, St Louis, 1996, Mosby.*

Another common oral manifestation of HIV disease is *hairy leukoplakia*, which is caused by Epstein-Barr virus. This lesion is important because it is strongly associated with an immunodeficient condition (e.g., HIV disease). The lesions are generally asymptomatic and found as incidental findings. Clinically the lesions present as white plaques with a flat or corrugated surface on the lateral borders of the tongue. The lesions do not scrape off. Microscopic evaluation reveals characteristic find-ings, including hyperparakeratoic folds ("hairs"), acanthosis, vacuolation of bands or clumps of prickle cells, and little associated submucosal in-flammation.[92] Because the clinical appearance is so characteristic, biopsy is rarely indicated. Leuko-plakic lesions are generally asymptomatic and do not require treatment.[93] Antiviral agents do pro-vide temporary regression of the lesions.

HIV-infected patients appear to be at in-creased risk for having unusual or severe forms of periodontal disease, including linear gingival erythema (LGE), necrotizing gingivitis, and necrotizing periodontitis. LGE is distinctly different from marginal gingivitis. Specifically, in the presence of marginal gingival inflammation, patients with LGE have a notable lack of plaque accumulation.[92,96,97]

Necrotizing gingivitis in the HIV-positive patient appears to be the same entity as seen in the HIV-negative patient.[96] Necrotizing gingivitis, also known as *acute necrotizing ulcerative gingivitis*, is characterized by rapid development of symptoms, including marginal gingival necrosis, spontaneous bleeding, fetid breath, pain, and possible fever or regional lymphadenopathy. A pseudomembrane composed of necrotic tissue, inflammatory cells, and microorganisms covers the gingiva. An increase in the proportion of fusiform organisms and spirochetes mark the condition. While superficially similar, necrotizing periodontitis can be differentiated from necrotizing gingivitis on the basis of longer duration of onset (weeks to months versus days) and the presence of bone loss and exposed, necrotic alveolar bone.

Both nonspecific ulcers (aphthous stomatitis, minor and major) and specific ulcers due to viruses are a significant problem for the HIV-positive patients. As with the patient undergoing chemotherapy for WBC disorders, the symptoms from the stomatitis can be debilitating. As successful treatment is based on the correct diagnosis, it is important to discriminate between nonspecific and specific oral ulcerations. Oral pain and localization of the lesions to nonkeratinized mucosal surfaces characterize aphthous or nonspecific oral stomatitis. Regional lymphadenopathy may be present. The etiology of aphthous stomatitis is unknown. The lesions are variable in size, covered by a necrotic pseudomembrane, and ringed with erythema. The diagnosis is commonly made by exclusion. Other causes include malignancy, bacterial infection (e.g., syphilis, cryptococcus), or viral infection. A biopsy or cytologic smear is indicated if the presentation is unclear.

Viral causes of oral ulcerations include herpes simplex and cytomegalovirus (CMV) infections. Primary *herpetic stomatitis* involves the lips and gingiva with lesions composed of blisters and ulcers. Fever, malaise, and regional lymphadenopathy are often present. Recurrent herpetic lesions tend to localize on keratinized surfaces such as the hard palate, attached gingiva, and lips. The diagnosis is based on history, physical examination, and culture. Varicella-zoster virus can cause oral and facial herpes zoster. The intraoral lesions can occur anywhere but usually are distributed in a unilateral manner. CMV infection can produce ulcers anywhere in the mouth, including the oropharynx and esophagus, producing mouth pain and dysphagia.[93] The diagnosis of CMV infection is based on biopsy. Uncommon lesions found in HIV+ patients include precancerous leukoplakia or erythroleukoplakia, lichen planus, white sponge nevus, leukoedema, and squamous cell carcinoma.[93]

Other oral diseases and conditions include xerostomia and salivary gland dysfunction, increased risk for dental caries, and tumors such as Kaposi's sarcoma and non-Hodgkin's lymphoma.[92,93,98,99] It is also suspected that HIV+ patients have a higher risk for complications from odontogenic infections and operative treatment.

The operative results following oral and maxillofacial surgical procedures, however, have been mixed. Some studies suggest that HIV+ patients have an increased risk for postoperative complications. One study found that the postoperative infection rate after the treatment of mandibular fractures was significantly higher in HIV-positive patients compared with HIV-negative patients.[100] Furthermore, a retrospective study found that when comparing HIV-positive and HIV-negative patients, HIV+ patients had an increased risk of postoperative infection after tooth extraction. In addition, the complication rates increased with the severity of HIV disease.[101]

Other studies, however, report no significant differences in postoperative complication rates between HIV-positive and HIV-negative patients after oral and maxillofacial surgical procedures. One study found that the overall complication rate for various dental procedures was 0.9% in HIV+ patients with a CD4 count less than 200 cells/mm^3.[102] Another study found no difference in infection rates after dental extractions when comparing HIV-positive and HIV-negative patients.[103] Also, prophylactic antimicrobials are probably not required for dental extractions in the HIV+ population.[98,104]

Dental Management

The treatment of oral candidiasis includes both topical and systemic antifungal therapy. Oral topical agents include clotrimazole and nystatin. An antifungal cream is useful in managing angular cheilitis. Systemic antifungal agents used in managing oral candidiasis include fluconazole and ketoconazole. The role for mouth rinses such as chlorhexidine in preventing recurrences of oral candidiasis is unclear, as recurrent fungal infections are common.[92,94]

Management of HIV-associated periodontal disease relies on mechanical, topical, and systemic therapy. To manage LGE, the patient should have a thorough scaling and root planing and crevicular irrigation with 10% povidine-iodine solution. There is a role for topical or systemic antifungal therapy if there is fungus associated with the gingival erythema. Home care includes brushing and flossing and topical chlorhexidine digluconate (0.12%) rinses.[96]

Treatment of necrotizing gingivitis and necrotizing periodontitis includes debridement of necrotic tissues and scaling and root planing. Local anesthesia is often necessary to perform the debridement adequately. After debridement, irrigate the involved tissues with 10% povidine-iodine solution. Patients with necrotizing periodontitis receive a short course (5 to 7 days) of a limited-spectrum antibiotic such as metronidazole. For patients taking antiviral therapy, the dentist should consult with the patient's physician regarding the use of metronidazole. Other choices for antibiotic therapy include clindamycin or amoxicillin.[92] Home care is similar to that for LGE.

The treatment of symptomatic oral ulcerations derives from the underlying diagnosis. Supportive care and the use of topical and systemic steroids provide symptomatic relief for nonspecific oral ulcerations.[105] These lesions often are unresponsive to topical steroids, and patients may need systemic prednisone in doses of 40 to 60 mg/day.[98] Thalidomide has been documented to be effective in treating oral aphthous ulcers in HIV+ patients.[106,107] Treatment of herpes simplex stomatitis and zoster includes supportive care and the use of antiviral therapy such as acyclovir (1 to 4 g in divided oral doses).[98] CMV infection that produces symptomatic oral ulcerations may respond to acyclovir.

The operative management of HIV+ patients is unclear. Earlier data suggest that HIV+ patients have better outcomes with closed reduction than with open reduction of their mandibular fractures, but better treatment of HIV+ patients is now available. HIV+ patients may have an increased risk for minor postoperative complications following tooth extraction. There are, however, no clear indicators of which HIV+ patients are at increased risk for postoperative complications.[108] In addition, HIV+ patients do not seem to be at increased risk for severe odontogenic infections.[109] As such, when treating HIV-positive individuals as outpatients, there seems to be little basis for treating them differently from HIV-negative individuals. HIV+ patients have a slightly increased risk of postoperative complications. In general, these complications are minor and easily managed. In addition, there seems to be little that can be done to prevent complications. As such, HIV+ patients require closer or multiple postoperative visits. There is, however, a low, but finite rate of idiopathic thrombocytopenia in HIV+ patients.[110] Therefore the dentist should exercise caution and look for evidence of bleeding problems, such as oral petechiae, ecchymoses, and spontaneous gingival hemorrhage, before surgical intervention.

SUMMARY

Dentists are in a unique position to diagnose and manage patients with hematologic disorders or immunosuppression. In addition, RBC disorders are common, and patients are surviving longer with both WBC disorders and HIV infection. These patients will be presenting to the dentist for evaluation and treatment of dental conditions. In many situations, only minor modifications of usual practice are necessary to accommodate these patients. The dentist plays a critical role in the prechemotherapy evaluation and management of patients with WBC disorders. In all these disorders, oral manifestations are common. The dentist's findings play an important role in the early diagnosis and appropriate referral of patients.

REFERENCES

1. Ziccardi VB, Lalikos JF, Sotereanos GC, Patterson GT: Retroperitoneal hematoma as a complication of anterior iliac crest harvest: report of a case, J Oral Maxillofac Surg 50:1113-1136, 1992.
2. Adamson J, Hillman RS: Blood volume and plasma protein replacement following acute blood loss in normal man, JAMA 205:609-612, 1968.
3. Cook JD, Lynch SR: The liabilities of iron deficiency, Blood 68:803-809,1986.
4. Worwood M: The clinical biochemistry of iron, Semin Hematol 14:3-30, 1997.
5. Finch CA, Huebers H: Perspectives in iron metabolism, N Engl J Med 306:1520-1528, 1982.
6. Dallman PR: Iron deficiency: does it matter? J Intern Med 226:367-372, 1989.
7. Hershko C, Peto TE, Weatherall DJ: Iron and infection, Br Med J Clin Res Ed 296:660-664, 1988.
8. Kalra L, Hamlyn AN, Jones BJ: Blue sclerae: a common sign of iron deficiency? Lancet 2:1267-1269, 1986.
9. Rector WG Jr, Fortuin NJ, Conley CL: Non-hematologic effects of chronic iron deficiency: a study of patients with polycythemia vera treated solely with venesections, Medicine 61:382-389, 1982.

10. Schrier SL: Anemia: blood loss and disorders of iron metabolism. In Dale DC, Federman DD, editors: *Sci Am Med* on CD-ROM, New York, 1996, Scientific American.

11. Boggs DR: Fate of a ferrous sulfate prescription, *Am J Med* 82:124-128, 1987.

12. Waller DG, Smith AG: Attitudes to prescribing iron supplements in general practice, *Br Med J Clin Res Ed* 294:94-96, 1987.

13. Schrier SL: Anemia: hemolysis. In Dale DC, Federman DD, editors: *Sci Am Med* on CD-ROM, New York, 1996, Scientific American.

14. Sirchia G, Lewis SM: Paroxysmal nocturnal haemoglobinuria, *Clin Haematol* 4:199-229, 1975.

15. Lewis SM, Dacie JV: The aplastic anaemia: paroxysmal nocturnal haemoglobinuria syndrome, *Br J Haematol* 13:236-251, 1967.

16. Rosse WF: Dr. Ham's test revisted, *Blood* 78:547, 1991 (editorial).

17. Hartmann RC, Jenkins DE Jr, McKee LC, Heyssel RM: Paroxysmal nocturnal hemoglobinuria: clinical and laboratory studies relating to iron metabolism and therapy with androgen and iron, *Medicine* 45:331-363, 1966.

18. Hartmann RC, Kolhouse JF: Viewpoints on the management of paroxysmal nocturnal hemoglobinuria (PNH), *Haematologica* 5:42-60, 1972.

19. Valentine WN: Enzyme abnormalities in red cells, *Br J Haematol* 31(suppl):11, 1975.

20. Potter CG, Potter AC, Hatton CS, et al: Variation of erythroid and myeloid precursors in the marrow and peripheral blood of volunteer subjects infected with human parvovirus (B19), *J Clin Invest* 79:1486-1492, 1987.

21. Baum KF, Dunn DT, Maude GH, Serjeant GR: The painful crisis of homozygous sickle cell disease: a study of the risk factors, *Arch Intern Med* 147:1231-1234, 1987.

22. Serjeant GR, Serjeant BE, Thomas PW, et al: Human parvovirus infection in homozygous sickle cell disease, *Lancet* 341:1237-1240, 1993.

23. Schmalzer EA, Lee JO, Brown AK, et al: Viscosity of mixtures of sickle and normal red cells at varying hematocrit levels: implications for transfusion, *Transfusion* 27:228-233, 1987.

24. Homi J, Reynolds J, Skinner A, et al: General anaesthesia in sickle-cell disease, *Br Med J* 1:1599-1601, 1979.

25. Jan K, Usami S, Smith JA: Effects of transfusion on rheological properties of blood in sickle cell anemia, *Transfusion* 22:17-20, 1982.

26. Lane F, Goff P, McGuffin R, et al: Folic acid metabolism in normal, folate deficient and alcoholic man, *Br J Haematol* 34:489-500, 1976.

27. Sears DA: The morbidity of sickle cell trait: a review of the literature, *Am J Med* 64:1021-1036, 1978.

28. Rachmilewitz EA, Shinar E, Shalev O, et al: Erythrocyte membrane alterations in beta-thalassaemia, *Clin Haematol* 14:163-182, 1985.

29. Bull BS, Brailsford JD: Red cell membrane deformability: new data, *Blood* 48:663-667, 1976.

30. Sokol RJ, Hewitt S, Stamps BK: Autoimmune haemolysis: an 18-year study of 865 cases referred to a regional transfusion centre, *Br Med J Clin Res Ed* 282:2023-2027, 1981.

31. Levi JA, Aroney RS, Dalley DN: Haemolytic anaemia after cisplatin treatment, *Br Med J Clin Res Ed* 282:2003-2004, 1981.

32. Kopicky JA, Packman CH: The mechanisms of sulfonylurea-induced immune hemolysis: case report and review of the literature, *Am J Hematol* 23:283-288, 1986.

33. Schrier SL: Anemia: production defects. In Dale DC, Federman DD, editors: *Sci Am Med* on CD-ROM, New York, 1996, Scientific American.

34. Modell B, Berdoukas V: *The clinical approach to thalassemia*, New York, 1984, Grune & Stratton.

35. Poynton HG: *Oral radiology*, Baltimore, 1982, Williams & Wilkins.

36. Goaz PW, White SC: *Oral radiology: principles and interpretation*, St Louis, 1982, Mosby.

37. Shaefer WG, Hine MK, Levy BM: *A textbook of oral pathology*, Philadelphia, 1983, WB Saunders.

38. Van Dis ML, Langlais RP: The thalassemias: oral manifestations and complications, *Oral Surg Oral Med Oral Pathol* 62:229-233, 1986.

39. Mitchell K, Ferguson MM, Lucie NP, MacDonald DG: Epithelial dysplasia in the oral mucosa associated with pernicious anaemia, *Br Dent J* 161:259-260, 1986.

40. Ferguson MM: Oral mucous membrane markers of internal disease. Part II. Disorders of the endocrine system, haemopoietic system and nutrition. In Dolby AE, editor: *The oral mucosa in health and disease*, Oxford, 1975, Blackwell.

41. Hjorting-Hansen E, Bertram U: Oral aspects of pernicious anaemia, *Br Dent J* 125:266-270, 1968.

42. Chanarin I: *The megaloblastic anaemias*, Oxford, 1969, Blackwell.

43. Jacobs A: The buccal mucosa in anaemia, *J Clin Pathol* 13:463-468, 1960.

44. Terezhalmy GT, Hall EH: The asplenic patient: a consideration for antimicrobial prophylaxis, *Oral Surg Oral Med Oral Pathol* 57:114-117, 1984.

45. Schrier SL: The leukemias and the myeloproliferative disorders. In Dale DC, Federman DD, editors: *Sci Am Med* on CD-ROM, New York, 1996, Scientific American.

46. Appelbaum FR: Hematopoietic stem cell transplantation. In Dale DC, Federman DD, editors: *Sci Am Med* on CD-ROM, New York, 1996, Scientific American.

47. Bearman SI: The syndrome of hepatic veno-occlusive disease after marrow transplantation, *Blood* 85:3005-3020, 1995.

48. Crawford SW, Hackman RC: Clinical course of idiopathic pneumonia after bone marrow transplantation, *Am Rev Respir Dis* 147:1393-1400, 1993.

49. Sanders JE: The impact of marrow transplant preparative regimens on subsequent growth and development, the Seattle Marrow Transplant Team, *Semin Hematol* 28:244-249, 1991.

50. Sanders JE, Buckner CD, Amos D, et al: Ovarian function following marrow transplantation for aplastic anemia or leukemia, *J Clin Oncol* 6:813-818, 1988.

51. Socie G, Henry-Amar M, Bacigalupo A, et al: Malignant tumors occurring after treatment of aplastic anemia, European Bone Marrow Transplantation–Severe Aplastic Anaemia Working Party, *N Engl J Med* 329:1152-1157, 1993.

52. Witherspoon RP, Fisher LD, Schoch G, et al: Secondary cancers after bone marrow transplantation for leukemia or aplastic anemia, *N Engl J Med* 321:784-789, 1989.

53. Sullivan KM: Graft-versus-host disease. In Forman SJ, Blume KG, Thomas ED, editors: *Bone marrow transplantation*, Boston, 1994, Blackwell.

54. Nash RA, Pepe MS, Storb R, et al: Acute graft-versus-host disease: analysis of risk factors after allogeneic marrow transplantation and prophylaxis with cyclosporine and methotrexate, *Blood* 80:1838-1845, 1992.

55. Sullivan KM, Agura E, Anasetti C, et al: Chronic graft-versus-host disease and other late complications of bone marrow transplantation, *Semin Hematol* 28:250-259, 1991.

56. Van Rhee F, Lin F, Cullis JO, et al: Relapse of chronic myeloid leukemia after allogeneic bone marrow transplant: the case for giving donor leukocyte transfusions before the onset of hematologic relapse, *Blood* 83:3377-3383, 1994.

57. Copelan EA, McGuire EA: The biology and treatment of acute lymphoblastic leukemia in adults, *Blood* 85:1151-1168, 1995.

58. Barrett AP: Oral changes as initial diagnostic indicators in acute leukemia, *J Oral Med* 41:234-238, 1986.

59. Brenneise CV, Mattson JS, Commers JR: Acute myelomonocytic leukemia with oral manifestations: report of case, *JADA* 117:835-837, 1988.

60. Weckx LL, Hidal LB, Marcucci G: Oral manifestations of leukemia, *Ear Nose Throat J* 69:341-342, 345-346, 1990.

61. Barrett AP: A long-term prospective clinical study of oral complications during conventional chemotherapy for acute leukemia, *Oral Surg Oral Med Oral Pathol* 63:313-316, 1987.

62. Rosenberg SW: Oral complications of cancer chemotherapy: a review of 398 patients, *J Oral Med* 41:93-97, 1986.

63. Bergmann OJ: Oral infections and septicemia in immunocompromised patients with hematologic malignancies, *J Clin Microbiol* 26:2105-2109, 1988.

64. Bergmann OJ: Oral infections and fever in immunocompromised patients with haematologic malignancies, *Eur J Clin Microbiol Infect Dis* 8:207-213, 1989.

65. Sheller B, Williams B: Orthodontic management of patients with hematologic malignancies, *Am J Orthodont Dentofac Orthop* 109:575-580, 1996.

66. Tai CC, Precious DS, Wood RE: Prophylactic extraction of third molars in cancer patients, *Oral Surg Oral Med Oral Pathol* 78:151-155, 1994.

67. Dreizen S, McCredie KB, Bodey GP, Keating MJ: Quantitative analysis of the oral complications of antileukemia chemotherapy, *Oral Surg Oral Med Oral Pathol* 62:650-653, 1986.

68. Wahlin YB: Effects of chlorhexidine mouthrinse on oral health in patients with acute leukemia, *Oral Surg Oral Med Oral Pathol* 68:279-287, 1989.

69. Ramirez-Amador V, Esquivel-Pedraza L, Mohar A, et al: Chemotherapy-associated oral mucosal lesions in patients with leukaemia or lymphoma, *Eur J Cancer Oral Oncol* 32B:322-327, 1996.

70. Spiers AS, Dias SF, Lopez JA: Infection prevention in patients with cancer: microbiological evaluation of portable laminar air flow isolation, topical chlorhexidine, and oral non-absorbable antibiotics, *J Hygiene* 84:457-465, 1980.

71. Addy M: Chlorhexidine compared with other locally delivered antimicrobials: a short review, *J Clin Periodont* 13:957-964, 1986.

72. Ferretti GA, Ash RC, Brown AT, et al: Chlorhexidine for prophylaxis against oral infections and associated complications in patients receiving bone marrow transplants, *JADA* 114:461-467, 1987.

73. Langslet A, Olsen I, Lie SO, Lokken P: Chlorhexidine treatment of oral candidiasis in seriously diseased children, *Acta Paediatr Scand* 63:809-811, 1974.

74. Sharon A, Berdicevsky I, Ben-Aryeh H, Gutman D: The effect of chlorhexidine mouth rinses on oral candida in a group of leukemic patients, *Oral Surg Oral Med Oral Pathol* 44:201-205, 1977.

75. Tardieu C, Cowen D, Thirion X, Franquin JC: Quantitative scale of oral mucositis associated with autologous bone marrow transplantation, *Eur J Cancer Oral Oncol* 32B:381-387, 1996.

76. Mattsson T, Heimdahl A, Dahllof G, et al: Variables predicting oral mucosal lesions in allogenic bone marrow recipients, *Head Neck* 13:224-229, 1991.

77. Borowski B, Benhamou E, Pico JL, et al: Prevention of oral mucositis in patients treated with high-dose chemotherapy and bone marrow transplantation: a randomised controlled trial comparing two protocols of dental care, *Eur J Cancer Oral Oncol* 30B:93-97, 1994.

78. Bergmann OJ, Ellermann-Eriksen S, Mogensen SC, Ellegaard J. Acyclovir given as prophylaxis against oral ulcers in acute myeloid leukaemia: randomised, double blind, placebo controlled trial, *BMJ* 310:1169-1172, 1995.

79. Barrett AP, Schifter M: Antibiotic strategy in orofacial/head and neck infections in severe neutropenia, *Oral Surg Oral Med Oral Pathol* 77:350-355, 1994.

80. Galili D, Donitza A, Garfunkel A, Sela MN: Gram-negative enteric bacteria in the oral cavity of leukemia patients, *Oral Surg Oral Med Oral Pathol* 74:459-462, 1992.

81. Besa EC: Recent advances in the treatment of chronic lymphocytic leukemia: defining the role of intravenous immunoglobulin, *Semin Hematol* 29:14-23, 1992.

82. Gale RP, Caligaris-Cappio F, Dighiero G, et al: Recent progress in chronic lymphocytic leukemia, International Workshop on Chronic Lymphocytic Leukemia, *Leukemia* 8:1610-1614, 1994.

83. Cheson BD, Bennett JM, Rai KR, et al: Guidelines for clinical protocols for chronic lymphocytic leukemia: recommendations of the National Cancer Institute–sponsored working group, *Am J Hematol* 29:152-163, 1988.

84. DePaola LG, Peterson DE, Overholser CD Jr, et al: Dental care for patients receiving chemotherapy, *JADA* 112:198-203, 1986.

85. Fraschini D, Uderzo C, Rovelli A, et al: Oral and dental status in leukemic children treated with bone marrow transplantation, *Bone Marrow Transplant* 8:64-65, 1991.

86. Sonis AL, Waber DP, Sallan S, Tarbell NJ: The oral health of long-term survivors of acute lymphoblastic leukaemia: a comparison of three treatment modalities, *Eur J Cancer Oral Oncol* 31B:250-252, 1995.

87. Cabrerizo Merino MC, Onate Sanchez RE, Garcia Ballesta C, et al: Dental anomalies caused by oncological treatment: case report, *J Clin Pediatr Dent* 22:261-264, 1998.

88. Sonis AL, Tarbell N, Valachovic RW, et al: Dentofacial development in long-term survivors of acute lymphoblastic leukemia: a comparison of three treatment modalities, *Cancer* 66:2645-2652, 1990.

89. Einsele H, Ehninger G, Schneider EM, et al: High frequency of graft-versus-host-like syndromes following syngeneic bone marrow transplantation, *Transplantation* 45:579-585, 1988.

90. Schubert MM, Sullivan KM: Recognition, incidence, and management of oral graft-versus-host disease, *NCI Monogr*, 1990, pp 135-143.

91. Epstein JB, Reece DE: Topical cyclosporin A for treatment of oral chronic graft-versus-host disease, *Bone Marrow Transplant* 13:81-86, 1994.

92. Greenspan D, Greenspan JS: Oral manifestations of human immunodeficiency virus infection, *Dent Clin North Am* 37:21-32, 1993.

93. Migliorati CA, Koller MM: HIV disease: medical and dental aspects and trends for the future, a literature review, *Schweizer Monatsschr Zahnmed* 104:565-577, 1994.

94. Migliorati CA, Migliorati EK: Oral lesions and HIV: an approach to the diagnosis of oral mucosal lesions for the dentist in private practice, *Schweizer Monatsschr Zahnmed* 107:860-871, 1997.
95. Dull JS, Sen P, Raffanti S, Middleton JR: Oral candidiasis as a marker of acute retroviral illness, *South Med J* 84:733-735, 739, 1991.
96. Barr CE: Periodontal problems related to HIV-1 infection, *Adv Dent Res* 9:147-151, 1995.
97. Murray PA: HIV disease as a risk factor for periodontal disease, *Compendium* 15:1052-1063, 1994.
98. Scully C, McCarthy G: Management of oral health in persons with HIV infection, *Oral Surg Oral Med Oral Pathol* 73:215-225, 1992.
99. Schiodt M: HIV-associated salivary gland disease: a review, *Oral Surg Oral Med Oral Pathol* 73:164-167, 1992.
100. Schmidt B, Kearns G, Perrott D, Kaban LB: Infection following treatment of mandibular fractures in human immunodeficiency virus seropositive patients, *J Oral Maxillofac Surg* 53:1134-1139, 1995.
101. Dodson TB, Perrott DH, Gongloff RK, Kaban LB: Human immunodeficiency virus serostatus and the risk of postextraction complications, *Int J Oral Maxillofac Surg* 23:100-103, 1994.
102. Glick M, Abel SN, Muzyka BC, DeLorenzo M: Dental complications after treating patients with AIDS, *JADA* 125:296-301, 1994.
103. Dodson TB: HIV status and the risk of post-extraction complications, *J Dent Res* 76:1644-1652, 1997.
104. Robinson PG, Cooper H, Hatt J: Healing after dental extractions in men with HIV infection, *Oral Surg Oral Med Oral Pathol* 74:426-430, 1992.
105. MacPhail LA, Greenspan D, Greenspan JS: Recurrent aphthous ulcers in association with HIV infection: diagnosis and treatment, *Oral Surg Oral Med Oral Pathol* 73:283-288, 1992.
106. Jacobson JM, Greenspan JS, Spritzler J, et al: Thalidomide for the treatment of oral aphthous ulcers in patients with human immunodeficiency virus infection, National Institute of Allergy and Infectious Diseases AIDS Clinical Trials Group, *N Engl J Med* 336:1487-1493, 1997.
107. Paterson DL, Georghiou PR, Allworth AM, Kemp RJ: Thalidomide as treatment of refractory aphthous ulceration related to human immunodeficiency virus infection, *Clin Infect Dis* 20:250-254, 1995.
108. Dodson TB: Predictors of postextraction complications in HIV-positive patients, *Oral Surg Oral Med Oral Pathol Oral Radiol Endod* 84:474-479, 1997.
109. Miller EJ, Dodson TB: The risk of serious odontogenic infections in HIV-positive patients: a pilot study, *Oral Surg Oral Med Oral Pathol Oral Radiol Endod* 86:406-409, 1998.
110. Rossi G, Gorla R, Stellini R, et al: Prevalence, clinical, and laboratory features of thrombocytopenia among HIV-infected individuals, *AIDS Res Hum Retroviruses* 6:261-269, 1990.

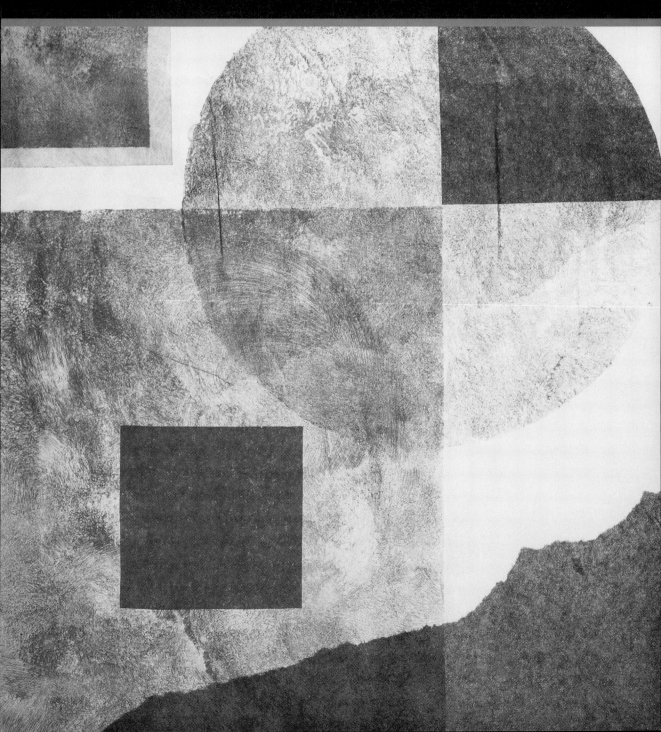

Special Populations and Issues IV

The Substance Abuse Patient

Steven J. Scrivani
Steven M. Roser

Substance abuse refers to a compulsive, persistent, or escalating consumption of a drug, involving uncontrollable drug-craving or drug-seeking behavior, with use for a nonmedical purpose, despite negative physical, psychological, and social consequences.[1] The abuse of drugs has reached epidemic proportions in the United States, and the cost to the economy is staggering. However, the cost in human suffering, damaged lives, and broken homes is beyond calculation.[2]

SUBSTANCE ABUSE IN THE UNITED STATES

Drug abuse in the United States has increased dramatically in the past 50 years. Not surprisingly, the legal drugs, alcohol and tobacco, are by far the most frequently abused substances. In 1990 a total of 167 million Americans over age 12 reported using alcohol at least once, and 103 million (51%) indicated that they had used alcohol in the past month. An estimated 147 million people had smoked cigarettes at least once, and 53.6 million (27%) had smoked in the past month.[3]

The estimated consumption of alcohol in the United States is 2.65 gallons of pure ethanol per person each year; however, only 10% of the drinking population consumes half the alcohol drunk in the United States each year.[4] Of high-school seniors, 91% have tried alcohol at least once, 66% use it once a month, and 5% use it daily.[6] Daily drinking is reported to be the same among college students; however, heavy and binge drinking is much higher, at 45%. Abuse of alcohol or other drugs is involved in 50% of youth suicides, and drinking is involved in 80% to 90% of automobile accidents among those aged 16 to 20.[5] The largest yearly cost of alcohol abuse in the United States is estimated to be $120 billion, the largest portion ($71 billion) of which is the indirect cost of reduced productivity and lost employment. The next most costly category is alcohol-related premature death, followed by medical treatment costs.[7] Although smoking is on the decline in the United States, 26.5% of adults still smoke (on the rise in females), and approximately 350,000 die from smoking annually. The costs of smoking-related health care and lost productivity amount to approximately $65 billion each year.[8]

The use of illicit drugs in the United States has been prevalent for centuries, but in modern times it reached its peak during the late 1970s and early 1980s. Estimates indicate that in the early 1960s, less than 5% of the population had ever tried an illicit drug. By the early 1970s, evidence suggested that 10% of Americans, primarily those less than 25 year of age, had used illicit drugs.[9] In 1982 an estimated 66% of high-school students had used an illicit drug.[10] More recent measures of population use of illicit drugs indicate a downward trend. There was a significant decrease in lifetime use of marijuana, hallucinogens, heroin, and cocaine among young persons between 1979 and 1990. Certain drug use patterns, however, continue to rise in specific locations and among certain population groups.

According to the 1990 National Household Survey on Drug Abuse, between 1985 and 1990, the number of illicit drug users decreased by 44%, from 23 million to 13 million people.[3] The most common illicit drug in America is marijuana. One third of the population over age 12 had tried marijuana at least once, 5.7% had used marijuana in the past month, and 2.7% reported using the drug once or more each week.[3] In comparison, 12% of the population had tried cocaine at least once, and approximately 1% had used the drug in the past month. Among American high-school seniors, 51% admit to having tried marijuana, and 4% use it daily; 17% admit to having tried cocaine, and 5% use it once a month.[6]

Although data in 1990 indicated that overall use of cocaine was declining, the frequent (weekly or more) use of cocaine has increased, suggesting that the heavy use of cocaine and crack cocaine is not showing a decline. The 1990 estimate was 500,000 users of crack cocaine, with 2 million current users of cocaine in any form in the United States.[3,9] Heroin use is more difficult to assess accurately, but data indicate that at least 1% of the population have tried heroin at least once, with approximately 500,000 people current users.[11] Hallucinogens and inhalants are estimated to be used by approximately 2% of the population under age 25, the group with the highest prevalence. In addition, an estimated 5.5 million Americans are dependent on prescription sleeping medications, tranquilizers, stimulants, and pain medications, with prescription drug abuse on the rise.[5]

SUBSTANCE ABUSE IN PATIENTS

It is estimated that one of every five patients seen by physicians is affected by alcohol or other drug problems. These patients make more office visits and require more frequent hospitalizations per year. Despite this, health care professionals recognize alcohol or other drug problems in fewer than 20% of patients who have them. The primary reason for this is inadequate substance abuse education in medical and dental schools. Medical education simply does not adequately prepare physicians to diagnose and care for patients with substance abuse problems and their families.[13] Of the 1% of time in the medical curriculum devoted to teaching substance abuse in United States medical schools, most consists of didactic lectures that address the medical complications of alcoholism. Schools are only recently offering clinical experience in managing the primary problem of substance abuse.[1] This educational deficit is more common in dental education and needs to be remedied.[14] This educational process is beginning to occur in dental school curricula, with specific educational guidelines for dental students and dental hygiene students at some schools.[14]

Dental professionals must be familiar with the profile of substance abuse, the substances commonly abused, and the decision-making ability to deal with this problem. Dentists should have the proper diagnostic skills to evaluate patients for potential substance abuse and should know the important dental implications of such abuse. Dentists must know the medical illnesses associated with substance abuse and the effects on dental treatment and patient safety. Most importantly, dental professionals need to know the warning signs of substance overuse and must be prepared to manage any medical emergency related to substance abuse.

CLASSIFICATION OF SUBSTANCE ABUSE

The motivation for using any psychoactive substance is related to the acute and chronic effects of these agents on mood, cognition, and behavior. In some individuals the subjective changes (e.g., euphoria, tension relief) that accompany substance intoxication are experienced as highly pleasurable and lead to repetitive use. Regular users may become psychologically dependent and therefore fit into a *psychiatric disorders* category. A reliable and valid diagnosis of psychiatric disorders in patients with drug problems has long been problematic. In the United States the standard instrument for psychiatric diagnoses has been the *Diagnostic and Statistical Manual of Mental Disorders* (DSM) of the American Psychiatric Association. The fourth edition, DSM-IV (1994), is a multiaxial framework for the classification of mental disorders developed for use in clinical, educational, and research settings.[1]

According to DSM-IV, a primary psychiatric disorder is diagnosed when "symptoms are not due to the direct physiological effects of a substance." A substance-induced disorder is diagnosed when criteria for a primary disorder are not met, but a prominent, persistent disturbance predominates the clinical picture, symptoms develop within a month of intoxication or withdrawal, and the symptoms cause clinically significant distress or impairment. Substance-induced disorders are differentiated from intoxication or withdrawal when "symptoms are in excess of those usually associated with the intoxication and withdrawal syndrome and when symptoms are sufficiently severe to warrant independent clinical attention"[15] (Boxes 28-1 and 28-2).

In using the DSM-IV criteria, the practitioner should specify whether substance dependence is with physiologic dependence or without physiologic dependence. In addition, patients may be variously classified as currently manifesting a pattern of abuse or dependence or as in remission. Those in remission can be divided into four subtypes (full, early partial, sustained, sustained partial) on the basis of whether any of the criteria for abuse or dependence have been met and over what time frame. The remission category can also be used for patients receiving agonist therapy or those living in a controlled drug-free environment.[16]

Box 28-1	*DSM-IV* Criteria for Substance Dependence

Substance dependence is manifested by three (or more) of the following, occurring within a 12-month period:
1. Tolerance, defined as a need for markedly increased amounts of the substance to achieve intoxication or the desired effect.
2. Withdrawal, as manifested by the characteristic withdrawal symptom for the substance.
3. Substance is often taken in larger amounts over a longer period than was intended.
4. There is a persistent desire or unsuccessful efforts to cut down or control substance use.
5. Much time is spent in activities necessary to obtain the substance.
6. Important social, occupational, or recreational activities are given up or reduced because of substance abuse.
7. Substance use is continued despite knowledge of having a persistent or recurrent physical or psychological problem that is likely to have been caused or exacerbated by the substance.

Box 28-2	*DSM-IV* Criteria for Substance Abuse

Substance abuse is manifested by one (or more) of the following, occurring within a 12-month period:
1. Recurrent substance use resulting in a failure to fulfill major role obligations at work, school, or home.
2. Recurrent substance use in situations in which it is physically hazardous (driving).
3. Recurrent substance-related legal problems.
4. Continued substance use despite having persistent or recurrent *social* problems caused or exacerbated by the effects of the substance.
5. Continued substance use despite having persistent or recurrent *interpersonal* problems caused or exacerbated by the effects of the substance.

The uncontrollable drug craving, drug seeking, and desire to secure its supply and use, regardless of the social, legal, or medical consequences, are the basis of all the functional impairments that characterize *addiction* and its consequences for individuals, their families, and society.[1]

NEUROBIOLOGY OF SUBSTANCE ABUSE

In any discussion of the cause of substance abuse, there arises the question, "Why do humans initiate and persist in such an obviously destructive and aberrant behavior?" Compulsive drug-seeking and drug-taking behavior poses two additional clinical questions: what is the cause and the perpetuating factors, and what can be done to modify the behavior to benefit the patient? Although the causes of substance abuse are complex and multifactorial, animal and human data suggest that a biologic basis exists for substance abuse and that the core for such a biologic basis is neurobiologic in nature.[17-19]

Numerous theories of the etiology of substance abuse have been discussed over the years, but currently there is no good consensus on the answer to the question of why certain people become substance abusers. There appears to be more compelling evidence to answer the question of why people become chemically dependent. A growing consensus of evidence considers substance abuse and chemical dependence as a disease or pathologic state.[20-22] Specific signs and symptoms and a predictable progression and course, if left untreated, characterize this disease. The disease model involves an interplay among biologic, psychological, and social factors that are manifested by a compulsion to use a drug, a loss of control over its use, and continued use despite adverse medical, psychosocial, and legal consequences.[22] Further, once individuals develop this disease, they cannot return to a controlled use of a psychoactive substance. This idea remains controversial, and this disease may be reversible with proper continued treatment programs.

People who do not try drugs do not become dependent or addicted. Many people who *do* try drugs do not like the effects and stop using the drug. However, others like the feeling of being under the influence of the drug and continue to use it without becoming addicted. Others eventually develop the disease of chemical dependency and addiction.[23]

Drug users learn quickly that use of a drug will produce a particular "feeling" that they desire, every time they use the drug. They learn to limit use or overuse a drug to produce a desired degree of a particular feeling. Drug use at this stage is generally referred to as *social use* and is often all that will occur in some individuals.[23] As drug use escalates, they develop some degree of tolerance and increase the quantity of drug use. They may also develop some medical problems and social behaviors considered abnormal. Tolerance increases to the point that very large quantities of a drug are required to produce the desired feelings. For many drugs, if the user stops taking the drug, withdrawal may occur. Users have severe craving for the drug and lose control of their drug use, and the compulsion to take the drug becomes overwhelming. Their abnormal behavior is masked by denial, and they suffer significant difficulty with physiologic, psychological, and social dysfunction.[22,23]

People become addicted to *feelings* rather than a drug itself, and *chemical dependence* is a repeated effort to achieve a certain feeling. Feelings originate in the limbic system in the brain and maintain the emotions and motivation to continue the production of those feelings, the "reward pathway" in the brain.[18] Drug addicts know that they are injuring themselves and hurting others, but once they develop dependence, driven by impulses from the limbic system, they continue to use drugs. As a result, addicts develop behaviors that enable them to continue to use drugs even in the face of multiple potential problems. Normally, guilt would reduce the persons craving for drug use, but at this stage, to protect the person from internal conflicts between degree of drug use and guilt, an elaborate *denial system* develops to reinforce and perpetuate the drug use. This denial system is defined as not recognizing or admitting a problem, even in the face of significant adverse consequences and despite the problem being clearly evident to others. The addict's denial, and often that of the family, is what keeps people addicted for many years.[22,23]

Addictive drugs that are abused by humans and that are self-administered by animals appear to possess reinforcing properties by virtue of their ability to reproducibly activate the reward pathway in the brain. This neural pathway consists of dopaminergic neurons in the ventral tegmental area (VTA) and their numerous projections, particularly those to the nucleus accumbens (NA) and the prefrontal cortex.[24] The *mesolimbic-dopamine system* appears to play a critical role in mediating the acute reinforcing actions of drugs of abuse. In addition, the mesolimbic-dopamine system may be one of the sites where drugs of abuse produce chronic adaptations that underlie the long-term changes in drug reinforcement mechanisms (e.g., craving), which are the core features of addiction clinically.[25] Thus the most important factor in the production of addictive behavior has been hypothesized to be the psychological or motivational aspects of *withdrawal*, which in humans may be manifested as dysphoria, anhedonia, and drug craving. These motivational and physical manifestations of withdrawal are thought to reflect long-term alterations in neural functioning occurring within specific areas of the brain, the mesolimbic-dopamine system.[18]

Drugs of abuse have many extracellular actions on receptor systems.[24,26,27] *Opioids* are hypothesized to activate the reward pathway by at least two mechanisms. First, opioid receptors exist on neurons in the limbic system, including the NA, where opiates can act directly. Second, opiates can activate VTA dopamine neurons via an indirect mechanism. VTA neurons are held in check tonically by inhibitory interneurons. These interneurons, in turn, possess opioid receptors. Since opiates are inhibitory, endogenous opioid peptides or opiate drugs inhibit the inhibitory interneurons and thereby disinhibit the dopamine neurons in the VTA pathway.[28]

Nicotine, *cannabinoids*, and *alcohol* produce brain reward by enhancing dopaminergic neurotransmission in the NA as well as directly through dopamine-independent mechanisms.[18] *Cocaine*, through increasing synaptic levels of dopamine, would activate all known subtypes of dopamine receptors throughout the brain. *Heroin* would activate the growing number of opioid receptors now known to be expressed in the brain. Alcohol initially interacts with such proteins as N-methyl-D-aspartate (NMDA) glutamate receptors, as well as the gamma-aminobutyric acid (GABA-A) receptor and the L-type calcium channels.[29,30] Clearly, these drugs of abuse produce very different effects in different brain regions and peripheral tissues, but growing evidence has shown that the actions of these drugs converge on the mesolimbic-dopamine system.

Adaptations in different brain circuits have different effects on the human behavior of drug abuse and addiction. Adaptations produce somatic dependence, psychological dependence, and sensitization and conditioned craving. Not all addictive drugs produce adaptations in brain regions that control somatic function. Alcohol and opioids produce somatic as well as psychological dependence; caffeine produces mild somatic dependence and very little psychological dependence. Adaptations in the brain reward pathway itself are hypothesized to underlie the motivational and emotional aspects of dependence and withdrawal for highly addictive drugs. Abnormal functioning in this pathway between drug use episodes or with attempts at cessation is hypothesized to cause the intense dysphoria that drives resumption of drug abuse.[24] These dopamine systems activated by drugs of abuse also appear to be involved in setting the strength and emotional valence of memories associated with certain repeated drug use. Drug-conditioned "cues" may initiate craving for many years. This aspect of addiction is particularly important clinically in causing relapses after initially successful detoxification.[31]

An adaptation of brain pathway that contributes to somatic dependence and withdrawal is that produced by opioids in the *locus caeruleus* (LC). Acute administration of mu-receptor opioid agonists inhibit LC firing by activating a potassium channel via intracellular second messenger systems and inhibiting a slowly depolarizing sodium channel pacemaker. Chronic opioid administration produces two compensatory adaptations: uncoupling of mu receptors from their ability to activate potassium channels and upregulation of the second messenger systems in the LC. With these adaptations, LC firing rates return toward basal levels despite continued opioid administration. Opioid withdrawal then unmasks the increase in intrinsic excitability of LC neurons, resulting in excessive firing, which correlates with the opioid somatic withdrawal syndrome.[32] In addition, an adaptation in the brain reward pathway is hypothesized to be linked to motivational aspects of withdrawal. The initial dysphoria that occurs during some withdrawal phenomena may be caused by compensatory increases in dynorphin peptide activation in the striatal regions of the brain.[26,28]

In addition to factors related to the drugs themselves, a complex set of factors related to the individual and the environment may affect the likelihood of becoming addicted. These factors may contribute to addiction by modifying the likelihood that drugs will be taken at all, taken repeatedly, and will initiate compulsive, uncontrolled use.[31] Genetic and developmentally related factors, psychiatric disorders (antisocial personality, mood, anxiety/depression), chronic pain, psychological stress, the user's goal, and the individual vulnerability to addiction may change over time. Environmental factors include drug availability in a particular setting, peer pressure or a subculture pressure, behavioral al-

ternatives to drug use, the settings in which drugs are used, and the presence of conditioned cues for drug use.

DENTAL IMPLICATIONS

Addiction to drugs is a persistent hazard in modern society, causing serious social and medical problems. Drug addicts have poorer health than the general population, with a higher prevalence of such diseases as endocarditis, hepatitis B and liver disease, infectious diseases, human immunodeficiency virus (HIV) disease, and acquired immunodeficiency syndrome (AIDS). Studies have also shown that there is a large gap in dental health between drug addicts and the general population. Several studies have pointed out that caries prevalence, periodontal health, oral hygiene, and patient compliance are poorer in drug addicts.[33] A Dutch study showed that 18% of drug abuse patients brushed their teeth less than once a day, 36% visited the dentist less than 1 year ago, and 25% had not visited the dentist in more than 5 years. Drug addicts had significantly more cervical plaque, diseased-missing-filled surfaces (DMFS), and bleeding of the gingiva.[34] Nutritional status was also suboptimal, with a higher sugar consumption, low calorie and protein intake, and high carbohydrate consumption. Almost half the addicts occasionally suffered from toothache, most of which went untreated. When in pain, more than one third did not go to the dentist, but instead ingested alcohol, drugs, or illicit analgesics.[34] Substance abusers score higher on the dental fear survey and were found to improve less with respect to specific dental fears and avoidance of dental care than non–substance abusers.[35]

Smoking and alcohol abuse are more common among all substance abusers and therefore place them at a higher risk for poor healing, localized infection, and oral cancer.[36-38] Alcohol abusers are additionally at risk of increased oral bleeding and poor healing with more complications after dental extractions.[39-41] Substance abusers are more likely to have abnormal liver metabolism of local anesthetics and sedative agents as well as most drugs prescribed by the dentist.[42] Cocaine users are at increased risk of labile fluctuations in blood pressure during dental procedures, with potential effects on bleeding after extractions.[41,43]

Treatment plans for addicted patients are less elaborate than those for nonaddicted patients.[44] For the addict, fillings are proposed more often than crowns or bridges and extractions more often than fillings. Drug-addicted patients do better with short visits with a maximum of 20 minutes. Psychoactive drugs can mask pain signals. During withdrawal the addicted patient has the severest dental pain, which can be difficult to manage effectively. Therefore dental treatment should be planned for just before or in the beginning of the withdrawal period or therapy.

Dental treatment should be integrated in addiction treatment programs to reduce drug-related harm and to improve re-socialization of drug addicts. Since there are differences in the medical and dental health of substance abuse patients, differences should also exist in dental management and treatment planning of these patients.[44]

EVALUATION AND ASSESSMENT

Evaluation and assessment of substance abuse depends mainly on the patient's medical, psy-

Health History Form | Medical Alert | Condition | Premedication | Allergies | Anaest. | Date

Name ______ (Last, First, Middle) Home Phone ( ) ______ Business Phone ( ) ______

Address ______ (P.O. Box or Mailing address) City ______ State ______ Zip Code ______

Occupation ______ Height ______ Weight ______ Date of Birth __/__/__ Sex ☐ M ☐ F

Emergency Contact ______ Relationship ______ Phone ( ) ______

If you are completing this form for another person, what is your relationship to that person? ______ (Name, Relationship)

For the following questions, please (X) whichever applies, your answers are for our records only and will be kept confidential in accordance with applicable laws. Please note that during your initial visit you will be asked some questions about your responses to this questionnaire and there may be additional questions concerning your health. This information is vital to allow us to provide appropriate care for you. This office does not use this information to discriminate.

Dental Information

Yes No Don't Know

- ☐ ☐ ☐ Do your gums bleed when you brush?
- ☐ ☐ ☐ Are your teeth sensitive to cold, hot, sweets or pressure?
- ☐ ☐ ☐ Have you had any periodontal (gum) treatments?
- ☐ ☐ ☐ Have you ever had orthodontic (braces) treatment?
- ☐ ☐ ☐ Do you have headaches, earaches or neck pains?
- ☐ ☐ ☐ Do you wear removable dental appliances?
- ☐ ☐ ☐ Have you had a serious/difficult problem associated with any previous dental treatment? If so, explain ______

How would you describe your current dental problem? ______

Date of your last dental exam ______ Date of last dental x-rays ______

What was done at that time? ______

How do you feel about the appearance of your teeth? ______

Medical Information

Yes No Don't Know

- ☐ ☐ ☐ Are you in good health?
- ☐ ☐ ☐ Has there been any change in your general health within the past year?

Do you have any of the following diseases or problems: **If you answer yes to any of the 3 items below, please stop and return this form to the receptionist.**

- ☐ ☐ ☐ Active Tuberculosis
- ☐ ☐ ☐ Persistent cough greater than a 3 week duration
- ☐ ☐ ☐ Cough that produces blood

- ☐ ☐ ☐ Are you now under the care of a physician? If so, what is/are the condition(s) being treated? ______ Date of last physical examination ______

Physician(s) ______ NAME PHONE ADDRESS CITY/STATE/ZIP

______ NAME PHONE ADDRESS CITY/STATE/ZIP

- ☐ ☐ ☐ Have you had any serious illness, operation, or been hospitalized in the past 5 years? If so, what was the illness or problem? ______
- ☐ ☐ ☐ Are you taking or have you recently taken any medicine(s) including non-prescription medicine? If so, what medicine(s) are you taking?
  Prescribed ______
  Over the counter ______
  Natural or herbal preparations ______
- ☐ ☐ ☐ Are you taking, or have you taken, any diet drugs such Pondimin (fendluramine), Redux (dexphenfluramine) or phen-fen (phentermine)?
- ☐ ☐ ☐ Do you drink alcoholic beverages? If yes, how much alcohol did you drink in the last 24 hours? ______ In the past month? ______
  If yes, ______ # of drinks per day for ______ # of years
- ☐ ☐ ☐ Are you alcohol and/or drug dependent? If so, have you received treatment? (Check one) ☐ Yes ☐ No
- ☐ ☐ ☐ Do you use drugs or other substances for recreational purposes? If yes, please list ______
  Frequency of use (daily, weekly, etc.) ______ Number of years of recreational drug use ______
- ☐ ☐ ☐ Do you use tobacco (smoking, snuff, chew)? If so, how interested are you in stopping? (Check one) ☐ Very ☐ Somewhat ☐ Not interested
- ☐ ☐ ☐ Do you wear contact lenses?

Allergies Are you allergic to or have you had a reaction to: (Please fill out both columns)

Yes No Don't Know

- ☐ ☐ ☐ Local anesthetics
- ☐ ☐ ☐ Aspirin
- ☐ ☐ ☐ Penicillin or other antibiotics
- ☐ ☐ ☐ Barbiturates, sedatives, or sleeping pills
- ☐ ☐ ☐ Sulfa drugs
- ☐ ☐ ☐ Codeine or other narcotics
- ☐ ☐ ☐ Latex
- ☐ ☐ ☐ Iodine
- ☐ ☐ ☐ Hay fever/seasonal
- ☐ ☐ ☐ Animals
- ☐ ☐ ☐ Food (Specify) ______
- ☐ ☐ ☐ Other (Specify) ______

To yes responses, specify type of reaction ______

Figure 28-1. Health history form. *Courtesy of The American Dental Association.*

chological, and social history. A patient's presentation and physical appearance and occasionally laboratory findings may be helpful in diagnosing substance abuse, either in the acute or chronic setting. In 1986 the American Dental Association (ADA) issued a policy statement recognizing chemical dependency as a medical disease, mandating that dentists have a responsibility to include questions related to a history of chemical dependency in the health question-naire (Figure 28-1). A positive response in the health questionnaire or in the medical interview may require the dentist to discuss the patient's substance problem with their primary care physician and may alter the treatment plan for the patient's dental care. This also prompted more education on substance abuse and chemical dependency in dental school curriculum. This familiarity with patients and their medical conditions will help prevent unwanted and untoward

Figure 28-1, cont'd. For legend see opposite page.

side effects, complications, and emergencies from dental treatment.

Questionnaires have been shown to be useful for evaluating patients for substance abuse.[15,45,46] These questionnaires are often cumbersome to use as part of the routine history-taking process and can be overwhelming and obtrusive to many patients. A thorough history and examination by dentists for specific signs and symptoms or changes that suggest drug abuse in their patients, particularly their young, otherwise healthy patients, may be more helpful than any standardized format. When such evidence is uncovered, the dentist should be encouraged to question the patient in a gentle, caring, and nonjudgmental manner. Even without such evidence, appropriate questions regarding use of licit drugs and illicit drugs should be a routine part of the patient evaluation and assessment.

If drug abuse is uncovered in the patient evaluation and assessment, the dentist should discuss with the patient the potential systemic health implications as well as the oral health implications. The dentist should not undertake treating the drug abuse problem but should be knowledgeable enough to inform the patient of available treatment programs for substance abuse and to refer the patient to the proper medical professional. The dentist should also discuss the potential oral complications of a particular substance abuse in depth and counsel patients on the signs and symptoms of oral disease related to their substance abuse. The dentist must also thoroughly discuss the potential interactions of the substance abuse and the patient's routine dental care needs, as well as any alterations in the treatment plan that may be necessary due to the substance abuse.

Patient History

A standard medical history should be taken with attention to specific issues related to substance abuse and medical problems related to substance abuse. As part of the personal history related to potential substance abuse, dental professionals should discuss specific substance use (alcohol and other drugs), psychological functioning, social functioning, family functioning, sexual functioning, sleep and diet.

Questions about substance abuse should begin with the least obtrusive and most morally and culturally acceptable questions and then more specific questions based on the previous answers. A patient's style of answer to questions can add pertinent information to the drug use history. Anger, resentment, evasiveness, and glib responses should be regarded as suspicious.[47] Additional and more focused questions should be raised about the extent of the substance abuse. The drug use history should probe the substance, nature, and extent of the abuse. The patient may be abusing one specific substance or may have the more common problem of abusing multiple substances. The most important questions relate to the extent that the substance abuse is altering the patient's life.

A variety of psychological and social findings may reveal a substance abuse problem. The social history should include questions about a patient's work, family life, interpersonal relations, sexual problems, and legal problems. Substance abusers are often troubled by insomnia, poor eating habits, anxiety, depression, and suicidal ideation or suicide attempts (Box 28-3).[22]

Family history may also give important information in the history. Alcoholism tends to run in families and may have a genetic predisposition. Family and environmental factors in families have also been implicated as causative factors in the development of substance abuse.[47]

The dentist's attitude during the interview is crucial. If he or she seems hurried, uneasy, or nervous about the questions, the patient is much less likely to be truthful. When both the dentist and the patient establish a positive rapport, the questioning will be easier and more productive, and the patient's answers should provide more accurate and useful information.[48]

Physical Examination

Numerous physical findings may indicate substance dependencies (Boxes 28-4 and 28-5).[22]

General Appearance

A patient's general appearance is usually unhelpful in distinguishing the drug abuser from the rest of the population. In American society, many "looks" often set people apart and cannot be equated with drug abuse. The traditional mores of a particular dress, employment status, level of education, and family background are not valid as good predictors of drug abuse. However, certain trends still appear to be associated with certain types of drug abuse and with a particular appearance. Therefore it is still important to begin with a "20 feet" examination of the patient's gait, posture, handshake, speech pattern, and communicative level before engaging in a comprehensive head-to-foot physical examination.

Box 28-3   Psychological and Social Findings in Patients with Chemical Dependence

Anxiety, insomnia, depression, suicide gestures or attempts
Social isolation
Change in mood, including unpredictability and impulsivity
Self-medication, regular or prolonged use of sleeping pills or tranquilizers or repeated requests for them
Repeated requests for narcotics or stimulants
Visiting many physicians, or "doctor shopping"
Divorce or separation
Interpersonal problems at work or school
Other job or school problems (tardiness, calling in sick, absenteeism)
Frequent job changes
Frequent moves to new areas (geographic cure)
Underemployment for educational level
Decreased school performance
Decreased goal-directed drives (amotivational syndrome)
Change in choice of friends or associates
Child or spouse abuse
Children doing poorly in school, disturbed or runaway children

Preoccupation with recreational drinking or using
Binge drinking
Gulping the first two or three drinks
Use of alcohol before any office visit
Loss of interest in nondrinking or nonusing activities
Drinking before a party
History of increased tolerance to alcohol or other drugs; loss of tolerance in older individuals
Repeated attempts to stop drinking or using (patients claim they can quit at any time)
Any alcohol-related or other drug-related arrests or driving under the influence
Blackouts (not remembering what happened during a drinking or using spell)
Loss of interest in personal hygiene or appearance
Complaints by family members about behavior related to use of alcohol or other drugs
Continued drinking or using despite medical, psychological, or social contraindications

From Milhorn HT Jr: *Chemical dependence: diagnosis, treatment and prevention,* New York, 1990, Springer-Verlag.

Box 28-4   Physical Findings in Patients with Alcoholism

ACUTE/CHRONIC USE
Nervous system: Sedation, confusion, disorientation, slurred speech, difficulty thinking, slowness of speech and comprehension, dizziness, poor memory, faulty judgment, narrowed range of attention, emotional lability, irritability, quarrelsomeness, hallucinosis, untidiness in personal habits, depression and suicide attempts, ataxia, impaired psychomotor performance, peripheral neuropathy, cerebellar degeneration, subdural hematoma, cerebral atrophy in a relatively young person, optic neuropathy, seizure disorder
Head, eyes, ears, nose, throat: Poor dentition, oropharyngeal lesions, hoarseness, plethoric faces, parotid enlargement, injected conjunctiva, flushed skin, head trauma, alcohol on breath
Chest: Repeated upper respiratory and bronchial infections, signs and symptoms of aspiration pneumonia, appearance of lobar pneumonias (particularly *Klebsiella* and *Pneumococcus*), tuberculosis, fractured ribs
Cardiovascular system: Cardiac arrhythmias, sinus tachycardia, hypertension, cardiomyopathy
Abdomen and gastrointestinal system: Nausea, vomiting, ascites, large or small liver, caput medusae, palpable spleen, abdominal tenderness due to gastritis, ulcers, duodenitis, esophagitis, ileitis, irritable bowel syndrome or pancreatitis, findings compatible with advanced liver disease such as loss of secondary sex characteristics, hemorrhoids, spider angiomata, or gynecomastia, positive stool test
Musculoskeletal system: Gout, especially if it is difficult to control, trauma, avascular necrosis of the femoral head in a young adult, myopathy primarily in shoulders and hips
Dermatologic system: Cigarette burns, bruises, seborrheic dermatitis, rosacea, palmar erythema
Genitourinary system: Impotence, menstrual disturbances, infertility, testicular atrophy, feminization in men, masculinization in women

OVERDOSE
Stupor, respiratory depression, coma, death

WITHDRAWAL
Insomnia, anxiety, tremor, nausea, vomiting, elevated blood pressure and pulse rate, agitation, sweating, hyperactive reflexes, grand mal seizures, delirium tremens

Box 28-5 Physical Findings in Patients with Drug Dependencies

CNS DEPRESSANTS

Acute/chronic use: Sedation, confusion, disorientation, slurred speech, ataxia, difficulty thinking, slowness of speech and comprehension, dizziness, impaired psychomotor performance, poor memory, faulty judgment, narrowed range of attention, emotional lability, irritability, quarrelsome, untidiness in personal habits, depression and suicidal gestures or attempts

Overdose: Shallow breathing, respiratory depression, hypotension, aspiration pneumonia, respiratory arrest and circulatory collapse, depressed sensorium to coma, death

Withdrawal: Insomnia, anxiety, panic attacks, tremor, nausea, vomiting, elevated blood pressure and pulse rate, irritability, agitation, sweating, hyperactive reflexes, pleading for drugs, grand mal seizures, confusion, delirium, psychosis

OPIOIDS

Acute/chronic use: Decreased pain, sleepiness, euphoria, nausea, vomiting, pupillary constriction, constipation, decreased libido and altered menstrual cycle, generalized itching, suppression of cough reflex, grand mal seizures

Overdose: Drowsiness, hypothermia, pinpoint pupils (may be dilated with meperidine), aspiration pneumonia, hypotension, respiratory depression, pulmonary edema, respiratory arrest, coma, death

Withdrawal: Lacrimation, rhinorrhea, yawning, irritability, sweating, restlessness, tremor, insomnia, piloerection, abdominal cramps, nausea, vomiting, diarrhea, muscle and bone pain, increased pulse and blood pressure, drug craving with drug seeking behavior

CNS STIMULANTS

Acute/chronic use: Euphoria with acute use/dysphoria with chronic use, increased energy with acute use/fatigue with chronic use, increased feelings of sexuality with acute use/decreased feelings of sexuality with chronic use, decreased appetite, insomnia, weight loss, excitement, tremor pupillary dilation, increased blood pressure and pulse rate, indifference to pain, rhinitis, nasal bleeding, sinus problems, dull frontal headache, hyperemic nasal turbinates, nasal spray abuse, septal perforation, hoarseness, difficulty swallowing, personal neglect, delusions, suspiciousness, paranoid pychosis

Overdose: Headache, flushed skin, tactile sensations (coke bugs), hallucinations, acute anxiety, agitation, confusion, malignant hyperthermia, tachycardia and hypertension, stereotypical repetitious behavior, bruxism and face picking, toxic psychosis, chest pain with cardiac arrhythmias, myocardial infarction, grand mal seizures, cerebral hemorrhages, hypothermia, circulatory collapse, coma, death

Withdrawal: Negativism, pessimism, lack of patience, irritability, depression, lack of energy, sleepiness, sleep disturbances, fear, paranoia, nervousness, diaphoresis, chills, hunger, drug craving

CANNABINOIDS

Acute/chronic use: Euphoria, decreased psychomotor performance, increased pulse rate, decreased pulmonary function, exacerbation of asthma, conjunctival injection; uveitis, pharyngitis, bronchitis, stuffy nose, dry mouth, sinusitis, disruption of menstrual cycle, perceptual delusions, paranoid feelings, mood shifts (joy to sorrow, fear to elation), sleepiness, heightened sexual arousal, anxiety to panic, amotivational syndrome with chronic use, angina in those with preexisting heart trouble

Overdose: Tachycardia, hypertension, delusions, hallucinations, seizures in epileptics, acute toxic psychosis

Withdrawal: Irritability, restlessness, nervousness, insomnia, mild tremor, mild body temperature elevation

PHENCYCLIDINE

Acute/chronic use: Increased blood pressure and pulse rate, increased respiratory rate, dizziness, lack of coordination, ataxia, slurred speech, vertical and horizontal nystagmus, paranoid delusions, delusions of superhuman strength, agitation, unpredictable behavior, nudity in public

Overdose: Vertigo, skin flushing, nausea, vomiting, auditory and visual hallucinations, hyperreflexia, rhabdomyolysis and acute renal failure, tremor bilateral ptosis, tachycardia, decreased respiration, grand mal seizures, acute toxic psychosis, fever, body rigidity, comalike state with eyes open and temporary periods of excitation, decreased pain perception, respiratory depression, hypertensive crisis, death

Withdrawal: Nervousness, anxiety, depression

Box 28-5	Physical Findings in Patients with Drug Dependencies—cont'd

HALLUCINOGENS

Acute/chronic use: Visual hallucinations, flushed face, pupillary dilation, fine tremor, increased blood pressure and pulse rate, increased body temperature, hyperreflexia, muscle weakness, tremor, dizziness, weakness, nausea, vomiting, paresthesia, labile mood, anxiety, panic attacks, depression, flashbacks

Overdose: Toxic psychosis, tachycardia, hypertension, cardiac arrhythmias, hyperpyrexia, shock, convulsions

Withdrawal: None known

INHALANTS

Acute/chronic use: Central nervous system effects (headache, euphoria, excitement, slurred speech, drowsiness, irritability, mental dullness, tremors, emotional lability, nystagmus, ataxia, polyneuropathies, permanent encephalopathies), intestinal effects (mucus membrane irritation, unpleasant breath odor, nausea, vomiting, gastric pain, anorexia, dyspepsia, chronic gastritis, hepatomegaly, weight loss), urinary dysfunction (renal tubular necrosis, renal failure), cardiovascular (irregular heart beat, increased pulse rate), other (eye irritation, rash around mouth or nose, cough, chemical pneumonia, muscle weakness and atrophy)

Overdose: Confusion, disorientation, cardiac arrhythmias, respiratory depression, decreased sensorium, loss of consciousness, sudden death

Withdrawal: Probably none

Mental Status

Drug abusers would be expected to arrange their schedule of drug use so that acute intoxication with evident drug effects would not coincide with a visit to the dental professional. Therefore an altered sensorium, with drowsiness, altered gait or speech pattern, and poor concentration with inappropriate answers, should be uncommon in the dental office. With the "fear of harm" in the dental office, however, some drug abusers may have recently used a particular substance to "get them through" the appointment.

The alcoholic patient may be partially intoxicated most of the time and may present with evidence of intoxication. The patient's breath may be the most telling sign of recent alcohol consumption and may coincide with an inappropriate behavior pattern. The cocaine abuser or psychostimulant abuser may have a heightened level of consciousness and may be profoundly anxious with rapid speech and confused awareness. The opioid abuser is also often under the influence of a drug and may present with the typical depressed level of consciousness, depressed mood, nodding, and withdrawn appearance.

In general the casual or intermittent drug abuser will probably not demonstrate any specific alteration in the level of consciousness, but the chronic abuser may present with typical signs of chronic drug use or acute intoxication. The dentist must be cautious in attributing any alteration in mental status or level of consciousness to substance abuse, since numerous medical conditions can present with these physical findings, and a potentially dangerous or life-threatening situation may be misinterpreted.

Vital Signs

The circumstances surrounding a patient's visit to the dental professional can often produce a certain level of anxiety and fear, and an alteration in the vital signs might be considered a physiologic response to a psychological stressor. These stressors should be taken into account when evaluating abnormalities in vital signs as possible indications of drug abuse. However, maintained alterations in vital signs throughout the dental visit should raise the suspicion of a recent drug use and should alert the dentist to question the patient further and even consider rescheduling the procedure.

Central nervous system (CNS) depressants often decrease heart rate, blood pressure, and respiratory rate. With certain drugs, these alterations in vital signs may be minimal due to tolerance and physiologic adjustment. Chronic opioid users often do not show the characteristic sign of respiratory depression unless they have recently ingested a large dose. Alcoholics in a stage of "drug need" at the dental visit may show the paradoxical vital sign changes of a withdrawal reaction, with increased heart rate and blood pressure. CNS stimulant use generally presents with increased heart rate and blood pressure. Cocaine users will often have labile swings in blood pressure with increased heart rate and, with overdoses and increased

Box 28-6	Physical Findings Related to Drug Injection

Skin tracks and related scars on neck, axilla, forearm, wrist, foot, ankle, under the tongue, and penile veins; new lesions may be inflamed

Needle puncture marks located over veins

Pockmark-like scars from subcutaneous injections, especially in deltoid, gluteal areas, abdomen, thigh, and shoulder

Wheals or hives at injection site

Abscesses, infections or ulcerations on the arm, thigh, shoulder, abdomen, chest, hand, or finger

Necrosis of the skin (spaceloderma)

Edema of the hand or irreducible finger flexion (camptodactylia); this occurs when drugs are injected into the veins of the fingers or the hands

Thrombophlebitis at possible injection sites

Accidental "tattoos" at injection sites; these result from carbon produced by heating needles to sterilize them

Dermatitis at injection sites

Allergic reactions (purpura, urticaria, pruritus)

Tourniquet pigmentation: this is a poorly defined linear mark above the antecubital space

Signs of hepatitis B (fever, jaundice, hepatomegaly, nausea, vomiting)

Signs of acute infective endocarditis (fever, mitral regurgitation murmur, septic pulmonary emboli, Roth's spots, Janeway's lesions, Osler's nodes)

Signs of septic arthritis or osteomyelitis (fever, local joint, limb, or back pain)

Signs of AIDS (fatigue, anorexia, weight loss, fever, diarrhea, lymphadenopathy, *Pneumocystis carinii* pneumonia, pulmonary aspergillosis, candidal esophagitis, tuberculosis, histoplasmosis, cryptococcal meningitis)

psychological anxiety, can present with chest pain, cardiac arrhythmias, respiratory depression, and sudden death.[41,49]

Temperature changes do not typically occur in uncomplicated drug abuse. When a patient is found to be febrile, a thorough work-up for a dento-alveolar/odontogenic cause must first be undertaken. The known or suspected drug abuser must be evaluated for a related infectious cause or foreign body reaction. Elevated temperatures in drug abusers may be caused by hepatitis, tetanus, sepsis, endocarditis, sterile or infected abscess, thrombophlebitis, or HIV infection. Elevated temperature may also result from adulterants used in the preparation of some drugs or used to "cut" certain drugs, which might be pyrogenic.[48]

Integument

The most common skin findings are with intravenous (IV) drug abusers. The signs of drug abuse often considered pathognomonic are the various skin punctures and complications of skin puncturing for drug administration (Box 28-6).[22] IV drug abusers generally develop progressive signs at the site of the vein used for injection. The mildest cutaneous signs of IV injection are fresh, healing puncture marks, frequently with minimal but distinct hyperpigmentation over the vein after an extended period. Chronic IV drug abusers frequently have skin signs known as "railroad tracks." These lesions are flat, atrophic, and sometimes pigmented scars traversed by multiple fine cross-marks that may extend over the course of a vein from 2 to 20 cm in length, the result of repeated punctures of the skin.[49,50]

Drugs on the street are frequently adulterated with inert compounds that are irritants. Drug abusers rarely use aseptic techniques, and the method of drug injection may cause both chemical irritants and infecting agents to enter the body at the injection site, with potential for local inflammation, infection, abscess, and acute thrombophlebitis. The lesions caused by subcutaneous injection or "skin popping" may be visible or hidden on the body. These lesions appear as puncture marks with underlying tissue involvement. In the early stages of skin involvement an untoward local reaction may occur with heat, swelling, and erythema of varying degree, progressing in some cases to obvious infection, abscess formation, and drainage.[49]

Skin lesions can occur with other drug abuse, but much less frequently than with IV abusers. Cigarette burns are common in users of CNS depressants (opioids, alcohol, benzodiazepines) due to the nodding or falling asleep with a lit cigarette. Marijuana and cigarette smokers may also have stains and burns on the fingers. Some CNS psychostimulants can cause skin flushing, and opioid abusers occasionally have skin flushing, rash, and itching.

Eyes

Miosis is a classic physical sign associated with opioid abuse. The failure of pupils to dilate in a well-lit room or on eye examination suggests recent opioid intake. Pinpoint pupils are generally seen only during acute intoxication, and the pupils will accommodate to normal quite quickly after drug detoxification. With tolerance to opioids in a chronic abuser, the pupillary effect will often habituate and lessen the degree of miosis.

Mydriasis occurs with psychostimulants and hallucinogens (except marijuana) and is a predictable pharmacologic effect of the sympathomimetic action of cocaine and amphetamines. Patients with sustained mydriasis may complain of photophobia and wear dark glasses in inappropriate settings. Pupillary changes do not typically occur with barbiturates, alcohol, and marijuana. Scleral injection can occur with frequent marijuana use, but this is not diagnostic. Scleral icterus in an otherwise healthy adolescent or young adult is highly suggestive of hepatitis or liver failure. Hepatitis may occur in IV drug abusers who share contaminated needles. Alcoholics may develop cirrhosis and liver failure with scleral icterus.

Nose

The vasoconstrictive properties of cocaine can present with the finding of an erythematous, ulcerated, or perforated nasal septum due to frequent cocaine sniffing. Nasal inflammatory and irritative lesions are also seen in sniffers of heroin, glue, and other caustic compounds. Chronic cocaine sniffers also frequently exhibit features of allergic rhinitis and sinusitis, with nasal secretions, stuffiness, and reddened mucous membranes.

Oral Cavity

Poor oral hygiene and dental decay may be a prominent finding in substance abusers due to alterations in diet, lack of commitment to dental and oral care, and potential alteration in salivary flow and composition. Alcoholics can have parotid gland hypertrophy secondary to an autonomic neuropathy and accumulation of zymogen granules in the acinar cells.[51] There may be an additional alteration in the flow rate with decreased saliva and an alteration in its chemical composition, which can lead to dry mouth, mucosal irritation, dental caries, and secondary microbial infections, mostly fungal.[51]

Mucosal lesions may be clues to substance abuse as well. Infectious diseases can occur in the oral cavity secondary to substance abuse and its complications. Fungal infections with *Candida* may be common in alcoholics and marijuana smokers. Secondary bacterial or viral infections may be potential markers for immunocompromise. IV drug abusers and alcoholics with liver disease may have secondary infections, frank gingival bleeding, or mucosal petechiae. HIV-positive and AIDS patients can present with more virulent infections, hairy tongue, and lymphadenopathy. Users of psychostimulants may have uncontrolled mandibular movements, with teeth grinding (bruxism) and muscle hyperactivity and hypertrophy. Squamous cell oral carcinoma may be seen, particularly in alcoholics and heavy smokers.

Pulmonary System

Physical examination and imaging of the pulmonary system is generally unremarkable, except with an inflammatory or infectious process from heavy sniffing of cocaine, crack smoking, or IV injection of irritants or infectious agents. Allergic asthmatic-like symptoms and signs may be caused by continued inhalation of substances or hypersensitivity reactions to an irritant or allergen. Pulmonary infection may be secondary to microorganisms injected or an immunocompromised patient. Tuberculosis, *Pneumocystis carinii* pneumonia, and *Mycobacterium* infection are common in the immunocompromised population. Heavy smokers may have findings of lung cancer.

Cardiac Function

Infectious *endocarditis* is a common finding in IV drug abusers. Endocarditis should be considered in an individual with fever of unknown origin or in an individual with no prior history or evidence of valvular or congenital heart disease. Right-sided endocarditis is highly suspicious for IV drug abuse and is often fungal in origin, with involvement of only the tricuspid valve and with septic pulmonary emboli and infarcts. The finding of a heart murmur should be further evaluated by the patient's primary care physician with transthoracic or transesophageal echocardiography.

Cardiac rhythm disturbances and electrocardiographic changes may be found in individuals abusing cocaine and psychostimulants. Abberant dysrhythmias with conduction defects can occur spontaneously and with administration of local anesthetics and sedatives, resulting in sudden cardiac collapse, as discussed earlier.

Abdomen

Liver disease is the most common finding in drug abusers. Physical examination may reveal an enlarged liver on palpation. The spleen may be enlarged, and patients with more advanced liver disease may have hepatic and abdominal tenderness, ascites, abdominal angiomata, and collateral periumbilical venous circulation.

Endocrine System

Most drugs of abuse have been found to produce some changes in endocrine system functioning. Marijuana reduces gonadotropin-releasing hormone, which results in decreased levels of luteinizing hormone (LH) and follicle-stimulating hormone (FSH) and a decrease in testicle and seminal vesicle weight in males and the potential for impotence and changes in ovulation in females.[52,53] Cocaine alters plasma prolactin and growth hormone levels and can alter thyroid gland responsiveness.[54] Long-term male alcoholics may suffer from feminization, with testicular atrophy, loss of male-pattern body hair, gynecomastia, alteration in fat deposition patterns, and skin pigmentation. Women alcoholics may have irregular menses and sterility.

Difficulties with pregnancy are also common in drug-abusing women. Due to chronic drug abuse, nutritional deficiencies, and inadequate hygiene and medical care, women may have subnormal rates of conception and elevated rates of spontaneous abortion, stillbirth, premature birth, small-for-gestational-age birth, and congenital malformation.[12]

Neurologic System

Specific neurologic abnormalities on physical examination are uncommon. The specific abused drug and the chronic CNS effects may manifest with some abnormal finding. In addition, acute intoxication can present with neurologic findings, particularly with overdose. Conversely, in withdrawal states, patients may present with neurologic findings typical for the particular drug. Alcoholics may develop peripheral neuropathies with neurosensory deficits, autonomic abnormalities, and pain. Cocaine and psychostimulants can produce tremors, twitches, and akinesia or akinesthesia.

Laboratory Evaluation

Routine laboratory studies are generally not diagnostic for substance abuse. Tests for drug screening are more specific and can be ordered in suspicious circumstances. Laboratory tests are ordered when the history is suspicious or positive for substance abuse. A history of alcohol abuse generally warrants laboratory evaluation given the specific physical findings or the treatment to be performed. Laboratory tests are not as helpful in diagnosing other drug abuse problems but may be necessary to confirm and evaluate specific levels, again given the physical examination findings and the anticipated procedures.

Numerous laboratory abnormalities are associated with alcohol use. Serum alanine transaminase (ALT, formerly SGPT) is thought to be the most sensitive indicator of liver disease but is elevated in only 31% to 70% of alcoholics.[55] ALT is an hepatic microsomal enzyme subject to induction and may indicate hepatic damage or induction by some other drug, typically the anticonvulsants. Serum aspartate transaminase (AST, formerly SGOT) may also be elevated in chronic alcohol abuse.

Alcoholics also may present with anemia and elevated mean corpuscular volume (MCV). Patients with folic acid and vitamin B_{12} deficiency may also present with anemia and abnormalities in the red blood cell (RBC) indices. Prothrombin time (PT) and the international normalized ratio (INR) may be prolonged due to liver disease and abnormality in clotting factors. Platelet and white blood cell (WBC) counts are also occasionally decreased because of bone marrow suppression by toxic effects of alcohol.

Since alcohol impairs gluconeogenesis, blood glucose levels may fall, especially in patients with poor nutritional status. If the pancreas becomes damaged, insulin secretion may be affected in response to a sugar load, and the blood glucose level may increase.[55]

Opioid use may produce a depressed testosterone level, a high fasting glucose level, and abnormal glucose tolerance test. Opioids may also cause false-positive tests for pregnancy or syphilis.[56] Abnormal arterial blood gases (ABGs) may be caused by depressed respiration from overdose or from pulmonary edema associated with heroin injection.[22] Vomiting caused by drug use or withdrawal may produce electrolyte abnormalities.

Other laboratory abnormalities are usually nonspecific and result from infections caused by parenteral drug use or immunocompromised states. Abnormal laboratory findings associated with infection include an elevated WBC count and differential and positive blood cultures. The hemoglobin and hematocrit may be decreased with infective endocarditis secondary to hemolysis. Typical abnormal laboratory values will be present with hepatitis B and HIV infection. There may be abnormal liver functions, decreased WBC counts, low absolute neutrophil counts, elevated lymphocyte counts, and abnormalities in specific immunologic studies for HIV disease.

Drug Screening

Laboratory tests for drug screening are classified as screening tests and confirmatory tests. *Screening tests* offer a high degree of sensitivity but have a low specificity. Most drug screens detect drugs in up to 99% of the specimens in which they are present in concentrations greater than a predetermined level. The number of false-positive results may therefore be high. *Confirmatory tests* are very specific and separate true positives from false positives with great accuracy.[57] Although a number of body fluids can be used for drug screening, urine is most often used. Urine is easy to obtain, collection is noninvasive, urine is simple and inexpensive to analyze, and it can be refrigerated and stored for future use. Drugs and their metabolites are usually found in higher concentrations in urine than in other body fluids because of the concentrating function of the kidney.[57]

Routine urine screening tests usually do not detect hallucinogens, alcohol, and many "designer drugs." Alcohol is best tested for in a blood sample. Laboratory drug screening tests provide no information about the pattern of drug use, the route of administration, or whether the patient is physically or mentally impaired by the drug.

False-negative results may result from a mixup of samples or testing for the wrong drug. More often, however, patients may adulterate their urine sample with other substances to cover up a particular substance. Patients may have taken the drug so recently that it may not have undergone renal excretion and may be detectable in the urine. Additionally, any medical condition with renal impairment might affect drug levels in the urine. The larger the dose, the longer a drug can be detected in the urine. In chronic drug users, after a drug has reached a peak blood level and steady state, it takes considerably longer to be completely excreted from the body. Some drugs, especially marijuana and barbiturates, are more fat soluble and will be bound to fat stores and detected in the urine a long time after stopping the drug. The cannabinoids (e.g., marijuana) can be detected in the urine for up to 60 days after patients stop heavy chronic use.[55,56] Barbiturates and methaqualone may be detected up to 7 days after use and PCP for up to 8 days. Most other drugs are not detected after 1 to 3 days, depending on the drug.[56]

SUBSTANCES OF ABUSE

 Alcohol

Ethyl alcohol (ethanol) is a sedative-hypnotic that is toxic to many organ systems. Medical complications of alcohol abuse include liver and cardiovascular disease; endocrine, hematologic, and gastrointestinal (GI) effects; malnutrition; and CNS disorders. Ethanol also readily crosses the placental barrier and can produce the fetal alcohol syndrome, a major cause of fetal morbidity and mortality.

Ethanol consists of small, water-soluble molecules that are absorbed rapidly and completely from the stomach and small intestine. After a person ingests alcohol on an empty stomach, it reaches its peak blood level within 30 to 40 minutes. Food in the GI tract delays alcohol's absorption. The distribution of alcohol is rapid, with tissue levels rapidly approximating the blood concentration. More than 90% of alcohol that a person consumes is metabolized in the liver; the remainder is excreted unchanged by the lungs and in the urine. The rate of alcohol metabolism is independent of the drug's concentration, and the typical adult can metabolize 7 to 10 g of alcohol an hour. However, the alcohol disappears from the body much more slowly in the patient with liver damage.

The main pathway for ethanol metabolism involves *alcohol dehydrogenase*, an enzyme that catalyzes the conversion of ethanol to acetaldehyde. A secondary pathway of ethanol metabolism is through the microsomal ethanol oxidizing system in the liver. At low concentrations of ethanol, alcohol dehydrogenase is the main oxidizing system, and at higher concentrations the microsomal ethanol oxidizing system plays a more significant role. During chronic alcohol consumption, ethanol oxidizing activity increases significantly due to enzyme induction. More than 90% of the acetaldehyde formed by these reactions is also metabolized in the liver. Aldehyde dehydrogenase is the main pathway for aldehyde oxidation; the product of this reaction is acetate, which is further metabolized and excreted as carbon dioxide and water.

The pharmacologic actions of alcohol vary widely, but the most acutely affected organ system is the CNS. Alcohol can cause relief of anxiety, slurred speech, sedation, impaired judgment, uninhibited behavior, and ataxia. Many people think alcohol is stimulating, but as with other CNS anesthetics, alcohol is a CNS depressant. The apparent stimulation at low doses results from the activity of various parts of the brain that have been freed from inhibition as a result of depression of the brain's inhibitory control mechanisms.[58] One of the most significant sites of action of alcohol is the *cell membrane*. Alcohol readily dissolves in the lipid layer, reducing the viscosity of the cell membrane. This membrane fluidization effect has been related to changes in specific membrane functions, including neurotransmitter receptors, various enzymes, and ion channels. Ethanol exposure has been reported to increase the number of GABA receptors, consistent with the ability of drugs that affect the GABA system receptor complex to mimic or intensify many acute effects of alcohol.[59]

The psychological and behavioral effects of various blood alcohol levels range from feeling warm and relaxed to death from respiratory depression with extreme toxicity. However, the individual reactions to any given blood level of alcohol can vary considerably. Tolerance due to persistent and excessive alcohol consumption increases the levels at which these reactions can occur; the effects are more marked when the concentration is rising than when it is falling.

The immediate effects of alcohol on the circulation are relatively minor. Blood pressure, cardiac output, and myocardial contraction do not change greatly in most people after they have consumed a moderate amount of alcohol. However, significant decrease in myocardial contractility has been observed in some patients.[60] Alcohol in moderate doses causes vasodilation, especially of the cutaneous vessels, which produces a warm and flushed skin. This vasodilation occurs partly from CNS vasomotor depression and partly from a direct vasodilating action of alcohol on blood vessels.[60,61]

Several studies have shown a negative correlation between alcohol ingestion in small amounts and the incidence of coronary artery disease. The protective effect was originally thought to occur because alcohol increased the concentration of high-density lipoproteins and decreased the concentration of low-density lipoproteins, but this hypothesis remains to be proven.[61]

Alcohol in about 10% concentration physically stimulates the salivary and gastric secretions, especially if an individual likes its taste. Alcohol may also stimulate the release of salivary and gastric secretions by directly stimulating sensory endings in the buccal and gastric mucosa. Alcohol may also stimulate gastric secretion by causing the release of gastrin. Drinks of higher alcohol concentration are very irritating to the gastric mucosa and cause congestive hyperemia and inflammation, besides the excess gastric secretions, and may result in erosive gastritis.

Alcohol exerts a significant diuretic effect on the kidneys, and although the large amount of fluid usually ingested with alcoholic beverages undoubtedly contributes to the increased urine flow, alcohol itself produces a marked diuretic response because of decreased renal tubular resorption of water. This effect likely results from a direct action of alcohol on the neuroendocrine axis that decreases the secretion of antidiuretic hormone (ADH).

After ingestion of alcohol, a feeling of warmth and increased sweating may occur because of enhanced cutaneous blood flow. The body therefore loses heat more rapidly than before alcohol ingestion, and the body's internal temperature tends to fall gradually. With the consumption of large amounts of alcohol, the central temperature-regulating system becomes depressed, and body temperature may fall precipitously, producing clinical hypothermia.

Health Consequences

Numerous health consequences may occur with persistent and excessive use of alcohol, involving virtually all organ systems. Besides the major effects on the CNS, more chronic and excessive alcohol intake affects the cardiovascular, GI, hematologic, musculoskeletal, and endocrine/metabolic systems, with the potential for development of carcinoma. In chronic alcoholics, any vitamin absorbed through the small intestine by active transport or stored in the liver may be deficient, including folate, pyridoxine (vitamin B_6), thiamine (vitamin B_1), niacin (vitamin B_3), and vitamin A. Significant thiamine deficiency causes Wernicke-Korsakoff syndrome. *Wernicke's encephalopathy* most often has an acute onset and is characterized by nystagmus, cranial nerve palsies and often paralysis, ataxia, and confusion. *Korsakoff's psychosis* associated with this deficiency usually follows years of drinking and is manifested by a memory disorder, psychological aberrations, and confabulation.

Another common neurologic manifestation of chronic alcohol abuse is peripheral polyneuropathies. These usually present with symmetric sensory impairment or loss of deep tendon reflexes and occasionally with motor dysfunction of the distal to proximal limbs, especially of the legs. The patient may have a burning pain in the feet with palpable muscle tenderness and areas of hyperesthesia. Pain and hyperalgesia may be followed by decreased tactile and deep sensation after a particular sensory loss pattern known as the "stocking glove distribution." Alcoholic peripheral neuropathies may also manifest in the trigeminal system and include sensory abnormalities of the face and head.

Alcoholic liver disease is responsible for 60% to 70% of patients with cirrhosis of the liver.[62] The three principal alcohol-induced liver disease lesions are designated alcoholic fatty liver, alcoholic hepatitis, and alcoholic cirrhosis. *Alcoholic fatty liver* is usually reversible on cessation of alcohol consumption and causes little liver disease. *Alcoholic hepatitis*, an inflammatory lesion characterized by infiltration of the liver with leukocytes, liver cell necrosis, and alcoholic hyalin deposition, is thought to be a precursor to cirrhosis. Subsequent healing accompanied by fibrosis distorts the normal lobular architecture, with formation of regenerative nodules. This may lead to loss of functioning hepatocytes, resulting in jaundice, edema, coagulopathy, and metabolic abnormalities. This fibrotic, cirrhotic liver with a distorted vascular pattern may cause portal hypertension and all its sequelae, including gastroesophageal varices, splenomegaly, ascites, and hepatic encephalopathy.

Chronic liver disease may also lead to a deficiency in the synthesis of hepatic proteins, especially vitamin K–dependent proteins. Vitamin K is a required cofactor for liver microsomal carboxylase, which is necessary to convert glutamyl residues in certain protein precursors to gamma-carboxyglutamates. The synthesis of plasma proteins, including most of the blood clotting factors (prothrombin; factors VII, IX, and X) are depressed in severe liver disease. This can result in problems with clotting after trauma, invasive procedures, and surgery.

Changes in the cardiovascular system secondary to chronic alcohol abuse include alterations in blood pressure, with a tendency for increased hypertension. *Alcoholic cardiomyopathy* should be considered in all patients less than 50

years of age who experience chronic heart failure. Arrhythmias are common, particularly after heavy bingeing, typically with referrals to atrial fibrillation, atrial flutter, premature ventricular beats, or other evidence of cardiac irritability without another cause.

Musculoskeletal system effects of alcoholism can include *myopathy*, with painful swollen muscles, proximal muscle weakness, and eventual muscle atrophy. With progressive damage to muscles and muscle cells, leakage of certain cellular enzymes may be manifest by elevations in serum creatine kinase (CK), lactate dehydrogenase (LDH), eventually with myoglobinuria and potential renal failure. Persistent and excessive consumption of alcohol can raise the serum uric acid levels and may precipitate attacks of gout or exacerbate preexisting gout.

The hematologic abnormalities encountered in alcoholics include *anemia* from hemorrhagic, hemolytic, hypoplastic, or some combination of these factors. This disorder usually presents as a folic acid or iron deficiency anemia, with a generalized macrocytosis of unknown etiology. Leukopenia can occur secondary to folic acid deficiency, hypersplenism with destruction of damaged WBCs, or direct bone marrow suppression. This leukopenia generally resolves in 2 to 3 weeks after discontinuation of the alcohol use and appropriate nutritional support. Coagulation disorders occur most often with cirrhosis because of the body's diminished production of the vitamin K–dependent coagulation factors. Decrease in platelet number and abnormal platelet function may also occur secondary to alcohol abuse. The immune system may also be affected, with decreased bacterial activity of certain WBCs and in particular, alveolar macrophages with the potential for localized infection (pulmonary infection) and life-threatening sepsis.

A variety of endocrine and reproductive disorders occur as a result of excessive alcohol consumption. After alcohol ingestion, ADH level falls, accounting for the diuretic effect of alcohol. Alcohol may interfere with gluconeogenesis and result in a decreased blood glucose level. In addition, depleted glycogen stores from abnormal nutritional patterns may contribute to the level of hypoglycemia. Alcohol also may be toxic to the testes, the pituitary, and the hypothalamus. Toxicity may result in abnormalities of hair pattern, loss of normal sexual drive, impotence, and abnormal sperm function in males.

A variety of metabolic abnormalities can result from excessive alcohol consumption, most notably *alcoholic ketoacidosis*, typically seen in heavy alcohol abusers. This may produce an overt metabolic acidosis, abnormal glucose regulation, and severe systemic illness that may culminate in coma and even death. Subtle abnormalities of magnesium, calcium, and phosphorus may produce a variety of symptoms associated with disorders in bone metabolism and neuromuscular function, fatigue and energy pattern disturbances, musculoskeletal complaints, and even severe delirium and coma. Alcohol, although highly caloric, contains primarily "empty calories" with very few vitamins, minerals, and amino acids. Alcoholics often present with weight loss and the potential for thiamine, riboflavin, niacin, and vitamin C deficiencies, with associated symptoms and signs. Alcohol also suppresses the normal appetite, both directly and as a result of gastric irritation, nausea, and vomiting, with the potential for additional damage to other organs of digestion, primarily the pancreas, liver, and small intestine. In advanced stages of alcoholism, many specific syndromes of nutritional deficiency may be evident.

Alcoholics have a greatly increased risk of developing cancer in numerous specific sites. Alcohol is a known carcinogen and is to be considered a co-carcinogen that enhances the effects of other known carcinogens, in particular smoking. The development of liver damage may also prohibit the body to adequately detoxify circulating carcinogens.[61] Numerous cancers of the digestive tract and digestive organs have been highly associated with alcohol abuse. Most notably, oral and esophageal cancers seem to be directly related to heavy alcohol consumption, as well as with smoking. Oral cancer is a particularly common problem in alcoholics, particularly those who also smoke, and often presents as a difficult and life-threatening disease when the diagnosis is finally made.[48,62]

Recognition and Assessment

Dentists are in a good position in the health care system to identify patients with substance abuse problems during the routine comprehensive history and physical examination process. In particular, dentists may readily be able to identify alcohol abuse by the numerous physical findings in the area of the head, face, and oral cavity. A comprehensive head, neck, and oral cavity examination may reveal the following clues to alcohol abuse: (1) arcus senilis, a ringlike opacity of the cornea; (2) acne rosacea or rhinophyma, a red and speckled nose; (3) alcohol smell on the breath; (4) telangiectasias and spider angiomas of the face; (5) generalized facial edema; (6) jaundiced skin or mucosa; (7) erythema of the oral mucosa; (8) changes in the pattern of the normal tongue architecture and topical papillae; and (9) angular cheilitis.[48,62,63]

Alcoholics and other substance abusers often display evidence of poor oral hygiene, extensive plaque and deposits of calculus, and advanced caries, especially with an increased rate of coronal and root caries. Heavy alcohol abusers may have a high incidence of tooth wear secondary to palatal erosion of the maxillary incisors due to regurgitation of gastric acid associated with alcoholic gastritis and episodes of vomiting. There is also a higher incidence of tooth loss due to trauma to the dentition (fighting and falls), caries, and periodontal disease.[64] The alcoholic is more likely to seek emergency dental treatment rather than having routine, regular dental evaluation and preventive care. This poor compliance with preventive measures and routine treatment and poor attendance at scheduled dental appointments make it difficult to monitor patients' dental health adequately.

Alcoholism is a primary cause of *sialadenosis*, an asymptomatic, generally bilateral enlargement of the parotid glands. It has been postulated that an autonomic neuropathy, manifesting as a demyelinating neuropathy, results in excessive stimulation or inhibition of acinar protein synthesis, clinically visible as parotid gland hypertrophy.[51]

Medical Issues

Treatment considerations for the alcoholic patient are primarily related to the liver disease, although numerous other system disorders can have an effect on certain types of dental procedures. The major considerations with liver dysfunction are related to drug metabolism/detoxification and hematologic abnormalities, primarily manifested as bleeding disorders.

Liver damage has a profound effect on drug metabolism. This phenomenon is directly related to the drug's competition with alcohol for the liver cytochrome P-450 enzyme system. The effect of acute versus chronic alcohol consumption has directly opposite effects, with different clinical signs and symptoms that directly affect treatment considerations. Drug metabolism is inhibited during acute administration of alcohol, leading to high blood levels of the concomitantly administered drug, whereas chronic alcohol intake induces the microsomal enzyme system and thus results in increased drug metabolism. Induction of the microsomal enzyme system also contributes to the metabolic tolerance of alcohol in chronic alcohol users.[40]

Not all drugs administered in dentistry need to be modified in patients with suspected or known alcoholic liver disease, but the effects of some drugs used in dentistry need to be considered. *Metronidazole* interferes with acetaldehyde dehydrogenase and has a disulfiram-like effect when combined with alcohol. Patients should refrain from consuming alcohol for at least 72 hours after discontinuing metronidazole.

In the analgesic group, most nonsteroidal antiinflammatory drugs (NSAIDs) can be used relatively safely in patients with liver dysfunction. The patient's hematologic status must be assessed before administering these agents because of the potential for gastric irritation and excessive bleeding.

Acetaminophen is not contraindicated but should be used with caution. Alcohol increases the isoenzyme associated with the formation of the toxic metabolite from acetaminophen. Alcohol preferentially interacts with this isoenzyme. However, when the patient ceases alcohol consumption in conjunction with acetaminophen administration, increased risk for liver toxicity results from acetaminophen metabolites. The recommended dose of acetaminophen may be decreased to 2 g in a 24-hour period, since therapeutic doses may be related to liver damage in a patient with potential liver disorder. Local anesthetics, with or without a vasoconstrictor, in doses used for routine dental treatment are generally unaffected by the liver dysfunction and are not associated with significant side effects.

The hematologic manifestations of liver dysfunction are related to coagulation abnormalities and platelet dysfunction. All the coagulation factors except factor VIII and von Willebrand's factor are produced by the liver cells. Vitamin K, an active and essential cofactor in coagulation, is stored in the liver and may be disrupted by liver disease. Platelet disorders may present as an increased number of platelets or as a platelet defect related to impaired aggregation of platelets. Thrombocytopenia may result from excessive consumption of abnormal platelets by the spleen or from folate deficiency and bone marrow alcoholic toxicity with decreased production of normal platelets. The most common platelet aggregation defect is caused by an abnormality of thomboxane A_2 and a disorder of platelet stickiness. This platelet aggregation disorder can be present even with normal numbers of platelets.

All platelet disorders may be exacerbated by the intake of aspirin, aspirin-related compounds, and other NSAIDs. Platelet abnormalities usually normalize after several days but can last for up to 2 to 3 weeks, depending on duration of alcohol consumption and degree of liver dysfunction.[40,63]

Dental professionals must consider both these sequelae of liver dysfunction before providing dental treatment. If patients present with acute alcohol intoxication, no dental treatment should be prescribed, and appropriate counseling should be given. Even emergency dental procedures should be postponed with acute alcohol intoxication until the effects of the intoxication have resolved. If treatment of the intoxicated patient is postponed, the dental office should ensure that the patient is not driving a vehicle.

In chronic alcohol abusers the dentist must consider evaluating liver function and hematologic status before providing dental treatment. Complete blood count, liver function testing, and coagulation parameters may be necessary before routine dental treatment and, most importantly, surgical treatment. PT, INR, and partial thromboplastin time (PTT) are most appropriate for evaluating the coagulation cascade. A platelet count must also be evaluated due to the risk of excessive bleeding secondary to any traumatic procedure. If PT, INR, or PTT is abnormal, the patient's physician must be consulted, with consideration of factor replacement and additional local hemostatic measures. Some patients may require hospitalization for these procedures, depending on the extent of the dental treatment necessary. With low platelet counts, particularly below 20,000 to 50,000/mm^2, traumatic dental treatment may be postponed, particularly surgical therapy, again with consideration of local hemostatic measures and physician consultation. In certain patients with platelet counts greater than 50,000/mm^2, dental procedures can be performed with atraumatic technique, topical hemostatic agents, and topical or systemic aminocaproic acid or other antifibrinolytic agent. If platelet counts are very low, hospitalization must be considered, with systemic administration of appropriate agents, including a platelet transfusion for surgical treatment.

The dentist must also consider other major organ systems affected by alcohol abuse when evaluating patients with disorders in the head, face, and oral cavity as well as before performing certain dental treatments. Neurologic involvement may present as alcoholic peripheral *neuropathy*, which may affect the trigeminal system and present as facial and toothache pain not of odontogenic/dento-alveolar origin. Trigeminal system neuropathies may also present as loss of normal sensation or loss of normal taste perception, similar to burning mouth/burning tongue syndrome. Acute and chronic alcohol abuse may present with abnormalities in mental status and normal cognitive ability. Any mental status change or alteration in consciousness contraindicates dental treatment, and appropriate referral for medical evaluation is necessary.

Alcoholics with a history of hypertension or cardiomyopathy must be appropriately evaluated with pretreatment and posttreatment vital signs, in particular blood pressure evaluation. Patients with poorly controlled hypertension and signs or symptoms of angina require appropriate referral, and most dental treatments should be postponed. No direct evidence indicates that alcohol abuse causes infection that can compromise the immunologic system.[40] With decreased platelet and WBC counts, however, delayed healing and localized infection are always risks.

The altered nutritional and metabolic status of chronic alcoholics may affect certain dental treatment considerations. Without a normal and nutritionally adequate diet, the patient may have vitamin deficiencies, abnormal blood glucose levels, and fluid and electrolyte imbalances. As in the diabetic patient, blood glucose level must be assessed before dental treatment that may alter the dietary intake ability.

As previously noted, risk of oropharyngeal cancer is greatly increased in alcohol abusers. Dental professionals, in performing their normal comprehensive oral and head and neck examination, must be overly rigorous in examination of the alcoholic patient. Examination of the oral cavity, with particular attention to areas prone to development of oral cancer (lips, lateral border of tongue, posterolateral oropharynx, retromolar trigone), and examination of the neck for lymphadenopathy are crucial. Any suspect intraoral area on history or examination must be evaluated further, most likely with close follow-up or biopsy. The appropriate dental or medical professional must further evaluate any lymphadenopathy in the neck.

 Nicotine

Nicotine is a highly physiologically active and psychoactive toxic agent, and its continued use usually leads to addiction.[65] The most common form of nicotine dependence is associated with the inhalation of cigarette smoke, although pipe and cigar smoking, use of snuff, and chewing of tobacco may also lead to nicotine dependence.[1] Cigarette smoking is the principal cause of preventable disease, disability, and premature death in the United States. Each year, however, more than 1 million American children and teenagers start smoking, and most established smokers have great difficulty quitting.[65] Recognition of tobacco use as an addiction and of nicotine as an addictive drug is essential for the effective health care of patients. Dental professionals in particular play a vital role in the identification and prevention of addiction as well as in smoking cessation efforts for their patients.

Cigarette smoke is composed of hundreds of substances and is pharmacologically active, antigenic, cytotoxic, and carcinogenic. These toxic substances can be divided into cigarette constituents (organic matter, nicotine alkaloids, additives) and pyrolysis products (carbon dioxide, carbon monoxide, tar).[22] Aldehydes, phenol, ammonia, and sulfur dioxide products are among the many surface irritants in cigarette smoke.

The average cigarette contains approximately 10 mg of nicotine. Most nicotine is concentrated in the oral cavity and pharynx, and a variable amount, probably 1 to 2 mg, is actually delivered to the lungs.[66] A puff of smoke results in a measurable blood level of nicotine in the brain within seconds. With regular use, nicotine accumulates in the body during the day and persists overnight. Nicotine readily crosses the blood-brain barrier, where it acts as an agonist on specific CNS cholinergic receptor systems.[67]

Through its direct effects on the brain, particularly in the medulla, nicotine causes a decrease in stomach contractions, with nausea and vomiting. In addition, many complex effects on other organ systems appear to be primarily mediated through catecholamine release.[67] Acute cardiovascular responses to nicotine include increases in systolic and diastolic blood pressure, heart rate, force of myocardial contraction, myocardial oxygen consumption, coronary blood flow, and peripheral vasoconstriction. Nicotine's effect on the endocrine system is a reduction in growth hormone, cortisol, and ADH and an increase in serum glucose concentration. Nicotine causes a generalized stimulating pattern of brain electrical activity.[66]

Nicotine can alter the activity of many drugs, usually by the induction of liver microsomal enzyme systems. Smokers may have reduced blood levels of certain drugs; in particular the rate of metabolism for coumadin may be increased. Therefore dosages of these drugs may need to be altered in heavy smokers. In women, smoking increases the potential for serious adverse effects when taking oral contraceptives.[68]

Health Consequences

The health consequences of smoking may be related to both active smoking and passive smoking, but the most troublesome consequences are directly related to active smoking. The most prevalent risks are cancers, cardiovascular disease, and pulmonary disease.

Cigarette smoking is associated with elevated rates of cancer of the lung, oral cavity, pharynx, larynx, esophagus, bladder, and kidney.[69,70] Smoking is the number-one risk factor associated with the development of oral squamous cell carcinoma.[62] Numerous cardiovascular problems are associated with long-term smoking, particularly the risk of coronary artery disease, angina, myocardial infarction, and debilitating peripheral vascular disease, most notably *thromboangiitis obliterans* (Burger's disease).[70] Long-term smoking causes significant pulmonary changes that are progressive and can lead to emphysema with chronic obstructive pulmonary disease and numerous recurrent lung infections. Smoking can cause a variety of changes in the upper aerodigestive tract, with decreased or abnormal smell and taste, particularly with alterations in tongue taste sensations. Vocal cord irritation may cause chronic cough and hoarseness.[22,68] In addition, chronic smoking can cause numerous changes in the overlying oral mucosa, with a greater incidence of mucous membrane and periodontal disease.[62,71]

Nicotine easily crosses the blood-placenta barrier, with an increased risk of fetal abnormalities. Heavy smokers have an increased risk of spontaneous abortion and are more likely to deliver babies small for gestational age; there is also an increased risk of giving birth to children with congenital abnormalities. Cigarette smoking has a harmful effect on a woman's chance of becoming pregnant, with fertility rate decreasing as the number of cigarettes smoked per day increases.[72] Chronic smoking has also been found to produce abnormal sperm counts and evidence of chromosomal damage in some males.[70]

Recognition and Assessment

In recent years, as patients have become more health oriented and medically informed, they are seeking advice, treatment, and support from dental professionals for oral problems that also affect their general health. In addition, dental professionals have become much more attuned to evaluating patient's oral health care needs in association with related general systemic health issues. Therefore it is vital that the dental professional have the knowledge and skills to confront the dental patient's smoking-related health problems from numerous perspectives. Dentists are in an ideal position to identify these disorders through new patient evaluation, oral health care maintenance and preventive treatment, and performance of routine dental care with regular follow-up visits. With routine vital signs assessment at each appointment, dental professionals may be the first to notice changes in blood pressure, heart rate, and respiratory status. Proper counseling and consultation with the patient's primary care physician may assist in the prevention of potential side effects of smoking.

A comprehensive head and neck examination with special attention to the oral cavity and a dental evaluation provide clues into the recognition of diseases associated with smokers. Smoking is the number-one risk factor associated with the development of oral squamous cell carcinoma, and long-time smokers should be closely followed with routine oral cancer screenings. Dental professionals are the ideal health care providers to evaluate oral and pharyngeal changes that may be precancerous lesions. Any area of erythroplakia (red) or leukoplakia (white) lesions must be appropriately documented and evaluated. Careful examination should be performed to rule out any suspected area of irritation to the local oral mucosa when a red or white lesion is found, and the area should be closely observed for 2 to 3 weeks to check for resolution. If any suspicious oral lesion persists, biopsy and histologic examination are mandatory.

Cigar and pipe smoking can particularly produce changes on the palatal mucosa, with palatal hyperkeratosis and inflamed accessory salivary gland duct orifices. This classic picture of *stomatitis nicotina* (smokers' palate) is produced by the caustic and irritating effects of smoke inhalation and is generally completely reversible after removal of the smoke and heat irritant. Smokeless tobacco in any form may also cause localized oral mucosal changes, especially localized hyperkeratosis in the buccal vestibule, where the smokeless tobacco is placed. Harmful effects of smoking on the periodontium are associated with an increased prevalence and severity of periodontal disease and a greater resistance to standard periodontal therapy.[71]

In recent years, dental professionals have become much more globally health oriented and medically informed about the role of dental health, dental and oral disease, and systemic disease. They are giving advice, treatment, and support for oral and dental problems that may affect systemic health. This is most evidenced by the role of smoking cessation training by dental professionals. Dental professionals can initiate smoking cessation programs in their offices in various ways. Reception areas can have written materials to increase patient awareness; hygienists can direct patient education; and dentists can provide reinforcement and advice and prescribe nicotine substitutes with other approved therapy. Dental professionals may be directly involved with more formal smoking cessation programs or may know of ongoing support systems for recovering smokers either in community-based smoking cessation programs or at medical center and academic institution programs. They can guide their patients to the appropriate and necessary treatment programs.

Medical Issues

Alterations in dental treatment for smokers are generally related to the amount, duration, and associated medical illnesses related to the patient's smoking. The dentist should assess the level of severity of systemic illness related to smoking, particularly any specific precipitants of an acute cardiopulmonary problem. Knowledge of the patient's medications for related systemic disease is also important before providing dental treatment.

 Sedative/Hypnotic (Benzodiazepines)

Sedative-hypnotics are CNS depressants that include the benzodiazepines, the barbiturates, and the many barbiturate-like drugs. The primary function of these drugs is to relax the patient or to induce sleep. The barbiturates were first synthesized in the late 1800s and were used to induce sleep. In the 1930s and 1940s the barbiturates were widely prescribed in the United States as "sleeping pills." Shortly thereafter, it was shown that the barbiturates were addicting and could cause withdrawal symptoms. Barbiturates became increasingly popular as sedatives and general anesthetics in the hospital setting, as well as in the outpatient surgical setting, particularly in dental care.[73,74] Despite a decline in their use in the 1960s, barbiturates were still widely prescribed and abused in the 1970s and 1980s. Currently, however, the barbiturates have been largely replaced by benzodiazepines for most medicinal uses and even for abuse potential.[75]

The use of the benzodiazepines in the United States steadily increased through the 1970s to a peak level in the mid-1970s as the most common drugs prescribed annually, with diazepam (Valium) the most frequently prescribed drug of any kind.[76,77] The benzodiazepines are virtually completely absorbed after ingestion. The parent drug and active metabolites bind to plasma proteins to an extent that correlates strongly with lipid solubility and ranges from about 70% for alprazolam (Xanax) to nearly 99% for diazepam. Rapid uptake of the benzodiazepines by the brain tissue occurs after ingestion because of this high lipid solubility and high profusion rate.[78] The benzodiazepines are metabolized by several different enzyme systems in the liver before excretion by the kidney. Most benzodiazepines have active metabolites with longer half-lives and durations of action than the original drug. Many long-acting benzodiazepines have half-lives up to several days.[78]

The benzodiazepines act on the CNS to produce sedation, hypnosis, decreased anxiety, muscle relaxation, alterations in sleep patterns, and anticonvulsant activity. These CNS effects are the primary reasons why benzodiazepines are prescribed in the medical setting. Their actions result from potentiation of neural inhibition, which is mediated by GABA. In therapeutic doses the drugs have little effect on the respiratory, cardiovascular, and GI systems.[22,78] Toxic doses of benzodiazepines may cause varying degrees of lightheadedness, lethargy, motor incoordination, ataxia, mental impairment, dysarthria, and even amnesia. In very large doses they may cause stupor or even coma, but they rarely cause death when taken alone. The benzodiazepines act synergistically with other CNS depressants, however, and may cause greater morbidity and even mortality when used together. With protracted use, patients can develop tolerance to the sedative effects of benzodiazepines, but tolerance probably does not develop to the drugs' antianxiety effects.[78,79]

The development of dependence to high doses or chronic administration of benzodiazepines is a well-known physiologic phenomenon. The type of benzodiazepine and duration of abuse determine the potential for dependence and the abstinence and withdrawal syndromes that may be identified. Benzodiazepines with shorter half-lives (alprazolam, lorazepam, oxazepam) appear to have the highest potential for abuse.[79,80]

The typical benzodiazepine abstinence syndrome is similar to that of the barbiturates and other CNS depressants. Symptoms may include intense anxiety, insomnia, sensitivity to light and sound, and irritability, which may progress to tremulousness, muscle twitching, tachycardia, elevated blood pressure, confusion, and seizures. Duration of symptoms varies from a few hours to several days and up to even a week or more depending on the half-life of the abused drug.[80] *Rebound phenomenon* occurs after discontinuation of short-term benzodiazepine use. This consists of an exacerbation of the original symptoms and lasts for only a few days. *Symptom reemergence* develops when the original symptoms recur after cessation of benzodiazepines. Unlike the rebound phenomenon, these symptoms persist, do not fluctuate, and are much more difficult to resolve.[80,81]

Health Consequences

Health consequences of benzodiazepine abuse, as with many other CNS drugs, are related to the type used, duration of use, and route of administration. In addition to producing sedation and decreased motivation, benzodiazepines can cause severe depression that may result in suicide attempts.[76] Significant sedation may lead to falls or other accidents, especially with driving or operating machinery. With long-acting benzodiazepines and particularly after chronic administration, there is an increased risk of seizures.[76,81] Although the IV route for benzodiazepines is not as common as for other abused drugs, the same complications can occur as with any IV drug of abuse.

 ### Cannabinoids

Cannabinoids are a derivative of the Indian hemp plant, *Cannabis sativa,* which contains more than 60 cannabinoids, of which *tetrahydrocannabinol* (THC) is the major psychoactive substance. *Marijuana* is the dried flowering top, leaves, and stems of this plant that are dried, chopped up, and smoked in cigarettes or pipes. *Hashish* is the resinous extract of the hemp plant obtained by boiling the plant parts covered with the resin in a solvent or by scraping off the resin. It is a very potent form, with a much higher THC content than marijuana. Marijuana is by far the most frequently used form of cannabis in the United States.[22,82]

In the United States, the THC content of most marijuana is only 1% to 2%, but selective breeding can yield marijuana plants with much higher THC concentrations. No more than 60% of the THC in a marijuana cigarette is actually absorbed from the lungs when smoked. Marijuana users inhale smoke as deeply into their lungs as possible and hold their breath for at least 30 seconds to extract as much THC from the smoke as possible.[22] With this technique for smoking, plasma concentrations reach their peak in 5 to 10 minutes, and the psychoactive effects may peak within 20 minutes, seldom lasting longer than 2 to 3 hours. Marijuana may be eaten but is only about one-half to one-third as effective as when smoked.[82]

A little THC is rapidly converted into an active metabolite, which produces effects identical to the parent compound. This metabolite is then converted to inactive metabolites and excreted in both the feces and the urine. After reaching its peak, the plasma THC level falls rapidly at first due to the distribution of this lipid-soluble drug to lipid-rich tissues, including the brain. This is followed by a much slower decline in plasma blood levels, reflecting the gradual metabolism and elimination of the drug.[82] Traces of THC can be detected in the urine for 2 to 3 days after isolated smoking of the drug. With heavy daily smoking a urine drug screen may be positive for up to 4 to 6 weeks.[22,83,84]

The mechanism of action of THC is presently unknown, and to date no specific receptor mechanism has been identified. Its mode of action is likely on the cell membrane itself, where THC exerts its most prominent effects on the CNS and the cardiovascular system. Smoking marijuana effects mood, memory, motor coordination, sensorium, sense of time and space, and self-perception. Marijuana typically produces an increased sense of well-being and euphoria, with feelings of relaxation and sleepiness. There may be a loss of short-term memory, with difficulty performing tasks that require multiple mental steps, and a sense of detachment from real-world parameters. The smoker may have impaired perception, attention, and information processing, with additional impaired psychomotor function and some balance and coordination difficulty. The senses of touch, taste, smell, and hearing may also be increased, with vivid visual imagery. The person often has an altered perception of time, which seems to pass more slowly, and a feeling of depersonalization with oneself and others.

Cardiovascular effects may include increased heart rate, increased systolic blood pressure in the supine position, and decreased blood pressure in the erect position, with lightheadedness and fainting on movements, particularly from the sitting to the standing position. Sodium retention and an expanded plasma volume may occur, along with muscle weakness, tremors, and increased deep tendon reflexes. Marijuana inhibits sweating, which leads to an increase in body temperature, especially in a hot environment.

Marijuana smoking causes dry mouth and dryness of the throat, with a risk for associated oral-mucous membrane changes as well as secondary lung disorders.[22,82,83]

High concentrations of THC can induce delusions, hallucinations, and paranoia; normal thinking becomes confused and disorganized. Chronic use of marijuana does increase the rate of metabolism of THC, although most of the tolerance that develops to marijuana is psychodynamic in nature, developing to changes in mood, tachycardia, decreased skin temperature, increased body temperature, and psychomotor impairment.[85] Those who stop smoking marijuana after chronic use of high doses become irritable, restless, and nervous and may have decreased appetite, insomnia, and an altered sleep pattern. These symptoms are relatively mild, beginning a few hours after drug use is stopped, and can last up to several days.[82,83]

Health Consequences

Over the years, many health concerns have been expressed regarding marijuana abuse, particularly since this is such a significant problem within the population. Inhaling marijuana smoke normally causes bronchodilation. For some individuals, however, the particles in the inhalant act as irritants and can cause bronchoconstriction and increased airway resistance. Pharyngitis, sinusitis, and bronchitis may also occur secondary to chronic smoke ingestion. Marijuana smoke contains numerous carcinogens, with the potential for development of oropharyngeal epithelial precursors to oral cancer. This phenomenon also suggests an increased risk of lung cancer in heavy marijuana smokers. Men who are heavy smokers may have decreased sperm counts and sperm mobility; both are reversible with discontinuation of the drug. Teratogenetic effects have been linked to marijuana use.

Marijuana increases heart rate and carboxyhemoglobin concentration, which can be particularly problematic in people with significant primary lung disease or cardiovascular disease. It is uncertain whether marijuana use suppresses cell-mediated immunity.[82,86,87] Some heavy marijuana smokers may develop an "amotivational syndrome," which consists of a loss of energy, lethargy, apathy, absence of ambition, loss of effectiveness, inability to perform activities of daily living, and problems with impaired memory and mental performance. It is also unclear whether this amotivational syndrome is a direct result of marijuana abuse or is a secondary phenomenon in some individuals with a preexisting persistent behavioral problem with psychiatric manifestations.[22]

Recognition and Assessment

If marijuana use is not elicited from the history, the diagnosis may be based on certain typical signs of marijuana intoxication. There may be the distinct smell of marijuana smoke on the breath, redness and injection of the conjunctiva, and an increased pulse rate and overall general arousal in an otherwise healthy person. Patients may also present either with the CNS effects of hyperarousal, anxiety, and agitation or with lethargy and somnolence, as in the acutely intoxicated, or "stoned," individual. A persistent dry mouth with dry mucous membranes or areas of hyperkeratosis or leukoplakia, without a history of cigarette smoking, should suggest marijuana use.

Medical Issues

The medical issues related to dental care of the marijuana abuser are first related to any behavioral issues that the patient may have with the providing of routine dental treatments. No treatment should be provided to a patient who appears acutely intoxicated or is in the anxious or the lethargic state. Medical issues relevant to providing routine dental care include frequent and comprehensive oro-pharyngeal and head and neck examination, given the potential for the development of precancerous or cancerous epithelial lesions. The pulmonary function abnormalities associated with chronic marijuana smoking may be relevant when providing long dental appointments in a particular patient position and using materials and substances that may potentiate the irritant effect on the upper respiratory tract. An allergic asthmatic-like attack and bronchoconstriction may occur in an acute hyperactive airway syndrome.

 Cocaine

Cocaine is a CNS stimulant and local anesthetic. It is a naturally occurring alkaloid extracted from the leaves of the *Erythroxylon coca* plant. Cocaine can be used in numerous forms: coca leaves, coca paste, cocaine hydrochloride, free-base cocaine, and crack cocaine. The most commonly used forms in the United States are cocaine hydrochloride and crack cocaine. Cocaine hyrdochloride is the purified form of cocaine extracted from the coca paste with hydrochloric acid. The powder is mixed with numerous adulterants before distribution or use. It most often is injected intravenously or snorted through the nose. With the aid of a volatile substance (e.g., ether, baking soda, ammonia) and heat, the mixture of cocaine forms small pieces of hard material that resemble rocks. Because these hard pieces of cocaine make a "crackling" sound when smoked, this form is known as crack cocaine.[22,88]

The rapidity of onset and duration of action depends on the form of cocaine used and its route of administration. The IV route is the most efficient method of cocaine administration. After IV injection, onset of action is in 15 to 30 seconds and duration of action 10 to 20 minutes. The quicker onset, shorter duration of action, and higher blood levels make IV injection more addictive than other methods of administration.[89] Intranasal cocaine use is very popular but suffers from the side effect of vasoconstriction of the nasal vessels, which limits absorption and effect as well as causing local complications. After intranasal administration the onset of action is within 2 to 3 minutes, with peak effect in 15 to 20 minutes and duration of 30 to 45 minutes.[89] The effects of smoking crack cocaine occur very rapidly and intensely because the free-base form has a lower temperature of volatilization. Also, a larger percentage enters the lungs, where the free-base cocaine has rapid access to the bloodstream. The crack form is also much more lipid soluble and allows quick passage into the CNS. The onset of action is 5 to 10 seconds after inhalation, with a duration of 5 to 10 minutes and peak effect in 1 to 2 minutes. Administration of the drug must be repeated every 20 to 30 minutes to maintain the euphoria and avoid any withdrawal symptoms.[88,89]

Cocaine has potent pharmacologic effects on the dopamine, norepinephrine, and serotonin neuron systems in the CNS, including alterations and blockade of cellular membrane transport and inhibited reuptake of biogenic amine from synaptic spaces. With acute cocaine use, synaptic transmission in the dopamine pathway is enhanced by specific blockade of dopamine reuptake, thus increasing the dopamine concentration at the synapse.[18] Repeated use of cocaine tends to decrease synaptic transmission by depleting dopamine stores through increased breakdown in the synaptic cleft. The dopamine depletion gives rise to the cocaine craving, withdrawal symptoms, and dysphoric reactions experienced with cocaine withdrawal.[90,91]

Cocaine use causes a variety of both acute and chronic effects similar to those produced by amphetamines and other CNS stimulants. Peripheral end-organ and CNS effects may produce severe and even life-threatening reactions and complications with overdose. Peripheral effects of cocaine include increases in heart rate, blood pressure, and respiratory rate; hyperactive reflexes; and muscle twitching or tremor. The danger of significant myocardial ischemia and cardiac arrhythmia is the main concern in patients who are acutely cocaine intoxicated. Patients who are "high" on cocaine should not receive dental treatment for at least 6 hours after the last administration of cocaine. Local anesthetics with vasoconstrictors must not be used during this waiting period after cocaine administration, because the cocaine potentiates the response of sympathetically innervated organs, which could result in a hypertensive crisis, acute myocardial infarction, and cardiac arrest.[39]

Health Consequences

The many health consequences of cocaine abuse are the result of either the type of cocaine abused and its route of administration or the direct toxic effects of cocaine itself. Numerous central and peripheral effects of cocaine must be taken into consideration when planning dental treatment.

Different routes of administration of cocaine produce varied side effects. Snorting cocaine can cause rhinitis, mucosal irritation, nasal bleeding, nasal septum perforation, sinusitis, hoarseness, and difficulty swallowing. Smoking cocaine can cause chronic cough, chronic bronchitis, hemoptysis, and altered pulmonary function with decreased pulmonary reserve. IV use may cause local infection at the sites of injection, development of hepatitis, bacterial endocarditis, and infectious transmittable diseases (e.g., AIDS).[92]

Acute cocaine intoxication can present as CNS overstimulation, with an agitated, anxious, energetic, and talkative patient who has moist, clammy skin and dilated pupils. Heart rate, respiratory rate, and blood pressure may be increased. Acute intoxication and overdose of cocaine may lead to an acute medical emergency. In this situation no treatment should be performed, and the patient should ideally be sent for emergency medical observation.

Recognition and Assessment

Recognition and assessment of cocaine abuse also primarily involves the signs and symptoms produced by the toxicity of the drug or from the route of administration.

Medical Issues

The medical issues related to providing dental care to the cocaine abuser primarily involve the systemic effects of cocaine and its potentiating effect on direct-acting sympathomimetics and other vasoactive compounds that act as substrates for neuronal amine reuptake. Sympathetic nervous system effects can put these patients at risk during dental treatment. The effect of local anesthesia with epinephrine can cause an increase in total plasma epinephrine concentration.[39] Combined with circulating cocaine, this excess sympathetic stimulation can have serious consequences. The dosage of cocaine is not critical, with dysrhythmias occurring at both low and high doses.[39,92] Also, unpredictable alterations may occur in heart rate and blood-pressure with administration of local anesthesia in these patients.[37] Toxic doses of stimulants such as cocaine along with local anesthesia with epinephrine may cause sudden death; cardiac dysrhythmias progress to ventricular fibrillation, convulsions, hyperpyrexia, and seizures.[39] In patients with a history of cocaine abuse, care must be taken not to provide dental treatment to the acutely intoxicated patient. In addition, local vasoconstrictor anesthesia should be used judiciously when the patient may have used cocaine in the past 24 hours.

Cocaine use may potentiate CNS effects, so drugs must be prescribed especially carefully to patients who use cocaine. Also, prescribed drugs may interact with cocaine and produce abnormally long clinical manifestations of CNS agents.

Other medical issues involve the particular route of cocaine administration. Respiratory complications may result from smoking crack cocaine and include hyperactive airway disorder and bronchospasm. This may be important when providing dental care in the supine position for long periods. As with any IV drug user, infectious disease may occur, either localized at the injection site or with the potential for infectious endocarditis. IV drug users also have a significantly greater risk for infectious disease, such as hepatitis B or C and AIDS.

 Opioids

Opioids have varying degrees of morphine-like properties. Opioids include naturally occurring, semisynthetic, synthetic, agonist-antagonist, and pure antagonist compounds. The various opioid drugs react with opioid receptors similar to the endogenous opioid peptides. At a specific receptor, a given opioid may act as an agonist, a partial agonist, or an antagonist. The receptors determine the actions of the drug and the potential side effects.[18,22,93] The three major categories of endogenous opioid receptors are designated as mu, kappa, and delta. The *mu receptor* is thought to mediate supraspinal analgesia, respiratory depression, euphoria, and physical dependence. The *kappa receptor* may mediate spinal anesthesia, miosis, and sedation. The dysphoria, hallucinations, and abnormal affective behavior often associated with opioid use are probably related to *delta* receptors.[93]

Most opioids are well absorbed from subcutaneous and intramuscular sites and the nose. Despite rapid absorption from the GI tract as well, some opioid drugs are much less potent when so absorbed because of a significant first-pass effect by the liver (e.g., morphine, hydromorphone, oxymorphone). On the other hand, some opioids do not undergo first pass effect, so their potency after oral dosing is similar to parenteral dosing (e.g., methadone, levorphanol, codeine). Opioids bind to plasma proteins with varying degrees of affinity; however, they rapidly leave the blood and localize in highest concentrations in tissues such as lungs, liver, kidneys, and spleen. These tissues serve as the major reservoir for the drug because of their varying bulk and distribution. Brain concentrations of opioids are usually relatively low compared with concentrations in these other tissues, but the effect on the brain and neuronal function is significant.[22,93] Opioids are converted largely by the liver to metabolites that are generally inactive and rapidly excreted by the kidneys. *Meperidine* is hydrolyzed by esterases in the liver to normeperidine, a toxic metabolite, and therefore should be used with caution in chronic administration.

The opioid analgesics cause a wide variety of pharmacologic effects on numerous systems in the body. The primary CNS effect of analgesia is the overwhelming reason why opioids are used in medical and dental practice. However, CNS effects of sedation, drowsiness, euphoria or dysphoria, impaired reflexes and incoordination, dizziness, and ataxia can also occur. Central effects may produce nausea and vomiting, in addition to the primary GI effects of opioids; increased tone and decreased propulsive movements of the intestines may exacerbate the problems of nausea and associated constipation. Opioids have only minimal cardiovascular effects, with a slight reduction in blood pressure and heart rate in the supine position and occasional orthostatic hypotension when changing positions or arising quickly. A major pharmacologic effect is decreased respiratory rate and depth due to both central and peripheral receptor effects. The endocrine and metabolic effects of opioids include increased release of ADH and prolactin and decreased release of LH and thyrotropin. Opioids generally produce a flushing and feeling of warmth, especially on the face, neck, and upper thorax, probably caused by histamine release. Itching and skin rash also may result from this same effect.

Health Consequences

The adverse health consequences of opioid abuse are related not only to the pharmacologic actions of the drugs themselves, but also to the methods used to administer them and to the lifestyles of the substance abuser. With respect to the pharmacologic actions of the opioids, overdose can result in respiratory depression, pulmonary edema, hypotension, circulatory collapse, and even death. Peripheral neural complications may include myelitis and plexitis, which may occur after periods of abstinence. These peripheral neuropathies may also occur in the face through the trigeminal system.

Depending on the route of administration, opioid abusers may develop serious infections because they lack aseptic techniques and may share needles and syringes for IV injections. Cellulitis, skin abscess, infectious endocarditis, pulmonary or intracranial abscess, hepatitis B or C infection, and HIV infection or AIDS are common in this population. Opioid abusers, particularly those who use the IV route, have high rates of sexually transmitted diseases, mostly from sexual promiscuity and prostitution. Opioid abusers develop higher tolerance and very low tolerance to many pharmacologic effects. Typically the abuser has a high tolerance to opioid, analgesic, euphoric, sedative, and mental-clouding effects and after a short period needs to increase the dose because of these physiologic effects. Physiologic and psychological dependence will occur with prolonged opioid use, and opioid abusers will have the "need" for these drugs to prevent withdrawal symptoms.

A withdrawal syndrome occurs approximately 6 to 8 hours after the last administration of opioid drug. The user usually experiences a runny nose, lacrimation, abdominal muscle cramps, chills, horripilation, hyperventilation, mydriasis, nausea, vomiting, diarrhea, muscle aches and twitching, and anxiety or hostility. About 12 to 14 hours after the last dose, opioid addicts may fall into a tossing, restless sleep from which they waken several hours later, more miserable than before.[22,94] Time of onset, intensity, and duration of the abstinence syndrome are related to the half-life of the specific drug. With short-acting drugs, withdrawal signs and symptoms start within 6 to 8 hours after the last dose, peak in 36 to 48 hours, then gradually subside. With long-acting drugs, many patients take several days to reach the peak of the abstinence syndrome, which may last as long as 2 weeks.[83]

Recognition and Assessment

The recognition of opioid abuse is primarily through a comprehensive review of the patient's medical history for clues of opioid abuse. There are two types of opioid abusers: the street abuser and the medical abuser. *Street abusers* have a high incidence of liver dysfunction, hepatitis, and infectious disease. IV drug abusers may also have a significantly greater risk of infectious endocarditis and valvular heart disease, requiring antibiotic prophylaxis before dental treatment.[48,63] *Medical abusers*, however, often have an undiagnosed chronic pain syndrome and may present to the dental practitioner with a history of facial pain.

Physical examination may reveal opioid abuse through CNS depressant effects (slurred speech, mental clouding, ataxia) and the finding of pinpoint pupils with minimal reactivity. Long-term abusers may exhibit multiple carious lesions in their teeth, particularly around the gingival margins, probably a result of the opioid-induced xerostomia with hypoglycemia, associated high intake of sweets, and lack of appropriate daily oral hygiene.

An abstinence syndrome with withdrawal signs and symptoms is likely in the physically dependent opioid abuser who has not "used" for some time. This patient may present to the dental practitioner, who can take precautions to avoid contributing to the physical dependence or the abstinence syndrome. NSAIDs with long-acting local anesthetics should be considered first to control any posttreatment discomfort. If severe pain is anticipated, it is appropriate to prescribe opiate analgesics, limiting the prescribed quantity and, if possible, verifying with the pharmacy that the patient has no similar prescription. The dentist may also want to consult with the practitioner managing the patient's substance abuse.

 Psychostimulants

The use of **psychostimulants** has a long history, and Chinese physicians have been using these compounds for more than 5000 years.

Amphetamines

Amphetamine proper was first synthesized in 1887 as part of a systematic program to manufacture amines for medical use. Early investigations of the properties of amphetamine focused on the peripheral effects and found that amphetamine was a sympathomimetic agent. Oddly, the CNS actions were not reported until the early 1900s, closely followed by the first reports of amphetamine abuse.[95] Amphetamines produce feelings of euphoria with relief from fatigue and improve performance on some simple tasks, increasing activity levels and producing anorexia. Chronic consumption of amphetamines results in stereotypic behavior, paranoia, and aggression. During the protracted withdrawal phase from amphetamine, individuals experience anhedonia and anergy, the result of long-lasting and probably permanent changes in the neurobiologic substrates that mediate the reward pathway in the brain.[96]

The amphetamines are direct catecholamine agonists, and administration results in the release of newly synthesized norepinephrine and dopamine.[97-99] Amphetamine administration also influences various neuropeptide systems. Peptidergic systems are associated with mesostriatal dopamine circuitry and are thought to play a modulatory role in dopaminergic activity within the brain. Neurotensin pathways also serve to modulate dopaminergic activity. These changes in neuropeptide levels may mediate some behavioral effects from repeated doses of amphetamine.[100]

The systemic administration of amphetamines generally results in a dose-dependent depression of the firing rate of catecholaminergic neurons and noradrenergic neurons in the brainstem LC.[101] One of the primary effects of the amphetamines and related stimulant compounds is CNS stimulation, which results in the characteristic activation of behavior. The major behavioral effects of acute and chronic administration of amphetamines are locomotor stimulation, stereotypic induction, aggression, and anorexia. These behavioral effects are mediated through potential neurosubstrates within limbic and basal ganglionic structures in the brain.

Health Consequences

Chronic, high-dose abuse of amphetamines results in toxic pathophysiologic changes, primarily mediated by long-term neurotransmitter (norepinephrine, dopamine, serotonin) depletion.[102-104] Changes in cerebral vasculature indicate that chronic amphetamine users are at high risk for cerebrovascular damage. High-dose amphetamines also induce hypertensive episodes associated with cerebral hemorrhage, with several deaths attributed to hemorrhages induced by chronic use.[105]

Amphetamines raise both systolic and diastolic blood pressure, and heart rate is reflexively slowed. Tachycardia and cardiac arrhythmias may occur after high doses. Catecholamines sensitize the myocardium to ectopic stimuli, thereby increasing the risk of fatal cardiac arrhythmias.[106] Amphetamines result in peripheral hyperthermia through activation of the sympathoadrenal system but produce hypothermia centrally, as mediated by the activity of the anterior hypothalamus.[107] Another major cause of death related to amphetamine abuse is hyperpyrexia, directly related to catecholamine effects. If not fatal in itself, hyperpyrexia leads to a cascade of convulsions, coma, and cerebral hemorrhage.[108]

Medical Issues

Despite the overwhelming abuse potential, amphetamines have several medical uses, with new uses in development. The U.S. Food and Drug Administration has approved amphetamines for narcolepsy and attention-deficit hyperactivity disorder (ADHD). The diagnosis of ADHD has become common, characterized by frequent fidgeting, difficulties in focusing on assignments, impulsivity, excessive talking and interruption of others, and repeated shifting from one activity to another.[109] First-line treatment for ADHD is use of psychostimulants, primarily the amphetamines, along with other non-stimulant-based pharmacologic treatments and numerous non-pharmacologic behavioral treatments.

Stimulants are also used as anorectic agents, which may be effective for weight loss at least for several months after treatment.[110] Besides abuse potential, only a small percentage of individuals maintain weight loss after cessation of anorectics. The stimulant-anorectic fenfluramine appears to work primarily on the serotonergic system without major psychostimulant effects.[111] Stimulants also are effective in senile and chronic brain syndrome patients, severely medically ill or post-stroke patients, depressed patients, and those with HIV-related neuropsychiatric symptoms.[112,113]

Phencyclidine

Phencyclidine (PCP, angel dust) was developed in the 1950s in a research program targeting general anesthetics. Patients anesthetized with PCP did not manifest the cardiovascular and respiratory depression typical of classic anesthetic agents. The PCP-induced anesthetic state differed sharply from the state of relaxed sleep induced by other general anesthetic agents. Patients appeared catatonic, open mouthed, and fixed, sightlessly staring with rigid posturing. It was inferred that without overt loss of consciousness, patients were sharply dissociated from the environment. PCP and other related compounds were thus classified as "dissociative anesthetics."[114,115] Despite its physiologic advantages over traditional anesthetics, PCP was removed from the market in 1965 and officially limited thereafter to veterinary applications.

PCP was originally ingested orally. Risk of overdose is greater with the oral form, however, so PCP is now more often smoked or snorted, allowing the user more control of dosage. Initial use is usually in a smoking form in conjunction with marijuana or tobacco. PCP is used by people from all socioeconomic backgrounds with and without formal premorbid psychopathology and is most often used as a social drug with other drug users.[116]

The CNS effects of PCP are initiated by binding of the drug to high-affinity PCP receptors. These receptors and PCP receptor ligands potentially inhibit neurotransmission mediated at NMDA-type glutamate receptors. Unlike other glutamate receptors, NMDA channels are permeable to calcium along with sodium. After NMDA receptor activation, NMDA-mediated calcium flux may lead to stimulation of multiple intracellular processes and second messenger pathways.[117,118] The behavioral effects of PCP respond partially to treatment with neuroleptics and may also be reversed by agents (e.g., glycine) that augment NMDA receptor–mediated neurotransmission.[119] Behavioral effects of PCP in rodents appear to result from interactions with dopamine terminal fields rather than with dopaminergic midbrain nuclei.[120]

Health Consequences

Overall, research has established a compelling case that PCP is a strongly addictive drug. Despite a paucity of controlled studies of tolerance and dependence in humans, PCP must be considered comparable to classic drugs of abuse in this respect. The range of clinical effects of PCP can be correlated with dose and serum PCP concentrations, as well as interactions with molecular target sites. PCP is difficult to eliminate from the body through the urine after large doses. The extremely large volume of PCP distribution implies that neither hemodialysis nor hemoperfusion would promote drug clearance.[121] At present, no drug has been shown to function as a PCP antagonist, making management of the acutely intoxicated state extremely difficult, if not impossible.

The majority of PCP-intoxicated patients manifest *nystagmus*, which may be horizontal, vertical, or rotatory. Nystagmus is one of the crucial signs that can help distinguish PCP intoxication from a naturally occurring psychotic state. Coma can occur at any point during intoxication. Dose-dependent neuronal hyperexcitability ranges from increased deep tendon reflexes through opisthotonos, to generalized or focal seizure states and status epilepticus.[122] Focal neurologic findings may result from cerebral vasoconstriction. Seizures can be managed with IV benzodiazepines.

A psychotic state may occur after even extremely low doses of PCP, and such cognitive and emotional alterations are the drug's threshold effects. Clinically urgent behavioral complications of PCP abuse do not result from the psychotic symptoms but rather from *behavioral disinhibition*, which may be coupled with severe anxiety, panic, rage, and aggression. Such reactions are more common at higher doses, and delirium and neurologic symptoms may also occur. These behavioral manifestations can severely compromise the clinician's ability to diagnose further and treat life-threatening medical complications of PCP intoxication. The disruption of sensory input by PCP causes unpredictable, exaggerated, distorted, or violent reactions to environmental stimuli. A cornerstone is therefore minimization of sensory inputs to PCP-intoxicated patients; they should be evaluated and treated in as quiet and isolated an environment as possible.

No specific PCP antagonist is available. The goal of therapy for PCP-induced behavioral toxicity is patient protection, sedation, and prevention of more life-threatening complications, using nonpharmacologic behavioral modalities or benzodiazepines.

DENTAL TREATMENT CONSIDERATIONS

With patients who are known substance abusers, the dentist must consider the following questions when planning dental treatment:

1. What is the substance abused, duration of abuse, amount and pattern of current use, and route of administration?

2. How will the substance use alter the patient's medical health?
3. What dental treatment is planned (emergency, examination, restorative, minor surgery, more extensive surgery), and what form of anesthesia is planned (none, local, IV sedation, general anesthesia)?
4. What information is necessary before performing treatment?
5. How will the substance abuse alter the treatment?
6. How can untoward reactions be prevented?
7. What considerations are necessary for the postoperative period?

Certain abused substances require little alteration in most forms of dental treatment; knowledge of the potential complications and how to prevent them is usually sufficient. Other abused substances will necessitate further evaluations and information before some forms of dental treatment and specific alterations in treatment and postoperative care. Prescription medications often given to patients (who do not abuse substances) in the emergency dental care situation or after treatment may need to be altered for substance abuse patients. Before instituting dental treatment for substance abusers, the dental professional must carefully evaluate all these considerations in order to provide safe, quality dental care.

Alcohol

1. Long-standing alcohol abusers should be considered to have some degree of liver dysfunction and may have significant liver damage and liver failure.
2. Liver dysfunction can cause alterations in production of coagulation factors and cofactors and can cause problems with coagulation and prolonged bleeding.
3. Liver dysfunction can alter the production of protein compounds, most notably albumin. This can alter fluid balance and may promote altered or delayed wound healing.
4. Liver dysfunction will alter the metabolism of many exogenous drugs given for dental treatment (e.g., local/general anesthetics, sedatives) and after treatment (e.g., antimicrobials, analgesics, antianxiety-sedative agents).
5. Heavy alcohol use can cause esophagitis, gastritis, and GI ulcerative disease. Prescribed drugs can exacerbate these conditions and may be extremely harmful (e.g., aspirin compounds, NSAIDs).
6. Heavy alcohol use is associated with oral mucous membrane disease and especially oral cancer. A comprehensive oral cavity and head and neck examination is mandatory.
7. Laboratory Evaluation: prothrombin time (PT), international normalized ratio (INR), partial thromboplastin time (PTT), total protein and albumin, liver function tests, complete blood count (CBC). This evaluation can be done in consultation with the patient's primary care physician. Alterations from normal laboratory values may necessitate replacement of deficient coagulation factors, platelets, red cells, or postponing treatment.
8. No dental treatment should be performed in acutely intoxicated patients.
9. No contraindication must exist to routine local anesthesia with or without a vasoconstrictor.
10. Amounts of certain IV sedatives and general anesthetics may need to be changed because of altered drug metabolism.
11. Local hemostatic agents and primary wound closure are used when possible, with good postoperative wound care.
12. Caution should be exercised with prescribing aspirin compounds and NSAIDs, which may predispose the patient to gastric bleeding; acetaminophen, which may lead to liver disease; and opioids, which may cause excessive sedation.
13. Caution should be exercised with prescribing CNS depressants (e.g., benzodiazepines).
14. Alcoholics who are admitted to the hospital are at risk for alcohol withdrawal syndromes. Early stages of withdrawal, left untreated, can progress to hallucinations and seizures. This late withdrawal is called *delirium tremens* and occurs in approximately 5% of patients with withdrawal symptoms. This is a potentially life-threatening condition with a 12% to 15% mortality rate.[41] The mainstay of treatment is prevention. Administration of prophylactic long-acting benzodiazepines, such as diazepam (Valium), chlordiazepoxide (Librium), or clonazepam (Klonopin), is the treatment of choice. Supportive treatment with either β-blockers or α-blockers may be necessary to prevent withdrawal symptoms.

Nicotine

1. Cigarette smoking does not have a significant impact on routine dental treatment.
2. There are no specific alterations in dental treatment planning.
3. Due to the carcinogenic potential of cigarette smoking, a comprehensive oral cavity and head and neck examination should be performed frequently in patients who smoke. Any suspicious white or red lesion that does not resolve should be closely followed and a biopsy performed for histopathologic analysis.
4. There is an association between cigarette smoking and increased risk for periodontal disease, with increased breakdown and poor healing.
5. There is also the potential for delayed healing with cigarette smoking and the potential for development of localized alveolitis ("dry socket") after surgical procedures and extractions.

Cocaine

1. The most problematic effects are caused by the significant adrenergic effects of these drugs. The effects on the sympathetic and central nervous systems cause the most significant problems and need to be considered before dental treatment.
2. The route of administration also warrants consideration for evaluation and treatment. Cocaine users that inhale (snort) may develop nasal mucosal lesions and perforation of the nasal septum. Those who inject cocaine are prone to local infections, abscesses, and poor IV access. IV abusers are also more prone to infectious disease (e.g., hepatitis, HIV infection). Crack cocaine smokers are prone to respiratory complications that include bronchospasm, pulmonary edema, and pneumonia.
3. A comprehensive oral cavity and head and neck examination is important to identify any lesions related to cocaine abuse or infectious disease. IV abusers may have liver disease and need to be evaluated for liver dysfunction. Thrombocytopenia can occur secondary to bone marrow suppression. Evaluation of liver function and CBC may be necessary.
4. Cocaine use can produce acute elevations in blood pressure (tachycardia) and a predisposition to ventricular tachyarrhyth-

mias and seizures.[41] Coronary artery spasm has been related to acute myocardial infarction in cocaine abusers.
5. No treatment should be performed in a patient with suspected acute intoxication. Treatment should also be delayed (if possible) if cocaine has been used up to 24 hours before the office visit.
6. Local anesthesia with a vasoconstrictor should be used with extreme caution in cocaine abusers.
7. Chronic use may be associated with catecholamine depletion, which may require alterations in the amount of anesthetic agents required for IV sedation and general anesthesia. These agents should be used with caution in this situation, since hypotension and a myocardial ischemic event may result.
8. Psychotropic drugs should be prescribed with caution due to the unpredictable interactions with stimulants.
9. When sympathetic hyperarousal symptoms occur, all procedures should be stopped and oxygen administered along with monitoring of vital signs. Supportive emergency care should be provided and further evaluation performed and/or emergency support summoned. If possible, IV access should be obtained and IV fluids administered. Chest pain should be treated with sublingual nitrates. Hypertension should be treated with β-blockers or calcium channel blockers. Seizures should be treated with diazepam (Valium) or midazolam (Versed).

Benzodiazepines/Barbiturates

1. Benzodiazepine and barbiturate abusers often obtain their drug by prescription and are often difficult to identify. Due to a social stigma associated with prescription drug abuse, they may go to great lengths to hide their abuse.
2. Benzodiazepines and barbiturates are metabolized in the liver and have chemically active, long-acting metabolites and are known for inducing hepatic microsomal enzyme metabolic systems, often reducing the effectiveness of other drugs metabolized by the liver.
3. No treatment should be performed in the acutely intoxicated patient.
4. There are no contraindications to local anesthesia without evidence of other abnormalities.

5. Chronic abusers are prone to developing a withdrawal syndrome similar to alcohol withdrawal. This may start within 24 hours of the last dose and may last up to 3 weeks. Seizures and delirium occur infrequently with benzodiazepines but are often seen with barbiturate dependence.[41]

6. Gradual withdrawal of these drugs over 1 to 2 weeks is recommended (when possible) before treatment. If more immediate or emergency treatment is needed, patients should be maintained on a substitute, long-acting compound, and consideration should be given to hospitalization.

Opioids

1. Opioid abusers may present to dental professionals with a complaint of facial pain or "toothache." They often display other drug-seeking behaviors that might alert the dental professional of opioid abuse.

2. Opioids interact at multiple opioid receptors, which are responsible for the analgesia, physical dependence, euphoria, and respiratory depression.

3. IV opioid abusers should be further evaluated for signs of liver dysfunction, infectious disease (e.g., hepatitis, HIV), and a history of infectious endocarditis. Screenings should be performed for liver damage, infectious disease, endocarditis, and hematologic disorders.

4. Other problems include a high tolerance to other pain medications, difficult IV access, withdrawal syndromes, skin infections, infectious diseases, and behavioral problems.

5. No dental treatment should be performed in an acutely intoxicated patient.

6. Patients with a history or physical findings of endocarditis or valvular heart disease should be given appropriate antibiotic prophylaxis before treatment. Patients with significant liver disease should be managed as a patient with liver failure.

7. Patients in need of IV sedation or general anesthesia may require higher doses of opioids, benzodiazepines, and other anesthetic. During anesthetic induction, hypotension may occur secondary to intravascular volume depletion and adrenocortical insufficiency secondary to low levels of circulating opioids.

8. Patients on methadone maintenance should take their daily dose of methadone before treatment. These patients usually need supplemental opioid or other analgesic for postoperative pain management.

9. Chronic opioid abusers can start to withdraw from opioids within 6 hours of the last use, and therefore a withdrawal syndrome can occur in the dental office or hospital setting during treatment. Opioid withdrawal syndromes are mediated by alterations in neurochemicals (physiologic dependence), and most harmful effects are mediated via upregulation of the sympathetic nervous system.

10. Symptoms include excessive lacrimation, salivation, rhinorrhea, diaphoresis, fever, tremor, muscle cramping, tachycardia, restlessness, and diarrhea. Although not necessarily life threatening, these symptoms are very uncomfortable and may exacerbate associated medical conditions.[41]

11. Management of opioid withdrawal syndromes focuses on symptomatic treatments. Low-dose, long-acting opioids should be administered. Methadone is often advocated due to its good oral absorption from the GI tract, long half-life, good oral potency, and few active metabolites. Prevention of the sympathetically mediated side effects can be treated with an α-agonist (e.g., clonidine). Partial agonists and agonist-antagonists should be avoided because they may precipitate a withdrawal syndrome.

Cannabinoids (Marijuana)

1. Marijuana users can present in a euphoric (high) state after acute intoxication.

2. No dental treatment should be performed on a stoned patient.

3. Heavy marijuana smokers may show hyperreactive airway symptoms and evidence of pulmonary dysfunction. Positional changes may be necessary if long treatment is anticipated.

4. There is no contraindication to local anesthesia.

5. There is no contraindication to routine dental procedures.

6. As with cigarette smoking, marijuana smoking may interfere with postoperative bleeding and wound healing.

REFERENCES

1. American Psychiatric Association: *Diagnostic and statistical manual of mental disorders*, ed 4, Washington, DC, 1994, American Psychiatric Association.

2. Leshner AI: Substance abuse, *Arch Gen Psychiatry* 54:691-694, 1997.

3. *National Household Survey on Drug Abuse*, National Institute On Drug Abuse, Washington, DC, 1990, US Government Printing Office.

4. *Epidemiology in alcohol and health*, DHHS Pub No (ADM) 87-1519, Rockville, Md, 1987, US Department Of Health And Human Services.

5. Van Cleave S, Byrd W, Revell K: The equal opportunity destroyer: the magnitude of the drug abuse epidemic. In *Counseling for substance abuse and addiction*, Waco, Texas, 1987, Wordbook.

6. Johnston LD, O'Malley PM, Bachman JG: *Drug use by high school seniors, class of 1986*, Rockville, Md, 1986, US Department Of Health And Human Services.

7. Stoudemire A, Wallack L, Hedenark N: Alcohol dependence and abuse. In Amler RW, Dull HB, editors: *Closing the gap: the burden of unnecessary illness*, New York, 1987, Oxford University Press.

8. Milhorn HT Jr: Nicotine dependence, *Am Fam Physician* 39:214-224, 1989.

9. Gfroerer J: Nature and extent of drug abuse in the United States. In *Drug abuse and drug abuse research: third triennial report to Congress*, National Institute on Drug Abuse, DHHS, Washington, DC, 1991, US Government Printing Office.

10. Drug abuse and drug abuse research, report to Congress from Secretary, Department Of Health And Human Services, Washington, DC, 1984, US Government Printing Office.

11. *Epidemiologic trends in drug abuse*. Vol 1. Community Epidemiology Work Group, National Institute On Drug Abuse, DHHS, Public Health Service, Washington, DC, 1998, National Institutes Of Health.

12. Winger G, Hofmann FG, Woods JH: *A handbook on drug and alcohol abuse: the biomedical aspects*, ed 3, New York, 1992, Oxford University Press.

13. Delbanco TL, Barnes HN: The epidemiology of alcohol abuse and the response of physicians. In Barnes HN, Aronson MD, Delbanco TL, editors: *Alcoholism: a guide for the primary care physician*, 1987, New York, Springer-Verlag.

14. Jones OJ: Substance education at the University Of Maryland Dental School, *Md State Dent J* 39:89-90, 1996.

15. Frances RJ, Miller SI, editors: *Clinical textbook of addiction disorders*, ed 2, New York, 1998, Guilford.

16. Practice guidelines for the treatment of patients with substance disorders: alcohol, cocaine, opiods, *Am J Psychiatry* 152(suppl), November 1995.

17. Lettieri DJ: Drug abuse: a review of explanation and models of explanation. In Stimmel B, editor: *Alcohol and substance abuse in adolescents*, New York, 1985, Haworth.

18. Hyman SE, Nestler EJ: *The molecular foundations of psychiatry*, Washington, DC, 1993, American Psychiatric Association.

19. Tarter RE, Alterman AI, Edwards KL: Neurobiological theory of alcoholism etiology. In Chaudron CD, Wilkinson DA, editors: *Theories of alcoholism*, Toronto, 1988, Addiction Research Foundation.

20. Lester D: Genetic theory: an assessment of the hereditability of alcoholism. In Chaudron CD, Wilkinson DA, editors: *Theories of alcoholism*, Toronto, 1988, Addiction Research Foundation.

21. Heath DB: Emerging anthropological theory and models of alcohol use and alcoholism. In Chaudron CD, Wilkinson DA, editors: *Theories of alcoholism*, Toronto, 1988, Addiction Research Foundation.

22. Milhorn HT: *Chemical dependence: diagnosis, treatment and prevention*, New York, 1990, Springer-Verlag.

23. Van Cleave S, Byrd W, Revell K: If drugs are so bad, why do people keep using them? How denial and guilt perpetuate drug abuse. In *Counseling for substance abuse and addiction*, Waco, Texas, 1987, Wordbooks.

24. Nestler EJ: Molecular neurobiology of drug addiction, *Neuropsychopharmacology* 11:77-87, 1994.

25. Nestler EJ: Molecular mechanisms of drug addiction. J *Neurosci* 12:2439-2450, 1992.

26. Nestler EJ, Duman R: G-proteins and cyclic nucleotides in the nervous system. In Siegel GJ, Albers RW, Agranoff BW, Molinoff P, editors: *Basic neurochemistry: molecular, cellular and medical aspects*, ed 5, Boston, 1994, Little, Brown.

27. Koob GF: Drugs of abuse: anatomy, pharmacology and function of reward pathways, *Trends Pharmacol Sci* 13:177-184, 1992.

28. Johnson SW, North RA: Opioids excite dopamine neurons by hyperpolarization of local interneurons, J *Neurosci* 12:483-488, 1992.

29. Morrisett RA, Swartzwelder HS: Attenuation of hippocampal long-term potentiation by ethanol: a patch-clamp analysis of glutamatergic and gabaergic mechanisms, J *Neurosci* 13:2264-2272, 1993.

30. Wafford KA, Burnett DM, Leidenheimer NJ, et al: Ethanol sensitivity of the GABA-a receptor expressed in xenopus oocytes requires 8 amino acids contained in the gamma-2l subunit, *Neuron* 7:27-33, 1991.

31. Self DW, Nestler EJ: Molecular mechanisms of drug reinforcement and addiction, *Annu Rev Neurosci* 18:463-495, 1995.

32. Aghajanian G: Tolerance of locus ceruleus neurons to morphine and suppression of withdrawal response by clonidine, *Nature* 267:186-188, 1978.

33. Shen EC, Fu E: Carious lesions in the heroin-addicted patient, J *Periodont* 69:938-940, 1998.

34. Molendijk B, Ter Horst G, Kasbergen M, et al: Dental health in Dutch drug addicts, *Community Dent Oral Epidemiol* 24:117-119, 1996.

35. Milgrom P, Weinstein P, Roy-Byrne P, Tay KM: Dental fear treatment outcomes for substance use disorder patients, *Spec Care Dent* 13:139-142, 1993.

36. Robb ND, Smith BG: Chronic alcoholism: an important condition in the dentist-patient relationship, J *Dent* 24:17-24, 1996.

37. Crossley HL: Management of the active or recovering chemically dependent dental patient, *Md State Dent J* 39:85-86, 1996.

38. Little JW, Falace DA: *Dental management of the medically compromised patient*, ed 3, St Louis, 1988, Mosby.

39. Johnson CD, Lewis VA, Faught KS, Brown RS: The relationship between chronic cocaine or alcohol use and blood pressure in black men during uncomplicated tooth extraction, J *Oral Maxillofac Surg* 56:323-329, 1998.

40. Glick M: Medical considerations for dental care of patients with alcohol-related liver disease, *JADA* 128:61-69, 1997.

41. Sampson D, Gordon N: The clinical management of the alcoholic and substance abuse patient, *Oral Maxillofac Surg Clin North Am* 10:385-399, 1998.
42. Fiset L, Leroux B, Rothen M, et al: Pain control in recovering alcoholics: effects of local anesthesia, *J Stud Alcohol* 58:291-296, 1997.
43. Johnson CD, Brown RS: How cocaine abuse effects post-extraction bleeding, *JADA* 124:60-62, 1993.
44. Ter Horst G, Molendijk B, Brouwer E, Verhey HG: Differences in dental treatment plan and planning for drug-addicted and non-drug-addicted patients, *Community Dent Oral Epidemiol* 24:120-123, 1996.
45. Selzer M, Vinkour A, Van Rooijen L: A self-administered Short Michigan Alcohol Screening Test (SMAST), *J Stud Alcohol* 36:117-126, 1975.
46. Ewing JA: Detecting alcoholism: the CAGE questionnaire, *JAMA* 252:1905-1907, 1984.
47. Arif A, Westermeyer J: *Manual of drug and alcohol abuse: guidelines for teaching in medical and health institutions*, New York, 1988, Plenum.
48. Sonis ST, Fasio RC, Fang L: *Principles and practice of oral medicine*, ed 2, Philadelphia, 1995, WB Saunders.
49. Norris LH, Pappageorge MB: The poisoned patient: toxicologic emergencies, *Dent Clin North Am* 39:596-619, 1995.
50. Shuster MM, Lewin ML: Needle tracks in narcotic addicts, *NY J Med* 68:3129-3133, 1968.
51. Mandel L, Hemele-Bena D: Alcoholic parotid sialadenosis, *JADA* 128:1411-1415, 1997.
52. Harclerode J: Endocrine effects of marijuana in the male: preclinical studies, *NIDA Res Monogr* 44:46-64, 1984.
53. Smith CG, Asch RH: Acute, short-term and chronic effects of marijuana on the female primate reproductive function. In Braude MC, Ludford JP, editors: *Marijuana effects on the endocrine and reproductive systems*, Washington, DC, 1984, US Government Printing Office.
54. DiPaolo TC, Rouillard M, Morissette D, et al: Endocrine and neurochemical actions of cocaine, *Can J Physiol Pharmacol* 67:1177-1186, 1989.
55. Milhorn HT Jr: The diagnosis of alcoholism, *Am Fam Physician* 37:175-183, 1988.
56. Schonberg SK, editor: *Substance abuse: a guide for health professionals*, Elk Grove Village, Ill, 1988, American Academy Of Pediatrics.
57. Mullen J, Brach HS: Toxicology screening: how to assure accurate results, *Postgrad Med* 84:141-148, 1988.
58. Ritchie JM: The aliphatic alcohols. In Gilman AG, Goodman LS, Rall TW, Murad F, editors: *Goodman and Gilman's the pharmacological basis of therapeutics*, New York, 1985, Macmillan.
59. Lee NM, Becker CE: The alcohols. In Katzung BG, editor: *Basic and clinical pharmacology*, Norwalk, Conn, 1987, Appleton & Lange.
60. Poley WG, Vibe G: Alcohol and its effects on the individual. In *Alcoholism treatment manual*, New York, 1979, Gardner.
61. Ende J: Nutritional status, cardiovascular, hematologic, reproductive, and musculoskeletal systems. In *Alcoholism: a guide for the primary care physician*, New York, 1987, Springer-Verlag.
62. Kumar V, Contran R, Robbins A, editors: *Pathologic basis of disease*, ed 6, Philadelphia, 1997, Saunders.
63. Rose LF, Kaye D, editors: *Internal medicine for dentistry*, ed 2, St Louis, 1990, Mosby.
64. Niquille M, Burnand B, Magnenat P, et al: Dental disease among alcoholic individuals, *J Gen Intern Med* 8:470-475, 1993.
65. US Public Health Service: *Report of the Surgeon General: Nicotine addiction*, Rockville, Md, 1988, US Department of Health and Human Services.
66. Shuckit MA: *Drug and alcohol abuse*, New York, 1984, Plenum.
67. Taylor P: Agents acting at neuromuscular junctions and autonomic ganglia, nicotine. In Hardman JG, Lambard LE, Milinoff PB, editors: *Goodman and Gilman's the pharmacologic basis of therapeutics*, ed 9, New York, 1996, McGraw-Hill.
68. Henningfield JE, Nemeth-Coslett R: Nicotine dependence: interface between tobacco and tobacco-related disease, *Chest* 93:37-55, 1988.
69. *AMA drug evaluations*, Philadelphia, 1986, WB Saunders.
70. Milhorn HT Jr: Nicotine dependence, *Am Fam Physician* 39:224, 1989.
71. Schwartz M, Lamster I, Fine J: *Clinical guide to periodontics*, Philadelphia, 1995, Saunders.
72. Howe G, Westhoff C, Vessey M, Yeates D: Effects of age, cigarette smoking and other factors on fertility: findings in a large prospective study, *BMJ* 290:1697-1700, 1985.
73. O'Brien R, Cohen S: Barbiturates. In *The encyclopedia of drug abuse*, New York, 1984, Facts on File.
74. Harvey S: Hypnotics and sedatives. In Gilman AG, Goodman LS, Rall TW, Murad F, editors: *Goodman and Gilman's the pharmacological basis of therapeutics*, New York, 1985, Macmillan.
75. Cohen S: The barbiturates: has their time gone? In *The substance abuse problems*. Vol 1, New York, 1981, Haworth.
76. Laux G, Puryear DA: Benzodiazepines: misuse, abuse, and dependency, *Am Fam Physician* 30:139-147, 1984.
77. *National Household Survey on Drug Abuse: main findings*, Pub No ADM 88-1586, Rockville, Md, 1985, Department Of Health And Human Services.
78. Hoobs WR, Rall TW, Verdoom TA: Hypnotics and sedatives: ethanol. In Hardman JG, Limbard LE, Milinoff PB, editors: *Goodman and Gilman's the pharmacologic basis of therapeutics*, ed 9, New York, 1996, McGraw-Hill.
79. Rickels K, Case WG, Downing RW, Winokur A: Long-term diazepam therapy and clinical outcome, *JAMA* 250:767-771, 1983.
80. Smith DE, Wesson DR: Benzodiazepine withdrawal syndromes, *J Psychoactive Drugs* 15:85-95, 1983.
81. Winokur A, Rickels K, Greenblatt DJ, et al: Withdrawal reaction from long-term, low-dosage administration of diazepam, *Arch Gen Psychiatry* 37:101-105, 1980.
82. Schwartz RH: Marijuana: an overview, *Pediatr Clin North Am* 34:305-317, 1987.
83. Jaffe JH: Drug addiction and drug abuse. In Gilman AG, Goodman LS, Rall TW, Murad F, editors: *Goodman and Gilman's the pharmacological basis of therapeutics*, New York, 1985, Macmillan.
84. Schwartz RH, Hawks RL: Laboratory detection of marijuana use, *JAMA* 254:788-792, 1981.
85. Hunt A, Jones RT: Tolerance and disposition of tetrahydrocannabinol, *J Pharmacol Exp Ther* 215:34-44, 1980.
86. Wu TC, Tashkin DP, Djahed B: Pulmonary hazards of smoking marijuana as compared with tobacco, *N Engl J Med* 318:346-351, 1988.
87. Morris RR: Human pulmonary pathophysiology changes from marijuana smoking, *J Forensic Sci* 30:345-349, 1985.
88. Vereby K, Gold MS: From coca leaves to crack: the effects of dose and routes of administration on abuse liability, *Psychiatr Ann* 18:513-520, 1988.
89. Bouknight LG: Cocaine: a particularly addicting drug, *Postgrad Med* 83:115-131, 1988.
90. Dackis CA, Gold MS: Psychopharmacology of cocaine, *Psychiatr Ann* 18:528-530, 1988.
91. Wyatt RJ, Carourn F, Suddath R, Hitri A: The role of dopamine in cocaine use and abuse, *Psychiatr Ann* 18:531-534, 1988.

92. Cregler LL, Mark H: Medical complication of cocaine abuse, N Engl J Med 345:1495-1500, 1986.

93. Jaffe JH, Martin WR: Opioid analgesics and antagonists. In Gilman AG, Goodman LS, Rall TW, Murad F, editors: *Goodman and Gilman's the pharmacological basis of therapeutics*, New York, 1985, Macmillan.

94. McCann MJ, Miotto K, Rawson RA, et al: Outpatient non-opioid detoxification for opioid withdrawal: who is likely to benefit? Am J Addict 6:218-223, 1997.

95. Caldwell J: The metabolism of amphetamines and related stimulants in animals and man. In Caldwell J, editor: *Amphetamines and related stimulants: chemical, biological, clinical, and social aspects*, Boca Raton, Fla, 1980, CRC Press.

96. Kalivas PW, Duffy P: Effect of acute and daily cocaine treatment on extracellular dopamine in the nucleus accumbens, *Synapse* 5:48-58, 1990.

97. Carlsson A: Amphetamine and brain catecholamines. In Costa E, Garattini S, editors: *Amphetamines and related compounds*, New York, 1970, Raven.

98. Carlsson A, Waldeck B: Effects of amphetamine, tryamine, and protryptyline on reserpine resistance amine-concentrating mechanisms of adrenergic nerves, J Pharm Pharmacol 18:252-253. 1966.

99. Carlsson A, Lindqvist M, Dahlstroem A, et al: Effects of the amphetamine group on intraneuronal brain amines in vivo and in vitro, J Pharm Pharmacol 17:521-524, 1965.

100. Hanson GR, Sonsalla P, Letter A, et al: Effects of amphetamine analogs on central nervous system neuropeptide systems. In Asghar K, De Souza E, editors: Pharmacology and toxicology of amphetamine and related designer drugs, NIDA Res Monoger Ser 94:259-269, 1989.

101. Graham AW, Aghajanian GK: Effects of amphetamine on single cell activity in a catecholamine nucleus, the locus coeruleus, Nature 234:100-102, 1971.

102. Seiden LS, Fischman MW, Schuster CR: Changes in brain catecholamines induced by long-term methamphetamine administration in rhesus monkeys. In Ellinwood E, Kilbey M, editors: *Cocaine and other stimulants*, New York, 1977, Plenum.

103. Lee T, Ellinwood EH: Time-dependent changes in the sensitivity of dopamine neurons to low doses of apomorphine following amphetamine infusion: electrophysiological and biochemical studies, Brain Res 483:17-29, 1989.

104. Ricaurte GA, Schuster CR, Seiden LS; Long-term effects of repeated methylamphetamine administration on dopamine and serotonin neurons in the rat brain: a regional study, Brain Res193:153-163, 1980.

105. Kalant H, Kalant O. Death in amphetamine users: causes and rates. In Smith DE, editor: *Amphetamine use, misuse, and abuse*, Boston, 1979, GK Hall.

106. Richards H, Stephens A: Sudden death associated with the taking of amphetamines, Med Sci Law 13:35-38, 1973.

107. Jellinek P: Dual effect of dexamphetamine on body temperature in the rat, Eur J Pharmacol 15:389-392, 1971.

108. Elinwood EH, Rockwell WJK: Central nervous system stimulants and anorectic agents. In Blackwell B, editor: *Meyler's side effects of drugs*, Amsterdam, 1988, Elsevier.

109. Henker B, Whalen CK: Hyperactivity attention deficits, Am J Psychol I44:216-223, 1989.

110. Scoville BA: Review of amphetamine-like drugs by the Food and Drug Administration. In Bray GA, editor: *Obesity in perspective*, Washington, DC, 1980, US Department of Health, Education and Welfare.

111. Gotestam KG, Gunne L: Subjective effects of two anorexigenic agents, fenfluramine and AN488, in amphetamine-dependent subjects, Br J Addict 67:39-44, 1972.

112. Satel SL, Nelson JC: Stimulants in the treatment of depression: a critical overview, J Clin Psychiatry 50:241-249, 1989.

113. Holmes VJ, Fernandez F, Levy JK: Psychostimulant response in AIDS-related complex patients, J Clin Psychiatry I50:5-8, 1989.

114. Johnstone M, Evans V, Baigel S: Sernyl (Cl-395) in clinical anesthesia, Br J Anaesth 31:433-439, 1958.

115. Corssen G, Domino EF: Dissociative anesthesia: further pharmacologic studies and first clinical experience with the phencyclidine derivative CI-581, Anesth Analg 45:29-40, 1966.

116. Peterson RC, Stillman RC: *Phencyclidine: a review*, National Institute on Drug Abuse, Pub No 1980-0-341-166/614, Washington DC, 1980, US Government Printing Office.

117. Michaelis EK: Glutamate neurotransmission: characteristics of the NMDA receptors in mammalian brain, Neurol Notes 2:3-7, 1996.

118. MacDermott AB, Mayer ML, Westbrook GL, et al: NMDA-receptor activation increases cytoplasmic calcium concentration in cultured spinal cord neurons, Nature 321:519-522, 1985.

119. Toth E, Lajtha E: Antagonism of phencyclidine-induced hyperactivity by glycine in mice, Neurochem Res 11:393-400, 1986.

120. Wang T, O'Connor WT, Ungerstedt U, French ED: N-methyl-D-aspartic acid biphasically regulates the biochemical and electrophysiological response of A10 dopamine neurons in the ventral tegmental area: in vivo microdialysis and vitro electrophysiological studies, Brain Res 66:255-262, 1994.

121. Baldridge EB, Bessen HA: Phencyclidine, Emerg Med Clin North Am 8:541-550, 1990.

122. McCarron MM, Schulze BW, Thompson GA, et al: Acute phencyclidine intoxication: incidence of clinical findings in 1,000 cases, Ann Emerg Med 10:290-297, 1981.

Adverse Drug Reactions Associated with Local Anesthesia

Paul A. Moore

A dentist's ability to safely administer regional anesthesia is essential for the outpatient dental practice. The sophisticated dental and surgical procedures provided in dental offices today are possible through the advances in local anesthesia that have occurred since the introduction of procaine anesthesia almost 100 years ago. Fortunately, significant hypersensitivity reactions to local anesthetic agents or other components of dental local anesthesia formulations are rare, particularly since the preservative methylparaben was removed from dental anesthetics in the 1980s. Similarly, dose-dependent reactions associated with local anesthesia administration are extremely infrequent, and when treated properly, do not result in significant morbidity or mortality.

PATHOPHYSIOLOGY

Local anesthetic solutions used in the United States for dental anesthesia are formulated with several components. The contents of a standard local anesthetic cartridge may include an amide or ester local anesthetic drug, an adrenergic vasoconstrictor, and an antioxidant. In susceptible patients, any of these components may induce systemic, dose-dependent adverse reactions. Although extremely rare, allergic reactions may also occur.

When the local anesthetic contained in a dental cartridge diffuses away from the site of injection, it is absorbed into the systemic circulation where it is metabolized and excreted. The doses of a local anesthetic used in dentistry are usually minimal, and systemic effects are therefore uncommon. However, if an inadvertent vascular injection occurs or when repeated injections are administered, blood levels of a local anesthetic may become elevated and excitable tissues of the central nervous system (CNS) and the cardiovascular system may be affected.

Because local anesthetics act primarily as neuronal membrane depressants, it should not be surprising that neurons within the CNS are most sensitive to the systemic effects of local anesthetics. As blood levels increase, excitatory reactions such as tremors, muscle twitching, shivering and clonic-tonic convulsions are initially seen.[1,2,3] These initial excitatory reactions to local anesthetic overdose are thought to be disinhibition phenomena resulting from selective blockade of small inhibitory neurons within the limbic system of the CNS. Whether this initial excitatory reaction is seen or not, a generalized CNS depression with symptoms of sedation, drowsiness, lethargy, and life-threatening respiratory depression follows as blood levels continue to rise.[4] With extremely high toxic doses, myocardial excitability and conductivity may also be depressed, particularly with highly lipid-soluble, long-acting local anesthetics, etidocaine and bupivacaine.[5] Cardiac toxicity to local anesthetic overdose is most often manifested as ectopic cardiac rhythms and bradycardia. With extreme local anesthetic overdose, cardiac contractility is depressed and peripheral vasodilation occurs, leading to significant hypotension.

With the possible exception of mepivacaine (Carbocaine, Polocaine) and prilocaine (Citanest), most local anesthetics induce some degree of vasodilation at the site of injection.[6] To limit systemic uptake and to prolong the duration of the anesthesia, vasoconstrictors are often added to local anesthetic formulations. A concentration as low as 1:200,000 epinephrine (0.005 mg/ml) improves the onset, profundity, and duration of regional anesthesia.

The vasoconstricting agents most commonly used in dental local anesthetic formulations, epinephrine and levonordefrin, have catecholamine structures and act by stimulating postsynaptic receptors of the sympathetic nervous system. Vasoconstriction at the site of injection is the therapeutic goal of adding adrenergic vasoconstrictors to local anesthetic solutions. Systemic epinephrine and levonordefrin have both α– and β–stimulating properties, thereby stimulating increases in cardiac heart rate and force of contraction, as well as inducing vasoconstriction in skin and vasodilation in muscle tissue.

After injection of one or two cartridges of a dental local anesthetic containing epinephrine, normal circulating levels of epinephrine may increase twofold or threefold.[7] While not appreciably altering mean blood pressure, this additional exogenous epinephrine has been shown to decrease peripheral resistance, increase cardiac output, and increase heart rate.[8] This cardiovascular response is generally well tolerated in healthy adults and is transient, lasting only a few minutes after inadvertent intravascular injection. Of greatest concern, particularly with a massive adrenergic vasoconstrictor overdose, are cardiac dysrhythmias, including premature ventricular contractions and ventricular fibrillation.

Methemoglobinemia is a unique dose-dependent reaction reported to occur after the administration of nitrates, aniline dyes, and some amide-containing medications. When administered in excessive doses, the dental anesthetics, prilocaine and benzocaine (and rarely lidocaine and articaine), may induce methemoglobinemia. These local anesthetics, as well as nitrogylcerin, nitrite preparations, and the antimicrobials, dapsone and sulfonamide, can cause the oxidation of the iron atom within hemoglobin, producing methemoglobin. Risk factors for this reaction include extremes of age, anemia, respiratory disease, deficiencies in glucose-6-phosphate dehydrogenase and methemoglobin reductase, and possibly combinations of oxidant drugs.[9] Reports of methemoglobinemia associated with the use of topical lidocaine/prilocaine (EMLA) for neonatal circumcisions are due to the reduced activity of erythrocyte methemoglobin reductase, an enzyme that does not reach adult levels until 3 months of age.[10,11]

With toxicity, clinical signs of cyanosis are initially observed as blood levels of methemoglobin reach 10% to 20%. Dyspnea and tachycardia are observed as methemoglobinemia levels reach 35% to 40%. Reports of methemoglobinemia after administration of prilocaine and benzocaine are most often associated with large doses. One case associated with a high dose of

prilocaine and concomitant sulfonamide therapy has been reported.[12]

The FDA required removal of methylparaben from dental local anesthetic formulations in the 1980s because of its reported allergenicity.[13] Since then, serious allergic reactions after local anesthesia administration in dentistry are almost never reported. Although a practitioner should be prepared to treat local anesthetic hypersensitivity reactions, most suspected reactions are psychogenic. Reports from allergy clinics suggest that most patients referred for local anesthetic allergenicity testing have been misdiagnosed.[14,15]

Concern has recently developed for possible dose-dependent reactions to the antioxidant sulfites used in the local anesthetic formulations that contain epinephrine or levonordefrin.[16] Sulfites are included in local anesthetic solutions to prevent nonenzymatic oxidation of the catecholamine vasoconstrictors, thereby prolonging the shelf-life of these formulations. Formulations that do not include vasoconstrictors, such as 3% mepivacaine and 4% prilocaine, do not include antioxidants in their formulations.

Antioxidant sulfites (sulfur dioxide, sulfites, bisulfites, and metabisulfites) have been found to sensitize some asthmatic patients when they are exposed to rather large amounts of sulfite preservatives. Large doses, such as previously used in restaurant salad bars and homemade wines, were linked to six deaths in 1984.[17] Five percent of the 9 million asthmatic patients in the United States may be sulfite-sensitive.[18] Reactions of urticaria, angioedema, bronchospasm, and anaphylactic shock have been reported. Although some concern and caution is justified when using local anesthetics that contain vasoconstrictors and sulfites, a documented reaction in dental practice has not been published, probably because the amount of this antioxidant sulfite in a dental formulation is too small to stimulate a significant life-threatening reaction.

DIFFERENTIAL DIAGNOSIS

Signs and symptoms of the various adverse reactions associated with local anesthetics are quite distinctive, permitting rapid diagnosis and treatment (Box 29-1). The case reports summarized here are quite rare, having been compiled over the last 20 to 30 years. It is a tribute to the expertise of dental practitioners and the inherent safety of dental anesthesia that so few reports of adverse drug reactions can be found in the literature, since over a million injections are

---

| Box 29-1 | Differential Diagnosis of Local Anesthesia Reactions |

LOCAL ANESTHESIA TOXICITY
Initial symptoms include tremors, muscle twitching, and convulsions. After the initial phase, respiratory depression, lethargy, and loss of consciousness are possible. Cardiovascular depression may induce hypotension at blood concentrations. Hypoxia secondary to respiratory depression can rapidly produce the most serious outcomes of cardiovascular collapse, brain damage, and death.

METHEMOGLOBINEMIA
Because the causative agent for methemoglobinemia is often metabolites of prilocaine, symptoms frequently do not occur for 1-3 hours after treatment. Cyanosis without signs of respiratory distress may be apparent when methemoglobin levels reaches 10%-20%. Vomiting and headache have been described. At higher blood concentrations of methemoglobin, dyspnea, seizures, stupor, coma, and death are possible.

VASOCONSTRICTOR REACTIONS
Initial signs of the sympathetic nervous system stimulation include palpitations, increased heart rate and elevated blood pressure. Anxiety, nervousness, and fear are often associated with the palpitations. With severe overdose, arrhythmias, stroke, and myocardial infarction are possible.

ALLERGIC REACTIONS TO LOCAL ANESTHETICS
Mild manifestations of allergy to systemic drugs include urticaria, erythema, and intense itching. More severe reactions may include angioedema and respiratory distress. Although extremely unlikely, one should be prepared for the life-threatening anaphylactic reactions of dyspnea, hypotension, and loss of consciousness.

SULFITE ANTIOXIDANT REACTIONS
Asthma-like signs of tachypnea, wheezing, bronchospasm, dyspnea, tachycardia, dizziness and weakness have been reported, usually after exposure to foods (salads, shellfish, wines) containing-sulfite antioxidants. Severe flushing, generalized urticaria, angioedema, tingling, pruritis, rhinitis, conjunctivitis, dysphagia, nausea and diarrhea have also been reported.

---

given each day in dental offices across the United States.

As illustrated in the following cases, overdose reactions resulting from local anesthetic administration in dentistry (Cases 1 and 2) are manifested by CNS excitatory and depressant responses.[19,20] A stress response to the injection procedure in a medically compromised geriatric patient (Case 3) is also described.[21] Adverse drug reactions related to methemoglobinemia are most frequently recognized by signs of cyanosis (Case 4).[22] Reactions induced by the vasoconstrictor contained in some anesthetic formulations are manifested by stimulation of cardiovascular responses (Case 5)[23] and reactions resulting from sulfite sensitivity are manifested by bronchial and respiratory responses (Case 6).[24] True allergic reactions to local anesthetics are extremely unusual and are most frequently characterized by skin reactions (Case 7).[25]

It is important to note that true toxicity reactions to local anesthetic in dentistry almost always occur in children. Careful dose calculations using weight-based maximum recommended doses (MRDs) can prevent this reaction (see

| CASE 1 | Overdose in a Pediatric Patient: CNS Toxicity |

A healthy 5-year-old girl, was scheduled for multiple extractions. The child, who weighed 36 lb, received N_2O/O_2 sedation via a nasal mask, followed by maxillary and mandibular injections of five cartridges of 3% mepivacaine (270 mg). Ten minutes later the child experienced "stiffening and shaking" of all extremities that lasted 10 seconds. Two more convulsive episodes occurred, and cardiopulmonary arrest ensued. Transport to a local hospital and resuscitation measures were unsuccessful. Death occurred 4 days later.

Adapted from Hersh EV, Helpin ML, Evans OB: *J Dent Child* 58:489-491, 1991.

Table 29-1). For example, the maximum dosage for mepivacaine for a child weighing 36 lb would be calculated as 2.6 mg/lb $\times$ 36 lb = 94 mg. Since this is approximately the amount of local anesthetic contained in two dental cartridges of 3% mepivacaine (108 mg), the administration of five cartridges as in Case 1 was clearly excessive.

<table>
<tr><td>CASE 2</td><td>Local Anesthetic Seizures during Pediatric Sedation</td></tr>
</table>

An 8-year-old girl weighing 50 lb was brought to a private dental office for multiple extractions of primary teeth. The child had no history of drug allergies or significant systemic illnesses. Sedation was initiated with oral promethazine 6.25 mg and nitrous oxide/oxygen sedation 25%/75%. Thirty minutes later, the child appeared to be inadequately sedated and the initial drug regimen was supplemented with intramuscular meperidine 50 mg and nitrous oxide concentration increased to 37.5%. Local anesthesia was administered for all four dental quadrants using six cartridges of 3% mepivacaine (324 mg). Five minutes after local anesthesia administration, the child had multiple seizures, followed by respiratory distress. Initial emergency medical management included 100% oxygen, subcutaneous naloxone 0.4 mg, and sublingual epinephrine 1 mg. On arrival, paramedics initiated oral intubation, provided positive pressure ventilation, and immediately transported the child to the local hospital. Further efforts for resuscitation were unsuccessful.

Adapted from Moore PA: *J Am Dent Assoc* 123:60-64, 1992.

Pediatric sedation regimens that include opioids may increase the risk of local anesthetic–induced convulsions, therefore requiring conservative dosing of local anesthetics.[26] The local anesthetic dose of 324 mg that was administered to the patient in Case 2 was excessive when compared with the calculated MRD of mepivacaine for a 50 lb child (2.6 mg/lb × 50 lb = 130 mg). The inclusion of an opioid in the pediatric sedation has been shown to decrease the convulsant threshold of the local anesthetic. This drug interaction, rated "1" in Table 29-2, is well documented and clinically significant.[3]

Extensive dental services are becoming more common for older, medically compromised and sometimes frail patients. In Case 3, a death occurred after local anesthesia was administered to an elderly patient with an extremely complex medical and drug history. Although the adverse outcome for this patient was primarily stress related and not a pure local anesthetic toxicity reaction, the administration of a relatively large dose (300 mg) of mepivacaine may have contributed to her disorientation. The MRD for this 100-lb patient is calculated to be 260 mg.

Because this reaction is often associated with prilocaine's metabolite toluidine, symptoms often develop after the patient has left the

<table>
<tr><td>CASE 3</td><td>Death after Local Anesthesia in a Geriatric Dental Patient</td></tr>
</table>

An 84-year-old woman weighing approximately 100 lb was scheduled for extraction of her remaining 18 teeth under local anesthesia. Her health history was significant for organic brain syndrome, renal failure, chronic cystic breast disease, iron deficiency anemia, rheumatoid arthritis, osteoarthritis, arteriosclerotic heart disease with congestive heart failure, chronic pyelonephritis, and multiple surgeries including a prosthetic hip replacement. Current medications included furosemide, bethanechol, ferrous sulfate, hydroxychloroquine, amitriptyline, and cephalexin. Nine tablets of amoxicillin 500 mg were prescribed for prophylaxis; six to be taken 1 hour before surgery and three tablets taken postoperatively. On the day of surgery, local anesthesia of the left and right mandibular and maxillary quadrants was induced using approximately 10 ml 3% mepivacaine. Shortly after, the patient

began to vomit and the procedure was aborted. She was dismissed from the office and on the ride home became so sick and disoriented that she was taken to the emergency room. X-ray revealed a collapsed lung that was treated with a chest tube. Her condition deteriorated, and she required intubation and mechanical respiration. Laboratory findings included a creatinine of 1.4, BUN of 49, and blood sugar of 115. ECG showed left axis deviation with right bundle branch block and left ventricular hypertrophy. The following day, intermittent partial seizures occurred that were attributed to hypoxic encephalopathy. Eight days later, the patient expired while still in the hospital. Postmortem examination revealed pulmonary fibrosis, bronchopneumonia, bronchiectasis, arteriosclerotic cardiovascular disease, brainstem infarct, cerebral cortical necrosis, and possible adrenal cortical nodular hyperplasia.

Adapted from Estabrooks LN: *AAOMS National Closed Claims Review,* Personal communication, 2000.

dental office (Case 4). A patient may experience dizziness, cyanosis, fatigue, and respiratory distress. As documented in Table 29-1, the MRD for prilocaine is 4.0 mg/lb up to a maximum of 600 mg. The prilocaine dose administered to the patient in Case 3 (560 mg) did not exceed this maximum.

This serious reaction has been repeatedly reported after dental anesthesia using prilocaine. Fortunately, fatalities after its use for dental anesthesia have not been reported. The reports suggest that the dose of prilocaine is the primary cause of the reaction and the use of concomitant drugs that increase the likelihood of methemoglobinemia is secondary. It is recommended that the dose of these local anesthetics be calculated carefully and that the weight-based recommended dose not be exceeded.

Reactions associated with the vasoconstrictor in a local anesthetic solution are usually seen as mild stimulation of the cardiovascular system; the resulting rises in heart rate and blood pressure are usually transient. In Case 5, the reported cardiovascular stimulation was exaggerated because the patient was receiving a nonselective β-adrenergic blocker. Generalized inhibition of the β-adrenergic response permits the α-adrenergic properties of the vasoconstrictor to be expressed uninhibited. As described in Table 29-3, adverse drug interactions associated with local anesthetic vasoconstrictors may potentially occur for several medications patients may be taking concomitantly.[27]

Although local tissue reactions have been reported, the most serious and most commonly reported reaction to sulfite exposure is bronchospasm (Case 6). Symptoms include wheezing, dyspnea, tachycardia, dizziness and weakness. Loss of consciousness and anaphylactic shock are also possible. As described in Case 5, severe gastrointestinal distress and hypotension may be the most prominent response after oral ingestion. Fortunately, the reaction is dose-dependent and few reactions have been attributed to the small amount of sulfite preservatives formulated in parenteral medications.

Although patients often report allergy to local anesthetics, confirmed responses of true allergy are extremely rare. Because alternatives to local anesthetics, such as diphenydramine injection, deep sedation and general anesthesia, are not ideal, a referral for allergy testing to confirm the diagnosis is recommended. Results of

---

CASE 4	Methemoglobinemia after Extraction of Third Molars

A 22-year-old woman weighing 127 lb arrives in a private dental office for extraction of four third molars. Local anesthesia was administered using 560 mg of prilocaine. Intravenous sedation was induced with methohexital (90 mg) and diazepam (10 mg). Dexamethasone (6 mg) was administered to control postoperative swelling. Five hours after surgery, the patient came to the emergency department complaining of dizziness. The emergency department physician noted perioral and nailbed cyanosis. Oral temperature was 99.1° F, pulse 108/min, respirations 20/min, and blood pressure was 130/90 mm Hg. Blood analysis determined methemoglobin levels of 27%. Oxygen was administered by full-face mask. Intravenous methylene blue 100 mg was administered over a 5-minute period. Recovery was rapid, and the patient was discharged 1 hour later.

Adapted from *MMWR* 43(35): 655-657, 1994.

CASE 5	Hypertension after Local Anesthesia

A fearful 32-year-old female with a medical history of alcohol abuse, controlled hypertension, mitral value prolapse, and episodes of cardiac arrhythmia was scheduled for dental rehabilitation with intravenous sedation. The patient was taking the nonselective β-adrenergic antagonist propranolol 60 mg/day. Lorazepam 2 mg was administered preoperatively. Nitrous oxide was administered before establishing intravenous access. Intravenous conscious sedation was established using diphenhydramine 25 mg, meperidine 25 mg, pentobarbital 175 mg, and methohexital 30 mg. Five minutes after the administration of 1.5 cartridges of 2% mepivacaine 1:20,000 levonordefrin, a transient (15 minutes) rise in systolic and diastolic blood pressure of 40 and 15 torr, respectively, occurred. A similar blood pressure response occurred 75 minutes later after the second dose of this local anesthetic. At a subsequent dental appointment, anesthesia was induced with 3% mepivacaine; no rise in blood pressure was noted.

Adapted from Mito RS, Yagiela JA: *J Am Dent Assoc* 116:55-57, 1988.

> | CASE 6 | Asthma Attack from Metabisulfite Sensitivity [26] |
> |---|---|
>
> A 34-year-old female developed dizziness, nausea, palpitations, hives, dysphagia, chest tightness, and dyspnea after a restaurant meal of salad, Italian dressing, and shellfish. Because she felt weak and faint, she was transported to a hospital emergency room and administered intravenous fluids, and kept under observation. In the emergency department, she was dyspneic, tachypneic, and extremely anxious. Blood pressure was 130/90 mm Hg, and heart rate was 160 beats/minute. Symptoms diminished over several hours without specific therapy. An oral metabisulfite challenge performed several weeks later induced weakness, dizziness, nausea, and a significant drop in blood pressure. The response to this challenge was considered consistent with a diagnosis of sulfite sensitivity.

Adapted from Schwartz HJ: *J Allergy Clin Immunol* 71(5): 487-489, 1983.

> | CASE 7 | Allergy to a Local Anesthetic |
> |---|---|
>
> A 33-year-old woman sought treatment of a broken down and painful left mandibular molar. She informed the dentist that she had experienced an allergic reaction to lidocaine after spinal anesthesia for a cesarean section with symptoms including urticaria and difficulty breathing. Treatment of her previous reaction included epinephrine and diphenhydramine. A referral to a board-certified allergist/immunologist had confirmed definitive wheal and flare reactions to lidocaine, mepivacaine, and procaine. The dental emergency was treated with diphenhydramine with epinephrine and deep intravenous sedation. To permit future dental treatment and to avoid intravenous sedation, further local anesthesia testing was recommended with the rationale that preservative supplements in the previous dental cartridge solutions may have induced the apparent allergic reactions. The pharmaceutical company provided 2% lidocaine and 4% prilocaine containing no epinephrine, methyparaben preservatives, or metabisulfite antioxidants. Using controls, dilutions of both lidocaine and prilocaine induced irrefutable sensitivity reactions to percutaneous testing.

Adapted from Seng GF, Kraus K, Cartridge G, et al: *Gen Dent* 44:52-54, 1996.

allergy testing most often rule out true allergy or identify a specific local anesthetic agent that can be used for dental anesthesia (Case 7).

PREVENTION
Medical and Drug Histories

A patient's health history and past experiences with medications may provide valuable information for preventing the adverse drug reactions associated with local anesthesia. Because acute drug reactions are physiologically stressful, the outcome of any emergency is more likely to be favorable if the patient is healthy. Medically compromised patients may require limiting dental treatments to immediate needs and creating treatment plans that avoid excessive anesthesia. Cardiovascular histories that indicate significant impairment may indicate limiting the use of vasoconstrictors. History of asthma, particularly if sulfite sensitivity is noted, may be important in selecting an anesthetic agent. Comprehending a patient's anxiety and fear of dental injections may provide useful information for recognizing psychogenic reactions as compared to true adverse drug responses. Sedation strategies that reduce the psychological and physiologic stress of dental treatment should be considered for both dental phobics and medically compromised patients.

Histories of adverse reaction to local anesthetics during previous dental treatment can prevent allergic and hypersensitivity reactions. Knowledge of medications currently being taken and drugs possibly being abused will guide a practitioner to avoid some of the significant adverse drug interactions associated with the administration of dental anesthesia (see Table 29-2). Additionally, as listed in Table 29-3, vasoconstrictors should be used with caution with patients currently taking tricyclic antidepressants, nonselective β-adrenoreceptor antagonists, cocaine, α-adrenergic blockers, adrenergic neuronal blocker, and thyroid hormones.[27]

Drug Selection and Dosage Recommendations

Selection of the safest anesthetic agent and proper dose is essential in preventing most adverse drug reactions. Understanding the relative toxicity of the amide local anesthetics used in dentistry (see Table 29-1) will permit procedures to be accomplished painlessly and safely.

True dose-dependent toxicity reactions to local anesthetics are most frequently reported in pediatric patients. Dosing calculations and systemic reactions to local anesthetics are dependent on body weight. Children may be at greater risk of toxicity reactions because their lower body weight does not represent a proportionate decrease in orofacial anatomy. Because the mandible and maxilla of a 50-lb child are not one-third the size of a 150-lb adult, there is an apparent need to use relatively larger volumes of local anesthetics when treating preschool children. The consequence of this disparity is that local anesthetic toxicity occurs more frequently in children, and systemic drug interactions involving local anesthetics and other CNS depressant drugs become a greater concern.[2,26]

The local anesthetic formulation of 3% mepivacaine plain appears to have been associated with a disproportionate number of local anesthetic toxicity reports.[19,28] This may be due to the absence of a vasoconstrictor, thereby allowing more rapid systemic absorption of the anesthetic. Additionally, the higher concentration used in its anesthetic formulation (3%) may result in the administration of larger relative doses. Pharmacokinetic studies by Goebel and colleagues demonstrated that peak anesthetic blood levels of 3% mepivacaine occur more rapidly and exceeded that of an equal volume of 2% lidocaine with 1:100,000 epinephrine by approximately threefold after maxillary infiltration injections (see Table 29-1).[29,30]

The 3% mepivacaine formulation may also be chosen for children because it is considered by some to have a shorter duration of soft tissue anesthesia, therefore limiting severe lip biting and oral trauma seen in children after dental local anesthesia. However, the results of one double-blind, randomized trial demonstrated that onset time, peak effects, and duration soft tissue anesthesia after mandibular block injections with 2% lidocaine 1:100,000 epinephrine, 3% mepivacaine plain, or 4% prilocaine plain were quite similar.[31] The selection of anesthetic formulations that do not contain a vasoconstrictor, such as 3% mepivacaine, may not be a clinical advantage for children.

The maximum volume of 3% mepivacaine plain for anesthetic injection (6 cartridges for an adult) is the most restrictive of any local anesthetic used in dentistry. In comparison, the maximum volume for 2% lidocaine with epinephrine (14 cartridges for an adult) permits the greatest volume for safe anesthesia injection. With chil-

dren, selection of 2% lidocaine with 1:100,000 epinephrine is the least likely to cause toxicity reactions if multiple injections are required.[20] Because of our desire to prevent oral trauma after dental anesthesia, the long-acting local anesthetics are generally not indicated for young children.[32]

The calculation of MRDs for children receiving local anesthetics is complicated by the conflicting published dosage recommendations found in the literature and the various units involved in the determination (e.g., milligrams, cubic centimeters, milliliters, kilograms, pounds, cartridges). The MRDs for dental local anesthetics recently published in the ADA *Guide to Dental Therapeutics* is possibly the most current authoritative source.[33] These values are summarized in Table 29-1.

A simplified alternative for calculating maximum safe doses of local anesthesia has been to establish a conservative recommendation that can be applied to *all* anesthetic formulations used in dentistry. This recommendation, "the Rule of 25," states that a dentist may safely use 1 cartridge of any marketed local anesthetic for every 25 lb of patient weight (i.e., 3 cartridges for a 75-lb patient, 6 cartridges for a 150-lb patient).[34]

Avoiding Drug Interactions

Significant adverse drug interactions associated with the use of dental therapeutics were the topic of a recent symposium sponsored by the American Dental Association, IADR, and ADEA. Medications commonly prescribed by dental practitioners (antibiotics, analgesics, anxiolytics, local anesthetics, and vasoconstrictors) were reviewed to determine the clinical significance of potential drug interactions. The symposium's findings for all categories of dental therapeutics have been recently published.[3,27,35-37] During this symposium, the severity of the interactions was identified by the following three categories:

Major: Potentially life-threatening or capable of causing permanent damage

Moderate: May cause deterioration of patient's clinical status and additional treatment or hospitalization may be necessary

Minor: Mild affects that are bothersome or unnoticed and should not significantly affect therapeutic outcome.

The strength of the documentation of the reported interactions was rated as *established*, *probable*, *suspected*, *possible*, or *unlikely*. The following

Table 29-1	Adult Dosage Guidelines for Local Anesthetics				
	MAXIMUM RECOMMENDED DOSE		**CARTRIDGES (NO.)**		
Anesthetic	**Dose**	**Mg/lb**	**Concentration**	**150 lb Adult**	**50 lb Child**
Lidocaine					
2% with epinephrine	500 mg	3.3 mg/lb	20 mg/ml	13.9	4.6
Mepivacaine					
3% plain	400 mg	2.6 mg/lb	30 mg/ml	7.4	2.5
2% with levonordefrin	400 mg	2.6 mg/lb	20 mg/ml	11.1	3.7
Prilocaine					
4% plain or epinephrine	600 mg	4.0 mg/lb	40 mg/ml	8.3	2.8
Articaine*					
4% with epinephrine	500 mg	3.3 mg/lb	40 mg/ml	6.9	2.3†
Bupivacaine					
0.5% with epinephrine	90 mg	0.6 mg/lb	5 mg/ml	10	—‡
Etidocaine					
1.5% with epinephrine	400 mg	2.6 mg/lb	15 mg/ml	14.8	—‡

From Yagiela J, Malamed SF, editors: Injectable and topical local anesthetics. In Ciancio SG, editor: *ADA guide to dental therapeutics*, Chicago, 1998, ADA Publishing.
*Cartridges are packaged with 1.8 ml except articaine, which is available as 1.7 ml.
†Some manufacturers use a lower dosage recommendation for articaine (2.3 mg/lb) for children 4-12 years of age.
‡The long-acting local anesthetics bupivacaine and etidocaine are not recommended for use in children younger than 12 years of age.

assessments determine the significance of an adverse drug interaction:
1. Major reactions that are at least suspected
2. Moderate reactions that are at least suspected
3. Minor reactions that are at least suspected
4. Major or moderate reactions that are possible
5. Minor reactions that are possible and all reactions that are unlikely.

The significant adverse drug interactions associated with local anesthetics and vasoconstrictors are summarized in Boxes 29-2 and 29-3.

Summation Response to More than One Local Anesthetic

Drugs with identical mechanisms of action and similar receptor sites will usually have additive effects when administered in combination.[3] This generalization is certainly true for local anesthetic toxicity. Summation drug interactions and local anesthetic toxicity becomes a concern when young children are being treated, when additional anesthetic is required for completing prolonged dental procedures, when excessive topical anesthesia of mucous membranes is necessary to supplement regional anesthesia, or when a long-acting local anesthetic such as bupivacaine is administered postoperatively for

pain management. MRD calculations must consider the total dose of the combination and whether sufficient time has been allowed for the elimination of the initial dose before additional anesthetic is administered. As shown in Box 29-2, combined use of local anesthetics at total doses that significantly exceed guidelines can cause classic local anesthetic toxicity reactions: CNS excitation, convulsions, respiratory depression and cardiac arrest. Fortunately, most dental practitioners are aware of this adverse interaction and prevent its occurrence by limiting total dosage of local anesthetics used.

Local Anesthetics Used with Opioid Sedation

During conscious sedation, the use of local anesthesia is essential for painless oral surgery procedures. No conscious sedation therapy can provide adequate analgesia to offset the need for profound local anesthesia. Unfortunately, the term *local* implies that local anesthetics have little or no systemic absorption and generalized effects. Local anesthetics are absorbed, and because they are membrane depressants, alter CNS and cardiovascular function. The systemic effects of local anesthetics and the possible in-

Box 29-2	Adverse Drug Interactions: Local Anesthetics	
DRUG INTERACTION		**SIGNIFICANCE RATING***
Local Anesthetics Example: Lidocaine with bupivacaine Local anesthetic toxicity is additive when given in combination; although combination therapy with local anesthetics is acceptable, total dose should not exceed combined MRDs.		1
Local Anesthetics with Opioid Sedation Example: Mepivacaine with meperidine Sedation with opioids may increase the risk of local anesthetic toxicity particularly with children. Reduce local anesthetic dose.		1
Local Anesthetic with Other Drugs that Induce Methemoglobinemia Example: Prilocaine with dapsone Methemoglobinemia is usually due to prilocaine dosing in excess of MRD. Increased risk may be possible when similar oxidizing drugs are administered.		4
Ester Local Anesthetics with Sulfonamide Antibiotics Example: Procaine with sulfamethoxazole Procaine is infrequently used; the procaine metabolite, *p*-amino benzoic acid (PABA), may transiently reduce sulfonamide antibiotic efficacy.		5
Amide Local Anesthetics with Inhibitors of Metabolism Example: Lidocaine with cimetidine Inhibition of local anesthetic metabolism has little effect on peak plasma levels when given as a single anesthetic injection.		5

From Moore PA: *J Am Dent Assoc* 130:541-554, 1999.
MRD, Maximum recommended dose.
*Significance ratings are specific to dental therapy (i.e., regional anesthesia within MRD): 1, *Major* reactions that are at least *suspected; 2, moderate* reactions that are at least *suspected; 3, minor* reactions that are at least *suspected; 4, major* or *moderate* reactions that are *possible;* or *5, minor* reactions that are *possible* and all reactions that are *unlikely.*

teractions with other CNS depressants are most evident when treating pediatric dental patients.

The use of an opioid such as meperidine (Demerol) as part of a pediatric sedation regimen is often associated with reports of local anesthetic toxicity reactions. The mechanism for this interaction is probably multifaceted. In part, synthetic opioids, such as meperidine and the previously available alphaprodine (Nisentil), have convulsant properties when excessive doses are administered.[2] Decreases in the convulsant thresholds of local anesthetics after pretreatment with opioids have been demonstrated in animal studies.[38,39] The opioid component of the sedation induces a mild respiratory acidosis that can decrease protein binding of local anesthetics, thereby permitting more unbound drug to distribute into the CNS.[40,41] Additionally, the elevation of arterial carbon dioxide tensions that occurs with opioid premedication is known to increase CNS sensitivity to local anesthetic convulsions.[42]

Classic local anesthetic overdose reactions, including CNS excitation, convulsions, respiratory depression, and cardiac arrest, have been reported. This frequently described interaction may be particularly significant in general practice settings, because convulsions and respiratory depression are life-threatening and difficult to manage in a dental office. Practitioners using drug therapies for pediatric sedation should be trained and prepared to manage the serious reactions that are possible. This complication is best prevented by adjusting the dose of the local anesthetic downward when sedating children with opioids.

Box 29-3	Adverse Drug Interactions: Vasoconstrictors

DRUG INTERACTION	SIGNIFICANCE RATING*
Vasoconstrictors with Tricyclic Antidepressants Example: Levonordefrin and imipramine Sympathomimetic effects may be enhanced.	1
Vasoconstrictors with Nonselective β-Adrenergic Antagonists Example: Epinephrine and propranolol Hypertensive and/or cardiac reactions are possible.	1
Vasoconstrictors with General Anesthetics Example: Epinephrine with halothane Increased possibility of cardiac arrhythmias exists with general anesthetics.	1
Vasoconstrictors with Cocaine Example: Epinephrine and cocaine Arrhythmias and hypertensive response possible.	1
Vasoconstrictors with α-Adrenergic Blockers Example: Epinephrine with chlorpromazine Hypotension resulting from overdose of antipsychotic agent may be worsened.	4
Vasoconstrictors with Adrenergic Neuronal Blocker Example: Levonordefrin with guanadrel Sympathomimetic effects may be enhanced.	4
Vasoconstrictors with Local Anesthetics Example: Lidocaine and epinephrine Multiple effects on systemic toxicity that may be self-limiting.	4
Vasoconstrictors with Thyroid Hormones Example: Epinephrine with thyroxine Summation effects possible when thyroid hormones are used in excess.	4
Vasoconstrictors with MAO Inhibitors Example: Epinephrine with phenelzine No substantial evidence of an interaction.	5

From Yagiela JA: *J Am Dent Assoc* 130:701-709, 1999.
MOA, Monoamine oxidase inhibitors.
*Significance ratings are specific to dental therapy (i.e., regional anesthesia within MRD): 1, *Major* reactions that are at least *suspected*; 2, *moderate* reactions that are at least *suspected*; 3, *minor* reactions that are at least *suspected*; 4, *major* or *moderate* reactions that are *possible*; or 5, *minor* reactions that are *possible* and all reactions that are *unlikely*.

Local Anesthetics with Other Drugs that May Induce Methemoglobinemia

Nitrates, aniline dyes, and amide-containing medications may induce methemoglobinemia. Most reports of methemoglobinemia after the administration of the local anesthetics prilocaine and benzocaine are associated with excessive doses. Methemoglobinemia has occurred in infants after the topical administration of EMLA, a eutectic mixture of prilocaine and lidocaine.[11]

The need to avoid these local anesthetics agents with patients taking other methemoglobinemia-inducing agents appears to be primarily a theoretical concern. Only one case associated with a high dose of prilocaine and concomitant sulfonamide therapy has ever been reported.[12]

Methemoglobinemia has been repeatedly documented after dental anesthesia using prilocaine, although fatalities have not been reported.[23] The reports suggest that the dose of prilocaine is the primary cause of the reaction, and the use of concomitant drugs that increase the likelihood of methemoglobinemia is secondary. It is recommended that the dose of these local anesthetics be calculated carefully and that the weight-based MRD not be exceeded.

Two additional drug interactions are sometimes found in the literature (see Box 29-2). Sulfonamide antibiotics act by preventing the bacteria from incorporating *p*-aminobenzoic acid (PABA) in the synthesis of folic acid. The breakdown of the ester local anesthetic procaine into PABA could theoretically reduce the efficacy of sulfonamides. Because ester anesthetics are infrequently used in dentistry, the concentrations of PABA are minimal and short-lived after local anesthesia, this competitive drug interaction is clinically insignificant. Similarly, drug interactions with lidocaine and metabolic inhibitors such as cimetidine and propranolol are important only when continuous intravenous infusions of lidocaine are administered to manage cardiac arrhythmias. After single dose administration of a local anesthetic, peak toxic concentrations are only minimally affected by drugs that inhibit metabolism. As shown in Box 29-2, these adverse drug interactions are unimportant after dental anesthesia.

Vasoconstrictor Drug Interactions

Practitioners must be alert to drug-patient interactions when using local anesthetics containing the vasoconstrictors epinephrine and levonordefrin. When considering a patient's tolerance to cardiovascular stimulation, there is little to indicate that epinephrine 1:100,000 or levonordefrin 1:20,000 differ substantially. As supplied in dental cartridges, the dose of vasoconstrictor is rather small and rarely causes any notable problems in healthy adults. Although rarely contraindicated, a common recommendation when there is a medical history that suggests a need for caution, is to limit the dose of epinephrine to 0.018 to 0.054 mg, the amount of epinephrine contained in one to three cartridges of 2% lidocaine with 100,000 epinephrine.[43]

As summarized in Box 29-3, many drug interactions have been associated with the adrenergic vasoconstrictors used in dental anesthetics. As described in Case 5, patients taking nonselective β-adrenergic antagonists such as propranolol may experience exaggerated cardiovascular responses to epinephrine or levonordefrin. The tricyclic antidepressants may also

enhance the systemic adrenergic response. Cocaine and the halogenated general anesthetics, most notably halothane, may increase the sensitivity of the heart to life-threatening arrhythmias after the use of adrenergic vasoconstrictors. Each of these interactions is clinically relevant and potentially life-threatening and carries the highest significance rating[27] (see Box 29-3). Other drugs that may adversely interact with adrenergic vasoconstrictors, such as α-adrenergic blockers (i.e., chlorpromazine), adrenergic neuronal blockers (i.e., guanadrel), local anesthetics, thyroid hormones, and monoamine oxidase (MAO) inhibitors are poorly documented and are probably clinically insignificant when dose guidelines are followed.

PRACTICAL MANAGEMENT OF LOCAL ANESTHETIC TOXICITIES
Local Anesthetic Toxicity

Obviously, compliance with local anesthetic dosing guidelines is the first and most important strategy for preventing an adverse event. Tonic-clonic convulsions are the most common reaction to true overdose reactions. Fortunately, local anesthetic–induced convulsions are usually transient. After a convulsive episode, loss of consciousness and severe, prolonged respiratory depression is likely.

Immediate treatment should address both the convulsions and the potential respiratory depression. The clinician must monitor vital signs (particularly respiratory adequacy), protect the patient from injury, place the patient in supine position, and maintain the airway. If the patient is unconscious, positive pressure oxygen is essential. Although rarely required, intravenous diazepam 5 to 10 mg is the definitive treatment if convulsions persist.

Methemoglobinemia

Although small quantities of methemoglobin may be produced after local anesthetic administration, excessive levels are rarely reported. The initial symptom is cyanosis; respiratory distress may follow if methemoglobinemia levels are higher than 25% to 30%. Treatment strategies are usually symptomatic. This drug reaction reverses itself within a few hours in healthy patients as the drug and/or its metabolites are eliminated. In general, if the patient is not in distress, treatment recommendations include monitoring cardiovascular and respiratory function, administering 100% oxygen via face mask, and transporting to the local emergency room. If cyanosis, hypoxia and respiratory distress are clinically significant, intravenous methylene blue (1 to 2 mg/kg), which rapidly reverts the methemoglobin to hemoglobin, is the definitive treatment.

Vasoconstrictor Reactions

The vasoconstrictors used in dental local anesthetic cartridges in the United States are currently limited to epinephrine and levonordefrin. Both are adrenergic sympathomimetics with cardiac and vascular-stimulating properties. Reactions to excessive or intravascular vasoconstrictor administration are palpitations and hypertension. Additionally, cardiovascular responses are usually transient, lasting only a few minutes. Fortunately, the symptoms are not life-threatening in most healthy patients. Careful medical histories can alert practitioners to cardiovascular impairments and possible drug interactions. Slow injections and careful aspiration can prevent rapid systemic absorption of epinephrine and levonordefrin.

If a reaction does result from local anesthetic administration, treatment recommendations include monitoring vital signs, explaining to the patient the cause of the symptoms and assuring the patient that the response will last only a few minutes. If a significant rise in blood pressure is noted, sublingual nitroglycerin should be administered and the patient should be immediately transported to the local hospital emergency department.

Allergic Reactions to Local Anesthetics

Allergic reactions to injected medications range from mild to severe. A rapid rate of onset of an allergic drug reaction should alert practitioners to a possible anaphylactoid response. Taking a complete drug history and avoiding allergy medications can prevent most allergic reactions. Mild skin responses are managed with an antihistamine such as diphenhydramine 25 to 50 mg and are administered either orally or intramuscularly. Frequently, a patient having an allergic reaction for the first time will be extremely anxious. If dyspnea, nausea, vomiting, hypotension, or other acute signs of anaphylaxis occur, immediate treatment is required. Recommended treatment includes basic life support, intramuscular epinephrine 0.3 to 0.5 mg, and transport to the local hospital emergency room. Additional therapy, including antihistamines and corticosteroids, may be required subsequent to the acute therapy.

Sulfite Preservative Reactions

Adverse reaction to sulfites occurs most frequently in patients with a history of atopic allergy or asthma. The most common reactions are wheezing and bronchospasm. Other symptoms of sulfite sensitivity include tachypnea, wheezing, dizziness, nausea, and weakness. Reactions usually occur within thirty minutes of oral ingestion. Severe respiratory distress and anaphylactic reactions should be treated immediately with epinephrine (see Chapter 11).

REFERENCES

1. Reynolds F: Adverse effects of local anesthetics, Br J Anaesth 59:78-95, 1987.
2. Moore PA, Goodson JM: Risk appraisal of narcotic sedation for children, Anesth Prog 32:129-139, 1985.
3. Moore PA: Adverse drug interactions in dental practice. IV. Interactions associated with local anesthetics, sedatives and anxiolytics, J Am Dent Assoc 130:541-554, 1999.
4. Covino BG, Vassallo HG: Local anesthetics: mechanisms of action and clinical use, New York, 1976, Grune & Stratton.
5. Liu PL, Feldman HS, Giasi R, Patterson MK, et al: Comparative CNS toxicity of lidocaine, etidocaine, bupivacaine, and tetracaine in awake dogs following rapid intravenous administration, Anesth Analg 62:375-379, 1983.
6. Lindorf HH: Investigation of the vascular effect of newer local anesthetics and vasoconstrictors, Oral Surg 48:292-297, 1979.
7. Yagiela JA: Local anesthetics. In Dionne RA, Phero JC, editors: Management of pain and anxiety in dental practice, Elsevier, New York ,1991.
8. Dionne RA, Goldstein DS, Wirdzek PR: Effect of diazepam premedication and epinephrine containing local anesthetics on cardiovascular and plasma catecholamine responses in oral surgery, Anesth Analg 63:640-646, 1984.
9. Wilburn-Goo D, Lloyd LM: When patients become cyanotic: acquired methemoglobinemia, J Am Dent Assoc 130:826-831, 1999.
10. Tse S, Barrington K, Byrne P: Methemoglobinemia associated with prilocaine use in neonatal circumcision, Am J Perinatology 12(5): 331-332, 1995.
11. Kumar AR, Dunn N, Naqvi M: Methemoglobinemia associated with a prilocaine-lidocaine cream, Clin Pediatr 36(4):239-240, 1997.
12. Jakobson B, Nilsson A: Methemoglobinemia associated with a prilocaine-lidocaine cream and trimethoprim-sulphamethoxazole. A case report, Acta Anaesthesiol Scand 29(4):453-455, 1985.
13. Larson CE: Methylparaben—an overlooked cause of local anesthetic hypersensitivity, Anesth Prog 24:72-74, 1977.
14. deSharo RD, Nelson HS: An approach to the patient with a history of local anesthetic hypersensitivity: experience with 90 patients, J Allergy Clin Immunol 63:387-394, 1979.
15. Incaudo G, Schatz M, Patterson R, et al: Administration of local anesthetics to patients with a history of prior adverse reactions, J Allergy Clin Immunol 61:339-345, 1978.

16. Seng GF, Gay BJ: Dangers of sulfites in dental local anesthetic solutions: warning and recommendations, J Am Dent Assoc 113:769-770, 1986.
17. New sulfite regulations, FDA Drug Bulletin 16:17-18, 1986.
18. Bush RK, Taylor SL, Holden K, et al: Prevalence of sensitivity to sulfiting agents in asthmatic patients, Am J Med 81:816-820, 1986.
19. Hersh EV, Helpin ML, Evans OB: Local anesthetic mortality: report of case, J Dent Child 58:489-491, 1991.
20. Moore PA: Prevention of local anesthesia toxicity, J Am Dent Assoc 123:60-64, 1992.
21. Estabrooks LN: AAOMS National Closed Claims Review, Personal communication, 2000.
22. Epidemiologic notes and reports: prilocaine-induced methemoglobinemia—Wisconsin, 1993, MMWR 43(35): 655-657, 1994.
23. Mito RS, Yagiela JA: Hypertensive response to levonordefrin in a patient receiving propranolol: report of case, J Am Dent Assoc 116:280-281, 1988.
24. Schwartz HJ: Sensitivity to ingested metabisulfite: variations in clinical presentation, J Allergy Clin Immunol 71(5):487-489, 1983.
25. Seng GF, Kraus K, Cartridge G, et al: Confirmed allergic reactions to amide local anesthetics, Gen Dent 44:52-54, 1996.
26. Goodson JM, Moore PA: Life-threatening reactions following pedodontic sedation: an assessment of narcotic, local anesthetic and antiemetic drug interaction, J Am Dent Assoc 107:239-45, 1983.
27. Yagiela JA: Adverse drug interactions in dental practice. V. Interactions associated with vasoconstrictors, J Am Dent Assoc 130:701-709, 1999.
28. Virts BE: Local anesthesia toxicity review, Ped Dent 21:375, 1999.
29. Goebel WM, Allen G, Randall F: The effect of commercial vasoconstrictor preparations on the circulating venous serum level of mepivacaine and lidocaine, J Oral Med 35:91-96, 1980.
30. Goebel W, Allen G, Randall F: Circulating serum levels of mepivacaine after dental injection, Anesth Prog 25:52-56, 1978.
31. Hersh EV, Hermann DG, Lamp CJ, et al: Assessing the duration of mandibular soft tissue anesthesia, J Am Dent Assoc 126:1531-1536, 1995.
32. Moore PA: Long-acting local anesthetics: a review of clinical efficacy in dentistry, Compend Cont Dent Ed 11:22-30, 1990.
33. Yagiela J, Malamed SF, editors: Injectable and topical local anesthetics. In Ciancio SG, editor: ADA guide to dental therapeutics, Chicago, 1998, ADA Publishing.
34. Moore PA, editor: Manual of local anesthesia in dentistry, ed 4, Rochester, New York, 1996, Eastman-Kodak.
35. Moore PA, Gage TW, Hersh EV, et al: Adverse drug interactions in dental practice. I. Professional and educational implications, J Am Dent Assoc 130:47-54, 1999.
36. Haas DA: Adverse drug interactions in dental practice. III. Interactions associated with analgesics, J Am Dent Assoc 130:397-407, 1999.
37. Hersh EV: Adverse drug interactions in dental practice. II. Interactions involving antibiotics, J Am Dent Assoc 130: 236-251, 1999.
38. Smudski JW, Sprecher RL, Elliott HW: Convulsive interactions of promethazine, meperidine and lidocaine, Arch Oral Biol 9:595-600, 1964.
39. Moore, PA, Burney RG: The interaction of morphine and meperidine with the analgesic, convulsant and lethal properties of lidocaine in mice, Tox Applied Pharm 49:279-282, 1979.
40. Tucker T, Mather LE: Clinical pharmacokinetics of local anesthetics, Clin Pharmacokinet 4:241-278, 1979.
41. Burney RG, DiFazio CA, Foster JA: Effects of pH on protein binding of lidocaine, Anesth Analg 57:478-480, 1978.
42. deJong RH, Wagman IH, Prince DA: Effect of carbon dioxide on the cortical seizure threshold to lidocaine, Exp Neurol 17:221-232, 1967.
43. Little JW, Falace DA, Miller CS, et al: Dental management of the medically compromised patient, ed 5, St Louis, 1997, Mosby.

Herbal Therapies

Michael T. Goupil

Over the past several years there has been an increased interest in the use of herbal remedies.[1-4] This interest has been fostered for a number of reasons. The increase in health maintenance organizations (HMOs) has led to the promotion of preventive medicine. Many patients are disenchanted with allopathic (versus homeopathic) medicine and are seeking alternative medicine techniques. Increased leisure time, increased medical costs, and a greater interest in health have led to the use of herbals and food supplements.

Many patients do not consider herbal drugs as true medications if these substances are not prescribed by their allopathic physician, or they may be embarrassed to discuss their use of folk medicine.[2] For this reason they may not indicate on a health history form that they are taking any herbals or food supplements. Thus health care providers are obligated to inquire about the use of nonprescription medications, over-the-counter medications, herbals, and food supplements. These supplements may be self-prescribed rather than under the direction of a qualified alternative medicine health care provider. The majority of herbs and alternative therapies are safe when used as prescribed or according to accepted guidelines. Many of these alternative medications and food supplements, however, can result in significant complications when taken in combination with more traditional Western medications.

This summary of herbal medicines can be used as a guide in obtaining a more complete health history. More importantly, it illustrates the many potential consequences of treating patients with an inadequate history.[2-8]

ADONIS

Indications. Because of the positive inotropic effect of adonis (*Adonis vernalis*), it is used for arrhythmias, nervous heart complaints, and cardiac insufficiency.

Interactions. Enhancement of the efficacy and side effects of adonis are increased when used simultaneously with quinidine, digoxin, calcium, saluretics, and extended therapy with glucocorticoids.

Other names. False hellebore, sweet vernal, oxeye.

ALOE

Indications. The use of aloe vera (*Aloe barbadensis/capensis/vera*) depresses the action potential generation and conduction at neuromuscular junction processes, which results in analgesic and antiinflammatory effects. It increases the collagen content of granulation tissue and the degree of cross-linking to contribute to wound healing. It is sometimes used to treat AIDS, diabetes, asthma, stomach ulcers, and general immune weakness. *Aloe barbadensis* is used for evacuation relief in the presence of anal fissures after recto-anal surgery. It is also used for the treatment of fungal diseases, constipation, colic, and worm infestations.

Interactions. The long-term use of aloe can lead to loss of electrolytes, especially potassium. This hypokalemic effect is enhanced when aloe is used in conjunction with thiazide diuretics, loop diuretics, licorice, and corticosteroids. This potassium loss can increase the action of cardiac glycosides and antiarrhythmic drugs.

Other names. First-aid plant, hsiang-dan, lu-hui, medicine plant.

ANGELICA, DONG QUAI

Indications. Angelica (*Angelica species*) is recommended for fevers and colds, urinary tract infection, and dyspeptic complaints. Other uses include the treatment of menstrual cramping, PMS, and hot flashes. It has been used for constipation,

461

hepatitis, high blood pressure, tiredness, palpitations, and Raynaud's disease.
Interactions. It may interact with warfarin (Coumadin) and increase the risk of bleeding. It potentially could interact with other blood-thinning drugs like aspirin and heparin.
Other names. Engelwurzel, root of the Holy Ghost, tang-kuei.

ARNICA

Indications. Arnica (*Arnica montana*) reparations have antiinflammatory, analgesic, and antiseptic effects when applied topically. Other applications are for inflammation of the oral and throat region, insect bites, phlebitis, and joint and muscle aches.
Interactions. The coumarin component of arnica may have an additive anticoagulation effect with warfarin. Arnica may also alter the effectiveness of antihypertension medications.
Other names. Leopard's bane, mountain tobacco, wolfsbane.

ASHWAGANDHA

Indications. The principal use of ashwagandha (*Withania somniferm*) is to improve the ability to withstand stress. It is also used to improve exercise ability, immunity, and sexual capacity; to prevent colds and flu; and to treat insomnia and anxiety.
Interactions. Some constituents of ashwagandha can make an individual drowsy, and thus it should not be mixed with sedative drugs.

ASTRAGALUS, HUANG-QI

Indications. Astragalus (*Astragalus species*) has been used in the treatment of respiratory infections, immune depression, cancer, heart failure, viral infections, liver disease, and kidney disease. Other proposed uses include hyperthyroidism, hypertension, insomnia, diabetes, genital herpes, AIDS, and the side effects of chemotherapy.
Interactions. It may potentiate the risk of bleeding when used in combination with other anticoagulant, antiplatelet, or antithrombotic agents. It is incompatible with opiates.
Other names. Superior Chinese astragalus, alvita astragalus root.

BASIL

Indications. Basil (*Ocimum basilicum*) is used for inflammation, pain relief, stomach ulcers, high blood sugar, appetite stimulation and digestion, and as a diuretic.
Interactions. When used medicinally, basil may increase the effectiveness of insulin and oral medications used in the treatment of diabetes.
Other name. St. Joseph wort.

BILBERRY

Indications. The principal proposed uses of bilberry (*Vaccinium myrtillus*) include poor night vision, cataract prevention, and the strengthening of blood vessels. It has also been used in the prevention and treatment of diabetes mellitus, complaints of the gastrointestinal tract, kidney and urinary tract problems, arthritis, gout, and dementia.
Interactions. Bilberry has a platelet aggregation inhibiting effect, and it may interact with other agents, such as aspirin and warfarin. It increases prothrombin time.
Other names. Huckleberry, whortleberry, blueberry, dyeberry, airelle.

BLACK COHOSH

Indications. The principal use for black cohosh (*Cimicifuga racemosa*) is for menopausal problems. It is also used for rheumatism, sore throats, and bronchitis. It is found in combination with St. John's wort for depressive moods associated with premenstrual and menopausal symptoms.
Interactions. Black cohosh can potentiate the effects of antihypertensive medications and when used with those drugs may lead to hypotension. It may lower blood sugar and could interact with drugs for diabetes.
Other names. Remifemin, black snakeroot, bugbane, cimicifuga, squawroot.

BLADDERWRACK

Indications. Bladderwrack (*Fucus vesiculosus*) is used internally for diseases of the thyroid, obesity, arteriosclerosis, and digestive disorders. It is used externally for sprains.
Interactions. This herb carries the danger of the induction or worsening of hyperthyroidism. It has a hypoglycemic effect and may interact with other hypoglycemic medications.

BOGBEAN

Indications. Bogbean (*Menyanthes trifoliata*) is used for constipation, fluid retention, rheumatism, and to stimulate the appetite. In Chinese medicine it is also used for the treatment of insomnia, headache, earache, and breathing difficulties.

Interactions.   It may increase the effects of heparin, Coumadin, and antiplatelet drugs, such as aspirin, clopidogrel (Plavix), and ticlopidine (Ticlid).

Other names.   Buck bean, bog myrtle, marsh clover, water shamrock.

BREWER'S YEAST

Indications.   Brewer's yeast (*Saccharomyces cerevisiae*) is used for dyspeptic conditions, eczema, furuncles, acne, and loss of appetite.

Interactions.   Brewer's yeast can trigger migraine headaches in susceptible patients. There may be an increase in blood pressure when taken in combination with MAO inhibitors.

BROMELAIN

Indications.   The primary use of bromelain is for the reduction of swelling and inflammation following surgery and athletic injuries, phlebitis, and dysmenorrhea. It has been proposed for use in the treatment of gout and hemorrhoids.

Interactions.   Because bromelain acts as a blood thinner, it will have an additive effect with Coumadin and heparin.

BROOM

Indications.   Broom (*Cytisus scoparus, Sarothamnus scoparlus*) relieves irregular heartbeat and is used for fluid retention. The herb is used for functional heart and circulatory disorders, as an adjunct in the stabilization of circulation, and to raise the blood pressure. In folk medicine the flowers are used for edema, rheumatism, gout, kidney stones, jaundice, liver disorders, and as a blood purifier.

Interactions.   It may enhance the effect of β-blockers, antihypertensives, and tricyclic antidepressants. Concurrent use with MAO inhibitors may cause a hypertensive crisis.

Other names.   Bannal, genista, hogweed, Scotch broom, Irish broom top.

BUCHU

Indications.   Buchu (*Barosma betulina*) is used as a diuretic and for the treatment for kidney and urinary tract infections.

Interactions.   Buchu may alter the effect of Coumadin.

Other names.   Agathosma, betuline, and bocco.

BUCKTHORN

Indications.   Buckthorn (*Rhamnus catharticus*) is used as a stool softener for constipation and for bowel movement relief in cases of anal fissures and hemorrhoids. It is also used as a diuretic and for poor digestion.

Interactions.   Resorption of other medications could be reduced due to the laxative effect of buckthorn. In cases of chronic use, potassium deficiency leads to an increase in the effect of cardiac gycosides as well as effecting heartbeat-regulating drugs.

Other names.   Herbal laxative, Herbalene, Neo-Cleanse.

BUGLEWEED

Indications.   Bugleweed (*Lycopus virginicus*) is used for the treatment of nervousness, insomnia, premenstrual syndrome, mild thyroid hyperfunction (Graves' disease), mastodynia, and functional and organic cardiac conditions.

Interactions.   *Lycopus* preparations disturb the administration of diagnostic procedures with radioactive isotopes.

Other names.   Virginia water horehound, gypsywort.

BURDOCK

Indications.   Burdock (*Arctium lappa*) is recommended for the relief of dry, scaly skin conditions such as eczema and psoriasis, and it may be used for acne. Burdock root preparations are used for gastrointestinal tract complaints and as a diuretic.

Interactions.   The effect of insulin and oral medications for diabetes may be enhanced by the use of burdock.

Other names.   Bardanam gobo, lappa, fox's clote, hardock.

BUTCHER'S BROOM

Indications.   Butcher's broom (*Ruscus aculeatus*) has been used for arthritis, fluid retention, hemorrhoids, and poor circulation in the legs.

Interactions.   It may interfere with the action of α-blockers for hypertension and MAO inhibitors.

Other names.   Box holly, pettigree, Curcu Capsules.

CASCARA SAGRADA

Indications.   Cascara (*Rhamnus purshiana*) is used for chronic constipation, relief of defecation with anal fissures, hemorrhoids, and as a recto-anal postoperative treatment. It is used as a tonic and for cleaning wounds, for rheumatism, and as a digestive aid.

Interactions. Prolonged use may lead to heart arrhythmias,465 nephropathies, edema, and accelerated bone deterioration. Long-term use leads to loss of electrolytes, in particular potassium. Thiazide diuretics, corticoadrenal steroids, and licorice root may potentiate potassium deficiency. Potassium loss may potentiate digitalis toxicity and arrhythmias when given comcomitantly with antiarrhythmic medications. Indomethacin decreases the effect of cascara.

Other names. Sacred bark, Bicholax, Cas-Evcac, Casvlium.

CAT'S CLAW

Indications. Cat's claw (*Uncaria tomentosa*) has been used for arthritis, birth control, inflammatory diseases of the intestinal tract, and rheumatism. It may have some antiviral, antiinflammatory, and immunostimulating properties.

Interactions. It may interfere with the effectiveness of antihypertension medications and Coumadin.

Other names. Samento, una de gato, Vegicaps.

CAYENNE

Indications. Cayenne (*Capsicum species*) is used for muscular tension and rheumatism. It is also used for painful muscle spasm in areas of shoulder, arm and spine, for frostbite, seasickness, stroke, and heart disease.

Interactions. Capsicum has been found to induce increased fibrinolytic activity and simultaneously cause hypercoagulability of blood. The bioavailability of aspirin and salicylic acid are reduced. Cayenne may increase the absorption of theophylline.

CELANDINE

Indications. Celandine (*Chelidonium majus*) is used in the treatment of cancer, biliary tract blockage, digestive disorders, and liver disease.

Interactions. Celandine may interact with digitalis, morphine and related drugs, oral drugs for the treatment of diabetes, and sulfa drugs.

Other names. Tettewort, felonwort, rock poppy, Cacau, Cytopure.

CHAMOMILE

Indications. Chamomile (*Matricaria recutia* [German], *Chamamelum nobile* [English]) has mild sedative effects. Various varieties of chamomile are used for cough/bronchitis, fevers and cold, inflammation of the skin, inflammation of the mouth and pharynx, wounds and burns. It is also used for inflammation and cramps in the gastrointestinal tract, teething symptoms, severe pain, and diarrhea and flatulence.

Interactions. Due to the content of hydroxycoumarin in chamomile, there may be an additive effect when taken with warfarin. Chamomile has weak anxiolytic properties at benzodiazepine receptor sites; thus concomitant use of alcohol and benzodiazepines should be avoided.

CHASTE TREE

Indications. Chaste tree (*Vitex agnus-castus*) is used for premenstrual syndrome and menopausal symptoms. It has also been used to suppress appetite, induce sleep, male sexual disturbances, and nervous depression.

Interactions. Chaste tree has a dopaminergic effect and reciprocal can occur with dopamine receptor agonists. It may effect the action of hormones such as oral contraceptives and bromocriptine.

Other names. Chasteberry, gatillier, hemp tree, monk's pepper.

CHINESE RHUBARB, DA-HUANG

Indications. Da-Huang (*Rheum palmatum*) is primarily used for constipation. It is also used as an appetite stimulant, painful teething, delirium, edema, and diarrhea.

Interactions. Long-term use leads to electrolyte loss, especially potassium. Electrolyte loss may lead to hyperaldosteronism and enhanced effects of cardioactive drugs. Long-term use may lead to arrhythmias, nephropathies, and bone loss.

COLCHICUM

Indications. Colchicum (*Colchicum autumnale*) is used in the treatment of gout and Mediterranean fever. It is also used for inflammation of the kidney and gastrointestinal tract, bodily secretions, and acute joint rheumatism.

Interactions. Colchicum drugs are severely poisonous. Long-term administration has led to kidney and liver damage, peripheral nerve inflammation, and bone marrow damage (leukopenia, thrombocytopenia).

Other names. Meadow saffron, autumn crocus, naked ladies, upstart.

COLEUS

Indications. Coleus (*Coleus forskohlii*) is used as a treatment for asthma, menstrual cramps, angina, irritable bowel syndrome, crampy bladder, and hypertension.

Interactions. It may interfere with the effects of blood pressure medications such as β-blockers, clonidine, and hydralazine. It may also alter the effects of anticoagulants such as Coumadin, heparin, and pentoxifylline (Trental).

CONDURANGO

Indications. Condurango (*Marsedenia condurango*) is used in the treatment of cancer, fluid retention, indigestion caused by tension, and as an appetite stimulant.

Interactions. It is not recommended for patients taking atropine, Epitol, Lanoxin, Norvir, Paxil, or Zoloft.

Other names. Eagle-vine bark, Conduran.

CORKWOOD

Indications. Corkwood (*Dubosia myoporoides*) may be used as an atropine substitute or a stimulant.

Interactions. Do not use it in combination with other anticholinergic drugs, β-blockers, Lanoxin, or tricyclic antidepressants.

Other name. Pituri.

COWSLIP

Indications. Cowslip (*Primula veris*) is used primarily for cough/bronchitis. It may also be used for anxiety, hysteria, insomnia, and irritability.

Interactions. Cowslip may alter the effectiveness of diuretics, antihypertensives, and sedatives.

Other names. Arteyke, fairy cup, keyflower, mayflower, paigle, password, plumrocks.

CRANBERRY

Indications. Cranberry (*Vaccinium macrocarpon*) is used to prevent bladder infections.

Interactions. It decreases the effectiveness of weakly alkaline drugs such as antidepressants and prescription analgesics.

DANDELION

Indications. Dandelion (*Taraxacam offinae/laevigatum*) is used primarily for dyspeptic conditions, urinary tract infections, liver and gallbladder complaints, and loss of appetite. It is also advocated in the treatment of fluid retention, constipation, rheumatism, and diabetes.

Interactions. Dandelion should not be used in combination with diuretics, antihypertensive agents, and oral hypoglycemics.

Other names. Lion's tooth, endive.

DIGITALIS

Indications. Digitalis (*Digitalis purpurea*) has been used to treat lower abdomen boils, headaches, abscesses, and paralysis. It is used for the treatment of cardiac insufficiency and migraine.

Interactions. The simultaneous administration of arrhythmogenic substances (e.g., sympathomimetics, methylxanthines, quinidine) increases the risk of cardiac arrhythmias.

Other names. Foxglove, dog's finger, witches' gloves, fairy caps.

ECHINACEA

Indications. Echinacea (*Echinacea species*) is commonly used for the common cold, cough/bronchitis, fevers, infections of the urinary tract, inflammation of the mouth and pharynx, wounds and burns.

Interactions. The immune-stimulating effect of echinacea may interfere with drugs that have immunosuppressant effects. Hepatotoxicity may occur with long-term use; therefore simultaneous use with other hepatotoxic drugs should be avoided.

Other names. American cone flower, black Susans, coneflower, Indian head, snakeroot.

ENGLISH HAWTHORN

Indications. English Hawthorn (*Crataegus laevigata*) is used for senile heart, chronic cor pulmonale, and mild forms of bradycardiac arrhythmias. It is also used for hypertension, cardiac ischemia, cardiac insufficiency, and angina pectoris. In Chinese medicine it is used for food stagnancy and blood stasis.

Interactions. In higher doses English Hawthorn can cause hypotension, cardiac arrhythmias, and sedation. It may potentiate the action of cardiac glycosides. It may cause a hypertensive effect when used in combination with β-blockers.

Other names. Leaves & Berries, HeartCare.

EPHEDRA, MA-HUANG

Indications. Ephedra (*Ephedra sinica*) is used as a central nervous system (CNS) stimulant, an appetite suppressant, a nasal decongestant, and in the treatment of bronchial asthma, the common cold, and headache. In Chinese medicine it has been used for severe febrile illnesses, bronchial asthma, joint symptoms, inability to perspire, edema and pain in the bones.

Interactions. Ephedra may alter the effects of monoamine oxidase inhibitors, ephedrine, β-blockers, phenothiazines, and Sudafed. Higher dosages may result in blood pressure and cardiac rhythm disorders. It has an additive effective in conjunction with caffeine, decongestants, and other central stimulants. It may result in heart rhythm disturbances when used with halothane.

Other names. Brigham tea, epitonin, joint fir, natural ecstasy, sea grape, yellow horse, Herbal Fen-Phen, Power Trim, Up Your Gas.

EVENING PRIMROSE

Indications. Evening primrose oil (*Oenothera biennis*) is used for neurodermatitis, premenstrual syndrome, hyperactivity in children and high cholesterol.

Interactions. It has a potential to decrease seizure threshold in patients with seizure disorders or those being treated with drugs that lower seizure threshold.

FENUGREEK

Indications. The primary use of fenugreek (*Trigonella foenumgraecum*) is for the management of diabetes and high cholesterol. It is also used for loss of appetite and inflammation of the skin. In Chinese medicine the drug is used to treat cold pain in the lower abdomen, impotence, and hernia.

Interactions. Fenugreek has a hypoglycemic effect. There is a potential for fenugreek to interact with hypoglycemic drugs used to treat diabetes and to enhance their effect, possibly causing excessively low blood sugar.

Other names. Bird's foot, trigonella, Fenu-Thyme.

FEVERFEW

Indications. Feverfew (*Tanacetum parthenium*) is used mainly for migraine, arthritis, and rheumatic diureses. It is also used as a stimulant, digestive aid, and blood purifier.

Interactions. There is a strong possibility that feverfew may interact with thrombolytics, anticoagulants, and platelet aggregation. It may reduce the effectiveness of NSAIDs.

Other names. Altamisa, bachelor's button, chamomile grande, nosebleed, wild quinine, Traditional Herb, Mygrafew.

FIGWORT

Indications. Figwort (*Scrophularia nodosa*) is used for digestive disorders, chronic skin conditions, lymphedema, chronic tonsillitis, and to stimulate the heart.

Interactions. Figwort should not be used in combination with digitalis, β-blockers, and calcium channel blockers.

Other names. Carpenter's square, scrofula plant, throatwort.

FRANGULA

Indications. Frangula (*Rhaminus frangula*) is primarily used for constipation. It is also used to ease bowel evacuation in the case of anal fissures and hemorrhoids.

Interactions. Long-term use of frangula leads to loss of electrolytes, especially potassium ions, which may lead to the enhancement of cardioactive steroids and arrhythmias.

Other names. Buckthorne, dog wood, black adder tree, arrow wood.

GARLIC

Indications. Garlic (*Allium sativum*) is used internally for elevated lipid levels and for the prevention of age-related vascular change and arteriosclerosis. It is also used for inflammatory respiratory conditions, gastrointestinal ailments, diabetes, constipation, and joint pain. Garlic appears to slightly improve hypertension and slow blood coagulation. Its regular use is proposed to help prevent cancer.

Interactions. A significant decrease in hematocrit values and plasma viscosity have been associated with garlic use. Concomitant use of garlic with anticoagulants such as Coumadin and antiplatelet drugs such as aspirin and dipyridamole could increase the effect of bleeding due to the effect of garlic on platelet aggregation and fibrinogen. Risk of bleeding is increased when taken in combination with ginkgo or high-dose vitamin E. Garlic may increase serum insulin levels.

Other names. Ail, da-suan, rustic treacle, Kwai, Kyolic, Sapec.

GINGER

Indications.   Ginger (*Zingiber officinale*) is primarily indicated for loss of appetite, travel sickness, and dyspeptic complaints. It is also used to treat colds, nausea, vomiting, and shortness of breath.
Interactions.   Ginger appears to have an antithrombotic effect and is not recommended for patients taking anticoagulants, antiplatelet drugs or those with bleeding disorders.
Other names.   Zingiber, Quanterra Stomach Comfort.

GINKGO, GINKGO BILOBA

Indications.   The primary use for ginkgo is for symptomatic relief of organic brain dysfunction, intermittent claudication, and vertigo and tinnitus of vascular origin. Ginkgo has been demonstrated to improve concentration and memory deficits. It is also used for asthma, hypertonia, erectile dysfunction, and angina pectoris.
Interactions.   Spontaneous bleeding has been associated with ginkgo due to its potent inhibitory effect on platelet-activating factor. Care should be used when used in combination with aspirin and other anticoagulant and antiplatelet agents. Hypertension may result from an interaction with thiazide diuretics.
Other names.   Ginkgo, ginkogink, rokan, sophium, tanakan, tebonin, Ginexin Remind, Quanterra Mental Sharpness.

GINSENG

Indications.   Ginseng (*Panax ginseng/quinquefolius*) is used internally for fatigue and debility, and for a decreased capacity for work and concentration. It is also used for loss of appetite, cachexia, anxiety, impotence and sterility, neuralgia, and insomnia.
Interactions.   Ginseng has been shown to have hypoglycemic effects. Hypotension resulting from ginseng abuse syndrome is associated with prolonged high-dose ginseng in combination with caffeine. It may have adverse effects when used in combination with oral hypoglycemics and MAO inhibitors. *P. ginseng* has antiplatelet activity and concomitant use with aspirin, NSAIDs, heparin, and warfarin should be avoided.
Other names.   Five-fingers, jintsam, seng and sang, tartar root, Bio Star, Cimexon, Chinese Red Panax.

GLUCOMANNAN

Indications.   Glucomannan (*Amorphophallus konjac*) may be used to treat constipation, lower cholesterol, reduce blood sugar, and to aid in weight loss.
Interactions.   Glucomannan may enhance the effects of oral hypoglycemics and cholesterol-lowering medications.
Other name.   Konjac.

GOAT'S RUE

Indications.   Goat's rue (*Galega officinalis*) is used as a diuretic and as supportive therapy for diabetes. It is also used to increase breast milk flow.
Interactions.   Goat's rue may have an additive effect when used in conjunction with hypoglycemic medications.
Other names.   French lilac.

GOLDENSEAL

Indications.   Goldenseal (*Hydrastis canadensis*) has been used for loss of appetite, gastrointestinal problems, and tinnitus. Mistakenly it has been used to hide illicit opiate drug use in urine tests.
Interactions.   Goldenseal can cause arrhythmias, including asystole and heart block. Goldenseal may alter the action and side effects of Coumadin, antihypertension medications, benzodiazepines, β-blockers, Lanoxin, and calcium channel blockers.
Other names.   Eye balm, ground raspberry, Indian dye, yellow paint.

GOTU KOLA

Indications.   Gotu kola (*Centella asiatica*) is used for rheumatism and skin diseases. It has been used for birth control, hypertension, chronic liver disease, and mental fatigue.
Interactions.   The use of gotu may result in altered action and adverse side effects when used in combination with hypoglycemic agents and cholesterol reduction medications. Large doses may result in sedation.
Other names.   Centella, Indian pennywort, talepetrako.

GREEN TEA

Indications.   Green tea (*Camellia sinensis*) has become a popular drink for cancer prevention. It may help prevent liver disease and dental caries.

Interactions. The vitamin K in green tea interferes with the effectiveness of Coumadin. It decreases the absorption of alkaline drugs.
Other name. Matsu-cha.

GUARANA

Indications. Guarana (*Paullinia cuanafor*) is used as a tonic for fatigue and to quell hunger and thirst, headache, digestion problems and as a diuretic. It has been used as an aphrodisiac and as an aid in weight and body-building.
Interactions. The diuretic action may result in hypokalemia and an increase in digoxin toxicity. The use of guarana in combination with fluoroquinolones and β-blockers may alter their action and side effects.
Other names. Brazilian cocoa, zoom.

HAWTHORNE

Indications. Hawthorne (*Crataegus species*) is used to strengthen and invigorate the heart and circulatory system.
Interactions. Hawthorne can cause hypotension, arrhythmias, and sedation. It may alter the effects and side effects of sedatives, tranquilizers, narcotics, cardiac glycosides, and antihypertensives.
Other names. Maybush, whitehorn, Cardiplant.

HENBANE

Indications. The primary use of henbane (*Hyoscyamus niger*) is for dyspeptic conditions. It is also used for various pain syndromes, particularly toothache and facial pain, stomach cramps, and lower abdominal pain.
Interactions. There may be an enhancement of the anticholinergic action of tricyclic antidepressants, amantadine, antihistamines, phenothiazines, procainamide, and quinidine.
Other names. Devil's eye, fetid nightshade, Jupiter's bean, poison tobacco.

HOPS

Indications. Hops (*Humulus lupulus*) are used as a mild sedative for restlessness, anxiety, and sleep disturbances.
Interactions. Hops may have an additive effect with anticholinergic, antidepressant, antihistamine, antipsychotic, and antianixety medications. Hops should not be used in combination with drugs that are metabolized by cytochrome P-450 system such as Coumadin, NSAIDs, and Tylenol.
Other names. Sedative Tea, Serene, HR133 Stress, Stress Aid.

HOREHOUND

Indications. Horehound (*Marrubium vulgare*) is commonly used for sore throat and cough. It may also be used as a digestive aid and for loss of appetite.
Interactions. Horehound may cause cardiac arrhythmias. It may also alter the action of antidepressants and migraine medications.
Other names. Marrubium, marvel, Hore Hound Tea.

HORSE CHESTNUT

Indications. The primary use of horse chestnut (*Aesculus hippocastanum*) is for the treatment of chronic venous insufficiency such as superficial and deep varicose veins. It is also used for posttraumatic and postoperative soft tissue swelling, sprains, hemorrhoids, and lumbar and low back pain.
Interactions. The leaf has a coumarin component that may interact with warfarin, salicylates, and other drugs with anticoagulant properties.
Other names. Aescin, Venostasin Retard, Venostat.

HORSETAIL

Indications. Horsetail (*Equisetum arvense*) is used for urinary tract infection, kidney and bladder stones, fluid retention, gout, indigestion, and rheumatism.
Interactions. It contains nicotine and may interfere with the use of smoking cessation products.
Other names. Bottle brush, Dutch rush, pewterwort, shave grass.

JAMAICAN DOGWOOD

Indications. Jamaican dogwood (*Piscidia erythnia*) is used in the treatment of asthma, insomnia, and migraine.
Interactions. It may cause drowsiness and increase the sedation effects of barbiturates, narcotics, muscle relaxants, sedatives, and tranquilizers.
Other names. Fishfuddle, fish poison tree, Willow-Meadowsweet Compound.

JAMBOLAN

Indications. Jambolan (*Syzygium cuminii*) is used for the treatment of diabetes, diarrhea, and inflammation of the mouth, pharynx and skin.

Interactions. It may alter the action or side effects of barbiturates, narcotics, muscle relaxants, sedatives, and tranquilizers.
Other names. Jambul, black plum, java plum, rose apple.

JIMSON WEED

Indications. Jimson weed (*Datura stramonium*) has been used for asthma, convulsive cough, pertussis, infection with high temperature, Parkinson's disease, and general states of pain.
Interactions. Jimson weed has an additive effect with other anticholinergic medications. It may alter the effects of antihistamines, phenothiazines, and tricyclic antidepressants.
Other names. Angel's trumpet, devil weed, green dragon, gypsyweed, locoweed, mad apple, stinkweed, zombie's cucumber.

KAVA

Indications. Kava (*Piper methysticum*) is primarily used for nervous tension, stress, agitation, depression, and insomnia.
Interactions. Dyskinesia and choreoathetosis of the limbs, trunk, neck and facial musculature have been reported. The simultaneous use with alprazolam has resulted in coma. The herb may potentiate the effectiveness of CNS depressants, such as barbiturates, and intensify the effects of psychoactive agents. It has been reported to antagonize the effect of dopamine.
Other names. Awa, kew, sakau, tonga, Aigin, Laitan, Mosaro, Potter's Antigian Tablets.

KELP

Indications. Kelp (*Laminaria digitara*) is used as an iodine source for thyroid function, to treat hypertension, and as a blood thinner.
Interactions. It should not be used in combination with antihypertensive medications, Coumadin, or aspirin.
Other names. Brown algae, horsetail, seaweed.

KHAT

Indications. Khat (*Catha edulis*) is used to improve appetite, and in the treatment of depression. It is said to have an aphrodisiac effect.
Interactions. It should not be used in combination with decongestants, antiarrhythmics, antihypertensives, β-blockers, and MAO inhibitors.
Other names. Gad, miraa, tschut.

KHELLA

Indications. Khella (*Amni visnaga*) is used for angina, to prevent and/or treat allergic reaction, asthma, and skin conditions such as vitiligo and psoriasis.
Interactions. Khella may affect the action and/or side effects of Coumadin, calcium channel blockers, and hypertension medications.
Other names. Ammi, bishop's weed, visnaga.

KOMBE SEED

Indications. Kombe seed (*Strophanthus hispidus*) is used for nervous cardiac complaints and cardiac insufficiency.
Interactions. The simultaneous administration of quinidine calcium salts, saluretics, laxatives, and glucocorticoids enhances the effects and side effects.
Other name. Arrow poison.

LAVENDER

Indications. Lavender (*Lavandula species*) is used as an appetite stimulant and to treat insomnia, restlessness, migraine, and muscle strain.
Interactions. Lavender may enhance the effects of benzodiazepines and narcotic pain medication.
Other names. Aspic, esplieg, spigo.

LICORICE

Indications. The primary use of licorice (*Glycyrrhiza glabra*) is for cough/bronchitis and gastritis. This herb is also used for appendicitis, constipation, to increase milk production, and micturation. Other uses include gastric ulcers, headache, sore throat, spleen disorders, and dehydration. It has been suggested as a treatment for chronic fatigue syndrome.
Interactions. Prolonged use may result in hypokalemia, hypernatremia, edema, hypertension, and cardiac complaints. Licorice has an additive effect with furosemide and thiazide diuretics. The hypokalemic effects may potentiate digitalis toxicity. Severe ventricular tachycardia of the torsades de pointes type has been reported with the concomitant use of antiarrhythmic agents. Licorice may prolong the half-life of cortisol increasing its effectiveness and its side effects.
Other names. Sweet root, Natural Artho-Rx, Tea with Mint

LILY-OF-THE-VALLEY

Indications. Lily-of-the-valley (*Convallaria majalis*) is primarily used for arrhythmia, cardiac insufficiency, and nervous heart complaint.

Interactions. The simultaneous administration with quinidine, digoxin, calcium salts, saluretics, laxatives, β-blockers, calcium channel blockers, and glucocorticoids enhances the effects and side effects of Lily-of-the-valley.

Other names. Jacob's ladder, lily constancy, male lily, muguet.

LOVAGE

Indications. Lovage (*Levisticum officinale*) is used as a diuretic, in the treatment of urinary tract infections and kidney and bladder stones, as a sedative, and for muscle spasms.

Interactions. Lovage may alter the effects of Coumadin.

Other names. Maggi plant, sea parsley, smellage.

LUNGWORT

Indications. Historically, lungwort (*Pulmonaria officinalis*) is used to treat lung diseases. It is also used for diarrhea, digestive tract bleeding, and hemorrhoids.

Interactions. Lungwort may prolong bleeding and it should not be used in combination with other blood thinners such as Coumadin.

Other names. Lung moss, comfrey, dage of Jerusalem.

MARIGOLD

Indications. Marigold (*Calendula officialis*) is used topically for skin injuries and inflammation. Orally it is used to treat mouth sores. It has been used as a digestive aid and to enhance milk production,

Interactions. Calendula may increase the sedative effect of sleeping pills and antianxiety medications.

Other name. Calendula.

MISTLETOE

Indications. Mistletoe (*Vicum album*) is used in the treatment of arteriosclerosis, depression, headache, hypertension, insomnia, nervousness, and tension.

Interactions. Mistletoe may enhance the effects of sedatives, narcotics, tranquilizers, muscle relaxants, antihypertensives, and MAO inhibitors.

Other names. Bird lime, devil's fuge, Viscum, Iscadore.

MOTHERWORT

Indications. Motherwort (*Leonurus cardiaca*) is used to treat heart conditions such as palpitations or nervous heart. It has also been advocated for hyperthyroidism and flatulence.

Interactions. Motherwort should not be used in combination with Coumadin, b-blockers, and digitalis.

Other names. Lion's ear, throwwort.

MOUNTAIN LAUREL

Indications. In homeopathic medicine, mountain laurel (*Kalmoa latifolia*) is used for rheumatism, shingles, nerve pain, rheumatic, and cardiac pain.

Interactions. Mountain laurel may produce bradycardia, cardiac arrhythmias, drops in blood pressure, eventual cardiac arrest and respiratory failure can occur. It is highly toxic and should not be used in the presence of other cardiovascular medications.

NETTLE

Indications. Nettle (*Urtica dioica*) is primarily used for infections of the urinary tract, kidney and bladder stones, and for rheumatic ailments. It is used widely in Europe for the treatment of benign prostate hyperplasia.

Interactions. Nettle enhances the antiinflammatory effects of diclofenac. In theory, nettle may interact with antihypertensive, sedative, and hyperglycemic medications.

Other name. Stinging nettle.

NIAULI

Indications. Primarily used for cough/bronchitis, Niauli (*Melaleucasea viridiflora*) is also used for rheumatism, neuralgia, and cystits.

Interactions. Nauli can cause the induction of liver detoxification enzymes, thus reducing or shortening the effect of other drugs.

NIGHT-BLOOMING CEREUS

Indications. Cereus (*Selenicereus grandiflorus*) is used for a wide variety of conditions, including anemia, angina, depression, fatigue, palpitations, Grave's disease, rheumatism, and prostate disease.

Interactions. Cereus should not be used in combination with many cardiac medications including digitalis, β-blockers, calcium channel blockers, and ACE inhibitors.
Other names. Sweet-scented cactus, vanilla cactus, cactus grandiflorus.

OAK

Indications. Oak (*Quercus rubor*) is primarily used for cough or bronchitis, diarrhea, inflammation of the mouth and pharynx, and inflammation of the skin. It may also be used for hemorrhagic stool and hemoptysis.
Interactions. Oak may reduce or inhibit the absorption of alkaloids and other alkaline drugs. It should not be used in combination with atropine, digoxin, and morphine.
Other name. Tanner's bark.

OLEANDER

Indications. Oleander (*Nerium oleander*) is used for functional disorders and diseases of the heart, as well as skin disorders.
Interactions. The simultaneous administration of oleander with quinidine, calcium salts, saluretics, laxatives, or glucocorticoids increases their efficacy and side effects. Numerous fatalities have been described.
Other names. Adelfa, laurier rose, rose bay.

PAPAYA

Indications. Papaya (*Carica papaya*) is used for gastrointestinal digestive complaints, athletic injuries, and herniated vertebral disks.
Interactions. Papaya has a fibrinolytic effect, and a tendency to bleed is possible when there is a predisposition to clotting delay. There is an interaction with warfarin and increased INR levels have been noted.
Other names. Melon tree, papain, pawpaw.

PARSLEY

Indications. Parsley (*Petroselinum crispum*) is used in the treatment of urinary tract infections, kidney and bladder stones, fluid retention, intestinal gas, muscle spasm, and digestive problems.
Interactions. It may affect the action of antidepressants and narcotic pain medication.
Other name. Insure herbal.

PASSION FLOWER

Indications. Passion flower (*Passiflora incarnata*) is used to reduce anxiety, insomnia, and nervous stomach.
Interactions. Passion flower may exaggerate the effect of other sedative medications.
Other names. Apricot vine, granadilla, maypop, water lemon.

PAU D'ARCO

Indications. Pau d'arco (*Tabebuia impetiginosa*) is advocated for a wide variety of ailments including AIDS, anemia, diabetes, headache, cancer, incontinence, rheumatism, and the common cold.
Interactions. Pau d'arco may potentiate bleeding when used in combination with blood thinners like Coumadin or in patients with coagulation disorders like von Willebrand's disease, thrombocytopenia, or severe liver disease.
Other names. Ipe, lapacho, roxo, trumpet bush, Advance Defense System Tablets, Ultra Multiple Vitamins, Wellness Formula Vitamin, Women's Ut Formula.

POPLAR

Indications. Poplar (*Populus alibi, P. tremulodes, P. nigra*) is used in the treatment of liver disorders, rheumatism, and the common cold. Other uses include hemorrhoids, burns, and micturition in benign prostate hypertrophy.
Interactions. Poplar may alter the effects of aspirin, Coumadin, and antiplatelet drugs like ticlopidine.
Other names. American aspen, quaking aspen.

PRICKLY ASH

Indications. Prickly ash (*Zanthoxylum americanum*) is used in folk medicine for toothache pain. It is used for intestinal gas, to promote circulation, and for rheumatism.
Interactions. Prickly ash may promote bleeding problems especially when used in combination with aspirin or other blood thinners.
Other names. Toothache tree, suterberry, angelica tree.

PSYLLIUM

Indications. Psyllium (*Plantago ovata*) is used in the treatment of constipation, diarrhea, and elevated cholesterol.

Interactions. The absorption of other drugs taken simultaneously may be delayed. Downward insulin dosage adjustment may be necessary.
Other name. Metamucil

QUEEN ANNE'S LACE

Indications. Queen Anne's lace (*Daucus carota*) has been advocated as an aphrodisiac, to lower blood sugar, and for fluid retention.
Interactions. Queen Anne's lace may alter the action of hypotensive medications, anxiolytics, sedatives, muscle relaxants, and pain medications.
Other names. Bee's nest, wild carrot, devil's plague.

QUININE

Indications. The primary use of quinine (*Cinchona pubescens*) is for loss of appetite and dyspeptic conditions. The bark is used for malaria, flu, enlarged spleen, muscle cramps, muscle pain, and gastric disorders.
Adverse reactions. There is a possibility that thrombocytopenia, an enhanced pseudohemophiliac condition, can occur.
Other names. Peruvian bark, Jesuit's bark, Cinchona.

RAUWOLFIA

Indications. Rauwolfia (*Rauwolfia serpentina*) is primarily used for hypertension, nervousness, and insomnia. It is also used for flatulence, vomiting, to encourage uterine contraction, local wound treatment, and snakebite.
Interactions. There is an increased drug effect with neuroleptics and barbituates. Severe bradycardia occurs in combination with digitalis glycosides. It should not be used in combination with sedatives, tranquilizers, narcotics, and muscle relaxants.
Other names. Snakeroot, Harmonyl, Serpasil.

SAW PALMETTO

Indications. Saw palmetto (*Serenoa repens*) is used for urination problems in benign prostate hyperplasia. It is also used for inflammation of the urinary tract, bladder and testicles, and mammary glands.
Interactions. Saw Palmetto is believed to exert estrogen, androgen, and α-adrenergic blocking effects.
Other names. Cabbage palm, sabal, American dwarf palm tree, Permixon, Strogen.

SCOPOLIA

Indications. Scopolia (*Scopolia carniolica*) is used for spasms and colic-like pain of the gastrointestinal tract, bile ducts, and urinary tract.
Interactions. It increases the effect of simultaneously administered tricyclic antidepressants, amantadine, and quinidine.
Other names. Scopola, Japanese or Russian belladonna.

SENEGA SNAKEROOT

Indications. Senaga (*Polygala senega*) is used for cough, chronic bronchitis, sore throat, graft rejection, multiple sclerosis, and to stimulate saliva production.
Interactions. It may alter the action and/or side effects of blood thinners, hypoglycemic agents, and central nervous system depressants such as sedatives, narcotics, and muscle relaxants.
Other names. Milkwort, mountain flax, rattlesnake root, Enhance, SN-X Vegitabs.

SENNA

Indications. Senna (*Cassia species*) is used for constipation and evacuation of the bowel before gastrointestinal tract diagnostic tests. It may also be used in the treatment of intestinal worms and skin disease.
Interactions. Long-term use leads to loss of electrolytes, particularly potassium. Enhancement of cardioactive glycosides and antiarrhythmics may occur with hypokalemia.

Concomitant use of indomethacin decrease the therapeutic effect of Senna. Therapeutic effects can be blocked with nifedipine.
Other names. Senekot, Senolax.

SHEPHERD'S PURSE

Indications. Shepherd's purse (*Capesella bursapastoris*) is used for bleeding disorders, hematuria, nosebleeds, premenstrual syndrome, headaches, and diarrhea.
Interactions. Shepherd's purse may alter the action and/or side effects of digoxin, antihypertension agents, beta-blockers, calcium channel blockers, and sedative/hypnotics.
Other names. Capsella, caseweed, shovelweed.

SIBERIAN GINSENG

Indications. Siberian ginseng (*Eleurherococcus senticosus*) is used as tonic for invigoration and fortification in times of fatigue and debility. In

Chinese medicine it is used for kidney pain, urine retention, impotence, sleep disturbance, loss of appetite, and as stimulation for the immune system.

Interactions. Use may result in elevated serum levels of digoxin, potentiate the effects of antidiabetic agents/insulin, and enhance the effects of anticoagulants/antiplatelets/antithrombotics.

SQUILL

Indications. Squill (*Urginea maritima*, *U indica*) is primarily used for cardiac insufficiency, arrhythmia, nervous heart complaints, and venous conditions. It is also used for reduced kidney capacity, bronchitis, asthma, and back pain.

Interactions. The concomitant use of quinidine, calcium, saluretics, laxatives, and extended use of glucocorticoids can result in the increased effectiveness of squill and its side effects. The simultaneous use of arrhymogenic substances increases the risk of cardiac arrhythmias. Squill potentiates the positive inotropic and negative chronotropic effects of digoxin.

Other names. Indian squill, sea onion.

ST. JOHN'S WORT

Indications. The primary use of St. John's wort (*Hypericum perforatum*) is for the treatment of anxiety, depressive moods, inflammation of the skin, blunt injuries, and wounds and burns. It may be effective in seasonal affective disorder. It has also been used for asthma, gall bladder disease, gout, and rheumatism.

Interactions. When used in combination with a MAO inhibitor, a hypertensive crisis may develop. St. John's wort has slight serotonin reuptake inhibitor properties and when used with other SSRIs toxicity may develop. It may decrease the effect of any critical medications such as digoxin, cyclosporin, protease inhibitors, Coumadin, and oral contraceptives. It should be avoided for concurrent use with other photosensitizers such as tetracycline and sulfonamides.

Other names. Amber, goatweed, mellepertuis, rosin rose, witches' brew, Hypercalm, Kira, Mood Support, Tension Tamer.

SROPHANTHUS

Indications. Srophanthus (*Srophanthus species*) is used for the treatment of arteriosclerosis, cardiac insufficiency, gastrocardial symptoms, hypertension, and neurodystonia.

Interactions. Effects and side effects are enhanced when used simultaneously with quinidine, calcium salts, saluretics, laxatives, and glucocorticoids.

Other name. Kombé

TONKA BEANS

Indications. Tonka beans (*Dipteryx odorata*) were used in the past for whooping cough. It may be used as an aphrodisiac, for nausea, stomach cramps, and in the treatment of lymphedema.

Indications. They may increase the effects of Coumadin.

Other names. Cumaru, tonquin bean.

TUMERIC

Indications. Tumeric's (*Curcuma longa*) primary use is for dyspeptic complaints and loss of appetite. It is also used to treat a variety of diseases including cancer, gallstones, intestinal gas, osteoarthritis, and rheumatoid arthritis.

Interactions. Tumeric may alter the action and/or side effects of Coumadin, NSAIDs, and immune system suppressants.

Other names. Indian saffron, jiang huang, red valerian.

UVA-URSI

Indications. The primary use of uva-ursi (*Arctostaphylos uva-ursi*) is for disorders of the urinary tract.

Interactions. Any substance that causes acidic urine reduces the antibacterial effect of uva-ursi. It may add to the gastrointestinal irritation of NSAIDs. It may decrease the effect of loop diuretics and thiazide diuretics.

Other names. Arberry, bear's grape, mountain cranberry, kinnicknick.

UZARA

Indications. Uzara (*X smalobium undulatum*) is used for the treatment of diarrhea and dysentery.

Interactions. This herb contains cardioactive glycosides and there is a potential for interaction with digoxin and other cardiac glycosides.

VALERIAN

Indications. Valerian (*Valeriana officinalis*) is used for restlessness, sleeping disorders, mental strain, lack of concentration, excitability, stress, headache, epilepsy, hysteria, and neuralgia.

Interactions. The long-term use of valerian can result in headache, sleeplessness, and cardiac function disorders. Valerian may potentiate the

Box 30-1	Herbals That Potentiate Anticoagulants*

Angelica (Dong Quai)   Khella
Arnica   Lovage
Astragalus (Huang-Qi)   Lungwort
Bilberry   Motherwort
Bogbean   Papaya
Bromelain   Pau d'arco
Buchu   Poplar
Cat's claw   Prickly ash
Coleus   Siberian ginseng
Feverfew   St. John's wort
Garlic   Tonka beans
Ginger   Tumeric
Ginkgo   Watercress
Ginseng   Willow
Horse Chestnut   Yarrow
Kelp

*These herbals may interact with warfarin (Coumadin), nonsteroidal antiinflammatory drugs (NSAIDs), and aspirin and have an additive effect on platelet activity and anticoagulation, resulting in increased bleeding problems.

effects of other CNS depressants. It has an additive effect with barbiturates and benzodiazepines.
Other names. Enchanter's herb, pigeon grass, purvain, wild hyssop, Nature's Root Nighttime, Quanterra Sleep.

WATERCRESS

Indications. The primary use of watercress (Nasturtium officinale) is for skin diseases such as acne, eczema, rashes, and infections.
Interactions. Watercress should not be used in combination with NSAIDs.
Other names. Garden cress, scurvy grass.

WILD YAM

Indications. Wild yam (Dioscorea villosa) is used for rheumatic conditions, gall bladder colic, dysmenorrhea, and cramps.
Interactions. Wild yam may decrease the antiinflammatory effect of indomethacin. It has an additive effect with estrogen.
Other names. Colic root, China root, Devil's bones, rheumatism root

WILLOW

Indications. The salicin component of willow (Salix species) is used in the treatment of fever, rheumatic ailments, headaches, and pain caused by inflammation.

Interactions. Caution should be used when used in combination with salicylates and other NSAIDs,
Other names. Willowprin, Aller g Formula.

WINTERGREEN

Indications. Wintergreen (Gaultheria procumbens) is used to treat muscle and joint pain, sciatica, and trigeminal neuralgia.
Interactions. Wintergreen should not be used simultaneously with aspirin or Coumadin.
Other names. Boxberry, Canada tea, deerberry, mountain tea, partridgeberry.

WORMWOOD

Indications. Wormwood (Artemisia absinthium) is used for loss of appetite, dyspeptic conditions, and liver and gall bladder complaints. In addition, in folk medicine, it is used for anemia, intermittent fever, and irregular menstruation.
Interactions. Wormwood may lower seizure threshold. Drugs that are used to control seizures have decreased effectiveness. It should not be used in combination with phenothiazides, Trazodone, and tricyclic antidepressants.
Other names. Green ginger, absinthe.

YARROW

Indications. The primary use for yarrow (Achillea millefolium) is as an appetite stimulant and liver

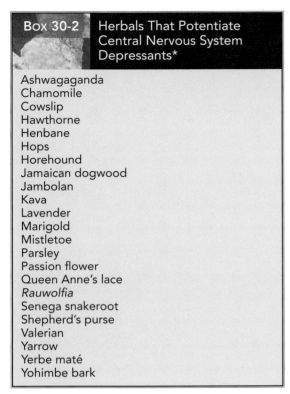

Box 30-2 Herbals That Potentiate Central Nervous System Depressants*

Ashwagaganda
Chamomile
Cowslip
Hawthorne
Henbane
Hops
Horehound
Jamaican dogwood
Jambolan
Kava
Lavender
Marigold
Mistletoe
Parsley
Passion flower
Queen Anne's lace
Rauwolfia
Senega snakeroot
Shepherd's purse
Valerian
Yarrow
Yerbe maté
Yohimbe bark

*These herbals may have an additive effect when used concomitantly with CNS depressants, including muscle relaxants, narcotic pain relievers, and benzodiazepines.

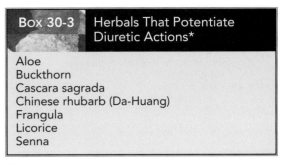

Box 30-3 Herbals That Potentiate Diuretic Actions*

Aloe
Buckthorn
Cascara sagrada
Chinese rhubarb (Da-Huang)
Frangula
Licorice
Senna

*These herbals act as diuretics and may produce hypokalemia and resultant cardiac sensitivity to sympathomimetics.

and gallbladder conditions. It is also used for digestive disorders, urinary tract problems, to stop bleeding from skin wounds, and eczema.

Interactions. Yarrow may alter the action and/or side effects of CNS depressants, antihypertensive medications, and Coumadin.

Other names. Bloodwort, milfoil, nosebleed, stanchgrass, Diacure, Rheumatic Pain Remedy.

YERBE MATÉ

Indications. Yerbe maté (*Ilex paraguariensis*) is used for diabetes, fluid retention, depression, hypertension, heart disease, and as an appetite suppressant.

Interactions. Yerbe maté may alter the action and/or side effects of Cipro, Tagamet, and CNS depressants such as sedatives, tranquilizers, muscle relaxants, narcotics, and barbiturates.

Other names. Armino, jaguar, Jesuit's tea, safira, union

YOHIMBE BARK

Indications. Yohimbe (*Pausinystalia yohimbe*) is approved by the FDA as a sympatholytic and mydriatic. It has been used to treat impotence. It is used as an aphrodisiac and for debility and exhaustion.

Interactions. Yohimbe can cause a marked increase in diastolic pressure. The overall analgesic effect of morphine may be enhanced. It may alter the action and side effects of antidepressants, including selective serotonin reuptake inhibitors, and tricyclics.

Other names. Aphrodien, corynine, quebrachine, Aphrodyne, Dayto Himbin, Yocon.

SUMMARY

A wide variety of herbal medicines are available in the marketplace. The question is not whether patients are taking herbal medicines or dietary supplements, but rather which ones they are taking. Many of these herbals have significant side effects of their own, and there can be serious consequences when they are taken in conjunction with other prescribed or over-the-counter medications (Boxes 30-1, 30-2, and 30-3). It is imperative that a thorough health history is taken that specifically inquires about the use of all medications and supplements.

REFERENCES

1. Crone CC, Wise TN: Use of herbal medicines among consultation-liaison populations, *Psychosomatics* 39:3-13, 1998.
2. Ko R: Adverse reactions to watch for in patients using herbal remedies, *West J Med* 71:181-186, 1999.

3. Miller LG: Herbal medicines, *Arch Intern Med* 158:2200-2211, 1998.

4. Murphy JM: Preoperative considerations with herbal medicines, AORN J 69:173-183, 1999.

5. *Alternative healing: what actually works*, Berkeley, Calif, 2000, Institute for Natural Resources.

6. Bratman S: *Your complete guide to herbs*, Roseville, Calif, 1999, Prima.

7. Fetrow CW, Avila JR: *The complete guide to herbal medicines*, New York, 2000, Simon & Schuster.

8. PDR *for herbal medicines*, Montvale, NJ, 2000, Medical Economics.

The Abused and Neglected Patient

Howard I. Mark

Violent behavior is on the rise in all segments of the American population. As the media, professional publications, and social agencies report, violence events are increasing. The term *domestic violence* includes child abuse, spousal abuse, and elder abuse,[1] as well as intentional and unintentional forms of neglect. There are no boundaries to this phenomenon; it crosses all ethnic and socioeconomic lines and is pervasive.

Dentists may be the first health professionals to come in contact with true and suspected cases of abuse and neglect.[2] Additionally, more than half of all cases of abuse involve head and neck injuries. Thus the dental staff must be competently trained to recognize the signs of abuse and neglect and to report their findings to the proper authorities for appropriate intervention. Early detection and intervention may present the only possibility for an abused and neglected victim to escape from a continuing cycle of violence and misuse.

THE PROFESSION'S ROLE IN ABUSE AND NEGLECT

The 1993 American Dental Association's House of Delegates amended the Principles of Ethics to state "dentists shall be obliged to become familiar with the perioral signs of child abuse and to report suspected cases to the proper authorities."[3] A further resolution extended the scope of the dentist's observation for abuse to include "all physical signs of child abuse that are observable in the normal course of a dental visit."[3] Continuing attention to other forms of abuse and neglect is being given by the profession to extend the dentist's responsibility to the diagnosis, treatment, reporting and referral of other victims of domestic violence: battered women, the elderly and the disabled. The American Academy of Pediatric Dentistry has defined den-

tal neglect as "the willful failure to seek and obtain appropriate treatment for rampant caries, trauma, pain, infections or bleeding."[4] Included in this definition is the failure to follow through with treatment once the parent or guardian has been informed that these conditions exist.[5,6] These same parameters with only minor modifications can also be applied to spousal and elder abuse and neglect findings that the dentist may encounter in varying degrees. The dental team's role is to identify and report cases of abuse and neglect and to add expertise in warranted cases when it can be used to the best advantage. Because these problems are highly complex by their very nature, they require the mobilization and activation of a cadre of well-trained professionals and support agencies. Many hospitals and services, such as child protective service (CPS) agencies, have formed teams of pediatricians, nurses, social workers, psychiatrists, psychologists, and attorneys trained and poised to intervene in all aspects of the presenting situation.

THE DENTIST AS MANDATED REPORTER

All fifty states and most of the territories have mandated that dentists report suspected cases of child abuse to appropriate agencies such as hospitals, social service organizations, or CPS (Figure 31-1).[7,8] The proponents of these child protection laws, cognizant of the ignorance, denial and confidentiality concerns that have made these laws necessary, devised certain provisions to reduce legal impediments to reporting. Among these are: statutory immunity from both criminal and civil liability for reports made in good faith; exemption from state laws protecting the confidentiality of patient information; reporting justification requiring only reasonable

Dentists as Mandated Reporters

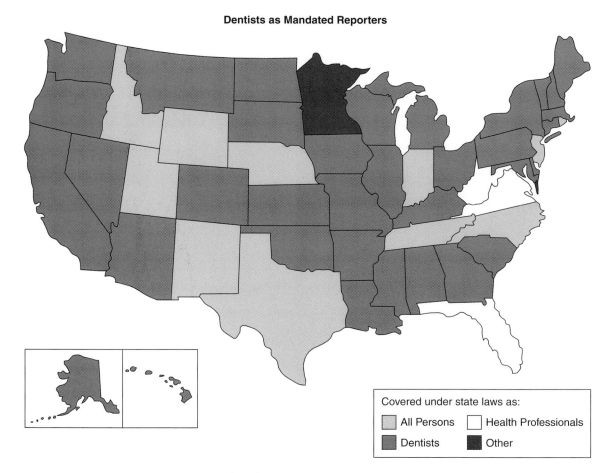

Figure 31-1. Dentists as mandated reporters. *From American Dental Association Council on Dental Practice 1995: The dentist's responsibility in identifying and reporting child abuse and neglect, ed 3, Chicago, 1995, The Council.*

suspicion or belief; anonymity provisions for reporters in some states; and assessment of civil and/or criminal penalties for failure to report.[9] The practitioner must review the statutes of concern in each state to become familiar with the exact terminology and requirements appropriate to the office location.

The dental hygienist, as a member of the dental team, has also been specifically mandated by most states to report suspected cases of abuse and neglect (Figure 31-2).[7] Suspicion of such findings may be discussed with other office personnel, but the report must be made promptly according to the laws of the jurisdiction in which the practice is located, not the one in which the victim lives or in which the injury occurred. The safeguards of reporting provisions cited above apply equally to the dental hygienist in these situations.

While these same statutes do not specifically refer to or outline the responsibilities of the dentist in regard to the other members of the dental team and his/her oversight of these situations, there is an implied obligation to ensure that the dental hygienist and other dental auxiliaries apprise him/her of their suspicions and concerns about possible abuse and/or neglect problems. Because these individuals come under the umbrella of office liability and malpractice policies in most jurisdictions, the practitioner should establish an appropriate protocol with guidelines for the office staff to follow as the most effective means for protecting victims. The recognition of the signs of abuse and neglect, the understanding of the necessity for reporting suspected cases, and the appreciation of the fact that this intervention may help break the cycle of violence, should effectively increase

Dental Hygienists as Mandated Reporters

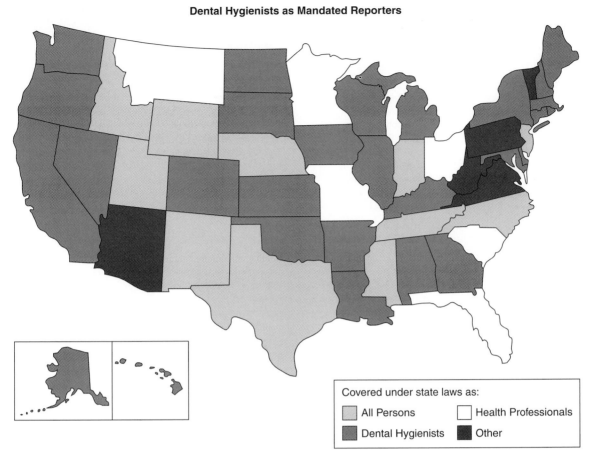

Figure 31-2. Dental hygienists as mandated reporters. *From American Dental Association Council on Dental Practice 1995:* The dentist's responsibility in identifying and reporting child abuse and neglect, *ed 3, Chicago, 1995, The Council.*

the numbers of cases reported to more acceptable levels.

CHILD ABUSE AND NEGLECT

Child abuse and neglect has become a national crisis of epidemic proportions. In 1995 more than three million cases of suspected child abuse and neglect were reported to social services and CPS agencies.[9] This is an appalling statistic and serves to point up the alarming and pervasive nature of the problem. More than one million of these reports were substantiated by authorities as actual occurrences.[9,10,11] A Minnesota study in 1992 found that 75.5% of all child abuse cases involved injuries to the head, face, neck and mouth, all of these areas falling within the observation of the dental professional.[12] These figures parallel earlier and subsequent

studies that clearly showed a serious upward trend in child abuse injuries from the 1970s to the 1990s.[13,14] Instances of child abuse and neglect can be categorized as follows: neglect as the most common, accounting for 52% of the reported cases; physical abuse approximates 25% of all reports; and some 13% of victims suffering sexual abuse, based on current reporting and substantiation. It is obvious that young children are the most vulnerable, being the most dependent and helpless, and more than half of all substantiated cases are under seven years of age.[9]

Recognition of Child Abuse and Neglect by the Dental Professional

Recognition of potential or suspected abuse and neglect victims requires basic knowledge by the dental professional and his staff (Box 31-1). This

| Box 31-1 | General Risk Factors for Child Abuse and Neglect* |

- History of drug or alcohol abuse within the family
- Severe stress—economic, lifestyle, or as a result of disasters
- Lack of a support network or isolation (e.g., single parent families; few close friends; no relatives nearby; geographic isolation; inability to, or fear of, interacting with neighbors)
- Other forms of family violence within the home (spousal or partner abuse, abuse or neglect of elders)
- History of a parent having been abused as a child

WARNING SIGNS
- Repeated injuries or injuries in various stages of healing
- Inappropriate behavior
- Neglected appearance or hygiene
- Parents that are extremely strict or super critical of the child

SOME CONDITIONS THAT MAY MIMIC ABUSE
- Accidental injuries, typically in similar stages of healing

- Birthmarks that do not heal and disappear, although they may fade after many years
- Bullous impetigo: Staphylococcal or streptococcal infections that respond to antibiotic regimens
- Folk medicine remedies, such as cupping, coin rubbing, or moxibustion, most common in families of Southeast Asian or Central American heritage
- "Port-wine stains" typical of Sturge-Weber Syndrome that do not change or disappear
- Slate-gray spots of infancy (formerly "Mongolian spots") that fade gradually over several years
- Epidermolysis bullosa: An autoimmune disease
- Idiopathic thrombocytopenia purpura may cause large contusions due to little or no injury
- Hemophilia: Clotting disorders with possible subcutaneous hemorrhage, often around joints
- Ehlers-Danlos syndrome: Congenital disorder resulting in improper collagen formation
- Menke's syndrome: Genetic disorder of copper metabolism resulting in friable hair

Courtesy Dr. Lynn Mouden, Jefferson City, Mo.
*This listing is not meant to be all-inclusive but is designed as a general guideline to the proper identification of child abuse or neglect. Clinicians are encouraged to seek additional information that will lead to proper diagnosis of suspected abuse or neglect.

should include awareness of the characteristics that can assist in the identification of children at high risk for abuse and neglect. Familiarity with the usual causes of childhood trauma is essential in making sound determinations of abuse/nonabuse injuries.[9] Since most abusive instances are considered not premeditated, the practitioner and staff should approach suspected problems with caution and attempt to rule out the typical, more accidental, forms of injury that are frequently found in this age group (see Box 31-1). Understanding the developmental capabilities of the injured child is most important in making these judgments on a more realistic basis. Contrasting the type and location of the injury, together with its appearance, may make the diagnosis a more positive one (Box 31-2).

A complete medical history, fully documented, will be useful in preventing mistakes in diagnosis. Certain disorders that are not uncommon in childhood may present in ways such as to mimic potential abuse injuries, unless previously noted or understood to be pre-existing,

and must be ruled out as not originating from an abuse situation (see Box 31-1).

Regardless of these findings, a 1995 study found only six states currently tracking numbers of dentists reporting. Of 201,944 reports filed in these states, 637 were from the dental community, or a .32% reporting rate.[15] The Prevent Abuse and Neglect through Dental Awareness (PANDA) program was initiated in the State of Missouri as a coalition of the Delta Dental plan of Missouri, the dental community, and social service agencies in 1992 to promote both the understanding of the problem by the dental profession and cooperation with appropriate health organizations.[16] CPS agencies were surprised to learn that dentists could become a valuable resource in preventing child maltreatment when this program was begun.[17]

The success of this campaign has been evidenced by dentists' increased reporting of child abuse and neglect cases since 1992. While total reports to CPS agencies increased by 16% between 1992 and 1996, the dental percentage grew by 160%, which speaks well for the impact

PHYSICAL INDICATORS

Physical Abuse

Unexplained bruises and welts:
- Face, lips, mouth
- Torso, back, buttocks, thighs
- In various stages of healing
- Clustered, regular patterns
- Reflecting shape of article used to inflict (e.g., buckle)
- On several different areas
- Regular appearance after absence, weekend, vacation

Unexplained burns:
- Cigarette, cigar burns, especially on soles, palms, back, buttocks
- Immersion burns (sock- or glove-like, circular, on buttocks or genitalia)
- Patterned burns: electric burner, iron
- Rope burns on arms, legs, or torso

Unexplained fractures:
- Skull, nose, facial structures
- In various stages of healing
- Multiple or spiral fractures

Unexplained laceration or abrasion:
- Mouth, lips, gingiva, eyes
- External genitalia

Physical Neglect
- Constant hunger, poor hygiene, inappropriate dress
- Consistent lack of supervision, especially in dangerous situations or for long periods

- Unattended physical problems or medical/dental needs
- Abandonment

Sexual Abuse
- Difficulty in walking or sitting
- Torn, stained, bloody underwear
- Pain or itching in genital area
- Bruises or bleeding on external genitalia, vaginal, or anal areas
- Venereal disease, especially in pre-teen
- Pregnancy

Emotional Maltreatment
- Speech disorders
- Lags in physical development
- Failure to thrive

BEHAVIORAL INDICATORS

Wary of adult contacts
Apprehensive when others cry
Behavioral extremes: aggressive, withdrawn, frightened of parents, afraid to go home
Reports injury by parents

Begging, stealing food

Extended stays at school, early arrival, late departure
Alcohol or drug abuse
Delinquency (e.g., thefts)
Constant fatigue, falling asleep in class

Says there is no caretaker

Unwilling to change for physical examination
Withdrawal, fantasy, or infantile behavior
Bizarre, sophisticated sexual knowledge or behavior
Poor peer relationship
Delinquency, runaways
Reports sexual assault by caretaker

Habit disorders (sucking, biting, rocking)
Conduct disorders (antisocial, destructive)
Neurotic traits (sleep disorders, inhibited play)
Psychoneurotic behaviors (hysteria, phobia, obsession, compulsion, hypochondria)
Behavior extremes: compliant, passive, aggressive, demanding
Overly adaptive behavior: inappropriately adult; inappropriately infantile
Developmental lags (physical or mental)
Attempted suicide

Courtesy Dr. Lynn Mouden, Jefferson City, Mo.

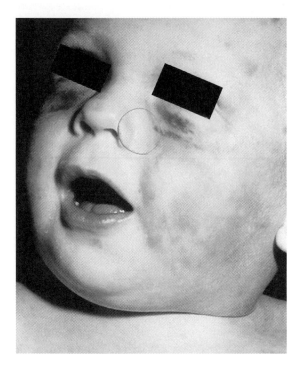

Figure 31-3. Multiple, bilateral injuries from abuse. *Courtesy Dr. Lynn Mouden, Jefferson City, Mo.*

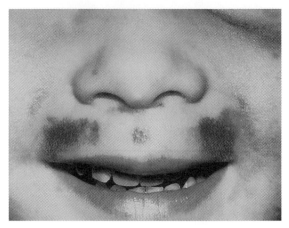

Figure 31-4. Contusions of the upper lip and cheek due to a beating. *Courtesy Dr. Lynn Mouden, Jefferson City, Mo.*

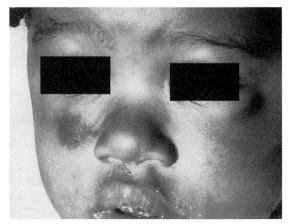

Figure 31-5. Multiple bruises in various stages of healing, although history given was that she had fallen once. Note bilateral facial injuries, extremely unlikely in a fall. *Courtesy Dr. Lynn Mouden, Jefferson City, Mo.*

training, increased knowledge, and deeper understanding of what is actually taking place, can make on a receptive profession.[17] The most common injuries relative to child abuse involve the head, perioral, and neck regions, as have been described. There is easy accessibility to these areas due to size considerations of the child versus the adult. The forms that oral injuries may take include, not only trauma to the teeth, but also to the surrounding oral tissues and bone. In 1979 a survey of pediatric dentists listed the principal injuries as follows: missing and fractured teeth (32%), contusions (24%), lacerations (14%), fractures (11%), and burns (5%)[18] (Figures 31-3 to 31-6).

Physical Signs of Child Abuse and Neglect

Torn frenal areas or soft tissue contusions in infants or young children can result from forced feedings, while palatal contusions may occur after forced oral sex[19] (Figure 31-7). Teeth can be displaced or luxated by a direct blow to the face or to the teeth themselves. The result of the trauma will be a lingual or palatal displacement of the injured tooth or teeth with resultant gingival or periodontal bleeding (Figure 31-8). At

times, teeth can be intruded, but this is a lesser finding.

Avulsive injuries with total displacement of the involved tooth or teeth from the alveolar bone can also occur, relative to the force and direction of the trauma and to the anatomy of the root(s). This is more often found in older children with more permanent dentition, due to the conical shape of the anterior maxillary tooth root structures. Tooth fractures per se are more likely to be the result of accidental injury, although the findings of root fractures or displaced roots on radiographic examination may indicate possible abuse. Any form of traumatic injury affecting

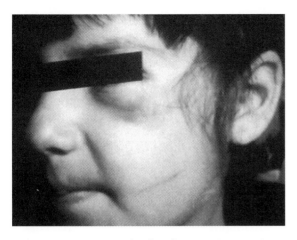

Figure 31-6. Large suborbital contusion. Patient said she had fallen off her bike; the mother said she had fallen down the stairs. Disparate histories often are pathognomonic of abuse. *Courtesy Dr. Lynn Mouden, Jefferson City, Mo.*

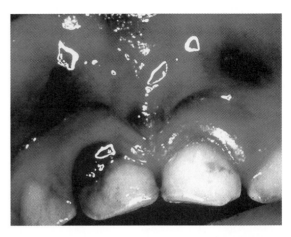

Figure 31-8. Multiple intraoral injuries from an open-handed slap to the face. Note laceration of upper lip, contusions of vestibule and frenum, and subluxation of central incisor. *Courtesy Dr. Lynn Mouden, Jefferson City, Mo.*

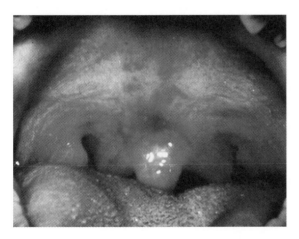

Figure 31-7. Victim of forced oral sex. Petechiae of hard palate; bruising of soft palate. *Courtesy Dr. Lynn Mouden, Jefferson City, Mo.*

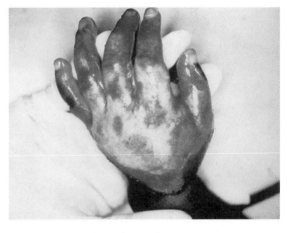

Figure 31-9. "Glove burn" from immersion in hot water. Note that some areas are spared where they are protected in making a fist. *Courtesy Dr. Lynn Mouden, Jefferson City, Mo.*

teeth is also more apt to involve supporting structures, including bone, so that periapical radiographs should be taken to rule out damage to adjacent teeth or alveolar bone.

Evidence of bruising or tearing at the commissures of the lips could point to the use of gagging to silence the victim. The tongue can be injured by trauma if it is in position between the teeth at the time of injury, as can be evidenced by the presence of jagged anterior or posterior indentations. Bruising noted on skin areas exposed to the observation of the dental profes-

sional can be further indications of abuse, especially if seen to be in different stages of healing, or if the explanation of these does not coincide with the known healing phase (see Figure 31-5).

Glove burns, named because they follow the immersion of one or both hands in hot water as punishment, can be easily detected by dental personnel and are definite indicators of child abuse. Portions of the hand may be spared if a fist is made, which protects the covered areas (Figure 31-9).

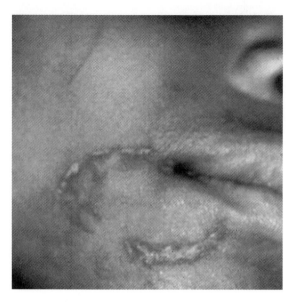

Figure 31-10. Bite mark to a boy's face. History given was a "dog bite." Identification was made of the father's dentition. *Courtesy Dr. Lynn Mouden, Jefferson City, Mo.*

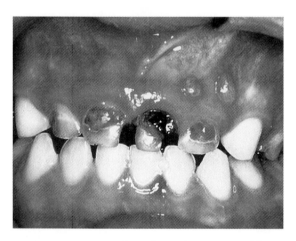

Figure 31-11. Dental neglect, characterized by multiple carious teeth and fistulae. Parents had resources available but did not think teeth were important. *Courtesy Dr. Lynn Mouden, Jefferson City, Mo.*

The presence of bite marks on the facial or neck regions should be highly suspect as well. Since most animal bites are of the tearing type, the more oval or circumscribed the appearance, the more these can be suggestive of the human variety (Figure 31-10).

Dental neglect may be more difficult to appreciate. When multiple carious teeth and fistu-

lae are noted, neglect should be suspected. While ignorance and dental phobias can play a decided role in this appearance, neglect is more probable if the parents or guardians appear to exhibit no noticeable financial constraints (Figure 31-11).

SPOUSAL ABUSE AND NEGLECT

Every 12 seconds in the United States a woman is beaten by someone she knows—a husband, a boyfriend, a relative.[20] This is termed *spousal abuse*, a violent behavior occurring between partners in an intimate relationship, regardless of the marital status.[21,22] This form of abuse has a direct correlation to the status of women in society, conditioned by sexism, racism, heterosexism, and classism.[23] It has been further defined as "the repeated subjection of a woman to forceful physical, social, and psychological behavior to coerce her without regard to her rights."[24,25,26] Spousal abuse can also include emotional and economic abuse, isolation, or sexual abuse.[27]

Estimates indicate that battered women abuse is much more common than abuse of children and the elderly.[28] Approximately 65% of the resultant injuries in these cases are found in the head and neck regions, clearly visible to the dental team.[29,30] Dental professionals must recognize that physical violence is not the only form that spousal abuse and neglect can take, and that they must be aware of other, more subtle, presentations. Mental and emotional abuse, and intimidation, become integral components of the abuse syndrome, potentially leading to repetitive patterns of the abuse and increased risk of death.[22]

The difficulty that health care providers have in clearly identifying victims of battering and spousal violence lies in the lack of specific demographic or diagnostic profiles of such victims.[22,31] When coupled with the reluctance of the injured partner to volunteer any substantiating information, this contributes to the low reporting rates encountered in these situations.[32] Direct and careful questioning in a non-threatening manner about suspected injuries may elicit information otherwise not forthcoming. Facial injuries and bruising noted in various stages of healing, coupled with obvious neglected dental and oral disease, can set the stage for the potential suspecting of spousal abuse and neglect. This questioning and review of the injuries should be done in quiet surroundings, well away from the victim's partner.[27,31]

Physical Signs of Spousal Abuse and Neglect

Injuries of any type, including lacerations, contusions, and fractures, may be seen. Periorbital ecchymoses, fractured noses, and fractured jaws are common occurrences.[1] The reporting of temporomandibular joint symptoms and pain should also trigger concern as to the causation. Presentations of bites, cigarette burns, and bruises in various stages of healing, affecting the face, cheeks, lips, and neck are potentially pathognomonic of spousal abuse.

The finding of multiple decayed and abscessed teeth in an otherwise healthy and responsive individual can also be indicative of purposeful neglect. While attributes of dental fear, cultural beliefs, and costs of care may be mitigating factors, careful and compassionate discussion of these findings may elicit the possible uncovering of spousal neglect.

Behavioral Indicators of Spousal Abuse and Neglect

Repetitive episodes of injury, accompanied by the seeming admission of being "accident-prone"; significant delay between the time of injury and the presentation for treatment; complaints of subjective pain without evidence of injury; and familiar excuses to explain away injuries should arouse suspicion as to the causative nature of the problem and to the likelihood of abuse. Stress-related health problems, such as asthma, insomnia, and anxiety, are found in greater numbers in these victims of abuse than most health providers would believe.[32] Characteristically, these victims do not voluntarily disclose environments of abuse and neglect to the treating professional.

RESPONSIBILITY OF THE HEALTH CARE PROFESSIONAL

Abused patients are often treated by health care professionals who fail to suspect abuse and neglect. Even when suspected, the compliance with state mandatory reporting laws varies widely.[22] This failure to report is well documented and can be attributed to a variety of causes such as uncertainty as to the clinical evidence, concern about the availability of protective services, and the fear of legal entanglements.[33] Minimal familiarity with specific state statutes can be a further deterrent to the reporting of these cases and reflects on the lack of education on this subject in both professional schools and in professional organizations.[34] A mail survey reported in the *American Journal of Public Health* in 1994 assessed responses from a group of dentists, dental hygienists, physicians, nurses, psychologists, and social workers. Both dental groups reported the least education in abuse, the lowest rate of suspecting and reporting abuse, and the greatest proportion who did not see themselves as responsible for intervening in situations of suspected abuse. These results, coupled with the known facts that injuries to teeth, jaws, facial areas, neck, and oral soft tissues can be common indicators of abuse and that dental professionals often have the first opportunity to observe these findings, reinforces dentistry's need for education in this important circumstance.[33,34] Those clinicians that had experienced professional training in the recognition and reporting of abuse and neglect cases do suspect abuse and neglect on a more frequent basis. All health care professionals have the responsibility of establishing the proper diagnosis, once abuse and neglect is suspected. The diagnosis requires the acknowledgment by the patient that the abuse situation does exist. Clinicians and their staffs need to be more supportive and nonjudgmental, and victims need to know that that they are not alone and that support groups are available for help. To ensure patient confidentiality and acquire more truthful answers from the suspected victim, any discussion relative to the problem should take place in a private setting away from the possible abuser. Any physical findings should be documented fully and photographs taken with the victim's consent. When the cause of injury is considered suspicious and the patient denies abuse, the term *suspected abuse* should be included in the record. The essential role of the clinician is to make the appropriate referral to supporting agencies or to a regional women's shelter. Even if the victim refuses to acknowledge abuse or neglect, the referral information and telephone numbers should be given for possible future use.[1] The goal of supportive intervention is to empower the victim to take control of the situation and to make the correct decisions as regards the future course of action.[27]

One method of communicating with patients suspected of being in an abusive situation is the use of SAFE Questions (Box 31-3). Developed by a physician, they demonstrate the health-giver's compassion and can bring the victim out of isolation, enabling her to acknowledge fears in a safe environment.[35]

Box 31-3	SAFE Questions

S—Stress/Safety: What Stress do you experience in your relationships? Do you feel Safe in your relationships/marriage? Should I be concerned for your Safety?

A—Afraid/Abused: Are there situations in your relationships where you feel Afraid? Has your partner ever threatened or Abused you or your children? Have you been physically hurt or threatened by your partner? Are you in a relationship like that now? Has your partner forced you to engage in sexual activities that you did not want? People in relationships/marriages often fight; what happens when you and your partner disagree?

F—Friends/Family: Are your Friends aware that you have been hurt? Does your Family know about this abuse? Do you think you could tell them and do you think they would be able to give you support? (Assess the degree of social isolation.)

E—Emergency Plan: Do you have a safe place to go and the resources you (and your children) need in an Emergency? If you are in danger now, would you like help in locating a shelter? Would you like to talk to a social worker/counselor/me to help develop an Emergency plan?

Another screening mechanism called the Partner Violence Screen, is composed of just three questions and has been found to be statistically valid in detecting 65% to 70% of domestic violence victims.[36] It consists of one question to assess physical violence and two questions to assess perceived safety. According to the authors, the physical violence question detects abuse almost as well as the three question combination. The questions are (1) Have you ever been kicked, hit, punched, or otherwise hurt by someone within the past year? If so, by whom? (2) Do you feel safe in your current relationship? and (3) Is there a partner from a previous relationship who is making you feel unsafe now? This review takes less than a minute, and can be performed in either the emergency department or in an office setting by any health professional.

ELDER ABUSE AND NEGLECT

The United States House of Representatives Select Committee on Aging defined elder abuse as "the willful infliction of injury, unreasonable confinement, intimidation, or cruel punishment with resulting physical harm, pain, or mental anguish; or willful deprivation by a caretaker of goods or services needed to avoid physical harm, or mental anguish or illness."[37] Elder mistreatment, defined as the abuse and neglect of older persons, includes physical, psychological, and sexual abuse; caretaker and self neglect; and financial exploitation. Fifty states and the District of Columbia have passed legislation to establish adult protective service (APS) programs; forty-two have mandatory reporting laws, with health care providers considered the major professional referral service.[38,39] Because of the high prevalence of dental disease and the need for ongoing dental care in this growing segment of the population, the frequency and the likelihood for any form of dental intervention is on the increase. This provides the dental team with multiple opportunities to observe, recognize, and report suspected instances of elder abuse and neglect. With current estimates of elder abuse indicating that nearly 10% of this group is affected, and realizing that this rate is on the rise, it is imperative that dentists develop a clearer understanding of the possible etiologies and know the physical and behavioral indicators of abuse and neglect that will confront them (Box 31-4).[40]

What must be kept in mind is the fact that elder abuse is easy to hide. In many instances, elders are embarrassed to admit someone they love could inflict any type of injury—physical, sexual, financial, mental—on them. Burns and bruises can be hidden by clothing; verbal abuse and intimidation may not be admitted; financial abuse will not be detected unless the provider is aware of the financial status of the victim; and sexual abuse is not likely to be discussed in a dental setting. Basic to the understanding and the prevention of elder abuse and neglect is the ability to appreciate potential causes. The American Medical Association Council on Scientific Affairs report on elder abuse in 1987 listed five possible situations that can lead to increased stress, presumed to be the most influential factor in elder abuse[41]:

Dependency
Lack of close family ties
Lack of financial resources
Psychopathology of the abuser
History of family violence

It is easy to appreciate the problems associated with dependency because of the various forms this can take, such as physical and men-

---

Box 31-4   The Rising Epidemic of Elder Abuse and Neglect

Most commonly seen as form of spousal abuse when the victim is over 60 or 65.

Many caregivers are unwilling or incapable of caring for the elderly, with little if any training or background.

Often elder abuse is a form of retribution abuse, "pay back" for a life of abuse when the child was young and defenseless.

CONTRIBUTING FACTORS TO ELDER ABUSE

Increasing elder population, especially those over 85.

A lower birth rate means fewer children to assist the elderly.

Increasing financial concerns for the family.

Increasing family mobility can mean the potential for less family support for the elderly.

Elder care can last many years longer than child rearing.

Elderly become more dependent with age and their care can be more demanding over time.

POSSIBLE SIGNS OF ELDER ABUSE AND NEGLECT

Injuries not treated or treatment is delayed.

Personal belongings or valuables are missing.

Confinement.

Malnourishment.

Property or savings that are mismanaged or stolen.

Inadequate clothing or personal items when the family's resources seem adequate.

Courtesy Dr. Lynn Mouden, Jefferson City, Mo.

---

tal impairments that necessitate constant care, placing severe burdens on caretakers in terms of the workload required for appropriate care. Neglect is even more likely when the patients are less able to care for themselves.

The other factors depend on a variety of subsets. Family members may be ill-equipped to care for a frail, dependent elder, and may opt not to be involved except indirectly, increasing the difficulties for those who may be incapable in themselves of providing the necessary care. Financial constraints may also be a factor because of the withholding of appropriate care by the caretaker on the premise that the victim is too old to receive it. This is even more certain when the caregiver has control of the patient's finances.[42]

Alcoholics and drug users share a propensity to become abusive caretakers, and may have mental disturbances, personal problems, or physical handicaps.[43] Other pathologic caretakers are those who, because of their own advancing ages, have become impaired mentally or physically, and who cannot respond correctly to the demands and needs of the older person. Surveys have shown that 75% of principal caretakers are older than 50 and 20% are older than 70.[44] It is also known that histories of previous family violence can play a significant role in the abuse of older persons. Individuals who were abused as children tend to become abusers themselves in adulthood. Researchers have postulated that an abusive behavior becomes a normative be-

havioral pattern in some families, with some members of these families practicing such behavior throughout their lives.[45]

Physical Signs of Elder Abuse and Neglect

While the enumerated physical signs may be present, they cannot be taken as positive indicators of elder abuse and neglect. Careful elicitation of supporting facts is vital to making the presumptive diagnosis of abuse and neglect. Recognition that self-neglect may play an important role in the physical appearance of the patient is extremely important to this process. Among these signs are uncombed hair, being unshaven, poor skin hygiene, dirty appearance, malnourished, dehydrated, bruises in various stages of healing, burns, injuries of an unexplained nature, and obvious lack of dental care.[46,47,48]

Behavioral Indicators of Elder Abuse and Neglect

The demeanor and affect of the elder victim may present as confused, frightened, withdrawn, depressed, helpless, disoriented as to time and place, evasive on questioning, and hesitant to talk freely about the circumstances for which he is being seen. These indicators may reflect emotional abuse being inflicted by threat, intimidation, humiliation, and isolation on the part of the caregiver.

Self-neglect must also be considered under behavioral indicators because of the prevalence of this finding among the elderly. A study conducted by the National Center on Elder Abuse in 1994 in 41 states showed that the majority of the confirmed cases or about one-third of all reports of elder abuse turned out to be self-neglect or self-abuse cases.[45] Because this form of neglect is so pervasive, the dental professional must not hasten to judgment but must be deliberative and thorough in making an assessment of the presenting conditions. Once again, careful questioning in a non-threatening manner, in a quiet environment, without the caregiver (if any) being present, is critical to the process.[49]

DOCUMENTATION OF ABUSE AND NEGLECT

There is no question that the types, indicators, and behavior patterns of abuse and neglect as seen in situations of child, spousal, and elder violence and neglect have differing aspects of appearance and involvement. Nevertheless, the overall need to document the findings and suspicions that can lead the health care provider to a conclusion of abuse and neglect is of vital importance, particularly if there is need for intervention by the appropriate state and local protective agencies, and the form that such documentation should take is approximately the same in all such cases (Boxes 31-5 and 31-6). It is imperative that the records be as complete as possible, that the examination of those areas visible and accessible in the dental setting be as thorough as it can be, and that answers to definitive questioning about the suspected abuse and neglect be specifically detailed. The process that needs to be followed includes the following:

1. Interview and examine the patient in a private area where confidentiality is assured, and be supportive during this time frame
2. Be certain that a staff person is present at all times to verify the findings noted and the answers to questions asked, with the inclusion of that individual's name in the record from a legal point of view
3. Record all statements as regards the history of the abuse or neglect in the patient's own words; including even those that may be inconsistent with the physical presentation
4. Keep a complete and accurate written description of any physical injuries, including an opinion that they may be inconsistent with the provided history if that appears to be the case.[22]

REPORTING AND INTERVENTION

Although all states have mandatory reporting statutes for cases of child abuse and neglect, they do vary widely when it comes to spousal abuse reporting. In this instance there is no question of the reporting of actual violence, involving the use of a weapon, but the specific provisions regarding the type of weapon or the seriousness of the injury that mandates reporting varies.[50] As for the reporting of elder abuse and neglect, a total of forty-two states, the District of Columbia, Guam, and the Virgin Islands operate mandatory reporting systems, covering dental personnel. On the other hand, in eight states the reporting is voluntary, so that suspected instances of elder abuse and neglect do not have to be reported.

In most areas of the country departments of social services maintain CPS and APS agencies and similar types of service arrangements that can assist the abused or neglected person. One valuable resource has been the advent of regional women's shelters that offer safety, counseling, vocational training opportunities, advocacy programs, and temporary facilities for children.

The National Organization for Victims Assistance maintains a 7 days-a-week, 24 hours-a-day crisis hotline number (1-800-TRY-NOVA) that can provide any health professional with the reporting information required for his state, with the name of the local agency dealing with these matters, and with the name of an area women's shelter. Local governmental listings in telephone books can be consulted for the APS agency, the Department on Aging, and for the CPS agency in their specific region. Other organizations that can assist include law enforcement agencies, hospitals and medical clinics, and mental health agencies.

It behooves the mandated reporter to become familiar with the state reporting statute covering the site of practice. When evaluating this statute for its reporting provisions, the following questions should be addressed[50]:

1. What is the purpose of the reporting statute?
2. What is to be reported?
3. Who makes the report?
4. What level of knowledge or suspicion is required?
5. Who receives the report and what is their response?
6. Are there penalties for failing to report?
7. Is there immunity from liability?
8. Are there provisions for confidentiality?

Box 31-5	Office Protocol for Identifying and Reporting Suspected Child Abuse and Neglect

STEPS IN IDENTIFICATION OF SUSPECTED CHILD ABUSE OR NEGLECT

1. **General physical assessment of the child.** Although general physical examinations may not be appropriate in the dental setting, be aware of obvious physical traits that may indicate abuse or neglect (e.g. difficulty in walking or sitting, physical signs that may be consistent with the use of force).
2. **Behavior assessment.** Judge the child's behavior against the demeanor of children of similar maturity in similar situations.
3. **Health histories.** If you suspect child maltreatment, it can be useful to obtain more than one history, one from the child and one separately from the adult.
4. **Orofacial examination.** Look for signs of violence, such as multiple injuries or bruises, injuries in different stages of healing, or oral signs of sexually transmitted diseases.
5. **Consultation.** If indicated, consult with the child's physician about the child's needs or your suspicions.

STEPS IN REPORTING SUSPECTED CHILD ABUSE OR NEGLECT

1. **Documentation.** Carefully document any findings of suspected abuse or neglect in the patient's record.
2. **Witness.** Have another individual witness the examination, note and co-sign the records concerning suspected child abuse or neglect.
3. **Report.** Call the appropriate CPS or law enforcement agency in your area, consistent with state law. Make the report as soon as possible without compromising the child's dental care. **The telephone number for reporting is _____.**
4. **Necessary information.** Have the following information available when you make the report:
- Name and address of the child and parents or other persons having care and custody of the child.
- Child's age.
- Name(s) of any siblings
- Nature of the child's condition, including any evidence of previous injuries or disabilities.
- Any other information that you believe might be helpful in establishing the cause of such abuse or neglect and the identity of the person believed to have caused such abuse or neglect.

Courtesy Dr. Lynn Mouden, Jefferson City, Mo.

Box 31-6	Dealing with Domestic Violence in the Dental Setting

ESSENTIAL ATTITUDES FOR PROFESSIONALS
Concern for the abused, for example:
- "I am concerned about your situation."
- "I don't want you to be abused."
- "I want to help you."
Respect for the abused, for example:
- "I don't blame you."
- "You don't deserved to be abused."

FIRST ESSENTIAL SKILL FOR PROFESSIONALS
Practice routine inquiry that is:
- Confidential
- Nonjudgmental
- Compassionate
Examples: "Have you ever been hit, kicked, punched or made afraid by someone who lives with you?" or "How are things at home?" (HATAH)

SECOND ESSENTIAL SKILL FOR PROFESSIONALS
AVOID questions that:
- Minimize the seriousness of the problem.
- Increase the patient's sense of shame and humiliation.

HELP VICTIMS UNDERSTAND THEMSELVES
- They do not deserve to be victimized.
- People do care about them.
- Health care professionals support their decisions.
- Patients can envision themselves in a non-violent environment.
- Resources and referrals are available.

JOBS FOR PROFESSIONALS
- Engage in conversations with women.
- Know the available resources.
- If you have a life of your own, realize that she can too!

Courtesy Dr. Lynn Mouden, Jefferson City, Mo.

9. Are provider-patient privileges specifically revoked?
10. Is there case law interpreting provider liability?

NEED FOR PROFESSIONAL EDUCATION

As the final statement, there is definitive need for further professional education of health care providers to enable them to become more aware of the problems of domestic abuse and neglect. The American Association of Dental Schools passed a resolution in 1994 adopting three policies on the subject of child abuse. These encourage all dental institutions and educators to (1) become familiar with all physical signs of abuse and the procedures for reporting suspected abuse, (2) instruct all students and staff in this area, and (3) monitor state and federal legislation and regulating activity on child abuse and make this information available to all students, faculty, and clinical staff. [51]

The American Dental Association has encouraged its members through amendments to its Principles of Ethics and Code of Professional Conduct to recognize and report instances of abuse and neglect, especially among children, although further emphasis is being placed on the other aspects of domestic violence, namely, spousal and elder abuse and neglect. All state dental organizations should also educate their members about these appalling problems.

REFERENCES

1. Dym H: The abused patient, Dent Clin North Am 39(3):621-635, 1995.
2. Meskin L: If not us, then who? Editorial, J Am Dent Assoc 125(1):10-12, 1994.
3. Minutes of the House of Delegates, November 6-10, 1993. In 1993 Transactions: 134th Annual Session, San Francisco, American Dental Association, pp 653-721.
4. Locchtan RM, Bross DC, Domoto PK: Dental Neglect in Children: definition, legal aspects and challenges. Pediatr Dent 8 (special issue 1):113-116, 1986.
5. Schmitt BD: Types of child abuse and neglect: an overview for dentists, Pediatr Dent 8 (special issue 1):67-71, 1986.
6. Schmitt BD: Physical abuse: specifics of clinical diagnosis, Pediatr Dent 8 (special issue 1):83-87, 1986.
7. Council on Dental Practice: The dentist's responsibility in identifying and reporting child abuse and neglect. Dentists as mandated reporters. Dental hygienists as mandated reporters, ed 3, Chicago, 1995, American Dental Association.
8. United States Department of Health and Human Services: Third National Incidence Study on Child Abuse and Neglect, 1996.
9. Persaud DI, Squires J: Abuse detection in the dental environment, Quint Intern 29:459-468, 1998.
10. Sfikas P: Does the dentist have an ethical duty to report child abuse? J Am Dent Assoc 127:521-523. 1996.
11. United States Department of Health and Human Services: National Child Abuse and Neglect Data System Report, 1995.
12. Fonseca MA, Feigal RJ, ten Bensel RW: Dental aspects of 1248 cases of child maltreatment on file at a major county hospital, Pediatr Dent 14:152-157, 1992.
13. Becker D, Needleman HL, Kotelchuck M: Orofacial trauma and its recognition by dentists, J Am Dent Assoc 97:24-28, 1978.
14. Cameron JM, Johnson HR, Camps FE: The battered child syndrome, Med Sci Law 6:2-21, 1996.
15. United States Department of Health and Human Services: Maternal and Child Health Bureau Report 40759, 1995.
16. Mouden LD: Oral injuries of child abuse. In Monteleone JA: Recognition of child abuse for the mandated reporter, ed 2, St. Louis, 1996, GW Medical Publishing.
17. Mouden L: How dentistry succeeds in preventing family violence, J Mich Dent Assoc 78(7):44-48. 1996.
18. Malecz RE: Child abuse, its relationship to pedodontics: a survey, ASCD J Dent Child 46:193-194, 1979.
19. Heitzler GD, Cranin AN, Gallo L: Sexual abuse of the oral cavity in children, NY State Dent J 60:31-33, 1994.
20. Jones RF, III: Domestic violence: let our voices be heard, Am J Obstet Gynecol 81:1-4, 1993.
21. Parker B, Schumacher DN: The battered wife syndrome and violence in the nuclear family of origin: a controlled pilot study, Am J Pub Health 67:760-761, 1977.
22. McDowell JD, Kassebaum DK, Stromboe SE: Recognizing and reporting victims of domestic violence, J Am Dent Assoc 123:45-46, 1992.
23. Connecticut Coalition Against Domestic Violence: Information material, May, 1994.
24. Chez N: Helping the victim of domestic violence, Am J Nurs 94(7):32-37, 1994.
25. Flitcraft AH, Hadley SM, Hendricks-Matthews MK, et al: Diagnostic and treatment guidelines on domestic violence, American Medical Association, 1992, Chicago.
26. Chez RA: Women battering, Am J Obstet Gynecol 158:1-4, 1988.
27. Gibson-Howell JC: Domestic violence: identification and referral, J Dent Hyg 70(2):74-79, 1996.
28. American Medical Association Council on Scientific Affairs: Violence against women: relevance for medical practitioners, JAMA 267:3184-3189, 1992.
29. Ochs HA, Neuenschwandr BA, Dodson TB: Are head, neck and facial injuries markers of domestic violence? J Am Dent Assoc 127(6):757-761, 1996.
30. Zacharides N, Koumoura F, Konsolaki-Agouridaki E: Facial trauma in women resulting from violence by men, J Oral Maxillofac Surg 48(12):1250-1253, 1990.
31. Sisley A, Jacobs LM, Poole G, et al: Violence in America: a public health crisis—domestic violence, J Trauma 46:1105-1113,1999.
32. McLeer SV, Anwar R: A study of battered women presenting in an emergency department, Am J Pub Health 79:65-66, 1989.
33. Tilden VP, Schmidt TA, Limandri BJ, et al: Factors that influence clinicians' assessment and management of family violence, Am J Pub Health 84:628-633, 1994.
34. Chiodo GT, Tilden VP, Limandri BJ, et al: Addressing family violence among dental patients: assessment and intervention, J Am Dent Assoc 125(1):68-75, 1994.

35. Ashur MS: Community oriented primary care approach to domestic violence. National Health Service Corps Educational Program for Issues in Primary Care, JAMA 269(18):2367-2368, 1993.

36. Feldhaus KM, Koziol-McLain J, Amsbury HL, et al: Accuracy of 3 brief screening questions for detecting partner violence in the emergency department, JAMA 277:1357-1361, 1996.

37. Hearings before the Elder Abuse Subcommittee, United States House of Representatives Select Committee on Aging: 99th Congress, 1st session, 1985.

38. Ehrlich P, Anetzberger G: Survey of public health departments on procedures for reporting elder abuse, *Pub Health Rep* 106(2):151-154, 1991.

39. Costa AJ: Elder abuse, *Prim Care* 20:317-327, 1993.

40. Jorgensen JE: A dentist's social responsibility to diagnose elder abuse, *Spec Care Dent* 12(3):112-115, 1992.

41. American Medical Association Council on Scientific Affairs: Elder abuse and neglect, JAMA 257:966-971, 1987.

42. Berrios DC, Grady D: Domestic violence risk factors and outcomes, *West J Med* 155(8):133-135, 1991.

43. Kelly MA, Grace EG, Wisnom C: Abuse of older persons: detection and prevention by dental professionals, *Gen Dent* 40(1):30-33, 1992.

44. Taler G, Ansello E: Elderly abuse, *Am Fam Physician* 32:107-114, 1985.

45. National Center on Elder Abuse: *Elder abuse: questions and answers. Information guide for professionals and concerned citizens*, ed 6, Washington DC, 1996, The Center.

46. New York Elder Abuse Coalition (NY EAC) Bulletin: Elder abuse definitions, signs and symptoms, January 1998, Http://www.ianet.org/nyeac/ea_signs.html.

47. California Department of Aging: Recognizing and reporting elder abuse, November 2, 1998, Http://www.cda.org/public/elder,html.

48. Lachs MS, Pillemer K: Abuse and neglect of elderly persons, N Engl J Med 332(7):437-443, 1995.

49. Rathbone-McCuan E, Fabian D: *Self-neglecting elders: a clinical dilemma*, Westport, Conn, 1992, Auburn House.

50. Hyman A, Schillinger D, Bernard LO: Laws mandating reporting of domestic violence: do they promote patient well-being? JAMA 273:1781-1787, 1995.

51. American Association of Dental Schools, House of Delegates Actions, 1994: *Bulletin of Dental Education* 27:1, 1994.

The Pregnant Patient

Leon A. Assael

U nderstanding the management of the pregnant patient is essential to the safe practice of dentistry. The pregnant dental patient may exhibit any medical, surgical or dental emergency. In addition, the pregnant patient is at risk for emergencies that are specific to pregnancy. Pregnancy produces a different mix of risk factors than in the non-gravid patient. Management of dental, surgical and medical emergencies during pregnancy depends on an understanding of both normal and abnormal pregnancy.

HEALTH DURING PREGNANCY

Three days after fertilization, implantation of the ovum into the endometrium of the uterus occurs. Estrogen, progesterone, prostaglandin, and other cytokines play a role in ovum transport through the fallopian tube. By 12 days after fertilization, the placenta is formed as well as embryonic mesenchyme. By 17 days, functioning maternal and fetal blood vessels are present. Human morphogenesis is now proceeding, and the fetal-placental unit is now established.

Although it is believed that infection, stress, or medication may play roles in inhibiting or over-accelerating implantation, precise mechanisms are not known. A patient seeking to become pregnant should maintain good general and oral health and avoid alcohol and tobacco, potentially harmful medications, and stressful dental procedures. The role of bacteremia, the inflammatory process, and the systemic activation of cytokines on early pregnancy are not unequivocal, the maintenance of good oral health and the prevention of infection may play a role in conception.

The transformation of embryo to fetus occurs with the completion of organ and limb morphogenesis at about 13 weeks of gestation. During this period, the fetus is most prone to teratogenic defects. Loss of pregnancy in the first trimester is most frequently due to abnormali-ties in the developing fetus. These birth defects include cleft lip and palate, limb malformation, and neural tube defects among others. Use of certain medications, administration of anesthesia, or the stress of illness or surgery may contribute to the formation of these defects. Fetal hypoxia may result in loss of pregnancy. Thrombosis of a fetal artery may result in hypoplasia, agenesis, atresia, or other structural abnormalities such as hemifacial microsomia. Elective surgical (including dental) treatment may be responsible for hypoxia, hypercoagulability, or chemically induced teratogenesis. Where delay of the procedure would not be detrimental, deferring invasive surgical and dental treatment until the middle trimester of pregnancy is advised.

Spontaneous abortions can occur due to many factors and it is possible that the physiologic and psychological stresses of a dental appointment, blood loss after oral surgery, pain, and the administration of certain drugs may increase the risk during medical/dental treatment. This occurs most frequently in the early stages of pregnancy. For this reason it is essential to determine if the patient is pregnant. One of the primary means of prevention of this emergency is through the detection of pregnancy before treatment is initiated. It is essential to ask each female patient of childbearing age at the time of dental treatment whether they are pregnant or could be pregnant. Patients who state that they could be pregnant but are unsure and are to be given potentially teratogenic drugs should be given a pregnancy test. β-HCG testing becomes positive in 98% of patients in approximately 10 days. This frequently coincides with the time of the expected menstruation. In a study of females, ages 12 to 21 years, presenting to a day surgery unit, 1 in 200 were found to be pregnant on routine, universal screening.[1] The potential consequences of undetected pregnancy are so severe that the cost of the service, the social issues involved, and the slowing of treatment

---

Box 32-1 Key Issues in Medication Use in Pregnancy

Is the drug teratogenic?
Does the drug affect mineralization?
Is the drug an inhibitor of CNS neurotransmission?
Does the drug inhibit placental blood supply?
Does the drug induce uterine contractions?
Does the drug produce clotting abnormalities?
Does the drug affect metabolism?
Can the drug inhibit respiration and oxygenation?
Can the drug cause maternal pulmonary aspiration of gastric contents?
Is the drug a hormone that may affect fetal growth and development?
Does the drug affect biosynthesis such as cholesterol synthesis in the liver?
Is the drug an antagonist of essential nutritional or vitamin functions such as Folate utilization?

Box 32-2 FDA Drug Classification

Category A: No known risk in the first trimester or later in pregnancy
Category B: Animal reproduction studies have not demonstrated fetal risk but there are no controlled studies in pregnant women or animal reproduction studies have shown an adverse effect but human studies have not confirmed adverse effect
Category C: Adverse effects are shown in animal studies but there are no controlled human studies available
Category D: There is evidence of human fetal risk but some use may be acceptable despite the risk to preserve the health of the mother
Category X: There is evidence of human fetal risk and the risk clearly outweighs any benefit in the pregnant mother.

---

caused by the pregnancy test would seem justified in most cases.

Box 32-1 contains some of the key issues in medication use during pregnancy.[2] These issues relate to harm to the fetus or mother. While drug formularies may list drugs that are not safe in pregnancy, it is up to the prescribing doctor to evaluate the need and the risk of the drug in the individual patient. These decisions are usually done with the participation of the patient's obstetrician.

In partial response to these issues, the Food and Drug Administration (FDA) has a classification system for drugs used during pregnancy (Box 32-2).[3]

On the FDA website's section on women's health, the online brochure for women patients states[4]:

If you are pregnant or nursing a baby, seek the advice of a health professional before taking any medication or diet supplement. Talk with your doctor, pharmacist or nurse. She/he will be happy to help you.

This FDA statement leaves the responsibility to the dentist to assure the safety of medications prescribed to pregnant patients. To supplement its classification system of category reporting the FDA launched a new initiative to gain more complete epidemiologic data on the safety of drugs used during pregnancy. The initiatives, Evaluation of Human Pregnancy Outcome Data (1999) and Establishing Pregnancy registries (1999), are currently under review for public comment.[4] Whenever possible, Category A drugs should be used for the pregnant patient. There may be circumstances when other categories of drugs may have to be administered, and the risks and benefits to the mother and developing fetus should be carefully considered.

MATERNAL PHYSIOLOGY IN PREGNANCY

The maternal pregnancy-state advances throughout the 275 days of gestation. Cardiovascular response to pregnancy is to increase the plasma volume and red cell mass. Because of dilution of the increased red cell mass, hematocrit of less than 35% is frequent although oxygen carrying capacity is not diminished. The heart enlarges due to hypertrophy. Increased cardiac blood flow produces a systolic ejection murmur and S_3. This murmur of pregnancy occurs in the majority of women and is not associated with any risk of congestive heart failure or risk of endocarditis.

Preeclampsia

Pregnancy-induced hypertension (PIH), or preeclampsia, is primarily a disorder of young women in their first pregnancy in the third trimester. The condition is characterized by elevated blood pressure, pathologic edema, and proteinuria. Seizures, renal failure, pulmonary

Box 32-3   Preeclampsia Therapy

Bed rest in the left lateral position
A moderate sodium-restricted diet
Antihypertensive therapy for those with
    persistent high blood pressure. The most
    frequently used drugs are hydralazine and
    labetalol
Consideration for hospitalization and
    induction of labor or cesarean section

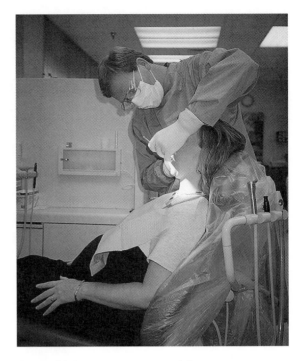

Figure 32-1. Proper position of the pregnant patient in the semiupright position for dental treatment.

edema, and thrombocytopenia may be associated with PIH and result in eclampsia. It is essential that any pregnant patient with hypertension, edema or abnormal weight gain be thoroughly evaluated for this condition before dental care. Pretreatment evaluation, normally done with the obstetrician, should include assessment of platelets and serum creatinine. The aim of pre-eclampsia therapy is to prevent maternal and fetal morbidity and mortality (Box 32-3).

If the patient is in the preeclampsia state, the stress of either dental infection or dental treatment may exacerbate the condition. Careful monitoring of blood pressure and organ function during the treatment period is necessary. To prevent an eclampsia emergency, the dentist should help ensure the patient's adequate but not excessive hydration, nutrition, oxygenation, and normotensive state during the dental treatment period.

Hypotension

Hypotension must be avoided during pregnancy. Compression of the inferior vena cava by the enlarged uterus may induce hypotension and syncope. A sustained episode of this type may result in fetal hypoxia and injury. Optimal patient position during dental treatment in pregnancy is important to ensure the comfort and safety of the mother and fetus. The supine position may be optimal for many dental procedures but it should be avoided whenever possible and particularly in the third trimester (Figure 32-1). The supine position may produce maternal and fetal hypoxia and hypotension due to compression of the inferior vena cava by the enlarged uterus compressing against the spinal column and elevation of the diaphragm due to the weight of abdominal contents. Compression of the vena cava may result in a loss of 30% of cardiac output. Prolonged compression may result in venous stasis and thromboembolism. Additionally, the supine position may promote silent, passive aspiration of gastric contents. While the dental procedure may seem to have passed uneventfully, an adverse outcome on maternal and fetal health may take days to become manifest.

Pregnant dental patients should be placed in a semi-reclined or upright position for dental treatment. The patient should draw up their right knee to turn their abdomen somewhat to the left, since the vena cava is in the right retroperitoneum. A folded blanket or wedge can be placed under the right hip to assist the patient in placement of their abdominal contents to the left (Figure 32-2).

If hypotension or syncope occurs during dental treatment of a patient in the third trimester, the patient should be placed with head at or below the level of the heart and with the abdomen rolled to the left. This is best done in the dental chair with the patient's right knee drawn up as the patient rolls to the left (Figure 32-3). Supplemental oxygen also is recommended during such episodes. If hypotension is associated with sustained bradycardia, administration of Atropine may be necessary. The use of α-adrenergic drugs such as Neosynephrine or mixed α- and β-adrenergic drugs such as

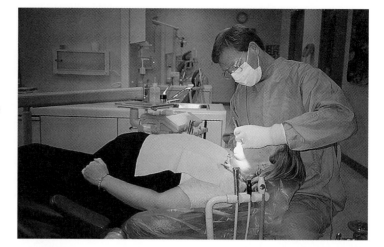

Figure 32-2. Improper position of the pregnant patient that may result in inferior vena cava compression.

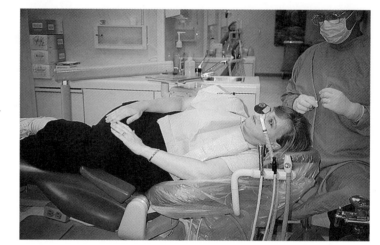

Figure 32-3. Repositioning of the pregnant patient during hypotension or syncope episode.

epinephrine should be avoided whenever possible, since their use results in placental hypoxia and potential death of the fetus.

Pulmonary Response

Pulmonary response of the third trimester is in part due to the elevation of the diaphragm, which results in tachypnea especially when reclining. Postural response often makes the patient wish to sit up with hands on knees, leaning forward with legs parted to accommodate the fetus. While this is not a good position for much dental treatment, sitting in the chair upright with legs hanging over either side in the third trimester offers the best position for ventilation.

The upper airway becomes capillary engorged and edematous late in pregnancy. This may make the patient less able to maintain her airway during dental treatment. In very late pregnancy, the patient will maintain her airway more comfortably in a "head forward" position. A pillow beneath the head to maintain a forward head position in a nearly upright patient position will help maintain unencumbered respiration. Upper airway engorgement may also make intubation more difficult in an emergency. Passive pulmonary aspiration may also occur due to upper airway engorgement, decreased gastrointestinal motility, and the pressure of the enlarged uterus.

Hematologic Response

The hematologic response of pregnancy is to produce a hypercoagulable state in the average patient due to inhibited fibrinolysis. There is an increased risk of deep vein thrombosis and pulmonary embolism from the first trimester. Compression of the inferior vena cava in the supine position, continuous flexing of the knees, or pressure to the back of the calves in the dental chair should be avoided. These can produce venous stasis which when combined with the hypercoagulability state can result in deep vein thrombosis.

DENTAL EMERGENCIES DURING PREGNANCY

Alterations in the immune response, elevated serum cortisol levels, elevated blood sugar and diminished home care may explain why odontogenic infection seems to occur so frequently during pregnancy. In some cultures, dental problems are expected during pregnancy. In folklore, the price of a new child is sometimes seen as the loss of a tooth. These infections may be periodontal, periapical or pericoronal in origin. They may result in deep space cervicofacial infection. Even minor infections may metastasize to the lung via aspiration or hematogenously to distant organs including the heart, brain, or placenta.

Periodontal infections are known to be a risk factor for systemic diseases. The American Academy of Periodontology[5] reports that "periodontal infections may influence pregnancy outcomes." A study of patients with premature low birth weight babies indicated a higher severity of periodontal disease when compared to parents of normal term babies.[6] This may be due to the systemic dissemination of inflammatory mediators present in periodontal disease such as prostaglandin E_2 (PGE_2) and tumor necrosis factor-alpha (TNF-α). These same substances are associated with the initiation of labor.

Women of childbearing age often have partially erupted third molars, which may be prone to pericoronitis. Vertical and distoangular impactions associated with the vertical ramus in patients from 16 to 25 years of age are most prone to pericoronitis (Figure 32-4). Clinical findings in pericoronitis include suppuration, swelling, trismus, fever and cervical lymphadenopathy. Pericoronitis may be more severe in the third trimester because of increased edema of the oral pharyngeal mucous membrane. Medical management of pericoronitis with appropriate antibiotic therapy and conservative surgical management with gentle debridement and irrigation is usually the first line treatment for pericoronitis during pregnancy. If the acute episode is controlled and hygiene is maintained, removal

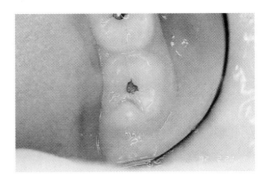

Figure 32-4. Pericoronitis is a common condition among pregnant women. *From Topazian RG, Goldberg M: Oral and maxillofacial surgery, ed 3, Philadelphia, 1994, WB Saunders.*

Box 32-4	Main Causes of Maternal Death During Pregnancy

Trauma
Bleeding
Embolism
Pregnancy-induced hypertension
Infection
Cardiomyopathy
Anesthesia

of the third molar can often be deferred until the postpartum period.

Periapical, periodontal or pericoronal infection may result in the need for dental extraction during pregnancy. In the presence of acute infection, systemic antibiotics are indicated before extraction. Necessary incision and drainage might precede extraction. If the tooth can be removed atraumatically as in a mobile tooth then the tooth may be extracted in the presence of acute infections. If a complex extraction is needed that might produce post-surgical edema and stress, the patient should be repeatedly assessed until all evidence of acute infection has subsided before extraction is performed. Attention to pain control in consultation with the obstetrician should be given to minimize maternal stress.

MATERNAL DEATH DURING PREGNANCY

A maternal death is the death of a woman from any cause while she is pregnant or within 90 days of delivery (Box 32-4).[7] The maternal death rate has dropped from 376 per 100,000 in 1940 to 7.5 per 100,000 in 1993.[8]

To avoid significant risk of maternal morbidity and mortality, the dentist should carry out therapeutic interventions that minimize the risk from the main causes of maternal death. Additionally, the dentist should avoid actions that might precipitate problems resulting in maternal death.

Trauma

Trauma during pregnancy occurs in 7% of patients and is the leading cause of maternal death in the United States. Maxillofacial or dental trauma in the pregnant patient may not appear in the level one trauma center where thorough evaluation according to American Trauma Life Support principles should proceed as a matter of course. When a pregnant patient appears after significant trauma including any resulting from a motor vehicle accident, assault, or fall, the patient should present to a trauma center for evaluation before definitive treatment of the oral injury.

Bleeding

Uterine bleeding during pregnancy and postpartum bleeding may result from structural abnormalities of the uterus combined with an acquired bleeding disorder such as thrombocytopenia or consumptive coagulopathy. Extensive oral bleeding resulting from oral surgery may consume clotting factors and make uterine bleeding more likely. For this reason (among others), procedures such as full mouth extraction should be deferred until several weeks postpartum.

Embolism

Poor patient position as noted previously may induce thromboembolism. In addition, pain, infection, extended immobilization, and other stress may play a role in venous stasis and thromboembolism. Expeditious, atraumatic, and low anxiety dental therapy and the prevention or prompt management of infection may play an important role in the prevention of embolism.

Cardiomyopathy

Heart failure during pregnancy may result from preexisting disease or the emergence of cardiomyopathy. Dental treatment in close cooperation with the obstetrician is indicated for these high-risk patients.

Anesthesia

Anesthesia carries both maternal and fetal risks. The main risks of maternal death during anesthesia are from failed intubation or pulmonary aspiration.[9] The risks to the fetus are hypoxia, preterm labor, and teratogenicity. The risk of teratogenicity may be the least of the three concerns since single exposure to the commonly used anesthetic agents have minimal risk of teratogenicity. There may actually be more concern about over-the counter analgesics, since certain medications may not be acceptable during specific stages of pregnancy. Most local anesthetics are considered relatively safe during pregnancy.

SURGICAL EMERGENCIES DURING PREGNANCY

While pregnancy itself is not shown to increase the maternal morbidity and mortality of surgery, delayed intervention may lead to a more complicated course of treatment (Box 32-5).[10-12] Reluctance of the patient to seek care and the reticence of the health care providers may cause delayed or incomplete treatment.

The risk of elective surgery appears to be lowest in the second trimester when organogenesis is complete, the pregnancy is established and the risk of premature labor is less.

INFLUENCE OF PREGNANCY ON THE DEVELOPMENT OF MEDICAL EMERGENCIES IN THE DENTAL OFFICE

As previously stated, the dentist must be aware of the presence of underlying complicating medical illnesses and their potential impact on the development of an adverse event. Several physiologic alterations and their potential contributing effect on medical emergencies have already been discussed. Other disease processes such as asthma have a high incidence within the popu-

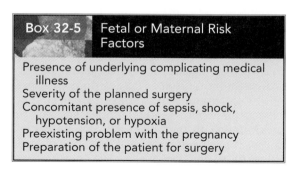

Box 32-5 | Fetal or Maternal Risk Factors

Presence of underlying complicating medical illness
Severity of the planned surgery
Concomitant presence of sepsis, shock, hypotension, or hypoxia
Preexisting problem with the pregnancy
Preparation of the patient for surgery

lation, so that it would be anticipated that a pregnant patient with a history of asthma may present for emergent dental treatment. Fortunately, the management of the pregnant asthmatic patient is similar to that of the nonpregnant patient. Alternatively, pregnancy has an impact on the diabetic patient and the epileptic patient. As discussed, these patients need to be appropriately evaluated and the dentist must understand that there may be an increased incidence of an adverse event occurring.

Hypoglycemia

Hypoglycemia is a potential problem in the pregnant female. This is secondary to several factors: increased use of glucose by the placenta and fetus, impaired glucose counterregulation with a decrease in hepatic glucose production, and altered recognition of hypoglycemic symptoms.[13] The risk is greatest in the type I diabetic patient. The dentist can prevent such an adverse event from occurring by monitoring the patient's glucose with a glucometer. If a hypoglycemic emergency were to occur in the dental office prompt treatment is required. Glucagon would be the recommended agent to administer in the unconscious patient.

Epilepsy

Pregnancy has a significant impact on the management of the epileptic patient. First there is the concern regarding the teratogenicity of the anticonvulsant medications. The risk of increased frequency and duration of seizure must be balanced against the risk of genetic defects. In those patients who have ceased their medication there will be an increased risk of a seizure. Second, is the ability to control and prevent seizures in the patient who will be maintained on her antiepileptic medications. The objective is to maintain blood levels of the antiepileptic medication that were effective before pregnancy. This varies between medications as metabolism is altered during pregnancy and has different effects on different medications. If the medications are maintained within a therapeutic level similar to what existed before pregnancy only 10% of the women will have a worsening of their epilepsy during pregnancy. Unfortunately, it is reported that up to 45% of women with epilepsy experience an increase in frequency of seizures during pregnancy. The dentist must be cognizant of this risk despite a patient who may be compliant with her medication.

The first step in preventing an emergency or minimizing the potential harm from an emergency is to obtain an accurate history. The second step is to be prepared and comfortable with the necessary interventions that may be required. Although benzodiazepines have been reported to be associated with an increase in craniofacial defects, this risk is associated with chronic use as opposed to use in an acute emergency. The dentist should be aware that the pharmacologic management of a seizure in the pregnant patient is similar to that in the nonpregnant patient. The hesitancy not to treat is not an option because the risk of maternal and fetal mortality is significantly increased if not managed in a timely and effective manner.

THE DENTIST'S ROLE IN THE PREVENTION OF EMERGENCIES DURING PREGNANCY

Dental treatment protocols are somewhat modified in the pregnant patient (Box 32-6). Good oral health is important to the prevention of emergencies during pregnancy. Maintenance of

---

Box 32-6   Guidelines for Dental Treatment During Pregnancy

ADULT FEMALE PATIENTS
1. Ask adult female patients if they are pregnant or if they could be pregnant.
2. If there is doubt, a pregnancy test needs to be performed before invasive treatment

PREVENTING INJURY TO THE PREGNANT PATIENT OR HER FETUS
1. In the pregnant patient, consult with the obstetrician before initiating care.
2. Consult with the obstetrician and a drug information resource before prescribing or administering any medication
3. On the day of dental treatment of a pregnant patient, review the current status of the pregnancy and perform vital signs

DENTAL EMERGENCIES IN THE PREGNANT PATIENT
1. Consult with the patient's obstetrician before initiating care.
2. Deliver care that will not unduly cause pain, stress, anxiety or fatigue.
3. Ensure that care is designed to minimize risk of adverse systemic effects, including sepsis, hypoxia, hypotension, or fluid or nutritional loss.

good oral health during pregnancy will support both maternal and fetal health. While good prospective studies remain to be completed, it now seems clear that prevention of oral infections through good dental maintenance programs will likely prevent some preterm low birth weight deliveries.

REFERENCES

1. Pierre N, Moy L, Redd S, Emns S, et al: Evaluation of a pregnancy-testing protocol in adolescents undergoing surgery, J *Pediatr Adolesc Gynecol* 11(3):139-141, 1998.
2. Hernandez-Diaz S, Werler M, Walker A, Mitchell A: Folic acid antagonists during pregnancy and the risk of birth defects, N *Engl J Med* 343:1608-1614, 2000.
3. Briggs GC, Freeman RK, Yaffe SJ: A *reference guide to fetal and neonatal risk: drugs in pregnancy and lactation*, Baltimore, 1994, Williams and Wilkins.
4. US Food and Drug Administration: http://www.fda.gov/womens/taketimetocare/Meds_Eng.html, December 2000.
5. Position Paper of the American Academy of Periodontology: Periodontal disease as a potential risk factor for systemic diseases, J *Periodontol* 69:841-850, 1998.
6. Offenbacher S, Katz V, Fertel G, et al: Periodontal infections as a risk factor for preterm low birth weight babies, J *Periodontol* 67:1103-1113, 1996.
7. Centers of Disease Control and Prevention: Pregnancy Related Mortality Surveillance System, Atlanta, 1990, CDC.
8. Hacker N, Moore J: *Essentials of obstetrics and gynecology*, Philadelphia, 1998, WB Saunders.
9. Kammerer W: Perioperative management of the pregnant patient undergoing nonobstetric surgery. In Merli G, Weitz H: *Medical management of the surgical patient*, Philadelphia, 1992, WB Saunders.
10. Sibai B: Surgery during pregnancy. In Gleicher N: *Principles and practice of medical therapy in pregnancy*, Norwalk, 1992, Appleton and Lange.
11. Leuzzi R: Nonobstetric surgery in the pregnant patient. In Merli G, Weitz H: *Medical management of the surgical patient*, Philadelphia, 1992, WB Saunders.
12. Cherry S: The pregnant patient: need for surgery unrelated to pregnancy, *Mount Sinai Med J* 58:81-84,1991.
13. Buchanan TA, Coustan DR: Diabetes mellitus. In Burrow JB, Ferris OL: *Medical complications during pregnancy*, ed 4, Philadelphia, 1995, WB Saunders.
14. Donaldson JO: Neurologic complications. In Burrow JB, Ferris OL: *Medical complications during pregnancy*, ed 4, Philadelphia, 1995, WB Saunders.
15. Newton E, Eckstein M: Chronic medical illness and pregnancy. In Rosen P, Barkin RM: *Emergency medicine: concepts and clinical practice*, ed 4, St. Louis, 1998, Mosby.

The Sedated Patient

Kevin J. Butterfield
Jeffrey D. Bennett

The practice of anesthesia has evolved to a point where a safe, predictable outcome is considered the standard of care. This standard can only be performed by those adequately trained in its administration, and more importantly, in management of its complications. Although proper preoperative patient selection and improved anesthetic technique have contributed to its current status, advances in anesthetic pharmacokinetics and pharmacodynamics and new pharmacologic agents have allowed anesthesia to be performed at a controlled, predictable level. However, adverse side effects secondary to an overdose or an inappropriate dosage may occur, most often resulting in respiratory depression, with secondary hypoxemia and hypercapnea. Less common potential adverse effects include both paroxysmal reactions to the drugs and cardiovascular side effects such as bradycardia or hypotension.

Initial management of these adverse situations (e.g., respiratory depression) follows the algorithms as described in prior chapters (e.g., chin-forehead lift, suction, 100% oxygen, positive-pressure ventilation). Additional management may also include the use of reversal agents for several common anesthetic drugs. These agents permit an improved margin of safety and control in administering anesthesia, allowing for correction of adverse side effects. The purpose of this chapter is to answer most questions that might arise when contemplating the administration of reversal agents in clinical practice.

FLUMAZENIL

Benzodiazepines, ubiquitous in current medical practice, have an impressive safety record and are extensively used in anesthesia and intensive care. They are naturally occurring substances found in wheat and potato[1] and are nearly ideal agents for conscious sedation (Box 33-1). Consequently, there has been a rapid, worldwide expansion of their use, and occasional abuse, in conscious sedation of both children and adults.[2,3]

Fortunately, benzodiazepines are rarely responsible for an overdose death,[4] partly because of their reversibility. However, even though benzodiazepine use for conscious sedation is an extremely safe procedure, it is still possible for an overdose to occur. In the past, attempts to terminate benzodiazepines' postoperative effects have focused on the use of physostigmine and aminophylline. Despite some success with these drugs, their slow onset of action, lack of true agonistic efficacy, and frequent side effects make them unacceptable for routine use in reversing the effects of benzodiazepine agonists.[5]

The approval of flumazenil by the U.S. Food and Drug Administration (FDA) in 1991[6] marked a turning point in conscious sedation, as this drug represented the first direct pharmacologic antagonist to benzodiazepines. Flumazenil is the only benzodiazepine-specific antagonist approved for clinical use in the United States. It was discovered while attempting to synthesize a more intensely binding gamma-aminobutyric acid (GABA) agonist, instead creating an intensely binding $GABA_A$ receptor–chloride channel antagonist.[1]

Pharmacokinetics

Flumazenil (Mazicon, Romazicon) is a 1,4-imidazobenzodiazepine structurally related to midazolam. It competitively inhibits the activity at the benzodiazepine recognition site on the $GABA_A$/benzodiazepine receptor complex. The $GABA_A$ receptor is a macromolecular complex consisting of five major binding regions together with an integral chloride ion channel. Binding regions include sites for GABA, benzodiazepines,

Box 33-1	Ideal Characteristics of Conscious Sedation Agents

Anxiolysis
Short-term amnesia
Ease of administration
Low cost
Rapid onset
Short duration of action
Predictable clinical effects
Reversibility

barbiturates, picrotoxin and anesthetic steroids, all of which modulate the receptor's response to GABA. The main function of the receptor complex is to mediate alterations in the chloride conductance of the neuronal membrane. Receptor conformational changes in response to GABA open the chloride channel, resulting in hyperpolarization of the cell and inhibition of action potential propagation. Flumazenil only acts at the benzodiazepine receptor. Many subtypes of benzodiazepine receptors exist. Peripheral benzodiazepine receptors are not coupled to GABA receptors and have different ligand specificity.[7]

Flumazenil is a weak partial agonist in some animal models of activity, but has little or no agonist activity in man. Its effects are surmountable by increasing the dose of the benzodiazepine agonist.[1] It competes with benzodiazepine agonists for the binding site, and a dose of 0.5 mg is required to occupy about 50% of the benzodiazepine receptors in the human brain.[8]

After intravenous (IV) administration, flumazenil has an initial distribution half-life of 7 to 15 minutes and a terminal half-life of 41 to 79 minutes. Protein binding is approximately 50%. Clearance of flumazenil occurs primarily by hepatic metabolism and is dependent on hepatic blood flow. Less than 1% of the administered dose is eliminated unchanged in the urine, and its pharmacokinetics are not significantly affected by gender, age, or renal failure; however, decreased clearance is reported in patients with liver dysfunction.[8]

Indications
Reversal of Benzodiazepine-Induced Sedation/Overdose

Benzodiazepine effects include drowsiness, sedation, confusion, dizziness, psychomotor and mental impairment, and anterograde amnesia. Signs and symptoms of an overdose include hypersomnolence, respiratory depression, and behavioral modifications, such as delirium, aggression, panic, and auditory/visual hallucinations. Cardiovascular alterations are rare, although hypotension has been reported.

Risk factors for the development of benzodiazepine overdosage include the following:

1. Presence of underlying hepatic or chronic pulmonary dysfunction.
2. Patient's age. There is less efficient drug elimination in elderly persons, and the pharmacodynamic response to a given dose of a benzodiazepine increases with advancing age, resulting in more pronounced CNS depressant effects.
3. Coadministration of other medications, which may depress the CNS or potentiate the effects of benzodiazepines (e.g., cimetidine, macrolide antibiotics, disulfiram).[7]

Reversal of Respiratory Depression and Laryngospasm

Flumazenil rapidly enters the central nervous system (CNS), and the beginning of recovery in terms of sedation score or conscious level is usually observed with one "arm-brain" circulation time, with subsequent return of the cough reflex and improved ventilation. Several studies have found evidence of improved ventilation among patients treated with flumazenil. In one randomized, double-blind, and placebo-controlled study by Flogel et al,[9] sedation was induced in 33 healthy male subjects with intravenous midazolam (mean dose 33 ± 1.3 mg) and reversal was achieved with either placebo or flumazenil (1, 3, or 10 mg). All flumazenil groups had full return of ventilatory status within 5 minutes of its administration, even the 1-mg group. The authors also found that there was no advantage to using flumazenil doses larger than 1 mg.

Flumazenil has been used to reverse midazolam-induced laryngospasm. Davis et al[10] reported on a 61-year-old male who received conscious sedation with midazolam for cardioversion in the emergency department. Ninety seconds after the IV administration of 3 mg of midazolam, the patient developed laryngospasm. This was treated with 0.4 mg flumazenil intravenously, with the onset of laryngospasm reversal within 60 seconds. Twenty minutes later, after no further midazolam administration, laryngospasm recurred and again was treated with a second similar dose of flumazenil. The patient subsequently required no further doses of flumazenil.

The use of a reversal agent for the management of laryngospasm is controversial. If pharmacologic intervention is required, an individual trained in general anesthesia would usually administer succinylcholine. Succinylcholine is a depolarizing neuromuscular blocking agent that has both rapid onset and short duration resulting in cessation of the laryngospasm. However, positive-pressure-assisted ventilation may be required, and if the clinician is not appropriately trained and skilled in the full scope of airway management, further adverse effects may develop. The rapid onset of flumazenil reverses the sedative effect of the medication, resulting in a more awake and alert patient with an improved respiratory drive once the laryngospasm ceases.

Reversal of Paradoxical Reaction

Benzodiazepine-induced paradoxical reactions are relatively rare disinhibitory events characterized by aggressive behavior, with restlessness, anxiety, euphoria, talkativeness, and hostility and rage.[11] There are numerous reports of benzodiazepine-induced paradoxical reactions reversed with flumazenil in the literature.[12-17] Ochs et al[15] reported on an 18-year-old female patient who was tearful and sobbing during the initial sedation and throughout the extraction of wisdom teeth. When questioned, she could not explain her reaction. However, on receiving 0.4 mg of flumazenil, she ceased crying and had a total change in her affect to being calm and comfortable. Rodrigo[16] also reported a case of paradoxical reaction during a surgical procedure. A 49-year-old female presented for dental implant placement with conscious sedation. She was reported to be extremely nervous before surgery. Midazolam, 4 mg, was administered initially, with an additional 8 mg administered in response to patient movement over the next 70 minutes. Suddenly, the patient's systolic blood pressure rose 30 mm Hg, and she became violent, requiring physical restraint. This reaction was reversed in 5 minutes with 0.5 mg of IV flumazenil. Sufficient residual sedation remained to allow completion of the surgical procedure. The paradoxical reaction did not recur. Thus flumazenil may selectively reverse a paradoxical reaction to midazolam without completely reversing its sedative effect.

Paradoxical reactions appear more readily with high IV doses of benzodiazepines and are more common in younger patients (i.e., 3 to 19 years old).[12,13] Roelofse et al[17] found a 23% incidence of paradoxical reactions in children between the ages of 2 to 10 years who had received 0.45 mg/kg of midazolam rectally as a premedication before dental extractions under general anesthesia. Another recent study[14] revealed that 1.4% of 2617 children receiving midazolam and meperidine experienced a paradoxical reaction that consisted of crying, combativeness, disorientation, dysphoria, tachycardia, agitation, and restlessness. The reaction occurred approximately 17 minutes after the administration of midazolam (0.3 mg/kg) and dissipated within 14 minutes of administration of flumazenil (0.01mg/kg).

It has been suggested that the disinhibiting effect of the benzodiazepines releases an "anxiety-bound" hostility in certain predisposed individuals, especially those who exhibit previous poor impulse control (e.g., history of violent or psychotic episodes).[11] These reactions appear to be greater in alcoholic or drug-using patients. It remains unclear whether the explanation for this increased agitation lies in the interaction or physiologic changes induced by the drugs and alcohol, an increased prevalence of underlying emotional or psychiatric disorders in this population, or higher doses of midazolam used to achieve adequate sedation.[12]

One of the major difficulties associated with paradoxical reactions is their protracted duration.[14] Some have been reported to last several hours, requiring constant monitoring and patient reassurance.[18] Therefore the dentist must remember, especially after giving large doses, that a patient may be developing a paradoxical reaction if abnormal talk and body movements persist after drug administration. At this stage, it would be better to stop administering the drug rather than to give more in attempts to stop the movements.

Dosage

Generally, doses of approximately 0.1 to 0.2 mg of flumazenil (corresponding to peak plasma levels of 3 to 6 ng/ml) produce partial antagonism, whereas higher doses of 0.4 to 1.0 mg (peak plasma levels of 12 to 28 ng/ml) usually produce complete antagonism in patients who have received the usual sedating doses of benzodiazepines. There is no advantage in giving additional flumazenil (>1 mg) to patients who do not respond to 1 mg or less after midazolam-induced ambulatory general anesthesia. The onset of reversal is usually evident within 1 to 2 minutes after the injection is completed. Eighty percent response will be reached within 3 minutes, with the peak effect occurring at 6 to 10 minutes. The duration and degree of reversal are related to the plasma concentration of the sedating benzodiazepine as well as the dose of flumazenil given. High-dose flumazenil has no agonist effects on resting ventilation or psychomotor performance in normal subjects and produces no serious adverse reactions, severe signs or symptoms, or clinically significant laboratory test abnormalities.[8]

Routes of Administration

Although flumazenil has been approved by the FDA only for IV administration, numerous other routes have been investigated and reported in the literature.[19] Heniff et al[20] report on a randomized, controlled, non-blinded, crossover canine trial in which four different routes of administration were investigated. The IV route was found to be significantly faster than the sublingual, intramuscular, and rectal routes, which did not differ significantly. Palmer et al[21] determined that administration of flumazenil via an endotracheal tube results in rapid attainment of therapeutic blood levels, without notable adverse effects. Several other studies[22-24] have reported on the administration of rectal flumazenil in a pediatric population. Carbajal et al[22] administered rectal flumazenil (29 μg/kg) to six patients, with an average age of 7.2 years, who had received an average midazolam dose of 0.39 mg/kg orally. Flumazenil required an average of 12.2 minutes for the patient to regain consciousness, and no resedations occurred. Lopez-Herce et al[23] reported on six patients, ages 1 month to 9 years, who were administered rectal flumazenil (15 to 30 μg/kg) to reverse midazolam-induced sedation. Initial effects were seen within 3 to 5 minutes after administration, with complete arousal between 5 and 15 minutes in three patients. The other three patients still had slight drowsiness 15 minutes after flumazenil administration, and a new dose of 10 μg/kg of flumazenil was administered that resulted in complete arousal within 5 to 10 minutes.

Amnesia Reversal

It has long been recognized that benzodiazepines impair the acquisition of new information but do not alter retrieval of information already in memory. In short, benzodiazepine-induced sedation is accompanied by *anterograde amnesia*, in that patients may appear to be fully aware of events and conversation but are found subsequently to have no memory of such occurrences. Dundee and Wilson[24] showed that 5 mg of IV midazolam caused dense anterograde amnesia for 5 to 15 minutes, followed by a variable period of less profound amnesia. The duration of such amnesia is dose dependent, and its reversibility with flumazenil has been studied extensively. Rosenbaum et al[25] performed a double-blind, placebo-controlled study that involved patients requiring dental extractions and found no reversal of amnesia with flumazenil administration after IV sedation with midazolam. Other studies have shown similar findings.[18,26,27] However, Ochs et al,[15] in their double-blind, crossover study of 31 patients requiring IV sedation for third molar extractions, found a significant difference in amnesia reversal between flumazenil and placebo at 5 to 60 minutes. Numerous other studies, including several large, multicenter investigations, have confirmed their results in both adults and children.[5,28,29] Finally, a well-designed, prospective, randomized, and double-blind crossover study by Ghoneim et al[30] that involved 72 subjects and seven separate memory tests found a significant, complete reversal of amnesic effects of midazolam at 5 minutes after flumazenil administration of either 1 or 3 mg intravenously.

Although still a controversial topic, the overwhelming evidence supports the concept that flumazenil does reverse midazolam's amnesic effects. This reversal is anterograde from the time that the flumazenil is administered, and there is no indication that flumazenil increases the recall of the procedure or that amnesia returns as part of minimal residual sedation, when appropriate doses of the agonist and antagonist are used.

Resedation

There is no dispute that after large doses of benzodiazepines, where high plasma levels are to be anticipated for a prolonged time (e.g., after benzodiazepine overdose), a single dose of flumazenil only generates a "window" of consciousness, after which previously dangerous levels of sedation can recur. Resedation after the administration of flumazenil for reversal of conscious sedation is due to its short half-life—approximately 1 hour compared with over 2 hours for midazolam, which has the shortest half-life of the benzodiazepine agonists. When the effect of flumazenil declines, the patient returns to a level of sedation, which would have been present had flumazenil not been given. Concern thus arises if resedation occurs after the patient has been transferred to an unmonitored environment where satisfactory observation and further access to flumazenil may not be available. In addition, it has been suggested that the availability of flumazenil may encourage the use of larger doses of benzodiazepine agonists, resulting in a potential increased risk to the patient. Several studies have investigated the incidence and risks associated with resedation after flumazenil administration. In a multicenter study without controls, 107 children were sedated with IV midazolam (0.18 mg/kg); the sedation was subsequently reversed with 0.01 mg/kg IV flumazenil, up to 1 mg total.[3] Overall, 6.5% of patients, 1 to 5 years of age, experienced resedation after initially responding to flumazenil, with a mean time to resedation of 24.6 ±11.3 minutes. For most studies, some level of resedation occurs after flumazenil administration, ranging from 13% to 30% over 115 to 180 minutes.[5,28,31] However, all patients remained responsive during the observation periods and reacted to pain by withdrawal of the appropriate limb and opening eyes when addressed.

The following factors determine the probability and onset of resedation after flumazenil administration.[32]

Inappropriate benzodiazepine used

- Prolonged half-life
- Active metabolites with a long duration of action
- Potential for enterohepatic circulation (e.g., diazepam, flunitrazepam)

Overdose

- Lack of knowledge of correct dose
- Variability of response to benzodiazepines in dose and time of onset (see below)
- Age and physical status of the patient
- Drug interactions
- Inadequate analgesia (see below)

Since the mean time of onset of the maximum effect of benzodiazepines administered intravenously is often in excess of 3 minutes and due to the individual variation in response, titration of the drug to a desired end point can be slow and tedious, particularly in the context of a busy clinic. Thus there is a tendency to hurry and use more than is required.

Benzodiazepines provide anxiolysis, sedation, amnesia, and muscle relaxation during conscious sedation and hypnosis during anesthesia. Care should be taken to avoid overuse secondary to poor analgesia.

Thus the use of flumazenil for reversal of conscious sedation always carries with it the risk of resedation. Fortunately, this risk has been shown not to be clinically significant. However, the clinician should assess the risk of resedation on a case-by-case basis and, when in doubt, should err on the side of safety and continue to observe the patient postoperatively.

Contraindications

Flumazenil is an extremely safe drug when used appropriately. Caution must be used in patients who receive chronic benzodiazepine therapy (especially with repeated high doses), those with a prior seizure disorder (particularly if the seizures are treated with benzodiazepine), and those who receive tricyclic antidepressants. Caution is also indicated for patients with known panic disorders, severe liver disease, or patients with head trauma. Flumazenil should be avoided in these patients.[11] Although it has no direct effect on the cerebral blood flow or cerebral metabolism, flumazenil does reverse the depression of cerebral hemodynamics caused by benzodiazepines.

Adverse Reactions

Flumazenil can safely and effectively reverse excessive sedation after administration of a benzodiazepine agonist. However, careful titration of the antagonist may be necessary to produce the desired clinical effect without producing untoward psychological sequelae and acute stress reactions (Box 33-2).

Seizure activity has been reported in certain high risk populations.[31,34] To minimize the likelihood of a seizure, it is recommended that

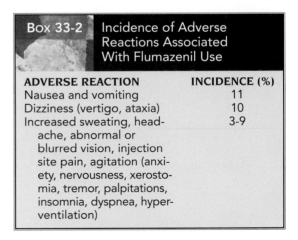

Box 33-2	Incidence of Adverse Reactions Associated With Flumazenil Use	
ADVERSE REACTION		**INCIDENCE (%)**
Nausea and vomiting		11
Dizziness (vertigo, ataxia)		10
Increased sweating, headache, abnormal or blurred vision, injection site pain, agitation (anxiety, nervousness, xerostomia, tremor, palpitations, insomnia, dyspnea, hyperventilation)		3-9

flumazenil not be administered to patients who have used benzodiazepines for the treatment of seizure disorders or to patients who have ingested drugs that place them at risk for the development of seizures, including cyclic antidepressants, cocaine, lithium, methylxanthines, isoniazid, propoxyphene, monoamine oxidase (MAO) inhibitors, buproprion, and cyclosporine. In addition, flumazenil may trigger opisthotonos in situations that predispose patients to seizure disorders, probably including local anesthetic toxicity. Therefore flumazenil is best avoided when the blood concentration of a local anesthetic may be toxic.

Anesthesia Techniques
Benzodiazepine Alone

Ochs et al,[15] in a double-blind, randomized study involving third molar extractions, found that reversal of IV midazolam (mean dose, 19.3 ± 3.9 mg) with intravenous flumazenil (mean dose, 0.8 ± 0.17 mg) resulted in significant improvements in alertness, psychomotor recovery, patient assessment, and observer assessment of recovery versus placebo for 5 to 60 minutes after flumazenil administration. In a double-blind, randomized, and placebo-controlled study by Clark et al[18] of dental extractions, patients received IV midazolam, reversed with IV flumazenil 0.2 mg every minute to a maximum of 1 mg. The authors report a significantly increased level of alertness in the flumazenil group versus placebo at 5 to 15 minutes but no difference beyond 15 minutes. Rodrigo et al,[35] in their double-blind, placebo-controlled, crossover study design for third molar extractions, had patients receiving IV midazolam (mean dose 6.2 ± 1 mg) reversed with IV flumazenil and found a significant difference for level of alertness 15 minutes after flumazenil versus placebo administration. Rosenbaum and Hooper[25] performed a double-blind, placebo-controlled study involving 40 patients who received IV midazolam to effect followed with reversal by flumazenil 0.4 mg IV or placebo for dental extractions. Flumazenil-group patients were found to be significantly less sedated, more cooperative, and better oriented versus placebo at 5 and 30 minutes after administration. In the largest series of multicenter, placebo-controlled studies carried out in the United States, flumazenil was shown to be highly effective in completely reversing IV benzodiazepine-induced conscious sedation in patients undergoing a variety of procedures. Out of 131 patients sedated with a mean dose of 10.6 mg midazolam and re-

versed with a mean dose of 0.7 mg flumazenil, 82% of patients demonstrated complete reversal of sedation within 5 minutes, compared with 15% of 65 placebo-treated patients.[5] Similarly, a mean dose of 0.73 mg flumazenil fully reversed 84% of 102 patients sedated with a mean dose of 26 mg diazepam, compared with 42% of 52 placebo-treated patients.[28] Several other studies have confirmed these results.[19,31,36,37]

Benzodiazepine and Opioid

The combined use of benzodiazepines and opioids has been recognized to produce synergistic effects on sedation scores. Finder et al,[38] in a randomized, double-blind, and placebo-controlled clinical trial of 30 patients receiving IV conscious sedation with a combination of fentanyl (1.5 μg/kg) bolus then diazepam to effect, found flumazenil to provide a clinically significant reversal of certain measures of cognitive and psychomotor impairment associated with the administration of benzodiazepine sedation. A recent multicenter, randomized, parallel, double-blind, and placebo-controlled study[26] that involved 179 patients sedated in the emergency department with a combination of IV fentanyl (2 μg/kg) and midazolam (0.05 mg/kg), found that patients in the flumazenil group showed a significant difference in return to baseline level of alertness versus placebo (11.1 minutes versus 24.8 minutes). In another study,[39] complete reversal of sedation was observed in 80% of 240 patients receiving a mean dose 0.7 mg of flumazenil, when sedation was induced by a mean dose of 9.2 mg midazolam combined with 0.2 mg fentanyl (63% of patients), 39.6 mg meperidine (33% of patients), or 4.2 mg morphine (4% of patients). When diazepam (mean dose, 22.2 mg) was combined with opioids—0.2 mg fentanyl (57% of patients), 50 mg meperidine (27% of patients), or 4 mg morphine (18% of patients)—a mean dose of 0.6 mg flumazenil resulted in 70% of 122 patients overall being completely awake and alert within 5 minutes.[29] Several other studies have found similar results.[22,27]

Reversal in Children

Reversal of conscious sedation theoretically has similar benefits in children as in adults. First, prompt reversal reduces the time and labor required to provide constant monitoring of the child who remains sedated after a procedure is completed. Second, in patients who have preexisting disturbances in mental status, reversal permits accurate assessment of central nervous system function by removing the influence of the sedating agent. Third, reversal agents can be used in patients who inadvertently receive excess sedation. Fourth, parent or caregiver anxiety is reduced by the rapid awakening of the sedated child. Collectively, these factors expand the benefits that flumazenil can provide to the child who requires conscious sedation.[3] Several studies and case reports on the pediatric administration of flumazenil are present in the literature. Jones et al[40] performed a randomized, double-blind, and placebo-controlled study involving 3- to 12-year-old males undergoing circumcision. Patients were sedated with oral midazolam (0.5 mg/kg) initially, then 0.5mg/kg intravenously to effect. Reversal was accomplished with 0.1 mg/kg flumazenil, followed by 0.05 mg/kg every minute until awake. The authors found a significant improvement in sedation reversal with four-times-faster waking (10.4 minutes versus 37.9 minutes) and three-times-faster self-identification (17.1 minutes versus 45.1 minutes) in the flumazenil group, with no cases of resedation. In a multicenter study[3] without controls, 107 children were sedated with IV midazolam (0.18 mg/kg) and subsequently reversed with 0.01 mg/kg IV flumazenil up to 1 mg total. Overall, 96% of patients returned to their baseline level of alertness within 10 minutes of flumazenil administration. The authors concluded that flumazenil produces consistent reversal of benzodiazepine-induced sedation in pediatric patients, without significant adverse effects.

NARCOTIC ANTAGONISTS

At present, opioid analgesics are used as primary or adjuvant anesthetics, sedatives, and postoperative analgesics. However, opioid analgesia, in clinically useful concentrations, produces a constellation of depressant and stimulant side effects.[26]

Opioids may be divided into three broad classes based on their pharmacodynamic effects: pure agonist (morphine, meperidine, fentanyl), pure antagonists (naloxone, naltrexone, nalmefene), and mixed agonist-antagonists (nalbuphine, butorphanol, buprenorphine, pentazocine). This review focuses only on pure opioid antagonists, specifically naloxone, which is most frequently used to reverse the opioid adverse effects associated with anesthesia.

Pure narcotic antagonists prevent or reverse the effects of opioids, including respiratory depression, sedation, and hypotension via competitive inhibition for opioid receptors. They do not produce respiratory depression, psychotomimetic effects, or pupillary constriction and essentially exhibit no pharmacologic activity when used in the absence of narcotics. However, all opioid antagonists, when used in the presence of physical dependence on narcotics, produce narcotic withdrawal symptoms.

It is important to remember that both the desirable and the undesirable effects of opioids are produced by similar pharmacologic mechanisms. Agonists like morphine or fentanyl probably interact with mu opioid receptors in the spinal cord, brainstem, and limbic cortex to produce most of their analgesic effects. In analgesic doses, all these opioids produce some degree of respiratory depression, which also results from their interaction with mu receptors in the medulla. It also stands to reason that reversal of respiratory depression normally entails some reversal of analgesia.

Opioid-Induced Respiratory Depression

Opioids cause medullary respiratory centers to become less sensitive to carbon dioxide (CO_2), even when there is no obvious change in respiratory rate. As administered doses increase, breathing slows and becomes deeper and eventually may become irregular or Cheyne-Stokes in nature.

Equianalgesic doses of all opioids produce equivalent degrees of respiratory depression. There is no convincing evidence that any analgesic is more or less dangerous than morphine in this regard. Both fentanyl and alfentanil have been reported to cause "recurrent" ventilatory depression. Episodes have been reported in which patients arrived in recovery areas, apparently breathing adequately, only to suffer respiratory arrest some time later.[41] This phenomenon is best explained by the relationship between arousal and drug effect. When a person given an opioid falls asleep, breathing is dramatically depressed. As long as such a patient is moved about and told to breathe, the patient will continue to do so until stimulation ceases. However, high doses of morphine or fentanyl have been reported to cause apnea in a patient who is still awake and responsive.

Naloxone

Naloxone (Narcan) is the prototypical pure opioid antagonist. It acts at all opioid receptors, but it has greatest affinity for mu receptors. Naloxone can reverse all the effects of opiates, including analgesia, sedation, respiratory depression, pruritus, biliary colic, and urinary retention. Because naloxone has lower affinity at the kappa receptor, larger doses are needed to antagonize such drugs as nalbuphine and butorphanol. Buprenorphine is unusual in that it binds to mu receptors with an affinity similar to that of naloxone. Even very large doses of naloxone cannot reliably reverse the effects of this drug.[42]

Use in Adults

For the partial reversal of narcotic depression after narcotic use during surgery, the dose of naloxone should be titrated according to the patient's response. Naloxone can be administered intravenously or intramuscularly, and there have been effective reported administrations via the submental[43] and intralingual routes.[44]

For the initial reversal of respiratory depression, IV naloxone should be injected in increments of 0.1 to 0.2 mg at 2- to 3-minute intervals to the desired degree of reversal (i.e., adequate ventilation and alertness without significant pain or discomfort). Larger-than-necessary dosage of naloxone may result in significant reversal of analgesia and increase in blood pressure. Similarly, too-rapid reversal may induce nausea, vomiting, sweating, or circulatory stress. Naloxone's competitive antagonism may be overcome by the administration of additional opioid agonist. Repeat doses of naloxone hydrochloride may be required within 1- to 2-hour intervals depending upon the amount, type (i.e., short or long acting) and time interval since last administration of narcotic. Supplemental intramuscular doses have been shown to produce a longer lasting effect.

Use in Children

The reversal of postoperative narcotic-induced respiratory depression is similar in children as for adults. Naloxone should be injected in increments of 0.005 mg to 0.01 mg intravenously at two- to three-minute intervals to the desired degree of reversal.

Adverse Effects

Use of naloxone, can have important hemodynamic consequences when reversing opioid activity.[45] Increases in blood pressure, heart rate, and norepinephrine/epinephrine release can oc-

cur. In animals this response is worsened by hypercarbia but can be seen in normocarbia, even in the absence of a surgical incision. In humans there have been several case reports of pulmonary edema and sudden death after naloxone administration. Sudden death has occurred in young, previously healthy individuals,[2] and pulmonary edema was described in a young man given only 100 μg of naloxone.[46] The etiology of this rare, catastrophic response is not known.

In general, opioid reversal should be used only when clearly necessary. It is almost always possible to titrate opioids to the point at which pain is tolerable but respiration is not compromised. However, the physician must always ensure adequate local anesthesia in order to provide the patient with a guaranteed level of comfort after potential overreversal of opioid-induced respiration with subsequent reversal of its analgesic effect.

CENTRAL ANTICHOLINERGIC SYNDROME

Central anticholinergic syndrome (CAS) is a condition that is not widely recognized after anesthesia and results from an imbalance in the widespread cholinergic pathways in the CNS. The term CAS was introduced by Longo[47] in 1966 to denote a group of symptoms associated with known anticholinergics and many other CNS-modifying drugs. CAS is caused by the use of drugs with anticholinergic properties that cross the blood-brain barrier, most often atropine and hyoscine. However, most anesthetic drugs probably interfere to some degree with central cholinergic transmission, and more than 500 drugs have been implicated in CAS, including antihistamines, antidepressants, benzodiazepines, antipsychotics, and antiparkinsonians.[53] In the vast majority of cases, CAS may simply be the result of the variable individual response to anesthetic drugs.

Clinical Manifestations

CAS involves alterations in the level of arousal and response to external stimuli and has both central and peripheral signs and symptoms.[49] Central manifestations include disorientation, agitation, hallucinations, illusions, ataxia, memory loss, seizures, and coma. Hallucinations are usually visual and tactile but may be auditory or in any combination. Peripheral effects include tachycardia, mydriasis, facial flushing, hyperpyrexia up to 41.5° C, urinary retention, dry mucous membranes, depressed or absent bowel sounds, and decreased sweating. In adults, CNS depression dominates, and somnolence, weakness, and coma may occur; however, seizures are uncommon. In children, CNS stimulation dominates, and agitation, hallucinations, ataxia, and athetosis may occur; seizures are common. CAS may occur without peripheral anticholinergic manifestations.

Epidemiology

CAS occurs in up to 3.3% of individuals after regional anesthesia with sedation[50] and 9.4% of patients after anticholinergic premedication and general anesthesia. CAS may be a contributory factor in a number of patients who show varying degrees of postoperative confusion in the recovery room.

Diagnosis

A diagnosis of CAS usually takes some time to reach and may only be made via a process of elimination. It is confirmed by the rapid response to physostigmine, usually 3 to 15 minutes after IV injection. Before diagnosing CAS, all other possible causes of an altered mental state must be excluded, such as prolonged action of anesthetics and other drugs; acid-base, respiratory, metabolic, or electrolyte disturbances; neurologic and psychiatric disorders; and hepatic and renal dysfunction.

Physostigmine

Physostigmine (Antilirium) is a centrally acting anticholinesterase that increases acetylcholine levels in the brain but has minimal effects elsewhere. It is an alkaloid originally obtained from the Calabar bean of West Africa. Unlike neostigmine, which contains a quaternary amine group, physostigmine contains a tertiary amine group and therefore is able to cross the blood-brain-barrier, increasing the amount of acetylcholine available for neurotransmission by reducing endogenous cholinesterase activity. It produces a wide range of effects, chiefly those of parasympathetic stimulation, including nausea, salivation, sweating, abdominal colic, and bronchospasm; however, these effects are reported to be minor. Central stimulation may cause bradycardia, hypertension, and convulsions. Therefore physostigmine should be used with caution in patients with epilepsy, diabetes, glaucoma, asthma, cardiovascular disease, peptic ulcer, and Parkinson's disease.

Physostigmine is usually obtained as a clear solution, does not require refrigeration, and has a shelf life of 2 years. It is available in 2-ml sterile vials containing 1 mg/ml. It should be diluted to 10 ml in dextrose in water or normal saline before administration. It has an onset of action of 3 to 8 minutes and a duration of action of approximately 45 to 60 minutes. The recommended initial dose is 0.04 mg/kg by slow IV injection, with no more than 1 mg/min and with electrocardiographic monitoring. Dosage may need to be followed by further doses at intervals of 10 to 30 minutes if the desired patient response is not obtained.

Rapid administration can cause bradycardia and hypersalivation, leading to respiratory difficulties and possible convulsions. Because of the possibility of hypersensitivity in an occasional patient, atropine sulfate injection should always be at hand since it is an antagonist and antidote for physostigmine. For pediatric administration the recommended dose is 0.02 mg/kg, intramuscularly or by slow IV injection, and should not exceed 0.5 mg/min. If the toxic effects persist and there is no sign of cholinergic effects, the dosage may be repeated at 5- to 10-minute intervals until a therapeutic effect is obtained or a maximum of 2 mg dosage is given.

Treatment

Although a relatively rare occurrence, all practitioners administering conscious sedation and general anesthesia must be able to diagnose and treat CAS. The physician should consider this possible diagnosis when faced with a confused or unexpectedly sedated patient in the recovery room, particularly when an anticholinergic premedicant has been given. If CAS is suspected, IV physostigmine should be used, and a dramatic return to normal consciousness may be anticipated with a correct diagnosis.

SUMMARY

Utilization of anesthetic agents in a clinical setting must only be performed by those highly trained in their administration. With the discovery and clinical utility of reversal agents, there is now an improved margin of safety in anesthetic practice. Subsequently, a more controlled environment equates into fewer complications and an improved anesthetic outcome. However, reversal agents are not a panacea and should not be regarded as such. Their indications and limitations must be respected, as with all anesthetic agents, so as to provide maximal patient benefit while avoiding adverse outcomes.

REFERENCES

1. Haefely WE: The story and activity of flumazenil (Anexate), Acta Anaesthesiol Belg 40(1):3-9, 1989.
2. D'Eramo EM: Mortality and morbidity with outpatient anesthesia: the Massachusetts experience, J Oral Maxillofac Surg 57(5):531-536, 1999.
3. Shannon M, Albers G, Burkhart K, et al: Safety and efficacy of flumazenil in the reversal of benzodiazepine-induced conscious sedation, the Flumazenil Pediatric Study Group, J Pediatr 131(4):582-586, 1997.
4. Midazolam—is antagonism justified? Lancet 2(8603):140-142, 1988.
5. Flumazenil in Intravenous Conscious Sedation with Midazolam Multicenter Study Group. I. Reversal of central nervous system effects by flumazenil after intravenous conscious sedation with midazolam: report of a multicenter clinical study, Clin Ther 14(6):861-877, 1992.
6. Benzodiazepine antagonist approved by FDA, Clin Pharmacol Ther 11(4):287, 290, 1992.
7. Whitwam JG, Amrein R: Pharmacology of flumazenil, Acta Anaesthesiol Scand Suppl 108:3-14, 1995.
8. Flumazenil Monograph.
9. Flogel CM, Ward DS, Wada DR, et al: The effects of large-dose flumazenil on midazolam-induced ventilatory depression, Anesth Analg 77(6):1207-1214, 1993.
10. Davis DP, Hamilton RS, Webster TH: Reversal of midazolam-induced laryngospasm with flumazenil, Ann Emerg Med 32(2):263-265, 1998.
11. Van der Bijl P, Roelofse JA: Disinhibitory reactions to benzodiazepines—a review, J Oral Maxillofac Surg 49(5):519-523, 1991.
12. Honan VJ: Paradoxical reaction to midazolam and control with flumazenil, Gastrointest Endosc 40(1):86-88, 1994.
13. Litchfield NB. Complications of intravenous diazepam—adverse psychological reactions: an assessment of 16,000 cases, Anesth Prog 27:175-183, 1980.
14. Massanari M, Novitsky J, Reinstein LJ: Paradoxical reactions in children associated with midazolam use during endoscopy, Clin Pediatr Phila 36(12):681-684, 1997.
15. Ochs MW, Tucker MR, Owsley TD, et al: The effectiveness of flumazenil in reversing the sedation and amnesia produced by intravenous midazolam, J Oral Maxillofac Surg 48(3):240-245, 1990.
16. Rodrigo CR: Flumazenil reverses paradoxical reaction with midazolam, Anesth Prog 38(2):65-68, 1991.
17. Roelofse JA, van der Bijl P, Stegmann DH, et al: Preanesthetic medication with rectal midazolam in children undergoing dental extractions, J Oral Maxillofac Surg 48(8):791-797, 1990.
18. Clark MS, Lindenmuth JE, Jafek BW, et al: Reversal of central benzodiazepine effects by intravenous flumazenil. Anesth Prog 38(1):12-16, 1991.
19. Andree RA: Sudden death after naloxone administration, Anesth Analg 59(10):782-784, 1980.
20. Heniff MS, Moore GP, Trout A, et al: Comparison of routes of flumazenil administration to reverse midazolam-induced respiratory depression in a canine model, Acad Emerg Med 4(12):1115-1118, 1997.
21. Palmer RB, Mautz DS, Cox K, et al: Endotracheal flumazenil—a new route of administration for benzodiazepine antagonism, Am J Emerg Med 16(2):170-172, 1998.
22. Carbajal R, Simon N, Blanc P, et al: Rectal flumazenil to reverse midazolam sedation in children, Anesth Analg 82(4):895, 1996.
23. Lopez-Herce J, Lopez de Sa E, Farcia de Frias E, et al: Reversal of midazolam sedation with rectal flumazenil in children, Crit Care Med 22(7):1204, 1994.
24. Dundee JW, Wilson DB: Amnesic action of midazolam, Anaesthesia 35:459-461, 1980.
25. Rosenbaum NL,Hooper PA: The use of flumazenil as an antagonist to midazolam in intravenous sedation for dental procedures, Eur J Anaesthesiol Suppl 2:183-190, 1988.
26. Chudnofsky CR: Safety and efficacy of flumazenil in reversing conscious sedation in the emergency department, Emergency Medicine Conscious Sedation Study Group, Acad Emerg Med 4(10):944-950, 1997.
27. Klausen NO, Juhl O, Sorensen J, et al: Flumazenil in total intravenous anaesthesia using midazolam and fentanyl, Acta Anaesthesiol Scand 32(5):409-412, 1988.
28. Flumazenil in Intravenous Conscious Sedation with Diazepam Multicenter Study Group. I. Reversal of central benzodiazepine effects by flumazenil after conscious sedation produced by intravenous diazepam, Clin Ther 14(6):895-909, 1992.
29. Flumazenil in Intravenous Conscious Sedation with Diazepam Multicenter Study Group. II. Reversal of central benzodiazepine effects by flumazenil after intravenous conscious sedation with diazepam and opioids: report of a double-blind multicenter study, Clin Ther 14(6):910-923, 1992.
30. Ghoneim MM, Block RI, Sum Ping ST, et al: The interactions of midazolam and flumazenil on human memory and cognition, Anesthesiology 79(6):1183-1192, 1993.
31. Saletin M, Muhlhofer H, Fischer M, et al: A randomised controlled trial to evaluate the effects of flumazenil after midazolam premedication in outpatients undergoing colonoscopy, Endoscopy 23(6):331-333, 1991.
32. Whitwam JG: Resedation. Acta Anaesthesiol Scand Suppl 92:70-74, 1990.
33. Davis CO, Wax PM: Flumazenil associated seizure in an 11-month-old child, J Emerg Med 14(3):331-333, 1996.
34. Spivey WH: Flumazenil and seizures—analysis of 43 cases, Clin Ther 14(2):292-305, 1992.
35. Rodrigo MRC, Chan L, Hui E: Flumazenil reversal of conscious sedation for minor oral surgery, Anaesth Intensive Care 20:174-176, 1992.
36. Chang AC, Solinger MA, Yang DT, et al: Impact of flumazenil on recovery after outpatient endoscopy—a placebo-controlled trial, Gastrointest Endosc 49(5):573-579, 1999.
37. Claffey L, Plourde G, Morris J, et al: Sedation with midazolam during regional anaesthesia: is there a role for flumazenil? Can J Anaesth 41(11):1084-1090, 1994.
38. Finder RL, Moore PA, Close JM: Flumazenil reversal of conscious sedation induced with intravenous fentanyl and diazepam, Anesth Prog 42(1):11-16, 1995.
39. Flumazenil in Intravenous Conscious Sedation with Midazolam Multicenter Study Group. II. Reversal of central benzodiazepine effects by intravenous flumazenil after conscious sedation with midazolam and opioids: a multicenter clinical study, Clin Ther 14(6):878-894, 1992.
40. Jones RDM, Lawson AD, Andrew LJ, et al: Antagonism of the hypnotic effect of midazolam in children: a randomized, double-blind study of placebo and flumazenil administered after midazolam-induced anaesthesia, Br J Anaesth 66:660-666, 1991.
41. Becker LD, Paulson BA, Miller RD, et al: Biphasic respiratory depression after fentanyl-droperidol or fentanyl alone used to supplement nitrous oxide anesthesia, Anesthesiology 44(4):291-296, 1976.
42. Barakat T, Lechat JP, Laurent P, et al: Ventilatory effects of flumazenil on midazolam-induced sedation, Anesthesiology 69(3A):A818, 1988.

43. Salvucci AA, Eckstein M, Iscovich AL: Submental injection of naloxone, *Ann Emerg Med* 25(5):719-720, 1995.
44. Maiio RF, Gaukel B, Freeman B: Intralingual naloxone injection for narcotic-induced respiratory depression, *Ann Emerg Med* 16(5):572-573, 1987.
45. Patschke D, Eberlein HJ, Hess W, et al: Antagonism of morphine with naloxone in dogs: cardiovascular effects with special reference to the coronary circulation, *Br J Anaesth* 49(6):525-533, 1977.
46. Partridge BL, Ward CF: Pulmonary edema after low-dose naloxone administration, *Anesthesiology* 65(6):709-710, 1986.
47. Longo VG: Behavioral and electroencephalographic effects of atropine and related compounds, *Pharmacol Rev* 18(2):965-996, 1966.
48. Martin B, Howell PR: Physostigmine—going . . . going . . . gone? Two cases of central anticholinergic syndrome after anaesthesia and its treatment with physostigmine, *Eur J Anaesthesiol* 14:467-470, 1997.
49. Richmond M, Seger D: Central anticholinergic syndrome in a child: a case report, *J Emerg Med* 3(6):453-456, 1985.
50. Cook B, Spence AA: Post-operative central anticholinergic syndrome, *Eur J Anaesthesiol* 14:1-2, 1997.

Occupational Health and Environmental Emergencies

Michael T. Goupil

M any emergency situations can arise in the dental office environment. Usually the anticipated emergencies deal with medical problems, such as syncope and cardiac disorders, but the dental environment also may be the site of other problems that may affect patients and staff.

Most dental procedures can result in an exposure to tissue fluids, especially blood. These same fluids can harbor bacteria and viruses that may present a significant health risk to both staff and patients. Dental supplies are usually considered to be safe and are not seen as a health risk, but unfortunately this is not always the case. Mercury and other metals, such as nickel, are well-known health hazards and potential allergens. Latex sensitivity reactions are occurring more frequently, especially among health care providers. Many medicaments, such as phenol and sodium hypochlorite are caustic in nature and can cause serious tissue damage. Even the air in the office has the potential for adverse health consequences. Airborne infections, autoclave exhaust pollution, and nitrous oxide all need to be considered as a potential for occupational health and safety emergencies for both patients and dental staff.

TISSUE FLUID EXPOSURE

Even with "universal precautions," the transfer of tissue fluid, especially blood products, between patients and staff continues to be a real possibility. Although many diseases can be transferred via this route, the disorders that have generated the greatest concern are *hepatitis* and *human immunodeficiency virus* (HIV). Both these should be considered as potential occupational emergencies and an office emergency plan is in-

dicated. *Syphilis* should also be added to this list. Even though syphilis rates are at that their lowest since Centers for Disease Control and Prevention (CDC) monitoring, this disease still reaches epidemic proportions in portions of the southern United States.[1]

The use of high-speed rotary instruments can easily spread blood and saliva from patients to office staff. Blood spatters that reach *intact* skin or mucous membranes usually do not pose a threat, and quick reaction may not be required, although the possibility of small cuts and abrasions must be considered. The area should be thoroughly washed as soon as possible, and an antibacterial agent such as Betadine should be considered. No seroconversions have occurred in more than 2000 cases of mucocutaneous exposures when the skin or mucosa was intact.[2]

Sharps

Careless or improper handling of sharp instruments and supplies ("sharps") can transfer diseased tissue fluid and should be considered an emergency health hazard. All sharps should be placed in a "sharps container" before an instrument tray is removed for the treatment area. This will help reduce the risk to personnel responsible for washing and sterilizing instruments. Heavy protective gloves should be worn when washing any instruments that have sharp surfaces or that may be contaminated with tissue fluid.

Needlesticks

Transfer of blood from patients to staff is most likely to occur with needle-stick injuries ("needlesticks"). Needlesticks may occur during patient care activities such as the administration of local anesthesia or starting an intravenous (IV) line. The risk of HIV transmission is estimated at 1 in 300 (0.3%) after a single percutaneous injury and 1 in 1000 (0.1%) after a mucous membrane exposure such as a splash.[3,4] Compliance with universal precautions has not demonstrated a decrease in the frequency of needlesticks.[5] Instrument transfer techniques involving sharp instruments or needles should be avoided. Needles should not be left uncapped on the instrument tray. Needles should be immediately discarded in the sharps container, or the needle should be recapped using an approved recapping technique (e.g., one handed) or a needle-capping device (Figure 34-1).

HIV and AIDS

This potential of transferring HIV contaminated blood is of great concern to both patients and staff and is, unfortunately, frequently emotionally driven. Needlesticks and other sharps injuries account for more than 80% of the occupational acquired cases of HIV in health care workers.[6] Though most personnel are concerned about the transmission of HIV, the greater health risk is from the potential transfer of one of the hepatitis viruses. The transmission of an HIV infection is estimated at 0.3% for percutaneous injuries, whereas the transmission of the hepatitis B virus from contaminated needles ranges from 3% to 30%.[7,8]

Even though the risk of HIV transmission to dental health care workers is quite low, the risk exists and represents a true occupational emergency to the health care worker that has been injured. The actual potential risk of HIV transmission to health care workers has been difficult to ascertain. Through September 1993, only 39 cases of documented HIV seroconversion and 81 possible occupational infections had been reported among health care workers.[9] No dental health care workers were in the documented seroconversion group, but six were in the "possible" occupational infection group. In 1991 the National Commission on AIDS reported that 190 dental workers had developed acquired immunodeficiency syndrome (AIDS) while working in health care or laboratory environments.[10] In 1993, however, Robert and Bell,[11] reported that only seven dental providers in the United States acquired HIV seroconversions through occupational exposure. According to the most recent CDC report, 22,218 health care workers were diagnosed with AIDS as of December 31, 1999.

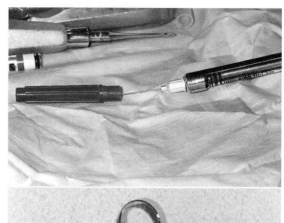

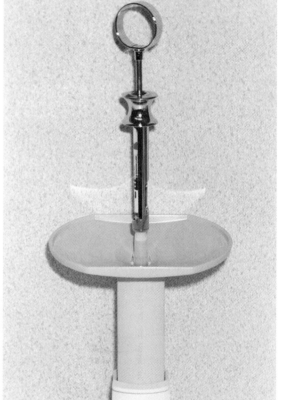

Figure 34-1. **A,** Single-handed needle recapping. **B,** Commercial needle-capping device.

Less than 500 of these were dental workers. The CDC has documented seroconversion from occupational-related exposure in only 56 health care workers, 25 of whom developed AIDS.[12] Thus the potential for seroconversion within the health worker community, especially the dental environment, appears to be extremely remote.

Even though the possibility of contracting AIDS in the dental office environment is low, providers and ancillary staff must be continually reminded of the importance of compliance with universal precautions. Eighty percent of occupational-acquired HIV infections are related to sharps injuries, especially needlesticks. The most common activity associated with sharp injuries are instrument cleanup procedures and linen disposal.[13] Another significant source of sharps injuries noted in the dental office are related to punctures from dental burs. Dental hand-piece mounts located underneath instrument delivery areas are a source of puncture injury, especially the thigh, when practicing sit-down dentistry.

The transmission of HIV is directly related to the amount of blood that is transferred from the source to the recipient. Thus the larger the bore or gauge of the needle, the more blood is transferred. A 20-gauge needle will transfer 30 times more blood than a 27-gauge needle.[14] Small-diameter needles should be used when administering local anesthesia. A 27-gauge needle may be more desirable than a 25-gauge needle. The same consideration should be made when initiating IV access. The amount of blood transferred is further decreased when a needle passes through a glove.[10] This further emphasizes the necessity of wearing gloves when starting IV lines and handling contaminated sharps.

Management

Sharps injuries continue to occur despite best efforts. When an injury does occur, prompt "emergent" action is required. Dilution and removal of the blood contamination should be accomplished as soon as possible. The contaminated area should be washed with a copious amount of regular hand soap and water.[15] For skin contamination the area should then be treated with a disinfectant solution. Mucous membranes, especially the eyes, should be thoroughly flushed with saline or water. Although the efficacy of these first-aid measures has not been proven, these are reasonable actions[16,17] (Figure 34-2).

The next phase of treatment is risk assessment. When the patient is still available, a detailed medical history is obtained to determine if the patient may be infected with HIV or hepatitis virus. At the same time the patient must be informed if blood may have been transferred from the health care worker to the patient. If the health care provider's HIV or hepatitis status is known, the patient must be told.

The amount of transferred blood should be estimated. If the injury was a result of a needle-

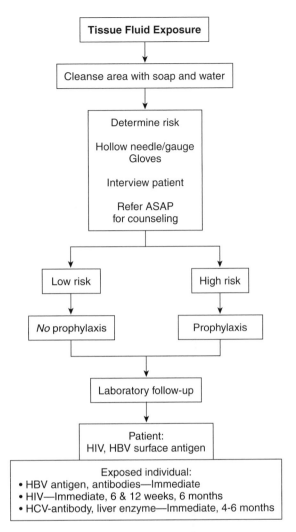

Figure 34-2. Treatment algorithm for tissue fluid exposure. HIV, Human immunodeficiency virus; HBV, HCV, hepatitis B, hepatitis C virus.

stick, it should be noted whether the health care worker was wearing gloves, the depth the needle penetrated, and what gauge or size of needle was involved in the injury and whether it was hollow.[16] All these factors determine the amount of blood that may have been transferred, and thus the degree of the risk factor. Further treatment recommendations depend on the HIV and hepatitis status of the source patient.

Both the patient and the health care worker should be tested for their HIV status as soon as possible after the incident occurred. The patient should be encouraged to participate on a voluntary basis. Testing requests should be made by a disinterested member of the health care team, such as the office manager, rather than the dentist or assistant, to avoid the impression of pressuring the patient. The costs of the tests are the responsibility of the dental office. Individual state laws should be consulted in advance to determine what legal options are available if the situation develops where the patient does not agree to voluntary testing.

Counseling

The most important phase of care that must be provided to the victim is qualified counseling (see Figure 34-2). The type and depth of counseling depend on the potential disease status of the source individual. The physician who will be responsible for prescribing medications and who is not a member of the dental office should provide counseling. If the risk of HIV transmission is low, the victim should be reassured that the potential for contracting AIDS is almost nonexistent, although further follow-up will be required. The victim should be followed serologically for at least 6 months with testing at the time of the exposure, at 6 weeks, 12 weeks, and 6 months.[4]

If the source patient is known to be HIV positive or is a member of high risk groups, the counseling becomes more important and must be carried out immediately on an emergent basis. Immediate counseling is required to afford the victim the choice of prophylactic treatment in a timely fashion. The primary prophylactic drug used to date has been *zidovudine*, which has been used as a single agent or in combination with other antiviral agents.[18,19] Although the U.S. Public Health Service could not recommend for or against postexposure prophylaxis in 1990, the use of zidovudine has increased significantly for exposed health care workers.[20-22]

Prevention

The efficacy of postexposure prophylaxis has not been proven. Animal studies have been inconclusive. There was a 67% reduction in the transmission of HIV to the babies of HIV-infected pregnant women in a prospective clinical trial testing zidovudine prophylaxis.[23] A major human study conducted by Burroughs-Wellcome was discontinued because of the low rate of seroconversion coupled with an increased demand by subjects for the prophylaxis as opposed to a placebo.[24,25] Most prophylaxis regiments have used zidovudine in the range of 200 to 250 mg every 4 to 6 hours for 4 to 8 weeks.[21,26] Because

the intracellular half-life of zidovudine is 3 to 4 hours, as opposed to its serum half-life of 1 hour, prophylactic dosing every 8 hours may be considered.[27,28] The most current CDC recommendation is a 4-week course of zidovudine and lamivudine for most exposures and to add a protease inhibitor, such as indinavir or nelfinavir, for higher risk situations.[4]

To optimize the potential prophylaxis effect, the drug administration should start as soon as possible after the HIV exposure. In the past the recommendation was made to initiate prophylaxis within 1 hour, but it is now advised to start prophylaxis as soon as possible, preferably within 24 hours, but no later than 7 days.[4,29]

If the source patient has been identified as HIV or AIDS positive, a further history should be taken to determine which antiviral drugs have been used for treatment. Failure of zidovudine prophylaxis has been related to virus mutation and resistance in source patients that have been treated with zidovudine. When source patients have been under active therapy, the recipient patient should be considered for combination antiretroviral prophylaxis. Zidovudine can be used in combination with didanosine, stavidine, zalcitabine, and interferon.[16,18,30]

The primary complaint of patients being treated with zidovudine prophylaxis therapy is nausea not responsive to antiemetics. Anemia is the most common objective side effect. These side effects appear to be dose related and are reversible when prophylaxis is discontinued.[20,31,32] Most health care facilities consider that the risk of contracting HIV is greater than the risk of long-term prophylactic treatment, and thus the cost of treatment is justified and cost-effective.[33]

Several recombinant envelope glycoprotein HIV-1 vaccines have been evaluated in human subjects, and prevention through vaccination is a possibility. These vaccines have proven to be safe and immunogenic, but whether they will prove to be effective in protecting health care workers against HIV infections is still unknown.[34,35]

Although exposure to HIV contaminated blood is possible, the *probability* is extremely remote. The potential contact with hepatitis-contaminated blood is more probable and a greater threat. The risk of being infected with *hepatitis B virus* (HBV) is essentially zero for health care workers who have developed immunity from the HBV vaccine. For the unvaccinated person the risk is highly variable, ranging from 6% to 30%, depending on the hepatitis Be antigen status of the source individual.[4] Virus transfer may occur from 1 in 3 percutaneous exposures.[16,17] Although only 3% to 5% of the general population are HBV positive, as many as 80% of these individuals have never been diagnosed. This high rate of undiagnosed HBV patients has resulted in 15% of general dental office team members seroconverting.[17] The complications of hepatitis seroconversion are significant; fulminant HBV infections have a fatality rate of 1.4%.

The risk of developing an infection after exposure to a cut or needlestick from *hepatitis* C *virus* (HCV)–infected blood is estimated at 1.8%.[4] HCV seroconversion is associated with hepatocellular carcinoma.[36]

Time is a critical factor in treating tissue fluid–induced emergencies, and thus an office plan must be developed in advance. When an exposure occurs, the wound should be immediately cleaned using regular hand soap and water. An antiseptic solution may then be applied. The source patient is then interviewed to determine the potential of HIV or hepatitis transmission. An individual not immediately involved in the incident should conduct this interview, such the office manager or nurse. This decreases the emotional overtone that could inhibit truth telling on the part of the patient. If the source patient is HIV positive or in a high-risk category for the virus, the exposed health care worker must receive appropriate counseling as to the potential of seroconverting and the risks and benefits of antiviral prophylaxis (see Figure 34-2).

Laboratory Tests and Follow-up

Laboratory testing is indicated whenever there is a possibility of tissue fluid transfer. The source patient should be tested for both HIV antibodies and HBV surface antigen. The exposed health care worker should be base line tested for HIV as well as for hepatitis B antigen and antibody and for hepatitis C antibody, along with an alanine transaminase (ALT) activity liver enzyme test.[4] If the exposed individual tests negative for hepatitis antibodies and antigen, vaccination should be initiated within 7 days. HBV immunoglobin (0.6 ml/kg) can be given immediately if the exposed person had not received hepatitis vaccination.

Follow-up testing is not required for HBV because current therapy is so effective. HCV antibody and liver enzyme testing should be reaccomplished 4 to 6 months after the initial exposure. HIV testing should be done periodically for 6 months.[4]

AIRBORNE DISEASE TRANSMISSION: TUBERCULOSIS

Another potential threat to both health care workers and to patients is the office air itself. For more than 30 years, there had been a steady decrease in the incidence of tuberculosis (TB) in the United States. Then in 1989 this trend reversed, and there is now an increase in the number of TB cases being reported to the CDC. This increase in reported cases has been attributed to an increase in high-risk populations, such as the homeless, IV drug abusers, and HIV-positive persons. Approximately one third of the world's population has been infected with TB, of whom 10 to 15 million live in the United States.[32,37,38] Hawaii, California, and New York rank as the most prevalent areas in the United States for TB.[39]

The increased prevalence of multiple-drug-resistant tuberculosis (MDR-TB) is of even greater concern.[40] MDR-TB is defined as a case of TB caused be a strain of *Mycobacterium tuberculosis* that is resistant to two or more antituberculosis drugs.[41] This MDR-TB increase is usually seen in larger population areas (e.g., New York City, San Francisco) but can occur anywhere in the United States. This MDR-TB at-risk group is composed mainly of HIV-seropositive individuals who are IV drug abusers and the homeless. In a California study, 1 in 12 homeless individuals was seropositive for HIV infection, and one third of these patients were infected with TB.

The prime reason for the development of MDC-TB is most likely related to the noncompliance of TB therapy. The patient may feel better within a couple of weeks of the initiation of therapy and then elect not to complete the full course of therapy due to the cost or difficulty in obtaining the drug. Lack of compliance and incomplete treatment results in resistant organisms. When a patient's medical history is positive for TB, the patient should be questioned further to determine whether they had been compliant with their TB therapy.

Health Screening

A screening health history should be taken on all at risk patients to determine the possibility of TB to decrease the risk of transmitting disease to office personnel and other patients in the area (Box 34-1). High-risk patients include the poor, the homeless, IV drug abusers, and residents and employees of long-term institutional settings such as nursing homes and correctional facilities.[42] Attention should be directed immediately

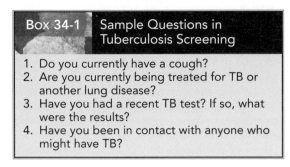

Box 34-1 Sample Questions in Tuberculosis Screening

1. Do you currently have a cough?
2. Are you currently being treated for TB or another lung disease?
3. Have you had a recent TB test? If so, what were the results?
4. Have you been in contact with anyone who might have TB?

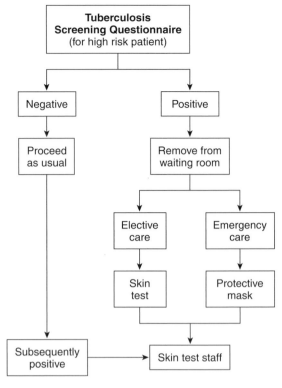

Figure 34-3. Treatment algorithm for tuberculosis.

to those that have a cough and have the potential of infecting others in the office environment. Patients that pose a potential health risk should be referred for further evaluation and TB skin testing before undergoing elective dental care.

Currently, no data are available on the risk of TB transmission in the dental office. The increase in TB prevalence in the community should lead to an increased risk in the dental office environment. The potential of TB transmission in the dental office may also be higher than in other health care settings because of the aerosolization of contaminated oral secretions.[43]

It is advisable to have office staff skin tested at least annually in those office environments where there is a high potential for providing care to undiagnosed TB carriers.[44] If care was provided to a patient who subsequently reports to be TB positive, a skin test should be provided to all staff members and patients who may have been in contact with the source patient. Patients presenting for emergency dental care should still be treated even if they could spread TB organisms. Special precautions can be taken to reduce the risk of contracting TB. The source patient should be removed from the waiting room environment to reduce the risk to other patients. Health care workers should wear protective airway respirators specifically designed to filter out the TB bacilli. Standard face masks are insufficient protection. Consideration should also be given to treating infected patients at the end of the day to further reduce the risk to other patients (Figure 34-3).

CHEMICAL INJURIES
Mercury

Contact with dental materials used daily may cause serious harm to both patients and health care workers. The long-term effects of mercury poisoning have changed the way amalgam is dispensed and used. Even in the absence of scientific evidence that amalgam restorations pose a health risk to patients, a minority of health care providers have advocated the replacement of mercury-containing restorations. When removing mercury restorations, for whatever reason, it is important to have a high-volume evacuation system engaged to prevent mercury contamination of the office environment.

There should be no risk of mercury spillage using currently accepted amalgam delivery systems. Amalgam and mercury constitute hazardous waste and should be disposed of safely. Mercury spills must be cleaned up immediately to ensure that there is no risk to the staff.

Chemical Spillage

Another potential emergency in the dental office is chemical spillage, especially caustic material. *Phenol* and *sodium hypochlorite* are frequently used in the dental office and may be extremely caustic. Extreme caution must be used with these materials because the potential exists for skin, mucosal, and eye burns.[45-47]

Immediate first aid is the treatment of choice. Most chemical agents cause tissue destruction by a direct chemical reaction, and the amount of destruction is determined by how long the agent is in contact with the skin or mucous membrane.[48] Copious irrigation of the affected area with saline or plain water is usually sufficient treatment.[49] The eye is particularly sensitive to alkaline chemicals. The chemical is absorbed by the protein structure of the corneal epithelium. A necrosis results, which in turn allows more of the chemical to penetrate and affect deeper tissue layers. The eye can be conveniently irrigated using a IV infusion line with a large-bore Teflon catheter attached to a liter bag of sterile saline. The eye should be washed for at least 15 minutes.[50] Phenol chemical spills to the skin should be irrigated with large volumes of water, swabbed with isopropyl alcohol, or treated with undiluted polyethylene glycol.[48,51,52] Therapy needs to be instituted immediately because phenol is rapidly absorbed by the skin or mucous membranes and causes systemic toxicity.

Injection

Injection of caustic material into the soft tissues of the body causes a very severe reaction. Severe pain, rapidly developing edema, hematomas, necrosis, and abscess formation have all been reported.[53] Hospitalization may be required for antibiotic, steroid, and analgesic management.

Air

The air in the sterilization area may also pose as a risk to health care providers. *Ethylene oxide* has been shown to cause mutations and chromosomal aberrations and may be a carcinogen.[3] Acute overexposure may cause conjunctiva, skin, and respiratory irritation, manifesting as headache, nausea, sore throat, cough, shortness of breath, and rhinitis.[54] The risks of nitrous oxide pollution are well known and include problems with female fertility and neurologic diseases.[55] Scavenger systems for polluting gases are mandatory, and offices should be well ventilated.

LATEX ALLERGY

One of the most common threats to the safety of both health care providers and patients is the growing problem of latex allergy. The first published report of an allergic reaction to latex gloves was in 1979.[22,56] Since that time, more than 1000 allergic reactions have been reported to the U.S. Food and Drug Administration (FDA) concerning latex containing products.[43,57-59] At

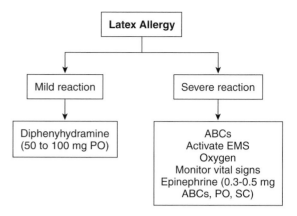

Figure 34-4. Treatment algorithm for latex allergy. PO, Orally; SC, subcutaneously; ABCs, airway, breathing, and circulation protocols; EMS, emergency medical services.

least 16 anaphylactic deaths have been attributed to latex products.[56,60]

Latex reactions described have been both type I and type IV allergic reactions (Figure 34-4).[61,62] *Type I latex reactions* are IgE mediated and include anaphylaxis. Clinical manifestations reported include urticaria, allergic rhinitis, asthma, angioedema, hypotension, and tachycardia. Introduction of the antigen into the circulatory system promotes a massive histamine release, resulting in vasodilation, hypotension, and plasma loss from the circulation. These types of reactions can be life threatening, and prompt emergency response is required.

Type IV latex reactions are represented by a contact dermatitis. These reactions are more likely related to the chemicals added to the rubber products during the manufacturing process rather than a reaction to the latex itself. Type IV reactions are characterized by erythema, inflammation, swelling, and eczema over the exposed sites. These reactions are delayed and usually occur 4 to 48 hours after exposure. Vesicle formation may be noted. (See Chapter 11.)

Epidemiology and Etiology

Several groups at risk for latex allergy have been identified. The majority of the anaphylactic reactions have been attributed to rubber-tipped barium enema applicators. Individuals who have been frequently exposed to latex products as part of medical diagnostic evaluations are at high risk. Latex product exposure occurs continually with health care workers on a daily basis. Exposure has increased significantly with the requirement for wearing protective gloves as part of universal precautions. Patients who have had multiple surgeries are also susceptible to latex allergy problems. Multiple surgeries are seen frequently in children with spina bifida or a history of recurrent genitourinary tract instrumentations.[18,58,63] Latex allergy in spina bifida patients has been estimated at 50%.[64]

An estimated 1% to 6% of the general population are at risk for problems related to latex products.[65] Latex sensitization increases to a range of 5% to 15% in health care workers.[59,66] For dental personnel, risk for latex allergy is estimated at 13% to 24%.[61,67,68] Yassin et al[69] reported that 38% of dental residents and dental assistants were positive when tested for latex sensitivity. Although the authors considered their sample size to be too low to establish a true prevalence, this does give an indication of the magnitude of the problem.

Anaphylactic reactions and deaths during medical and surgical procedures that were attributed to medications may have represented severe latex reactions.[70,71] Respiratory problems among health care workers have been attributed to the cornstarch on surgical gloves. These pulmonary problems are now thought to be more likely related to latex proteins carried in the air by glove powder.[72,73] Airborne particles from powdered gloves represents a serious threat to patients and health care workers with a latex sensitivity.

There are a number of reasons for the increase in adverse latex reactions being reported to the FDA. Universal precautions require that heath care workers wear protective gloves. Until recently most protective gloves were latex based, and thus both patients and health care providers had an increased exposure to latex products. There has also been an increased concern among the population about sexually transmitted disease, especially HIV, and this has led to an increase in condom usage.[19,63,67,69] Recommended condoms are manufactured from latex. Finally, now that latex allergy has been recognized as a significant risk, allergic reactions that previously were believed to be caused by other allergens are now being more properly attributed to latex allergy.[71,72]

Management

If patients or office staff exhibit any manifestations of a type I or type IV allergic reaction, a latex allergy should be considered. All latex products should be removed from the immediate area to reduce further exposure to the allergen.

Subsequent treatment is based on the type of reaction that has developed.[56] A type IV reaction is best treated by avoiding further contact with any latex product. Steroid creams and antihistamines may be considered depending on the severity of the reaction. Mild reactions may be treated only with antihistamine therapy, such as diphenhydramine, 50 to 100 mg orally. A more severe type I reaction, which may manifest as anaphylaxis, will require prompt recognition and treatment. Epinephrine, 0.3 to 0.5 mg for adults, is administered subcutaneously. Along with standard measures of airway, breathing, and circulation (ABCs) of life support, supplemental oxygen is provided and the patient's vital signs monitored. The local emergency medical services (EMS) system should be activated immediately. Further treatment within the office is dependent on the patient's reaction to initial treatment and how rapid the EMS system responds (see Figure 34-4).

Once the allergic reaction has been treated, the patient or health care employee must be evaluated for the precipitating allergen. Skin testing is a sensitive, inexpensive, and reliable method of testing.[6,56,73,74] Unfortunately there are no commercially available latex test antigens, and the skin-prick test carries a high risk of complications, including anaphylaxis.[61,74-76] The *radioallergosorbent test* (RAST) is an in vitro test specific for IgE antibodies toward a specific antigen. Currently the RAST is not sensitive enough to detect all true latex allergy patients. Also, no clear relationship exists between the severity of the allergic reaction and the RAST values.

Prevention

Every effort should be directed toward avoiding a latex allergy response. The medical health history must include questions that will uncover a potential allergy.[35,63,73] Inquiry should be made about a history of spina bifida, multiple urogenital surgical procedures, anaphylactic reactions from previous surgeries, reactions to common latex products (swollen lips from balloons, condom reactions), atopic allergy or allergy to multiple antigens, and allergy to certain foods (bananas, avocados, kiwi, chestnuts). Spina bifida patients are considered to be at such high risk that they are assumed to have a latex sensitivity.[59,77,78] All latex products should be avoided when treating this high-risk group.[79]

Once the possibility of a latex allergy is established, a latex-free environment must be provided. This type of environment is very difficult to establish. Gloves that are labeled as "hypoallergenic" does not mean that they are latex free.[57,62,80,81] The hypoallergenicity refers to the removal of chemicals used during the manufacturing process that are likely to elicit a type IV reaction. All products need to be carefully evaluated to determine whether they are made from latex or contain latex components. Rubber dam isolation is now available as a silicon product or can be fabricated from a silicon glove. "Prophy cups" are also available that are not made from rubber. Medication syringes, local anesthetic carpules, multidose vials, and nitrous oxide administration devices all contain rubber components.

When treating latex-sensitive patients, the dentist should schedule them as the first patients of the day. The use of latex surgical gloves throughout the day results in the air becoming contaminated with glove powder containing latex allergens.[77] Outer garments such as smocks, gowns, and lab coats will also become contaminated with the same powder. Providing a latex-free environment becomes a real challenge since not all rubber-containing products may be labeled as to the latex components. Even gutta percha has been implicated in one latex sensitivity report.[82]

To help reduce the frequency of latex problems, the National Institute of Occupational Safety and Health (NIOSH) has made several recommendations for health care employees. Nonlatex gloves should be worn when the possibility of contact with infectious material is minimal. When latex gloves are required, powder-free gloves should be worn. Oil-based hand creams and lotions should not be used when wearing latex gloves, and hands should be washed with mild soap after gloves are removed. The workplace should be frequently cleaned to removed latex-contaminated dust; this also includes frequent changing of ventilation filters and vacuum cleaner bags.[65]

Office staff must be prepared in advance to recognize and treat potential latex reactions. Staff must try to identify potential patients at risk through good history taking. Treatment protocols must be established and practiced frequently. Emergency drugs must be available, and staff must be briefed in their proper use.

OTHER HAZARDS
Lasers

Lasers have found increased uses in dentistry, but they also have become another source for potential hazard to both patients and office staff. Extra safety precautions are required to avoid fires and burning the patient and staff. Eyewear specific for the type of laser being used is necessary to prevent eye injury and must be worn by the staff and the patient. The laser smoke plume may contain malignant cells as well as viable bacteria and viruses.[3] These viable cells, bacteria, and viruses are capable of causing disease if inhaled. Laser masks are available to help protect against airborne bacteria and viruses. A high-volume smoke evacuator should be used to protect against the smoke plume. The laser room must be clearly marked with identification signs on the doors to prevent access by unauthorized personnel during laser procedures.

Electrical Devices and Burns

All electrical devices have the potential to harm. Almost everyone has experienced the unpleasant effects of artificial electricity. Current passing through the heart or thorax can cause direct damage to the myocardium and dysrhythmias. The first priority is to shut off the power or remove victim from the power source. Basic life support is initiated if spontaneous respiration or circulation is absent.[83]

Other than cardiac arrest, burns are the most devastating injuries resulting from electrical injuries. In children these burns most often occur in the oral region. Immediate referral to a specialist with an expertise in electrical injuries is indicated.[84] Electrical appliances should be routinely checked for frayed wires and broken contacts. All devices should only be used according to the manufacturers' direction, and grounding should be used when indicated.

All minor burns should be cleansed with sterile saline, then covered with Bacitracin ointment and retreated every 6 hours after cleansing the area. The wound can be recleansed with dilute soap and water. Prophylactic antibiotics are not recommended, but tetanus prophylaxis should be considered.[48,52]

SUMMARY: THE OFFICE ENVIRONMENT AS EMERGENCY

When considering the potential of emergencies occurring in the office setting, the dental practitioner is usually concerned with the potential of drug reactions and adverse responses to underlying systemic diseases. Although rare, emergencies arising from the office environment itself also may occur. Toxic reactions to various chemicals found in the office must also be considered. Adequate ventilation will help prevent the long-term consequences of breathing nitrous oxide and chemical exhaust fumes.

Care must be taken to ensure that complete medical histories are obtained on each patient. Patients with communicable diseases (e.g., TB) must be identified. These infections may be transmitted to office staff and other patients.

Health histories must also include the ability to identify patients with latex sensitivity. The increased use of latex products among health care workers has resulted in a higher incidence of latex sensitivity. The office staff must be prepared to recognize and quickly treat anaphylactic reactions. Provisions must be made to provide a latex-free environment for high-risk patients. This provision may include referral to an office environment known to be free of latex.

Even with the use of universal precautions, blood contamination exposures and needlesticks will still occur. Office staff should be protected against hepatitis through the administration of a hepatitis prevention vaccine. A protocol needs to be established in advance to handle blood exposure incidents. The patient history needs to be updated to determine potential risk. This information is sensitive and must be kept confidential. The exposed person must receive counseling as to the potential risk of HIV infection. If there is a potential risk of HIV contamination, the exposed individual must be given the opportunity to initiate prophylactic chemotherapy within 24 hours of exposure.

Even though the risks of occupational health and safety emergencies are rare, they must be considered. Contingency plans must be available for preventing emergencies such as providing a latex-free environment. The office staff must be prepared to treat emergencies that require immediate response, such as anaphylaxis and chemical spills. Arrangements must be available to quickly handle exposure to communicable infections. Advance planning and office procedure protocols are paramount to preventing emergencies and to responding rapidly should they occur.

REFERENCES

1. Primary and secondary syphilis—United States, 1997, MMWR 47(24):493-497, 1998.
2. Robinson P, Challacombe S: Transmission of HIV in a dental practice: the facts, Br Dent J, Nov 20, 1993, pp 383-384.
3. Babich S, Burakoff RP: Occupational hazards of dentistry: a review of literature from 1990, NY State Dent J, Oct 26-31, 1997.
4. US Department of Health and Human Services: Exposure to blood: what health-care workers need to know, Washington, DC, 1999, US Public Health Service.
5. Gerberding JL: Does knowledge of human immunodeficiency virus infection decrease the frequency of occupational exposure to blood, Am J Med 91(suppl 3B): 308S-311S, 1991.
6. Allenius H: IgE immune response to rubber proteins in adult patients with latex allergy, J Allergy Clin Immunol 93:859-863, 1994.
7. Head KC, Bradley-Springer L, Sklar D: The HIV-infected health care worker: legal, ethical, and scientific perspectives, J Emerg Med 12(1):95-102, 1994.
8. Torkas JI et al: Surveillance of HIV infection and zidovudine use among health care workers after occupational exposure to HIV-infected blood, Ann Intern Med 118(12):913-919, 1993.
9. Beckmann SE, Henderson DK: Managing occupational risks in the dental office: HIV and the dental profession, J Am Dent Assoc 125:847-852, 1994.
10. National Commission on AIDS: Preventing HIV transmission in health care settings, AIDS Patient Care 7(3):138-156, 1993.
11. Robert LM, Bell DM: HIV transmission in the healthcare setting, Infect Dis Clin North Am 8(2):319-329, 1994.
12. Centers for Disease Control and Prevention: Surveillance of health care worker with HIV/AIDS, Atlanta, 2000, CDC, http://www.cdc.gov/hiv/pubs/facts/hcwsurv.htm.
13. McCormick RD, Meisch MG, Ircink FG, et al: Epidemiology of hospital sharps injuries: a 14-year prospective study in the pre-Aid and AIDS eras, Am J Med 91(suppl 3B):301S-307S, 1991.
14. Shirazian D, Herzlich BC, Moktarian F, et al: Needlestick injury: blood, mononuclear cells, and acquired immunodeficiency syndrome, Am J Infect Control 20:133-137, 1992.
15. McKee JM: Human immunodeficiency virus: healthcare worker safety issues, J Intravenous Nurs 19(3):132-140, 1996.
16. Gerberding JL, Henderson DK: Management of occupational exposure to bloodborne pathogens: hepatitis B virus, hepatitis C virus, and human immunodeficiency virus, Clin Infect Dis 14:1179-1185, 1992.
17. Leonard RH, Eagle Jr JC: Developing an effective occupational exposure policy for the dental office, Gen Dent 40(5):379-381, 386, 388, 1992.
18. Malcome JA, Dobson PM, Sutherland DC: Combination chemoprophylaxis after needlestick injury, Lancet 34:112-113, 1993.
19. Mansell PI, Reckless JPD, Lovell CR: Severe anaphylactic reaction to latex rubber surgical gloves, Br Med J 308:246-247, 1994.
20. Polder JA et al: Public Health Service statement on management of occupational exposure to human immunodeficiency virus, including considerations regarding zivovudine post exposure use, MMWR 39(RR-1), 1990.
21. Ramsey SD, Nettleman MD: Cost-effectiveness of prophylactic AZT following neddlestick injury in health care workers, Med Decis Making 12:142-148, 1992.
22. Tomazic VJ, Withrow TJ, Fisher BR, et al: Latex-associated allergies and anaphylactic reactions, Clin Immunol Immunopathol 64(2):89-97, 1992.
23. National Institute of Allergy and Infectious Diseases, Division of AIDS: Zidovudine for the prevention of HIV transmission from mother to infant, MMWR 43(16): 26-28, 1994.

24. Burroughs-Wellcome: Prophylactic use of Retrovir (zidovudine) in health care workers exposed to human immunodeficiency virus (HIV), Oct 27, 1994.

25. Jeffries DJ: Zidovudine after occupational exposure to HIV, BMJ 302:1349-1350, 1991.

26. McLeod GX, Hammer SM: Zidovudine: five years later, Ann Intern Med 117:487-501, 1992.

27. Haas DW, Des Prez RM: Tuberculosis and acquired immunodeficiency syndrome: a historical perspective on recent developments, Am J Med 96:439-450, 1994.

28. Volberding PD: Perspectives on the use of antiretroviral drugs in the treatment of HIV infection, Infect Dis Clin North Am 8(2):303-307, 1994.

29. HIV seroconversion after occupational exposure despite early prophylactic zidovudine therapy, Lancet 34:1077-1078, 1993.

30. Mildvan D, Berge P: Prophylactic zalcitabime and interferon-alpha for a large-bore needlestick exposure to human immunodeficiency virus, J AIDS 7(4):426, 1994.

31. Lancaster DJ, Lancaster LL: Antiretroviral therapy on HIV-infected adults, Postgrad Med 95(1):47-50, 1994.

32. Tynes LL: Tuberculosis: the continuing story, JAMA 270(21):2616-2617, 1992.

33. Sacks HS, Rose DN: Zidovudine prophylaxis for needlestick exposure to human immunodeficiency virus: a decision analysis, J Gen Intern Med 5:132-137, 1990.

34. Belshe RB et al: Neutralizing antibodies to HIV-1 in seronegative volunteers immunized with recombinant gp 120 from the MN strain of HIV-1, JAMA 272:488-489, 1994.

35. Mascola JR, McNeil JG, Burke DS: AIDS vaccines: are we ready for human efficacy trials? JAMA 272(6):488-489, 1994.

36. Dana F, Becherer PR, Bacon BR: Hepatitis C virus: what recent studies can tell us, Postgrad Med 95(6):121-130, 1994.

37. Centers for Disease Control and Prevention: The deadly intersection between TB and HIV, Atlanta, 2000, CDC, http://www.cdc.gov/hiv/pubs/facts/hivtb.pdf.

38. US Department of Health and Human Services. TB facts for health care workers, Washington, DC, 1993, US Public Health Service.

39. Centers for Disease Control and Prevention, CDC-NCHSTP-DTBE, http://www.gov.cdc.gov.nchstp/tb/surv/surv.htm.

40. Neville K et al: The third epidemic: multidrug resistant tuberculosis, Chest 105(1):45-48, 1994.

41. Riley LW: Drug-resistant tuberculosis, Clin Infect Dis 17(suppl 2):542-546, 1993.

42. Zolpoa AR et al. HIV and tuberculosis infection in San Francisco's homeless adults: prevalence and risk factors in a representative sample, JAMA 272(6):455-461, 1994.

43. Shearer BG: MDR-TB: another challenge from the microbial world, J Am Dent Assoc 125:43-49, 1994.

44. Federal Bureau of Prisons, Indian Health Service, Dental Services Branch: Self-reported tuberculin skin testing among Indian Health Service and Federal Bureau of Prisons dentists, MMWR 43(11):209-211, 1993.

45. Ehrich, DG, Brian JD, Walker WA: Sodium hypochlorite accident: inadvertent injection in to the maxillary sinus, J Endod 19(4):180-182, 1992.

46. Gatot A, Arbelle J, Leiberman A, Yanai-Inbar I: Effects of sodium hypochlorite on soft tissue after inadvertent injection beyond the root apex, J Endod 17(11):573-574, 1991.

47. Jaffee E: Complication during root canal therapy following accidental extrusion of sodium hypochlorite through the apical foramen, Gen Dent 39(6):460-461, 1991.

48. Edlich RF, Moghtader JC: Chemical injuries. In Rosen P, Barkin R, editors: Emergency medicine: concepts and clinical practice, ed 4, St Louis, 1998, Mosby.

49. Ingram JA III: Response of the human eye to accidental exposure to sodium hypochlorite, J Endod 16(5):235-238, 1990.

50. Cyr D, Johnson SB: First aid for eyes, University of Maine Cooperative Extension, http://cdc.gov/niosh/nasd/doc3/me97007.html.

51. Spiller HA, Quadrani-Kushner DA, Cleveland P: A five-year evaluation of acute exposures to phenol disinfectant, Clin Toxicol 31(2):307-313, 1993.

52. Dimick AR, Wagner RG: Burns. In Schwartz GR, editor: Principles and practice of emergency medicine, ed 4, Baltimore, 1999, Williams & Wilkins.

53. Becking AG: Complication in the use of sodium hypochlorite during endodontic treatment, Oral Surg Oral Med Oral Pathol Oral Radiol Endod 71:346-348, 1991.

54. Weaver VM: Chemical hazards in health care workers, Occup Med Rev 12(4):655-667, 1997.

55. Suruda A: Health effects of anesthetic gases, Occup Med Rev 12(4):627-634, 1997.

56. Hancock I: Latex allergy: prevention and treatment, Anesth Rev 21(5):153-163, 1994.

57. Council on Dental Materials, Instruments, and Equipment; Council on Dental Therapeutics; Council on Dental Research: Reactions to latex in health care settings: dealing with patient/worker concerns, J Am Dent Assoc 124:91-92, 1993.

58. Harman C, Sullivan K: Latex sensitivity in dentistry, Operatory Infect Control 2(2):1-7, 1994.

59. White paper: Latex allergy, Franklin Lakes, NJ, 1993, Becton Dickinson.

60. Nelson LP, Soporowski N, Shusterman S: Latex allergies in children with spina bifida: relevance for the pediatric dentist, Pediatr Dent 16:18-22, 1994.

61. Hamann CP: Latex hypersensitivity: an update, Allergy Proc 15:17-20, 1994.

62. Rankin KV, Jones DL, Rees TD: Latex glove reactions found in a dental school, J Am Dent Assoc 124:67-71, 1993.

63. Barton EC: Latex allergy: recognition and management of a modern problem, Nurs Practitioner 18(11):54-58, 1993.

64. Yip L et al: Skin prick test reactivity to recombinant latex allergens, Int Arch Allergy Immunol 121:292-299, 2000.

65. National Institute of Occupational Safety and Health: NIOSH alert: preventing allergic reactions to natural rubber latex in the workplace, 1997, DHHD (NIOSH) Pub No 97-135, http://www.cdc.gov/niosh/latexalt.html.

66. Phillips VL, Goodrich MA, Sullivan TJ: Health care worker disability due to latex allergy and asthma: a cost analysis, Am J Public Health 89(7):1024-1028, 1999.

67. Dougherty HL: Allergy to rubber (an increasing dental practice problem), Am J Orthodon Dev Orthop 104(2):23A-24A, 1993.

68. McCann D: Allergic reactions to latex on the rise: researchers target protein chemicals, ADA News, Oct 3, 1994, pp 30-31.

69. Yassin MS et al: Latex allergy in hospital employees, Ann Allergy 72:245-249, 1994.

70. Kelly KJ et al: A cluster of anaphylactic reactions in children with spina bifida during general anesthesia, J Allergy Clin Immunol 94:53-61, 1994.

71. Warpinski JR, Folgert J, Cohen M, Bush RK: Allergic reaction to latex: a risk factor for unsuspected anaphylaxis, Allergy Proc 12(2):95-102, 1991.

72. Rubak ME: Allergic reactions to latex among health-care workers, Mayo Clin Proc 67:1075-1079, 1992.

73. Gonzalez E: Latex hypersensitivity: a new and unexpected problem, *Hosp Pract*, Feb 15, 1992, pp137-151.

74. Wrangston K, Osterman K, van Hage-Hamsten M: Glove-related skin symptoms among operating theater and dental care unit personnel, *Cont Derm* 30:139-142, 1994.

75. Charous BL, Hamilton RG, Yunginger JW: Occupational latex exposure: characteristics of contact and systemic reactions in 47 workers, *J Allergy Clin Immunol* 94:12-18, 1994.

76. Kelly K, Kurup VP, Reijula KE, Fink J: The diagnosis of natural rubber latex allergy, *J Allergy Clin Immunol* 93(5):813-816, 1994.

77. Slater JE: Latex allergy, *J Allergy Clin Immunol* 94:139-149, 1994.

78. Snyder HA, Settle S: The rise in latex allergy: implications for the dentist, *J Am Dent Assoc* 125:1089-1097, 1994.

79. Rankin KV, Seale NS, Jones DL, Rees TD: Reported latex sensitivity in pediatric dental patients from hospital- and dental school-based populations, *Pediatr Dent* 16:117-120, 1994.

80. Rosen A, Issacson D, Brady M, Corey JP: Hypersensitivity to latex in health care workers: report of five cases, *Otolaryngol Head Neck Surg* 109:731-734, 1993.

81. Wolf BL: Anaphylactic reaction to latex gloves, *N Engl J Med* 329(4):279-280, 1993.

82. Boxwe MB, Grammer LC, Orfan N: Gutta percha allergy in a health care worker with latex allergy, *J Allergy Clin Immunol* 93:943-944, 1994.

83. Cummins RO, editor: *Advanced cardiac life support*, Chicago, 1997, American Heart Association.

84. Cooper MA: Electrical and lightning injuries. In Rosen P, Barkin R, editors: *Emergency medicine: concepts and clinical practice*, ed 4, St Louis, 1998, Mosby.

Legal Implications of Emergency Care*

James R. Hupp
Roger L. Eldridge

Fortunately, dentists other than oral-maxillofacial surgeons are not regularly required to manage medical emergencies due to their relative infrequency in dental practice. Therefore an awareness of legal considerations related to the provision of such care is uncommon among dentists and most other health care providers. However, even though this is a rarity, a lawsuit may be filed against a dentist due to an untoward outcome allegedly resulting from causation or mismanagement of an emergency. This makes it important for dentists to be familiar with legal ramifications in this area of clinical care.

A dentist's risk of legal consequences as a result of managing or allegedly causing emergencies primarily depends on the nature of the dentist-patient relationship. If a dentist is treating a patient and that patient suffers an emergency because of or coincident with the dentist's care, it is clearly incumbent on the dentist to provide the care necessary to prevent or mitigate any lasting sequelae from the emergency. If a dental emergency is foreseeable, the legal system may expect the dentist to take steps to prevent or lessen the chances of the emergency occurring.

If the patient currently receiving care from the dentist has an emergency unrelated to the dental care, the dentist is still obliged to provide some assistance. Again, if the nondental emergency is foreseeable, a court or jury may believe that the dentist should have taken rea-sonable steps to prevent or lower the possibility of the problem.

It is a traditional legal principle that the dentist-patient relationship is voluntary in nature, and either party may choose whether or not to enter the relationship and may refuse to enter it for a variety of reasons. The dentist managing a medical emergency in a patient with whom the dentist has had no previous relationship rarely faces legal problems as a consequence of the emergency treatment. In fact, in many cases the legal system gives individuals providing care in such emergency situations special protection against lawsuits or other legal actions. In other circumstances, however, dentists forfeit their right to refuse to enter a dentist-patient relationship, such as if they agree to be "on call" for an emergency department (ED). In this situation, dentists may have a legal obligation to provide certain types of care even if they prefer *not* to provide care to specific individuals in the ED.

The legal exposure a dentist incurs when providing (or not providing) emergency care usually stems from the legal "duty" the dentist may owe to the person being assisted. If a duty is owed, other elements are required to create liability and become relevant in deciding if a legal cause of action exists.

Because so much depends on the nature of the duty owed to another individual when a dentist is trying to determine if and how to act in an emergency, the chapter first provides a general discussion of the elements of tort law. Then the various types of dentist-patient relationships are examined with particular attention to legal liability. The issue of informed consent is also discussed. The chapter concludes with a set of recommendations for risk management as related to the management of emergencies in the dental office.

---

*The information in this chapter is general in nature and not designed to be relied on when making legal decisions. Dentists needing legal advice should confer with their malpractice carrier or personal attorney.

Box 35-1   Four Elements of Tort Law

1. Duty
2. Breach of duty
3. Damages
4. Causation

TORT LAW

Tort law relates to alleged or real injuries a party accuses another individual of causing due to a negligent act or a failure to act. *Malpractice* cases are a form of tort in that a patient or family accuses a physician or other health care professional of providing care that was beneath the standard of care, which caused bodily, mental, and/or monetary damages. The belief by the patient or the person's representatives that the dentist did not intend to harm the patient keeps this type of case within the *civil law* system, rather than being considered a criminal case. In a *civil tort* case the patient and often the family become the plaintiff(s), and the dentist and often any corporation or health care facility in which the patient was being treated become the defendant(s).

A plaintiff's successful case must satisfy four requirements or elements (Box 35-1). If any of these elements is not proven to be more likely than not to the judge's or jury's satisfaction, the defendant will prevail. In most situations the initial burden of proof is on the plaintiff to provide evidence that each of the elements is satisfied. Once the plaintiff provides the proof, the defendant has the burden to refute the plaintiff's evidence with her or his own information.

If the legal case makes it to trial, a jury of 6 to 12 individuals will decide whose proof is more persuasive and will help determine the extent of damages if the plaintiff prevails. Any issue requiring an interpretation of the law, such as deciding if a case falls under any Good Samaritan law or whether a certain piece of evidence is admissible, is decided by the judge.

In medical/dental malpractice cases involving emergency care, *duty* is the first element a plaintiff must show. The plaintiff must provide evidence that the defendant dentist had the type of relationship with the patient or with the facility in which the patient was receiving care that required the physician to care for the patient's emergency.

Duty

A *duty* for a dentist to provide care for an individual can arise in two fundamental ways. The first situa-

tion occurs when a patient seeks out a particular dentist for advice or care. In these cases the duty to treat does not occur unless the dentist agrees, by verbal or written means, to accept the person as a patient or signals such an acceptance through actions the reasonable person would interpret as a dentist accepting responsibility for the patient's care. Simply seeing a patient for a consultation does not usually establish a duty to treat.

The second means of establishing a duty occurs when a patient chooses or is taken to a facility that offers care to patients using dentists chosen by the facility. Those practitioners have a contractual obligation to manage patients accepted by the facility. This contractual obligation arises by (1) agreeing to be "on call" to see emergencies, (2) being employed to see emergency patients for that facility, or (3) agreeing to cover on-call responsibilities for another dentist having some obligation to see emergency patients. For example, a patient presents at an ED for treatment of an emergency. The dentist working for the ED or on call to that ED has a duty to manage patients assigned to the physician or to make reasonably certain that another appropriate person takes on the duty to help the patient.

The duty imposed on the dentist is not boundless. Rather, the duty established relates to health problems the reasonable person would consider within the dentist's expertise. Thus a dentist accepting a patient with serious liver disease needing comprehensive dental care has a duty to provide appropriate dental care. However, the dentist does not take on any duty to manage the liver problem, except as to how that hepatic disorder may affect dental care or with respect to how the dental care may impact the liver problem. In the case of a medical emergency occurring while a patient is undergoing dental care, a dentist has a duty to protect the patient, as much as is reasonable, from harm while using the dentist's knowledge and skill to manage the emergency. It is also expected that the dentist will continue to assist the patient until care can be transferred to other providers capable of managing the emergency.

Breach of Duty

Once it has been established that a dentist had a duty to help the patient, the second tort element of *breach of duty* becomes important. This is the point in a tort case when the issue of the standard of care becomes relevant. Each jurisdiction has its own definition of the standard of care, but most use language that sets the *standard of care* as that treatment other similarly

Box 35-2   Case Studies—Determining Liability

The following specific circumstances will help illustrate how various tort elements come into play when determining liability.

DUTY

The first circumstance involves dentist A from an unrelated office, waiting in the reception area of dentist B's office for B to finish surgery on a patient under sedation, before A and B go to lunch. Dentist B calls for A's assistance in reviving a patient who has suddenly stopped breathing. In this case B has a clear duty to the patient to manage the problem, whereas A has no duty to the patient and could have refused to help without being held liable for any sequelae, even if the patient's death were due to dentist A's refusal to help.

BREACH OF DUTY

The second circumstance is a case where a patient with known coronary artery disease experiences chest discomfort while having dental care. The dentist gives the patient a nitroglycerin tablet or spray from an emergency kit, but when the patient shows no improvement after the third dose, the dentist notices the nitroglycerin is out of date. The patient goes on to suffer a cardiac arrest. In this case the plaintiff's lawyer is likely to find an expert who will testify that having out-of-date nitroglycerin is a breach of the duty (standard of care) owed to the patient, especially when he was identified as having coronary artery disease.

DAMAGES

The third circumstance relates to damages. A patient with a known allergy to penicillin has a severe odontogenic infection compromising her airway. As part of the treatment a dentist gives a large dose of intravenous ampicillin. No allergic reaction occurs, but the patient develops a short-lived "red-man rash" typically associated with ampicillin. Even though it is a breach of the standard of care for a dentist to give ampicillin to a penicillin-allergic patient, since no damages occurred, there is no cause of action.

CAUSATION

A final circumstance illustrates how causation (or lack thereof) can impact the outcome of a tort case. Assume evidence shows that a dentist had a duty to provide care for a patient and that using contaminated instruments (ones not sterilized after use on the previous patient) breached the standard of care. Further assume that the patient on whom the contaminated instruments were used suffered damages by being found to be infected by the human immunodeficiency virus soon after the dental visit, but that the serologic testing of the patient the dentist saw before the plaintiff was proven not to be HIV positive. This inability by the plaintiff to show a causal connection (linkage) between damages occurring after the dental visit and the dentist's breach of duty would lead to a finding of "no negligence" on the defendant's part since the causation element of tort was not satisfied.

---

trained individuals would provide under similar circumstances. In medical/dental tort cases, medicodental experts are often used to explain what the standard of care is to the jury and give an opinion as to whether the defendant(s) breached the standard of care. Opinions are given with the understanding that they are more likely true than not within a reasonable degree of medical/dental certainty. This allows experts to be as little as 51% sure of their opinion, as opposed to criminal cases, where many decisions need to be "beyond a shadow of a doubt."

Damage

If the elements of duty and breach of duty are shown, the plaintiff must then show that some *damages* have occurred. This disallows suing out of spite when no damages occurred. Plaintiffs' damages can include costs of further care, loss of time from employment, disruption of family life, and other factors.

Causation

The final element that must be satisfied in a tort case is that any damages proven to exist are indeed due to a breach of duty by the defendant(s). This *causation* element is important since other intervening events may have occurred that either caused or worsened the damages, thereby eliminating or lessening the dentist's liability (Box 35-2).

One means of avoiding the need to prove causation or breach of duty is the application of the doctrine of *res ipsa loquitor*; however, it rarely plays a role in dental negligence cases. The phrase roughly translates into "the circumstances speak for themselves." In other words, the reasonable person without any particular expertise could use common sense and common knowledge that a particular circumstance would likely lead to patient injury and the questions of standard of care and causation are irrelevant. Thus, if a dentist is shown to have personally given penicillin to a patient who had a well-documented history of anaphylactic reactions to that drug for treatment of a minor periapical abscess, and if the patient suffered damages after an anaphylactic reaction, the doctrine of *res ipsa loquitor* could conceivably be used. This relieves the plaintiff of producing a medical expert to educate the jury on the standard of care related to giving penicillin to such a patient.

DUTY TO TREAT

The presence or absence of a duty to treat another individual controls a dentist's legal obligation to render care. This duty arises based on whether a dentist-patient relationship is in place. If a dentist has accepted a patient based on a written or verbal agreement between the patient and the physician that the dentist will care for some or all of a patient's dental problems, a duty to provide care is established. This duty continues until the dentist-patient relationship ceases to exist. Termination of the relationship may be based on transfer of the patient to another dentist's care or termination of the relationship by the usual means, such as repeated failure of a patient to appear for appointments after receiving notice that such failures will terminate the relationship.

However, note that the duty to treat one's patient is not all encompassing. For example, if a patient calls the dentist complaining of chest discomfort, the dentist has a duty to refer that patient to an emergency facility or the patient's personal physician. The dentist in this case has no duty to see the patient to assess the situation or to try to manage such a problem that is out of the realm of general dental practice. On the other hand, if one's patient calls with an urgent situation relating to care provided by the dentist or within the usual scope of dental expertise, the dentist has a duty to either provide emergency care or ensure that another dentist with appropriate skills cares for the patient in a timely manner.

ETHICAL CONSIDERATIONS

Dentists have both ethical and legal duties to patients. The American Dental Association (ADA) *Principles of Ethics and Code of Professional Conduct* states that the dentist has several affirma-

tive duties toward patients and the public at large. The code states that a dentist has a duty to protect the patient from harm, the ethical principle of *nonmalfeasance*, by keeping knowledge and skills current, knowing one's limitations, and knowing when to refer to a specialist or other professional. The ethical principle of *beneficence* is included in the code when it states that professionals have a duty to act for the benefit of others, "with due consideration being given to the needs, desires and values of the patient." This is also an expression of the ethical duty to respect patients' rights of self-determination, the *autonomy* principle. Dentists are obligated to "make reasonable arrangements for the emergency care of their patients of record." Moreover, the code expressly states that when a dentist is consulted in an emergency by a patient with whom the dentist does not have a relationship, the dentist must also make reasonable arrangements for that individual's emergency care.

Members of the ADA voluntarily agree to abide by these ethical principles as a condition of membership. Failure to do so may result in censure or suspension from membership in the association, which may come to administrative or judicial notice in the event of a complaint to a state licensing board or a malpractice suit. The legal system frequently recognizes these ethical principles, formally in state dental practice acts and regulations, as well as informally in the common law precedents developed in malpractice litigation.

Despite these very broad ethical obligations, a dentist is generally under no legal obligation to accept a patient for treatment in the private practice setting. Traditional common law tort doctrine encompasses the idea that a person has no duty to help strangers in distress. A dentist may refuse to enter a treatment arrangement for any reason, subject to some limitations. The ADA code recognizes that dentists "may exercise reasonable discretion in selecting patients for their practices." However, refusal to enter into a practitioner-patient relationship based on discrimination is proscribed by many federal and state statutes, including the Americans with Disabilities Act of 1990. Dental practices are considered places of "public accommodation," in which discrimination is prohibited. Until a dentist-patient relationship is established, the ethical and legal duties owed a patient do not prevail. The current trend in the judicial system, however, is to recognize the establishment of practitioner-patient relationships when as little as a simple phone conversation, which includes professional advice, occurs. Nevertheless, until circumstances establish a dentist-patient relationship, the dentist is not legally obliged to provide anything other than minimal assistance to any individual.

MULTIPROVIDER GROUPS

Practices with several dentists present a special situation with respect to liability for providing emergency care. Typically, dentists in such groups work under the umbrella of a "professional corporation" or "professional association," or they are unincorporated partners. In such circumstances the patients of any one dentist may be legally considered to actually be a patient of the group. In this case, if the dentist the patient usually sees is unavailable, one of the other members of the group has the duty to assist that patient in the event of an emergency. Dentists either must manage it themselves if they have the appropriate training or must assist the patient the best they can while they arrange for a properly skilled person or facility to take over the patient's management.

DENTIST LIABILITY FOR EMPLOYEES

A dentist's office staff serves as the dentist's agent for essentially all activities related to their employment by the dentist or the dentist's corporation. As an agent, the dentist is responsible for most of the agents' actions or inactions while they work for the dentist. As with other legal issues, this liability through agency is not all encompassing. The dentist is responsible for hiring properly trained staff, providing appropriate training, and supervising the staff. However, if a staff member does something to injure a patient that no reasonable dentist would be able to foresee, the dentist's liability for any damages might dissolve. Thus, if staff members decided on their own, against their training and against the orders of the dentist, to try to do something for a patient, such as administer a nonprescription drug, that causes an injury, and it was not foreseeable by the dentist that the staff member would perform such an act, the court might declare that the dentist was not liable for the act.

In most cases, however, staff do serve as the dentist's agent or the dentist's corporation's agent, and the physician should take reasonable measures to do proper background checks during hiring and keep their staff properly trained and supervised. For emergency care assistance, dental office staffs can be kept trained by ongoing basic life support certification and by conducting mock emergency drills on a periodic basis.

EMERGENCIES

The dentist in a dentist-patient relationship has certain expectations imposed by society with respect to managing, preparing for, and preventing emergencies.

Prevention

Preventing dental or medical emergencies is sometimes possible. Medical emergencies are usually preceded by previous known medical conditions. Thus taking and regularly updating the medical history of patients is important. If a patient has a medical condition that tends to be difficult to tightly control, such as diabetes mellitus, the dentist is wise to assess how well the patient's medical condition has recently been in control. If, for example, a patient with a history of coronary artery disease has an increasing frequency of angina, or if an asthmatic patient has required several emergency room visits recently, the dentist may benefit from conferring with the patient's physician before providing complex dental care.

The other major means of preventing emergencies in the dental office is to take appropriate steps to deliver care safely. This is based primarily on (1) avoiding toxic levels of drugs, (2) not giving medications to which a patient is known to be allergic, (3) minimizing patient anxiety, and (4) monitoring a patient's well-being during care. Emergency prevention also often depends on giving good instructions to patients on prescribed medications and other postprocedural information and providing patients with a list of symptoms that should trigger a call to the dentist, such as prolonged bleeding or a fever.

Finally, emergency prevention includes designing and maintaining an office facility in a manner that lessens the risks of accidents by patients or staff. Marking and quickly drying slick wet floors is an obvious example.

Preparation

The dentist-patient relationship also creates a duty for dentists to prepare themselves, their staff, and their facilities to manage common emergencies. This typically includes regular basic life support training for dentist and dental staff, a well-equipped emergency cart, regular

| Box 35-3 | Advance Directives: Characteristics of Legal Documents |

A person who attains the age of majority automatically has *legal* capacity and is presumed to have sufficient decision-making capacity to make health care decisions. In the absence of a court's finding to the contrary, no other person may give consent to health care procedures for the patient unless the person designates another to make those decisions.

Advance directives are statements made by patients to direct the course of their health care in the event of their disability, before the need for that direction arises. Generally, the patient executing the advance directive must have legal capacity and reasonable decision-making capacity at the time the documents are executed.

With notable differences, all 50 states allow an adult of reasonable decision-making capacity (sound mind) to execute at least one of the following advance directives.

DURABLE POWER OF ATTORNEY
A document in which a person (the principal) appoints another person as his agent (attorney-in-fact), with wording that indicates that his attorney-in-fact has authority to act on behalf of the principal, and with authorities enumerated in the document. A power of attorney is durable when the document creating it indicates that the attorney-in-fact may act notwithstanding the latter disability of the principal. Some states may require the document to specifically enumerate health care decisions among those powers conveyed by the document.

HEALTH CARE PROXY
A document similar to a power of attorney in which a patient designates a surrogate decision maker who has the authority to decide health care issues for the patient when the person becomes too incapacitated to make them. Several states recognize health care proxies.

MEDICAL DIRECTIVE
A document which expresses the patient's wishes regarding the types of health care to be rendered under different circumstances, if the patient becomes disabled and unable to decide the course of treatment personally.

LIVING WILL
A document executed by an individual to govern withholding or withdrawing various life sustaining treatments in the event that the individual is incapacitated, or the individual's condition is irreversible or incurable, and likely to cause death in a relatively short time. No other person is authorized to decide for the individual. Living wills are permitted in most states.

continuing education on recognizing and managing medical emergencies, and office protocols on how emergencies can be handled. Private offices should also have the telephone numbers to hospital EDs, emergency medical services (EMS) groups, or others with expertise in handling medical emergencies on hand or programmed into speed dialers.

If a medical emergency that threatens the patient's life occurs in the dental treatment setting, it is important for the dentist to know whether the patient has a living will, a durable power of attorney, or an advance directive, three types of legal documents with unique characteristics (Box 35-3). This is an important example of an opportunity to prevent medicolegal complications before they arise. When a dentist has a patient with serious or chronic life-threatening or terminal medical problems, the dentist must obtain copies of any such documents at the outset of the treatment relationship and must include them in the patient's record. Dentists should consult their personal or corporate attorney to determine the impact of such documents, before treatment is initiated. It is also advisable that patient records are marked with prominent notice, visible to all providers, when the patient or a legally empowered party has specified any limitations on life support measures.

If a medical emergency that requires cardiopulmonary resuscitation should occur, the dentist should be aware of such directives as "no CPR." Commensurate with the ADA code's ethical duty to provide care within the desires and values of the patient and legal principles of informed consent, the dentist should make every effort to comply with any advance directive or the wishes of the person designated by the patient for those decisions. In the instance when such resuscitation efforts may be required and the practitioner is unaware of such documents, however, after a good faith effort to discover them at the outset of the treatment relationship, the dentist should take all measures necessary to preserve the patient's life and health.

Similarly, if a patient with reasonable decision-making capacity, at that moment when a medical emergency occurs, expresses a refusal to receive emergency treatment, the dentist must seriously consider the situation and the patient's decision-making capacity. If the dentist is able to determine objectively that the patient is making a reasonable decision based on the patient's values, the dentist should respect the patient's wishes and abstain from providing the emergency treatment. It is critically important, however, that patients have been advised of all the material risks of their refusal of emergency care. Such risks should be enumerated to the patient, and the dentist should ask if the patient understands them. If the patient's refusal is unflappable, the dentist should document it in the patient's record and have the patient sign that informed refusal of care. However, if there is any reasonable doubt about the patient's decision-making capacity at the moment of the emergency situation, the dentist does not have to rely on patient consent to emergency treatment procedures, within the dentist's abilities, which would prevent serious bodily harm or death of the patient.

Management

Properly managing emergencies is a logical extension of being prepared for emergencies. Regular updating of knowledge and skills in emergency management is the cornerstone of this concept, since fortunately, most emergencies are rare. "Refresher" training is useful. If an emergency occurs, the dentist is expected to use accepted techniques to mitigate the problem. The extent of care necessary depends on the nature of the problem. If the dentist possesses the appropriate knowledge and skills, she should implement them. If it is likely that additional help will be needed, calls for that assistance should be made as early during the scenario as possible. In many cases, definitive management of the emergency will be beyond the skills or licensure bounds of the dentist. In that case the dentist should do as much as possible to protect the patient from serious harm while awaiting emergency medical technicians or others with special skills and equipment for managing medical emergencies to take over the patient's management. The dentist should only do what he thinks is reasonably necessary to save the patient from serious irreversible harm if the dentist is performing procedures beyond his training or license.

COVERING FOR ANOTHER DENTIST OR AT AN EMERGENCY FACILITY

A duty to assist a patient having a dental emergency or a dental-related medical emergency can arise if a dentist has agreed to "take call" for another dentist, is "on call" to an emergency facility, or has agreed to serve as a "team dentist" for a sporting activity. This duty requires the dentist "taking call" for another dentist to provide similar care. The dentist either must completely manage those problems within the on-call dentist's training or must ensure that someone with appropriate expertise accepts and begins managing the patient.

Referring Patients

In the event of a medical emergency that requires referral of the patient to another health professional, the dentist should carefully document that referral in the patient record. The dentist should always determine the outcomes of any referrals and document them. An example of this is the management that should be pursued for a patient in whom a dental instrument (e.g., endodontic file) or an extracted tooth is accidentally dropped into the patient's throat, becoming irretrievable by normal means. Although the patient may not experience any distressful signs or symptoms, the person should still be referred to a medical radiologist for chest and abdominal films to locate the object definitively. A radiologist's report that the object has lodged in the respiratory tree requires another referral of the patient by the dentist to a specialist for bronchoscopy and retrieval of the object. Likewise, location of the object in the gastrointestinal tract dictates a referral to a gastroenterologist or surgeon. The dentist's failure to make these appropriate follow-up referrals may result in the patient later developing much more serious sequelae, which will increase the dentist's culpability and liability.

In the unlikely event that a patient fails to pursue the referral, the dentist should make every effort to persuade the patient of the importance of medical attention and the material risks that may occur as a result of the patient's neglect. Similarly, in the unlikely event that a medical specialist refuses to perform diagnostic tests or treatment requested by the dentist, a conference between the two practitioners should take place. The dentist should consider referral to another practitioner if the physician is steadfast in refusing to treat the patient without appropriate medical justification. Although a medical practitioner's improper or counterproductive advice to a patient in these circumstances may lead the patient to ignore the problem, any medical complications that the patient may subsequently experience would be considered caused by the dentist's negligence. Any negligence of the physician would not sufficiently supersede the causative nature of the initial accident to insulate the dentist from liability.

Obtaining Consent

It is important that a covering (substituting) dentist attempt to obtain the patient's consent to receive emergency care if the nature of the emergency permits. Even obtaining a verbal consent witnessed by another person unrelated to the patient is better than omitting the consent process. Obtaining consent in these circumstances should not create delays that would tend to worsen the emergency situation.

Legal Exposure of Taking Call

The legal exposure created by "taking call" for another dentist makes it important that the dentists participating in covering for each other make the relationship as formal as possible. This can be by written agreement specifying the dates and times the covering dentist is to be responsible for the absent dentist's patients. A telephone "sign out" to the covering dentist is helpful to alert the dentist to any patients who may have a greater chance of having an urgent problem due to recent surgery or an ongoing infection.

If on call to an ED, the dentist has a duty to treat or appropriately triage patients for whom consultation has been made. It is appropriate in some emergency circumstances for the dentist to rely on the ED's professional staff for information about the patient's status when deciding if the situation requires the dentist's presence or referral to a person with expertise the on-call dentist does not possess. However, in emergencies that are primarily of a dental nature, such as a continuously oozing dental socket, the patient will probably be best served by the on-call dentist's direct care. A less clear situation with respect to a duty to assist in an emergency presents if a dentist happens to be in an emergency facility or hospital for reasons other than being on call at that facility and responsible for helping manage emergencies. Several court cases have concluded that a physician does not have a duty to help a patient having an emergency, such as participating in basic or advanced cardiac life support, under these circumstances. However, the law does not prohibit offering assistance and even seeks to encourage participation through "Good Samaritan" acts (see following discussion). As in other situations, the dentist should limit assistance to those procedures for which the dentist has training and those within the scope or licensure, and do only what is necessary to abate the emergency sufficiently to stabilize the patient until those with appropriate training can take over.

GOOD SAMARITAN STATUTES

The final situation involves coming upon or being called to assist in emergency care for a patient with whom the dentist has no relationship, outside of a health care facility. The dentist, except in rare circumstances, has no duty to provide emergency treatment in this type of situation. Therefore situations such as a motor vehicle accident scene or injuries at a sports event do not create a duty for a dentist to help with an emergency. However, as mentioned earlier, society benefits from dentists and others volunteering to assist when emergencies occur. Good public policy places the advantages of encouraging health care providers to offer assistance over the benefit that may be derived by individuals seeking to sue those individuals for alleged malpractice.

This recognition of societal benefits is evidenced by legislatures passing Good Samaritan acts to minimize the chance that anyone will be deterred from helping another in trouble because of the fear of incurring legal problems, if the outcome is not favorable. The essence of these acts is to preclude those being assisted by those not owing them a duty from holding the assistor liable for any damages caused by her assistance. Box 35-4 provides examples of the language in such an act. This relatively broad immunity from liability is usually interpreted as providing protection even if the emergency care provided was found to breach the standards of care.

However, Good Samaritan statutes do not provide complete freedom from liability. They are usually interpreted as permitting the person seeking its liability protection to do only what is necessary to stop the emergency or provide assistance until those with greater expertise or

Box 35-4	Examples of Language in Good Samaritan Acts

"No licensee, who in good faith renders emergency care at the scene of an emergency, shall be liable for any civil damages as the result of any acts or omissions by such person in rendering the emergency care."

"Any dentist or any person licensed as a dentist in any other state or territory in the United States who in good faith provides emergency care without a fee to a victim of an accident at the scene of an accident shall not, as a result of his or her acts or omissions, except willful or wanton misconduct on the part of such person, in providing such care, be liable for civil damages."

"Failure to obtain a patient's informed consent may constitute malpractice. However, a patient's consent is not necessary when an emergency arises and treatment is necessary to protect the patient's health and it is impossible or impracticable to obtain consent either from the patient or from someone authorized to consent for him."

having a duty to manage the emergency can take over the patient's management. Good Samaritan acts usually provide coverage unless there is a wanton disregard for the patient's best interests. This means that if a jury can be convinced by the evidence, including expert opinion testimony, that the dentist provided willful or wantonly poor or grossly negligent care under the circumstances, Good Samaritan protection is lost. Also, if the person suffering the emergency expressly refuses care from an individual, and that individual nonetheless proceeds to deliver care, the protection of these acts usually dissolves. Furthermore, these acts assume that the care being provided is given for humanitarian reasons. Therefore, if the dentist providing care attempts to or actually bills the patient, the family, or others for any care delivered, Good Samaritan status is typically in serious jeopardy.

Good Samaritan statutes do not automatically give dentists the same liability waiver as is provided to physicians. Many state statutes specifically mention "medical practitioners" or those licensed to practice medicine and surgery. The immunity granted has usually been ex-

tended to nonphysician health care providers, including nurses and dentists, but they may be restricted to rendering care covered by their respective licenses. Since Good Samaritan statutes are state specific, the reader is urged to review the particular state's act and, if the language is unclear, confer with an attorney on this issue. In the majority of cases, however, the provision of assistance by dentists to those in need of emergency care is protected by Good Samaritan acts in most states.

DOCUMENTATION AND CONSENT

While managing an emergency, or as soon after the emergency has abated as possible, the dentist should carefully document the events leading up to the situation and its management in the patient's dental record. This information may be useful to physicians who subsequently treat the patient. If any legal action arises from the case, contemporary documentation will typically be helpful. In addition, if the emergency may have been caused by the dental care delivered, or if the emergency is serious, the dentist may find it useful to notify his malpractice carrier. If an employee, the dentist should notify his or her supervisor or employer.

For the most part, the provision of care during an emergency does not require prior *informed consent* if it would be impractical to obtain such permission. However, hospitals and other health care facilities routinely mention the issue of providing emergency care without additional patient consent in blanket admission consent forms and on consent forms for surgical procedures. Dentists may find it useful to consider inclusion of such language in materials provided to new or existing patients in their practices or on treatment plan or procedure consent forms.

SUGGESTED READINGS

Axelrod RB: Application of standard of care to particular facets of practice, *Florida Jurisprudence Medical Malpractice*, 36 §19, 1996.

Brown JL: Statutory immunity for volunteer physicians: a vehicle for reaffirmation of the doctor's beneficent duties, absent the rights talk, *Widener Law Symp* J 1:425, 1996.

Rothenberg KH: Who cares? The evolution of the legal duty to provide emergency care, *Houston Law Rev* 25:21, 1989.

Stomos JJ, Fintzen SS: Emergency medicine cases, *Ill Inst Cont Legal*, March 1996.

Veilleux DR: Construction and application of "Good Samaritan" statutes, *Am Law Rep* 68:294, 1989.

Wakeen LM: Dental office emergencies: do you know your legal obligations? *J Am Dent Assoc* 124:54-58, 1993.

Index

Beneficence, code of ethics and, 528

Benign essential tremor, description of, 331

Benzamide, nausea and vomiting treated with, 273

Benzocaine, methemoglobinemia caused by, 448, 456

Benzodiazepine
  abuse of, 432-433
    dental care and, 441
  anesthesia techniques with, 506
  anterograde amnesia associated with, 504
  delirium treated with, 262
  flumazenil for reversal of, 506
  health consequences of, 433
  hyperventilation treated with, 110, 111
  hypotension associated with, 157
  nausea and vomiting treated with, 273
  opioid drugs used with, 506
  overdose of, 505
    risk factors for, 502
  paradoxical reaction to, 503
  psychotic disorders treated with, 262
  sedation with, 501
    reversal of, 502
  seizure treated with, 52-53, 69, 235
  stress relieved with, 269

Benzodiazepine receptor complex, gamma-aminobutryric acid and, 501-502

Benzoic acid, diabetes mellitus management with, 349

Benztropine, Parkinson's disease management with, 330

Bernard-Soulier disease, description of, 287

Beta cell, insulin production and, 341

β-adrenergic blocker drugs
  hyperthyroidism treated with, 367
  thyrotoxicosis management with, 372

β-agonist drugs
  palpitations caused by, 128
  wheezing treated with, 91

β₂-agonist drugs, 54-55

β-blocker drugs
  bradycardia caused by, 132
  paroxysmal supraventricular tachycardia treated with, 137

Bethanechol, multiple sclerosis treated with, 334

BGM; see Blood glucose monitoring

Biguanide drugs, diabetes mellitus management with, 349

Bilberry, description and interactions of, 462

Bipolar disorder, 259-260

Biotin-dependent multicarboxylase deficiency, hyperventilation associated with, 107

BIPP; see Bismuth iodoform paraffin paste

Birth defect, spontaneous abortion of pregnancy and, 493

Bismuth iodoform paraffin paste, epistaxis management with, 298

Bisulfite, asthmatic reaction to, 448

Bite mark, child abuse indicated by, 484

Black cohosh, description and interactions of, 462

Bladder, cancer of, cigarette smoking associated with, 431

Bladder function, change in, altered mental status assessment and, 207

Bladderwrack, description and interactions of, 462

Bleeding
  gingival, child abuse as cause of, 482
  maternal death during pregnancy caused by, 498
  oral, chemotherapy and, 400
  periodontal, child abuse as cause of, 482

Bleeding disorder, 283-291

Blindness
  diabetes mellitus associated with, 352
  glaucoma associated with, 309
  retinal artery occlusion associated with, 309

Blood
  acute loss of, 389-390
  alcohol level in, effects of, 426

Blood—cont'd
  disorders of, 389-408
  drug screening by testing of, 425
  glucose level in, 49, 341
  hepatitis infection from, 516
  human immunodeficiency virus contamination in, 514
  oxygen-carrying capacity of, anemia and, 389
  oxygenated, 153
  volume of, in child, 66t

Blood cell
  defects in production of, 395-396
  membrane defects in, 391-392
  red
    disorders of, 389-398
    impaired production of, 395
    normal value of, 390t
    stimulation of production of, 395
  white
    disorders of, 398-402
    normal value of, 390t

Blood clot, normal, 285

Blood component therapy, 287-288

Blood dyscrasia, epistaxis and, 304

Blood glucose, level of, evaluation of palpitation and, 129

Blood glucose monitoring, diabetes mellitus management and, 348

Blood pressure
  altered mental status assessment and, 208
  amphetamine abuse and, 438
  arterial, 141
    regulation of, 154f
  assessment of, 5, 153
  baseline, 153
  cardiac arrest and, 15
  chest pain assessment and measurement of, 117
  in child, 65
  classification of, 142t
  diastolic, 36
    cardiovascular risk prediction and, 141
  effects of cannabinoids on, 433
  effects of cocaine on, 435
  elevated
    pregnancy-induced hypertension indicated by, 494
    stress as cause of, 145
    substance abuse assessment and, 421
  hemorrhage diagnosis and, 283
  increased, respiratory distress and, 87
  measurement of, 35-36
  normal ranges of, 10t
  normal variation in, 153t
  in older adult, 73
  opioid drug use and, 436
  pediatric, 65t
  reduction of, 147
  regulation of, 143f
  stroke and, 226-227
  systolic, 36
    cardiovascular risk prediction and, 141
    determination of, 153
    older adult and increase in, 73

Blood supply, illness level assessment and, 9

BLS; see Basic life support

Blue bloater, chronic obstructive pulmonary disease and, 99

Blurred vision, type 2 diabetes mellitus associated with, 347

BMT; see Bone marrow, transplantation of

Body dysmorphic disorder, 251

Body temperature, assessment of, 5

Body weight, anesthetic drug dosage calculation and, 453

Boerhaave's syndrome, esophageal rupture and, 122

Bogbean, description and interactions of, 462-463

Bone marrow
  failure of, platelet disorder associated with, 287

Bone marrow—cont'd
  immunogenesis and, 163
  transplantation of, 398

Bone marrow aplasia, anemic associated with, 396

Bone wax, hemostasis with, 284

Borrelia burgdorferi, Guillain-Barré syndrome associated with, 335

Bowel function, change in, altered mental status assessment and, 207

Bradyarrhythmia, description of, 320

Bradycardia, 320
  altered mental status assessment and, 208
  altered mental status caused by, 204t
  arrhythmia and, 127
  atropine for, 187
  causes of, 132
  in child, 65
  definition of, 132, 155
  dental emergency indicated by, differential diagnosis of, 4b
  emergency treatment of, 136f
  management of, 134
  palpitations with arrhythmia associated with, 128
  presyncope phase and, 184
  status epilepticus and, 237
  stroke associated with, 220
  treatment of, 156
  vasovagal syncope and, 156

Brain
  abscess in, headache and, 242, 246
  arteries of, 214f
  atrophy of, 75
  blood flow to, 213
  effect of aging on, 75
  effects of nicotine on, 430
  infarction of, 214
    altered mental status caused by, 201
  infarcts in, dementia associated with, 75
  intracerebral processes and, 189
  lower, level of consciousness and, 189
  oxygenation of, 213
  pathophysiology of, 213
  right-sided heart failure and, 318
  substance abuse and adaptation of, 414

Breach of duty, tort law and, 526-527

Breath
  acetone, hyperglycemia indicated by, 197
  odor of, altered mental status assessment and, 209
  shortness of
    anaphylaxis indicated by, 172
    hyperventilation associated with, 109
    serious illness indicated by, 10b

Breath sounds, 14
  assessment of, in resuscitation plan secondary survey, 17
  dyspnea assessment and, 103

Breathing, 13-14
  abdominal, in child, 63
  abnormal, stroke and, 220
  airway obstruction and, 85
  assessment of, 23
    in child, 61
  diaphragmatic, in child, 63
  effort of, description of, 98
  forced, hyperventilation treated with, 110
  hyperventilation and assessment of, 106
  Kussmaul, 112
  maintenance of
    seizure treatment and, 235
    stroke survival and, 219
  management of, altered mental status and, 202
  pain in, hyperventilation associated with, 109
  physiology of, 97
  voluntary, 97

Breathlessness, iron deficiency anemia indicated by, 391

Bretylium, pediatric advanced life support and, 67t